Haemophilia and other Inherited Bleeding Disorders

Haemophilia and other Inherited Bleeding Disorders

Edited by

CHARLES R RIZZA
MD, FRCPE
Formerly Consultant Physician and Director
Oxford Haemophilia Centre, Churchill Hospital
and Clinical Lecturer in Haematology
University of Oxford, Oxford

GORDON DO LOWE
MD, FRCP
Professor of Vascular Medicine
University of Glasgow
Consultant Physician
Co-Director, Haemophilia Centre
Glasgow Royal Infirmary, Glasgow

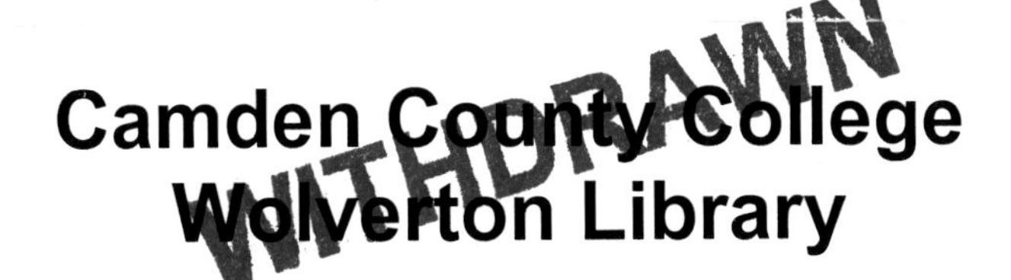

W B Saunders Company Ltd
London Philadelphia Toronto Sydney Tokyo

W. B. Saunders Company Ltd 24–28 Oval Road
London NW1 7DX

The Curtis Center
Independence Square West
Philadelphia, PA 19106-3399, USA

Harcourt Brace & Company
55 Horner Avenue
Toronto, Ontario M8Z 4X6, Canada

Harcourt Brace & Company, Australia
30–52 Smidmore Street
Marrickville, NSW 2204, Australia

Harcourt Brace & Company, Japan
Ichibancho Central Building, 22-1 Ichibancho
Chiyoda-ku, Tokyo 102, Japan

This book is printed on acid free paper

A catalogue record for this book is available from the British Library

ISBN 0-7020-1755-8

Typeset by Florencetype Ltd, Stoodleigh, Devon
Printed in Great Britain by The University Press, Cambridge

Contents

Contributors

Professor Louis M Aledort
The Mary Weinfeld Professor of Clinical Research in Hemophilia, Department of Medicine, Mount Sinai Medical Center, New York, USA

Dr Trevor W Barrowcliffe
Head, Division of Haematology, National Institute for Biological Standards and Control, South Mimms, Hertfordshire, UK

Dr Bruce Bennett
Department of Medicine, Aberdeen Royal Infirmary, Foresterhill, Aberdeen, UK

Professor Robert B Duthie
Nuffield Professor of Orthopaedic Surgery, Nuffield Orthopaedic Centre, Oxford, UK

Mary L Fletcher
HV Clinical Nurse Specialist, The Churchill Hospital, Oxford Haemophilia Centre, Headington, Oxford, UK

Dr Paul LF Giangrande
Consultant Haematologist, Director, Oxford Haemophilia Centre, The Churchill Hospital, Headington, Oxford, UK

Professor Francesco Giannelli
Professor of Molecular Genetics, Paediatric Research Unit, Division of Medical and Molecular Genetics, Guy's Hospital, London, UK

Professor Ian A Greer
Muirhead Professor of Obstetrics, Head, Department of Obstetrics and Gynaecology, Glasgow Royal Infirmary, Glasgow, UK

Dr Margaret W Hilgartner
Department of Paediatrics, Cornell Medical Centre, New York, USA

Dr Peter Jones
Haemophilia Centre, Royal Victoria Infirmary, Newcastle, UK

Dr Christine A Lee
Director, Haemophilia Centre and Haemostasis Unit, Royal Free Hospital, Consultant Haematologist and Honorary Senior Lecturer, Royal Free Hospital School of Medicine, London, UK

Profesor Gordon DO Lowe Professor of Vascular Medicine, University of Glasgow, Consultant Physician, Co-Director, Haemophilia Centre, Glasgow Royal Infirmary, Glasgow, UK

Dr Christopher A Ludlam Consultant Haematologist, Director, Haemophilia Centre, Royal Infirmary of Edinburgh, Edinburgh, UK

Ms Kathy B Matthews Senior Chief MLSO, Oxford Haemophilia Centre, The Churchill Hospital, Headington, Oxford, UK

Dr Charles R Rizza Formerly Consultant Physician and Director, Oxford Haemophilia Centre, Clinical Lecturer in Haematology, University of Oxford, Oxford, UK

Dr Harold R Roberts Kenan Professor of Medicine, Director, Centre for Thrombosis and Hemostasis, University of North Carolina at Chapel Hill, Chapel Hill, North Carolina, USA

Miss Rosemary JD Spooner Research Assistant, Oxford Haemophilia Centre, The Churchill Hospital, Headington, Oxford, UK

Dr Isobel D Walker Consultant Haematologist, Co-Director, Haemophilia Centre, Glasgow Royal Infirmary, Glasgow, UK

Dr Henry G Watson Consultant Haematologist, Director, Haemophilia Centre, Aberdeen Royal Infirmary, Foresterhill, Aberdeen, UK

Preface

The last fifteen years have seen a massive growth in our knowledge of normal and abnormal haemostasis. The purpose of this book is to give an easily readable, up-to-date account of these advances and we hope it will be of value to those involved in the day-to-day care of patients with haemorrhagic disorders especially haemophilia A, haemophilia B and von Willebrand's Disease. Emphasis is given to clinical management. The various therapeutic materials available, treatment options and complications of transfusion therapy are discussed in detail.

As will be seen there are differences of opinion expressed in several places, but on the whole these are minor and we have made no attempt to harmonise the different views. Nor have we attempted to remove some of the overlap between some chapters. Finally we should like to express our gratitude to the contributors for their help and to the staff of WB Saunders for their assistance in the preparation of this book.

CR Rizza
GDO Lowe

1 Normal Haemostasis

BRUCE BENNETT

Evolution has conferred upon man the necessity to defy gravity by walking upright, to survive for many years before reproducing and to develop specific organs to fulfil different functions among many other complex processes. This in turn has required the evolution of the cardiovascular system to transport nutrients, minerals, gases, waste products, humoral and other messages around this set of organs. To fulfil this function adequately the contents of the cardiovascular system must remain fluid, the system must maintain sufficient internal pressure to allow flow around it and must therefore not leak excessively when subjected to the hazards of daily life.

In order to prevent leaking, evolution has conferred upon us the systems that promote platelet plug and fibrin formation to secure closure of injuries to the cardiovascular system, to stop loss when injuries occur, to maintain blood volume and thus allow the circulation of blood that is so crucial to life. Too frequent or widespread dissemination of platelet and fibrin formation throughout the vascular system beyond the sites of injury would clearly impair the fluidity of blood necessary to continue its varied roles by virtue of its circulation. As a result a complementary system of mechanisms checking or restraining platelet aggregation and fibrin formation has also evolved, as have mechanisms ensuring removal of fibrin when its wound-sealing role is fulfilled. These mechanisms will be reviewed in this chapter.

The penalty for too efficient formation of haemostatic plugs in blood vessels is clearly a propensity for intravascular thrombosis. This increases with age and the accumulation of environmental injuries to the blood vessels and it is now a major cause of death in the developed world. Evolution is indifferent to this problem as continuation of the species does not require survival to an age beyond that necessary for the production and initial nurture of the next generation. Thereafter our genes ignore the problems caused in the cardiovascular system by an efficient haemostatic mechanism.

Vascular Response to Injury

Injury to small vessels is accompanied by vasoconstriction mediated by the contraction of the smooth muscle layer in arterial walls. Vein walls contain much less well developed muscular layers and capillaries none at all. Blood flow through injured arterioles is thus reduced and this may allow the processes of platelet plug formation and fibrin formation discussed subsequently to proceed more easily. The factors promoting vasoconstriction after injury are not well defined. Platelet-derived thromboxane A_2 (TXA_2) is a powerful vasoconstrictor released during platelet plug formation in response to injury. The endothelium-derived peptides, the endothelins, have a similar powerful vasoconstrictor effect (Yanagisawa et al, 1988; Randall, 1991). Bradykinin, released during contact factor activation, causes smooth muscle contraction (Ratnoff and Saito, 1979) as does fibrinopeptide B, released from fibrinogen by thrombin (Colman & Osbahr, 1967). Serotonin released from platelets at the site of injury also has vasoconstrictor properties.

These agents are opposed by substances such as prostacyclin (PGI_2) derived from the arachidonic acid pathway and nitric oxide (NO). Both these endothelial products are very powerful vasodilators.

The interaction between vasoconstrictor and vasodilator substances obviously has a significant effect on blood flow in vascular beds. How, or whether, these agents contribute to haemostasis itself is not known.

Platelets: General Aspects

These anuclear cells, produced from the megakaryocyte by the process of budding, circulate in blood at concentrations of approximately $150-400 \times 10^9/l$. Megakaryocytes, cells with large lobulated nuclei and present characteristically in the bone marrow and lung, develop from the pluripotent haemopoietic stem cells (Hoffman, 1989). Maturation is regulated by several agents, including interleukins 3 and 6 (IL3, IL6) and megakaryocyte colony-stimulating activity in the early phases and thrombopoietin, the above interleukins and granulocyte–macrophage colony-stimulating factor at later stages of maturation; transforming growth factor β (TGFβ), platelet-factor 4 (PF4) and certain of the interferons may inhibit colony formation. Erythropoietin itself promotes megakaryocyte maturation though it does not alter the platelet count in human recipients (Ishibashi et al, 1987; McDonald et al, 1987). Thrombopoietin, the agent that specifically promotes megakaryocytic development and differentiation, has recently been identified and cDNA cloned by several different strategies (Bartley et al, 1994; de Sauvage et al, 1994; Lok et al, 1994).

Normal platelets circulate for approximately 9–11 days as detected by labelled platelet studies using isotopes such as chromium 51 or indium 111. The shape of the isotope decay curve after reinjection of random (mixed population) labelled platelets is not quite linear as if a small number of platelets are used daily to maintain the security of the vascular endothelium (Hanson and Slichter, 1985) though quite how this occurs is unclear. One-fourth of platelets are sequestered in the spleen at any time and may be mobilized from here (Heyns et al, 1985) and another pool appears to exist in the lungs (Bierman et al, 1952). Ultimate sequestration of senescent platelets occurs in the spleen and to an extent in liver and marrow (Davey, 1966; Aster, 1969; Heyns et al, 1980, 1982). Platelet volume was originally thought to be a function of platelet age, as platelets released after a period of thrombocytopenia were larger than normal (McDonald et al, 1964). However, this is now regarded as unlikely as others have shown that volume does not vary throughout platelet life-span (Thompson et al, 1983).

Platelets, though lacking a nucleus, are metabolically and structurally complex. The membrane is a typical lipid bilayer rich in arachidonic acid. The cells contain mitochondria, smooth endoplasmic reticulum structures, storage granules of several types (protein storage, amine storage, lysosomes and peroxisomes), microfilament networks and microtubules together with an open canalicular system linking extracellular to intracellular areas (White, 1995). Contractile proteins such as actin, myosin and tubulin modify cell shape.

Many of the functions of platelets are directly related to the control of blood loss and maintenance of vessel wall integrity, and these subjects are addressed here. Other functions are clearly subserved by these cells and agents released by the platelet influence processes other than haemostasis (Crawford and Scruttons, 1995)

Many platelet reactions are initiated by the occupation of surface membrane receptors by appropriate agonists. Examples of such membrane glycoprotein receptors are listed in Table 1.1. Lower-density receptors exist on platelet membranes for many other excitatory or inhibitory agents such as thromboxane, prostacyclin, 5-hydroxytryptamine (5HT), etc. Such signals are transmitted to the intracellular compartment and trigger morphological and other changes. Platelets lose their discoid shape and become more spherical, intracellular organelles are rearranged and surface extensions appear forming pseudopodia. Concurrent with these events are the synthesis and release of metabolites such as thromboxane or prostaglandins and the release of granular contents, some of which are essential for the haemostatic process, the most obvious being the processes of platelet adhesion to subendothelial collagen structures and aggregation of individual platelets into platelet masses by direct cell to cell reactions.

While some proteins such as fibrinogen (Harrison, 1992) may enter platelets by receptor-mediated endocytosis, most of the contents of granules are conferred upon the platelet by the megakaryocyte rather than synthesized by the platelet itself. The platelet thus contains no rough endoplasmic reticulum. It does, however, possess an intracellular dense tubular system with features of a smooth endoplasmic reticulum and associated metabolic properties including calcium storage and the essentials for arachidonic acid release.

The platelet granules store proteins many of which modify haemostasis such as fibrinogen, von Willebrand factor, PF4, β-thromboglobulin (β-TG),

Table 1.1 Glycoprotein platelet membrane receptors

GPIa/IIa	Collagen
GPIb/GPIX	von Willebrand factor (vWF) receptor (adhesion to subendothelium) Thrombin
GPIc/IIa	Fibronectin
GPIIb/IIIa	Fibrinogen (platelet aggregation) von Willebrand factor (vWF) Thrombospondin Fibronectin
GPIV	Collagen Thrombospondin

plasminogen activator inhibitor-1 (PAI-1), basic platelet protein, platelet-derived growth factor and thrombospondin. Discrete granules store amines such as adenosine triphosphate (ATP), adenosine diphosphate (ADP) and 5HT (Table 1.2).

Platelet Role in Haemostasis

Platelets may play a role in the vascular reactions occurring immediately after injury. For example, in their dense bodies they contain 5-hydroxytryptamine (serotonin) which may contribute to vasoconstriction. Additionally they produce and secrete thromboxane A_2 during platelet plug formation, which also has a powerful vasoconstrictive property. None the less, as indicated above, since the role of vasoconstriction in haemostasis is uncertain, the contribution of platelets here must be similarly ill defined.

The major role of platelets is the production of the platelet plug which initially secures cessation of bleeding from injuries to tiny vessels. This process, sometimes referred to as primary haemostasis, has several components.

1. The initial injury disrupts the endothelium, exposes subendothelial collagen and may release tissue factor into the blood. The first two of these processes initiate platelet plug formation; the third ultimately generates thrombin, further enhancing this and, by producing fibrin, ensuring wound seal production.

2. There then follows the process of platelet adhesion. Among the agents exposed by endothelial disruption is subendothelial collagen. Polymeric forms of von Willebrand factor are specifically absorbed from plasma or adjacent endothelium onto collagen and form the link between it and the platelet surface

Table 1.2 Platelet storage structures

Protein storage (α granules)	Fibrinogen von Willebrand factor Platelet factor 4 β-thromboglobulin Platelet-derived growth factor Thrombospondin Factor V Plasminogen activator inhibitor-1 Plasminogen Fibronectin Platelet factor XI inhibitor
Amines (dense bodies)	5 Hydroxytryptamine Adenosine diphosphate Adenosine triphosphate Calcium
Lysosomes, perioxisomes	β-glucuronidase β-galactosidase β-N-acetyl glucosaminidase Cathepsins Collagenase Catalase Elastase

glycoprotein Ib (GPIb) (Stel et al, 1985; Turrito et al, 1985). This serves as the initial event in starting accretion of platelets at the site of injuries (Sixma, 1987). Deficiency in the process is responsible for the prolonged bleeding time in von Willebrand's disease (vWD) where the plasma agent is abnormal and in Bernard–Soulier syndrome where the platelet receptor (GPIb) is abnormal. Factors such as viscosity and shear rate influence the process and its requirements for von Willebrand factor (vWF) appears restricted to areas of high shear rate.

3. Adhesion to collagen is followed by aggregation, a process whereby platelets coalesce, bonding one to another, thus increasing the size of the platelet plug and further blocking the rupture in the vessel wall. This process is initiated in adherent platelets by, or concurrent with, another process known as the platelet release reaction, in which platelet calcium rises and granules fuse with the open canalicular system membranes and secrete or discharge their contents through this into the immediate environment (Holmsen, 1987). Released reagents include ADP, serotonin, PAI-1, β-TG, platelet-derived growth factor (PDGF), thrombospondin, von Willebrand factor, fibrinogen and fibronectin, all of which are biologically active and may take part in

haemostatic or other reactions (Coller, 1984; Marcus, 1991). The ADP, for instance, enhances further platelet aggregation, as, of course, does ADP from other sources. Many agents from outwith the platelets themselves, some generated by injury, will stimulate the release reaction and platelet aggregation as well. Collagen itself and thrombin may be the biologically important ones here but adrenaline, platelet-activating factor (PAF) and immune complexes are also relevant. Most act initially by specific binding to platelet surface receptors (Ruoslahti and Pierschbacher, 1987; Phillips et al, 1988). During these processes further platelet surface proteins, glycoproteins IIb and IIIa, undergo conformational change and act as receptor for fibrinogen, which binds the platelet plug together (Shattil and Bennett, 1981; Bennett et al, 1982; Nachman et al, 1984; Ginsberg et al, 1988). Absence of this receptor on platelets results in the prolonged bleeding time of Glanzmann's disease.

4. A parallel phenomenon is occurring to these events. Platelet phospholipases are activated by agonists such as collagen and release arachidonic acid from the platelet membrane. This is subsequently oxygenated by platelet cyclooxygenase and cytoplasmic lipoxygenase resulting in the formation of unstable prostaglandins (prostaglandins G_2 and H_2). From these, thromboxane A_2 is generated by platelet thromboxane synthetase (Fig. 1.1) and discharged into the environment. This agent is a powerful platelet aggregant and vasoconstrictor. The action of thromboxane on platelets is via inhibition of platelet adenylate cyclase with consequent reduction of platelet cyclic adenosine monophosphate (cAMP); this in turn mobilizes platelet calcium which exerts an important effect on platelet aggregation. While thromboxane A_2 is a most potent platelet aggregating agent, it too is labile with a half-life of only a few seconds. Multiple interactions occur between agents promoting aggregation. Synergism occurs between thrombin and collagen in inducing aggregation, between ADP, collagen and adrenaline and between thromboxane and collagen. These complex interactions, incompletely understood, will provide routes by which different stimuli may amplify platelet responses (Marcus, 1991).

The processes of vascular damage, platelet adhesion followed by the release reaction and platelet aggregation with binding of the aggregate by fibrinogen result in the formation of the platelet plug that initially staunches bleeding from injuries to small vessels. The function of platelets in haemostasis, however, does not end here as the modified platelets in the platelet plug expose membrane lipoprotein which contributes the phospholipid surface on which many of the reactions discussed later in the coagulation pathway (prothrombin, factor X and factor XII activation) may take place (Marcus et al, 1966; Nurden, 1994), thus shielding them, at least in part, from the effect of the plasma protease inhibitors. This property of platelets has been referred to as PF3 activity. Platelet factor 4 released modifies anticoagulant activity of glycosaminoglycans. Further, platelets carry with them into the platelet plug large quantities of PAI-1, which modifies the subsequent susceptibility to lysis of the platelet plug (Robbie et al, 1995a).

Unlike their anuclear cousins the red cells, platelets contain contractile proteins in their cytoskeletons, e.g. actin, myosin and tubulin (Coller, 1984), responsible

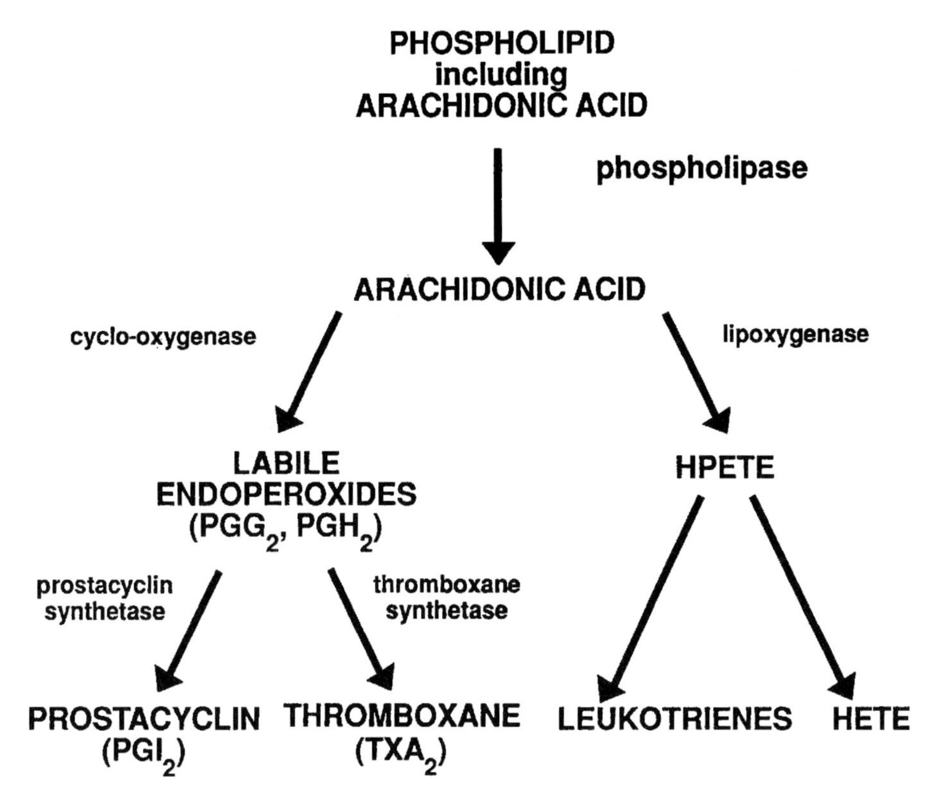

Figure 1.1 The arachidonic acid pathway. PGG_2, prostaglandin G_2; PGH_2, prostaglandin H_2.

for the platelet's ability to undergo striking shape change from their usual circulating discoid shape to the spherical form with pseudopodia production that takes place immediately after adhesion while the secretory process is occurring. Additionally, these proteins are subsequently responsible for the phenomenon of clot retraction (Widmer and Moake, 1976), whereby the clot formed in the test tube shrinks in upon itself and condenses after fibrin formation is complete, a process that is assumed in the body to contribute to the sealing of wounds.

Control of Platelet Reactivity

In the laminar flow occurring in blood vessels, erythrocytes usually occupy the axial part of the stream and platelets occupy the more peripheral and slow-moving layers of the moving blood; thus platelets are located in sites adjacent to the endothelium. While their function is mainly to control or initiate repair of rupture to vessel walls, mechanisms are in place to discourage excessive activity. The haemodynamic pattern at any location will influence the facility with which platelets are deposited locally, while, as platelets are negatively charged, the glycosaminoglycans on the endothelial surface repulse them by virtue of their own negative charge.

At least two major biochemical systems further discourage excessive platelet accretion on normal endothelium. One of these is the endothelial processing of the products of arachidonic acid metabolism (Fig. 1.1). Whereas the platelet generates thromboxane from the unstable prostaglandins produced by this pathway, the endothelium processes these agents differently and produces prostacyclin (PGI_2) (Moncada, 1982; Moncada et al, 1987; Samuelsson et al, 1987). This agent elevates platelet cyclic AMP, prevents calcium mobilization and thus inhibits platelet accretion to endothelium. It additionally is a powerful vasodilator and might be seen as the endothelium's response to the tendency of platelets to aggregate via this pathway. The arachidonic acid pathway, it is established, is sensitive to the inhibitory effect of aspirin which inhibits thromboxane synthesis more efficiently than that of prostacyclin. However, other mechanisms inhibit platelet accumulation on the endothelium by aspirin-independent routes.

Nitric oxide (NO) produced by vascular endothelial cells and circulating leucocytes powerfully relaxes smooth muscle, causes vasodilatation and inhibits platelet aggregation and adhesion (Furchgott and Zawadzki, 1980; Ignarro, 1989; Moncada et al, 1988, 1989). This is achieved, in contrast to prostacyclin, via elevation of cyclic GMP. Nitric oxide is produced from L-arginine and several stimuli promote its release including acetylcholine, bradykinin and ADP.

A further mechanism by which the endothelium may modify platelet reactions is via its nucleotidases, enzymes that hydrolyse the nucleotides, ADP, etc., responsible for platelet agglutinating reactions. Hydrolysis of these agents and adenosine metabolism by endothelial cells will therefore remove this stimulus from the platelet microenvironment efficiently and reduce the propensity for accumulation (Marcus et al, 1980; Gordon, 1986). A lipoxygenase product of linoleic acid, 13-hydroxoctadecadienoic acid (13-HODE), has been proposed as a further endothelial and polymorphonuclear leucocyte product inhibiting platelet aggregation (Buchanan & Bastida, 1988).

The processes of platelet adhesion to subendothelium, release of granule contents, arachidonic acid pathway activation and platelet aggregation all overlap and occur rapidly to produce the platelet plug and initial cessation of bleeding. However, fibrin is necessary for the longer-term cessation of bleeding and its formation occurs in parallel with platelet plug production.

Fibrin Formation

Coagulation depends ultimately on conversion of fibrinogen to fibrin by thrombin. Fibrinogen is present in solution in plasma in high concentration, normally 2–4 g/l. However, as an acute phase reactant, higher quantities are noted in response to challenges such as inflammation, trauma or malignancy. It comprises three polypeptide chains (αA, Bβ and γ) coordinately controlled at the level of gene expression (Crabtree and Kent, 1992) and each fibrinogen molecule represents a dimer of the three. During fibrin formation, thrombin splits fibrinopeptide A from each A α and fibrinopeptide B from the B β chain at their amino-terminal segments to produce soluble fibrin monomer (Blomback & Blomback, 1972). Fibrinopeptide A is released first and this allows polymerization of the monomers. Polymerization by end-to-end and side-to-side links of monomer molecules produces insoluble fibrin (Budzynski et al, 1983; Doolittle, 1984).

Fibrin so produced, though insoluble in plasma, is easily redisolved in solvents such as urea or monochloroacetic acid and is very susceptible to digestion by plasmin until the final reaction forming covalent bonds between fibrin molecules occurs. This requires the activation of factor XIII by thrombin. Activated factor XIII forms gamma-glutamyl ϵ-lysine bonds (Chen and Doolittle, 1969, 1971) between the γ and, later, α chains of fibrin (Folk and Finlayson, 1977; McKee et al, 1970). Alpha$_2$-antiplasmin is also cross-linked to fibrin by factor XIII along with fibronectin (Sakata and Aoki, 1980) and this confers plasmin resistance on the stabilized fibrin molecules.

Factor XIII in plasma is inert, consisting of twin pairs of subunits, a and b. Platelets contain only subunit a. Thrombin cleaves a small peptide from each subunit, the a and b subunits dissociate in the presence of calcium, exposing the transaminase active centre on the a subunit. This contains cystine at its active site unlike the serine of the other coagulant enzymes (Schwartz et al, 1973; Lorand et al, 1980). The active enzyme then cross-links fibrin as described above.

Pathways Leading to Fibrin Formation

Fibrin formation, deposition in wounds and other damaged tissues and its persistence there until healing processes are underway so that further blood loss is prevented, is central to the human haemostatic mechanism. In the 19th century (Morawitz, 1905, 1958), three agents were identified in plasma, namely fibrinogen, calcium ions and prothrombin, that were necessary for coagulation. Thrombokinase, now known more prosaically and practically as tissue factor, was the contribution made by solid tissues or the cellular elements of the blood,

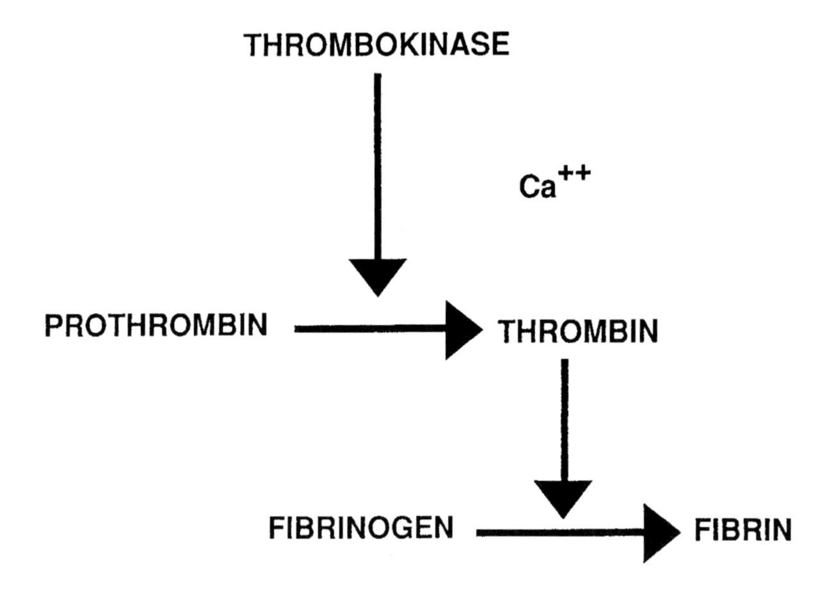

Figure 1.2 The early concept of fibrin generation.

platelets and leucocytes. Released on injury, this agent was thought to generate thrombin from prothrombin and this in turn generated insoluble fibrin from the circulating, soluble plasma fibrinogen (Fig. 1.2). Deficit in this series of interactions was identified by the one-stage prothrombin time (Quick et al, 1935) in which concentrated tissue factor was added to plasma, generating thrombin and thus a fibrin clot if the known agents were present. Fibrin strands enmeshed the cellular elements of the blood in the initial wound seal, which prevented further blood loss and provided a skeleton on which wound healing could progress.

In the decades from 1940 to 1960, several additional plasma agents were postulated and later identified, mainly by virtue of their functional deficiency or absence from the blood of patients with a variety of (usually) haemorrhagic disorders. The agents now known as factors VIII, IX, XI and XII were so identified (Ratnoff, 1991) though the last-mentioned was discovered by the study of plasma that coagulated poorly in vitro but came from an individual, Mr John Hageman (Ratnoff and Colopy, 1955), who showed no sign of bleeding at all and indeed ultimately died of pulmonary embolism. The problem facing workers at that time was the fact that plasma completely deficient in any one of these agents produced fibrin normally in the prothrombin time test. New concepts were required and took the form that two separate and discrete pathways existed leading to thrombin and fibrin formation. The first was the tissue factor or extrinsic pathway and the second the intrinsic pathway (Fig. 1.3) which did not require tissue factor but in which activity was initiated when blood came into

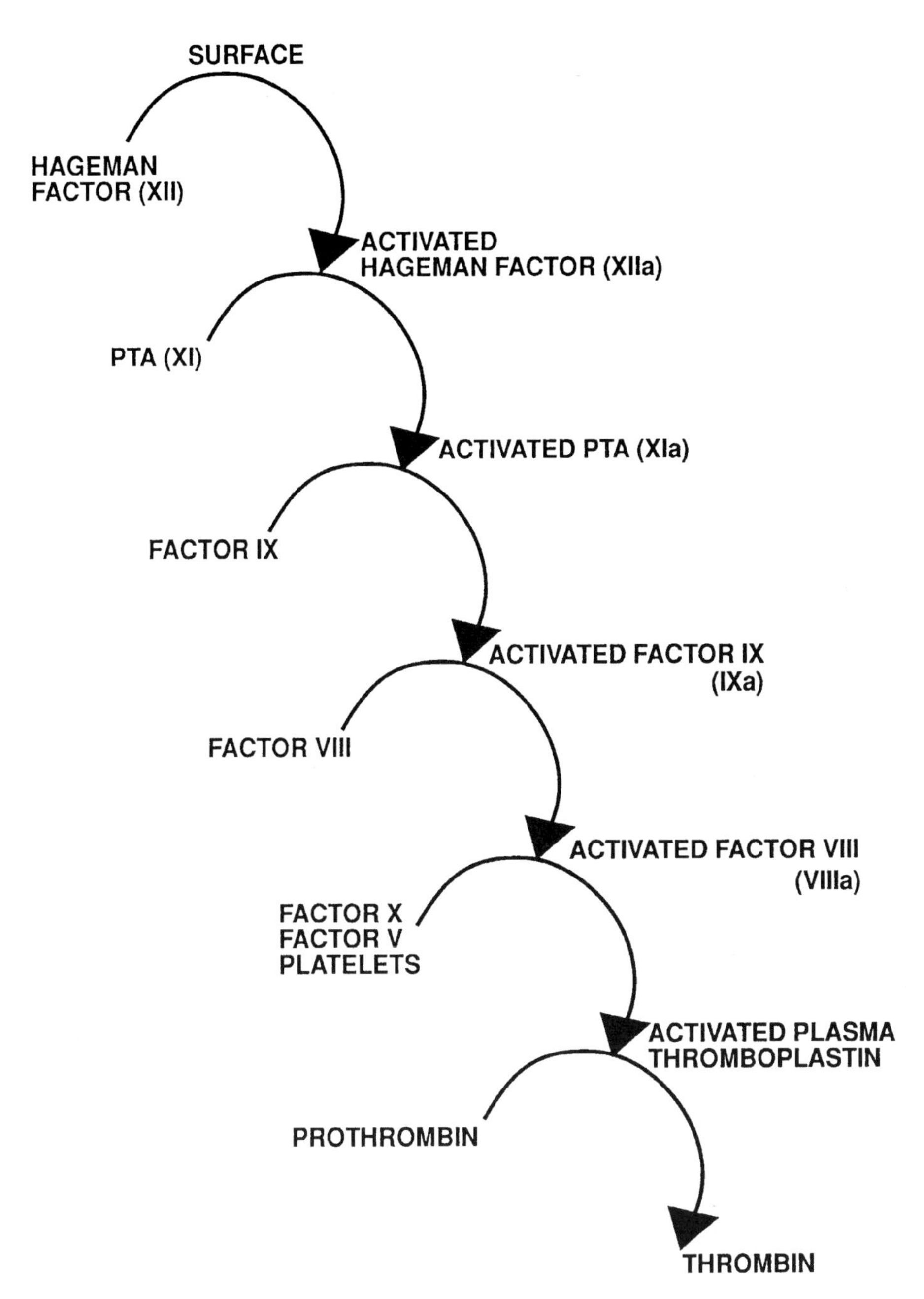

Figure 1.3 The intrinsic path to thrombin generation.

contact with foreign, negatively charged surfaces that activated factor XII. Ultimately this pathway's integrity became screened by the partial thromboplastin time in which plasma was exposed to negatively charged surfaces, usually particulate kaolin, that initiated its activity and a sequence of reactions occurred finally generating thrombin and so fibrin from fibrinogen.

Clearly as both pathways generated thrombin, and thus fibrin, they had to share final steps. Two further agents, additional to prothrombin, were found necessary and common to each pathway, again by studying rare deficiencies in haemorrhagic patients. These were factors V and X. An additional factor operating entirely in the unique part of the extrinsic pathway was also identified, namely factor VII.

In the early 1960s the concept of two pathways characterized by sequential proenzyme to enzyme conversions and likened to a waterfall, or cascade, was proposed in Britain and in the USA (Macfarlane, 1964; Davie and Ratnoff, 1964). At this time it was not possible to purify the agents completely and many questions about their interactions remained unanswered. Phospholipid was regarded as providing a surface for the interaction of these proteins and was provided by platelets activated in the process of aggregation or platelet plug formation at wound sites in vivo. Ionic calcium was necessary for the binding of these proteins to the phospholipid.

In the years since, the strict sequence of proenzyme to enzyme conversions initially conceived has been modified; factors VIII and V, for instance, do not partake directly as individual players occupying a step of their own, but rather function as co-factors, factor VIII by enhancing the activation of factor X by factor IXa and factor V, that of prothrombin by factor Xa (Fig. 1.4). Despite the fact that they do not function as active enzymes themselves, both require minor proteolysis by thrombin to exert their co-factor role.

Several proteins active in haemostasis require vitamin K for their production, examples of these are the procoagulant factors II, VII, IX and X and the anticoagulant agent proteins C and S (see below). Linkage of the coagulant proteins in the vitamin K-dependent group to phospholipid is a calcium-dependent phenomenon occurring at gamma carboxyglutamic acid (Gla) residues near the amino-terminal end of these molecules (Chung et al, 1975). These residues are formed by vitamin K-dependent modification of glutamic acid residues on the individual protein skeletons which are themselves produced entirely independent of this vitamin by the liver (Fujikawa et al, 1974a,b; Nelsestuen et al, 1974; Stenflo et al, 1974; Magnusson et al, 1975a,b)

These coagulation factors in their native form may be single chain (factors VII, IX, II and protein S) or two chain (factor X and protein C) molecules. They all undergo some degree of proteolysis, with the exception of protein S, on activation in the cascade.

These advances came from techniques available in the 1960s and 1970s such as protein purification, gel electrophoretic analysis, amino acid sequencing and so on. More recently, molecular biological methods have resulted in cloning of the coagulation agents such as the three fibrinogen chains (Chung et al, 1983a,b;

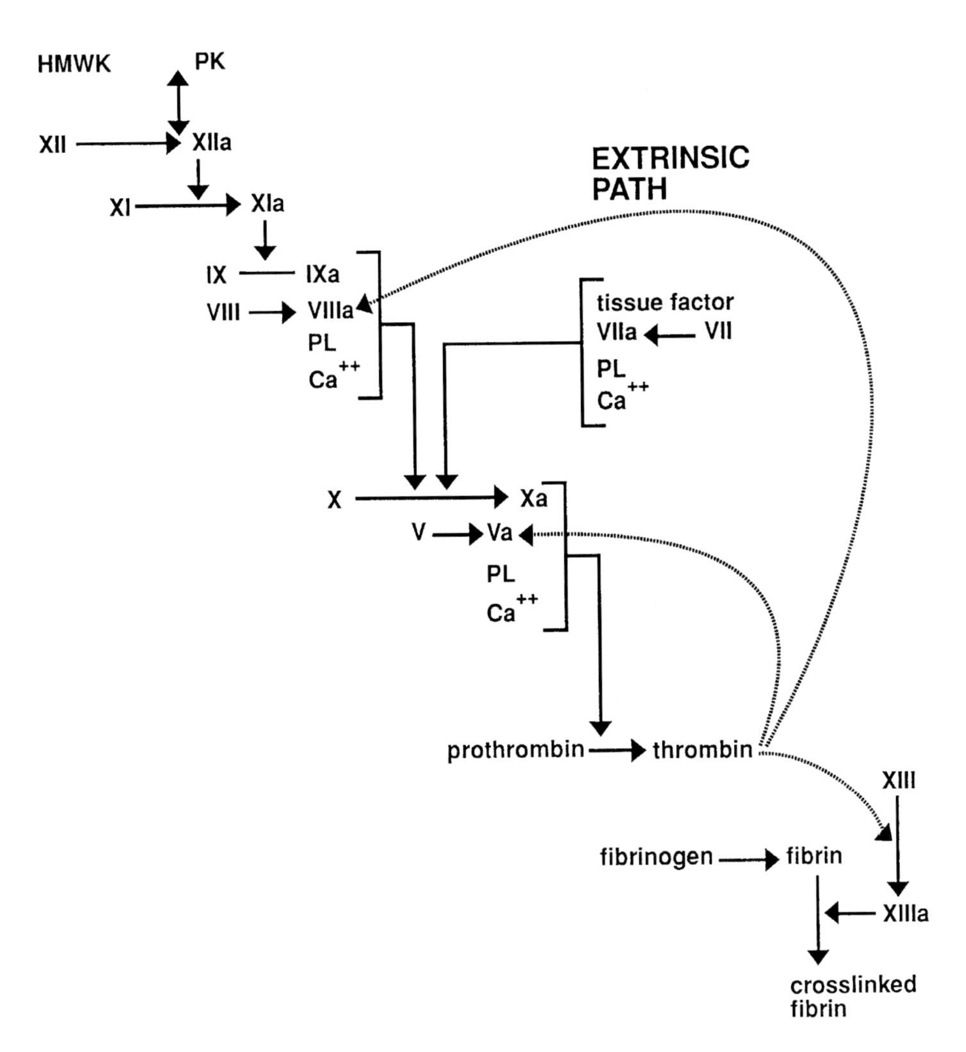

Figure 1.4 The intrinsic and extrinsic pathways of thrombin generation. HMWK, high-molecular-weight kininogen; PK, prekallikrein; PL, phospholipid.

Table 1.3 Human coagulation factors

Protein (factor)	Approximate molecular size (kDA)	Chromosome	Approximate half-life (hours)
Fibrinogen (I)	340	4 (α, β, γ chains)	100–150
Prothrombin (II)	70	11	50–80
Tissue factor (III)	40	1	—
Factor V	330	1	24
Factor VII	50	13	6
Factor VIII	330	X	12
Factor IX	55	X	24
Factor X	59	13	30–60
Factor XI	160	4	40–80
Factor XII	80	5	50–70
Factor XIII	320	6 (a subunit) 1 (b subunit)	150

Rixon et al, 1983), prothrombin (MacGillivray et al, 1980; Degan et al, 1983), factor VIII (Gitschier et al, 1984; Toole et al, 1984), factor IX (Kurachi and Davie, 1982; Anson et al, 1984; Yoshitake et al, 1985) and factor X (Leytus et al, 1984; Fung et al, 1985). A vast amount of information on the nature of the molecules and their interactions has become available as a result (Table 1.3).

The Intrinsic Pathway of Thrombin Generation

Contact activation

Initiation of activity in the intrinsic pathway is achieved via the contact of plasma with negatively charged foreign surfaces. This induces interaction between four agents: factor XII (Hageman factor), factor IX (plasma thromboplastin antecedent, PTA) prekallikrein (Fletcher factor) and high-molecular-weight kininogen (HMWK, Fitzgerald, Flaujeac or Williams factor).

Hageman factor, factor XII, was initially identified as the agent deficient in individuals with Hageman trait (Ratnoff & Colopy, 1955). In these individuals severe coagulation abnormalities are present in the intrinsic pathway in vitro but no bleeding disorder is evident and Mr Hageman ultimately died of a pulmonary embolism.

Factor XII is an 80 kDa glycoprotein encoded by a gene on chromosome 5. The N-terminal portion binds to negatively charged surfaces and the C-terminal possesses enzymic activity (Revak and Cochrane, 1976). Activation of factor XII is achieved by kallikrein as described below. This can convert the single chain molecule to a two chain form by limited proteolysis and this retains coagulant activity (alpha XIIa). Further proteolysis results in the production of beta XIIa which loses the ability to activate factor XI losing the surface binding site (Revak et al, 1978) but is a powerful activator of prekallikrein.

Factor XI, deficient in the plasma of a small number of patients with a mild hereditary bleeding disorder (Rosenthal et al, 1953), is a 160 kDa protein comprising two identical polypeptide chains controlled by a gene on chromosome 4 (Bouma and Griffin, 1977; Kurachi and Davie, 1977), which circulates in plasma in a complex with high molecular weight kininogen (Thompson et al, 1977). It is cleaved to factor XIa by factor XIIa in the presence of high molecular weight kininogen. The activated protein comprises two light and two heavy chains, the light chain possessing active serine sites. The function of factor XIa is to activate factor IX, a conversion that requires calcium but no other agent. The relative importance of this reaction as opposed to activation of factor IX by factor VIIa is discussed below. XIa in vitro can attack other agents including factor XII, high molecular weight kininogen, fibrinogen and plasminogen but the significance of these interactions is doubtful.

Prekallikrein, the factor deficient in the plasma of an asymptomatic disorder characterized by severe coagulation abnormality in vitro, was initially described as Fletcher factor (Hathaway et al, 1965). This was subsequently identified with prekallikrein (Wuepper, 1973). Prekallikrein has a molecular size of approximately 85 kDa and circulates in plasmin complexed with high molecular weight kininogen (Mandle et al, 1976) which is absorbed onto negatively charged surfaces. Prekallikrein is converted to kallikrein by factor XIIa cleavage. This produces a two chain molecule, the active serine site residing in the light chain while the heavy chain contains the binding site for high molecular weight kininogen (Mandle and Kaplan, 1977). Kallikrein activates factor XII in addition to releasing kinin from high molecular weight kininogen. The interaction with factor XII appears to be reciprocal (Cochrane et al, 1973; Revak et al, 1977).

High molecular weight kininogen (HMW kininogen), a single chain glycoprotein, acts as a co-factor in the contact activation system. It was initially identified as doing so when plasma deficient in the agent was identified in several families: Fitzgerald (Saito et al, 1975) Flaujeac (Wuepper et al, 1975) or Williams (Colman et al, 1975). They all shared markedly prolonged partial thromboplastin time but bleeding was not a major problem. It has a molecular weight of 120 kDa and circulates in a complex with either prekallikrein or factor XI. It functions as a surface binding protein linking these agents to foreign surfaces and so speeds contact activation (Wiggins et al, 1977). Additionally it contains the braydkinin fragment, released by kallikrein, with vasoactive properties.

When exposed to negatively charged surfaces, all four of these agents are bound to them; factor XII binds directly while factors XI and prekallikrein are bound via the high molecular weight kininogen complex. Binding of factor XII makes it more susceptible to cleavage (Griffin, 1978) and it is converted to factor XIIa by limited proteolysis (Revak et al, 1977). Factor XIIa, as indicated above, activates conversion of surface-bound prekallikrein to kallikrein by cleavage of a bond and this in turn reciprocally converts factor XII to factor XIIa (Cochrane et al, 1973). Ultimately when sufficient XIIa is formed, surface-bound factor XI is converted to factor XIa. Autoactivation of factor XII can occur but reciprocal activation by kallikrein predominates. High molecular weight kininogen acts as a co-factor in this process, speeding activation of prekallikrein and factor XI by surface-bound factor XII and of factor XII by kallikrein. During the course of these reactions, bradykinin may be released from this molecule. The nature of the first molecular change that initiates this cycle of events remains unclear. It has been suggested that a conformational change in factor XII occurs on binding, which initiates events (Ratnoff and Saito, 1979) but other suggestions exist such as the possibility that zymogen factor XII contains a very low inherent level of enzymatic activity, enough to initiate the reciprocal interaction with prekallikrein on binding (Griffin & Beretta, 1979). Just as it is difficult to identify the initial event in producing activation in the extrinsic pathway, so a similar question here remains unresolved.

Platelets participate in the contact phase of coagulation, thereby promoting the interaction between the reagent proteins and assembling contact factors on their surface (Walsh, 1987). Additionally, platelets contain factor XI, high molecular weight kininogen, C1 inhibitor and may participate in the contact phase by virtue of these.

Several plasma agents exert a controlling influence on the contact phase of coagulation, some by occupying binding sites on negatively charged proteins, others by direct action on the enzymes themselves. For instance, C1 inhibitor inhibits factor XIIa, factor XIa and kallikrein, alpha$_1$-antitrypsin inhibits factor XIa and alpha$_2$-macroglobulin inhibits prekallikrein.

The contact phase of blood coagulation has recently been extensively reviewed in detail (Saito, 1995).

Factor IX

Factor IX, deficient in Christmas disease, is a 55 kDa single chain protein of established sequence and gene structure (Kurachi and Davie, 1982; Yoshitaki et al, 1985). It is one of the vitamin K-dependent factors, but unlike the others the gene occurs on the X chromosome. Activation involves rupture of two bonds with release of 10 kDa glycopeptide (Thompson, 1986) and production of a two chain molecule. Its conversion may be achieved by factor XIa, a reaction requiring no co-factors, or by factor VIIa, which requires tissue factor and calcium (Thompson, 1986; Osterud and Rapaport, 1977). Which mode of conversion is dominant is disputed (Walsh et al, 1984; Warn-Cramer et al, 1986; Nemerson, 1988).

Factor IXa converts factor X to its activated form cleaving the ^{52}Arg–^{53}Ile bond of the heavy chain of factor X. This requires the presence of factor VIII, phospholipid and ionic calcium, the phospholipid binding the coagulants to its surface approximating and enhancing their interaction in a manner similar to its function in conversion of prothrombin to thrombin by factor Xa (Furie and Furie, 1988; Mann et al, 1988). Endothelial cells, platelets or monocytes can also provide phospholipid (Stern et al, 1984; Rosing et al, 1985; McGee and Li, 1991).

Factor IXa activity is principally controlled by the action of antithrombin III enhanced by the heparin effect (Rosenberg et al, 1975).

Factor VIII

Factor VIII, like factor IX, is produced by a gene located on the X chromosome, which has been recently cloned (Gitschier et al, 1984; Toole et al, 1984; Wood et al, 1984). It is the procoagulant agent defective in classic haemophilia (Patek and Taylor, 1937). It is the largest procoagulant molecule in plasma, with a size of over 300 kDa, and it circulates there in a complex with another large protein, von Willebrand factor (vWF). Factor VIII is produced in the liver (Wion et al, 1985) and several other tissues. Unlike factor V, with which it has considerable sequence homology, it has no intrinsic enzyme activity but enhances activation of factor X by factor IXa as a co-factor, apparently interacting with both light and heavy chains of factor IXa (Vehar and Davie, 1980; Frazier et al, 1989; Nishimura et al, 1991). Its molecular conformation is modified by thrombin (Rapaport et al, 1963; Eaton et al, 1986; Kane and Davie, 1968; Mann et al, 1988). This enhances its co-factor function but in this form it is susceptible to inhibition by activated protein C, also generated by thrombin activity.

Von Willebrand Factor (VIIIR Ag, VIIIR Co)

Von Willebrand factor (vWF), the agent deficient in von Willebrand's disease (vWD), acts as a carrier for factor VIII in the circulation but has no coagulant activity itself (Girma et al, 1987). Synthesized by endothelial cells (Jaffe et al, 1973) and megakaryocytes (Sporn et al, 1985), it exists in plasma as a series of multimers, the basic unit being of 250 kDa. The largest of the multimers (10 000 kDa) maximally promote adhesion of platelets to subendothelium (Sixma et al, 1984). Unlike factors VIII and IX, the gene encoding this agent is located on an autosomal chromosome, number 12. The clinical pattern of the von Willebrand disease (vWD) subtypes varies according to the pattern of loss or the abnormality of these multimers (Sadler, 1995). Deficiency is responsible, by virtue of impaired adhesion mechanisms, for the prolonged bleeding time characteristic of von Willebrand's disease (vWD).

Factor X (Stuart–Prower Factor)

Factor X was identified as a result of a specific deficiency in the 1950s (Telfer et al, 1956; Hougie et al, 1957). It occupies a crucial position central to the pathways of thrombin generation. It is a vitamin K-dependent glycoprotein with a molecular weight of 59 kDa and is a double chain molecule. It is formed in the liver under the influence of a gene on chromosome 13. Like the other vitamin K-dependent proteins it undergoes gammacarboxylation and other post-translational changes in hepatocytes. Its activation involves release of a glycopeptide from the N-terminal end of the heavy chain (Fujikawa et al, 1974a). Its activation by the extrinsic pathway is achieved when factor VII bound to tissue factor complexes with membrane phospholipid of several cell types in the presence of calcium. The presence of this complex vastly accelerates the conversion of factor X to factor Xa by factor VII. A regulation loop whereby factor Xa positively enhances factor VII to VIIa conversion at low concentrations while at higher concentrations it cleaves and inactivates factor VIIa has been described (Radcliffe & Nemerson, 1975). The first part of the loop, namely the activation of factor VII, is thought to be a key early step in the tissue factor dependent pathway (Rao & Rapaport, 1988). As described above, the intrinsic pathway also converts factor X to factor Xa in a qualitatively similar manner, requiring factor IXa, phospholipid, calcium and factor VIIIa in a complex with factor X, and the presence of all these agents in the complex vastly accelerates the rate of production of Xa.

Prothrombin

Prothrombin, a single chain "kringle"-containing 70 kDa glycoprotein, is encoded by a gene on chromosome 11 (Royle et al, 1987). It is, along with factors VII, IX and X, a vitamin K-dependent protein produced in the liver (Jackson et al 1974, 1975; Jackson, 1995). In this site the gamma carboxy-glutamic acid (Gla) residues are attached to the N-terminal end of the molecule and confer the ability to bind calcium and thus to attach to phospholipid. Without these residues these factors (PIVKA – proteins induced by vitamin K

Table 1.4 Influence of thrombin on several facets of the haemostatic mechanism

Coagulation		
Fibrinogen	→	Fibrin
Factor XIII	→	Factor XIIIa
Factor V	→	Factor Va
Factor VIII	→	Factor VIIIa
Protein C	→	APC
Platelets		
Platelet release of granular proteins		
Platelet aggregation		
Endothelium		
PGI_2 production		
von Willebrand factor (vWF) production		
APC production via thrombomodulin		
PAI-1 production		

absence) do not bind thus and have severely diminished coagulant properties. Factor Xa itself splits two peptide bonds in prothrombin to produce thrombin at a slow rate. Enormous acceleration of this conversion occurs in the presence of phospholipid, calcium ions and factor Va (Jackson and Suttie, 1977). This occurs as factor Xa and prothrombin bind via calcium to the phospholipid through their Gla residues while factor Va binds to phospholipid and prothrombin (Esmon et al, 1973). In this "prothrombinase" complex these agents in close proximity interact more readily, protected from the influence of inhibitors (Teitel and Rosenberg, 1983; Furie and Furie, 1988; Mann et al, 1988). Activated platelets, leucocytes or endothelial cell membranes (Tracy et al, 1983) may localize the phenomenon to sites of injury. Activation to thrombin can occur via two different pathways according to the order in which cleavage of arginine-containing bonds occurs and different subunits are released. These intermediates may be either prethrombin 2 and fragment 1/2 or meizothrombin (Stenn and Blout, 1972; Esmon et al, 1974; Jackson et al, 1974; Owen et al, 1974; Magnusson et al, 1975; Morita et al, 1976).

Thrombin, once formed, not only generates fibrin from fibrinogen but has a vast number of other functions. Those affecting the haemostatic mechanism are outlined in Table 1.4.

Factor V

Factor V, encoded by a gene on chromosome 1 and produced by liver endothelial cells, megakaryocytes and smooth muscle, is a large protein (about 250 kDa; Kane and Davie, 1988) which, like factor VIII, acts as a co-factor in the conversion of one vitamin K-dependent coagulation factor by another in a multimolecular complex. In this case the conversion concerned is that of prothrombin by factor Xa. Circulating factor V has little activity but minor proteolysis by traces of thrombin (Rapaport et al, 1963; Kane and Davie, 1988; Mann et al, 1988) promotes its co-factor activity enormously. The activated form binds to factor Xa via both its light and heavy chains (Freeman et al, 1977), to prothrombin via its heavy chain (Esmon et al, 1973) and to phospholipid via its light chain (Guinto and Esmon, 1981). Like factor VIII, factor Va is inhibited by activated protein C.

The Extrinsic Pathway Factor VII and its Extended Role

A problem in interpreting the physiological significance of the intrinsic pathway lay in the fact that patients with factor XII deficiency, though their blood coagulated abnormally in the test tube, did not bleed and neither did patients with high molecular weight kininogen or prekallikrein deficiency. Additionally, patients deficient in the next stage involving factor XI bled only slightly in marked contrast to those with deficiencies of factor IX and factor VIII, which occupy subsequent steps of the pathway, who had major and spontaneous lifelong haemorrhage. The fact that these deficiencies lay in steps apparently unique to the intrinsic path alone led to its dominating thinking about coagulation mechanisms for many years. The clinical frequency of congenital factor VIII and IX deficiencies enhanced this attitude. However, factor VII deficiency, if severe, produces a major bleeding disorder but this deficiency is exceedingly rare so the extrinsic path, though the first to be identified, received relatively less attention as exciting observations were being made elsewhere and involved the common hereditary bleeding disorders. Recently attention has returned to examination of the extrinsic pathway and the role of tissue factor and factor VII in maintaining haemostasis. The fact that adding tissue factor to plasma deficient in factors VIII and IX resulted in a normal rate of coagulation indicated that the effect of these deficiencies could be bypassed under some circumstances. Early clues suggested that extrinsic and intrinsic pathways might be linked by additional interactions; in particular, suggestions were made that tissue factor or products of its pathway might substitute for the products of the contact

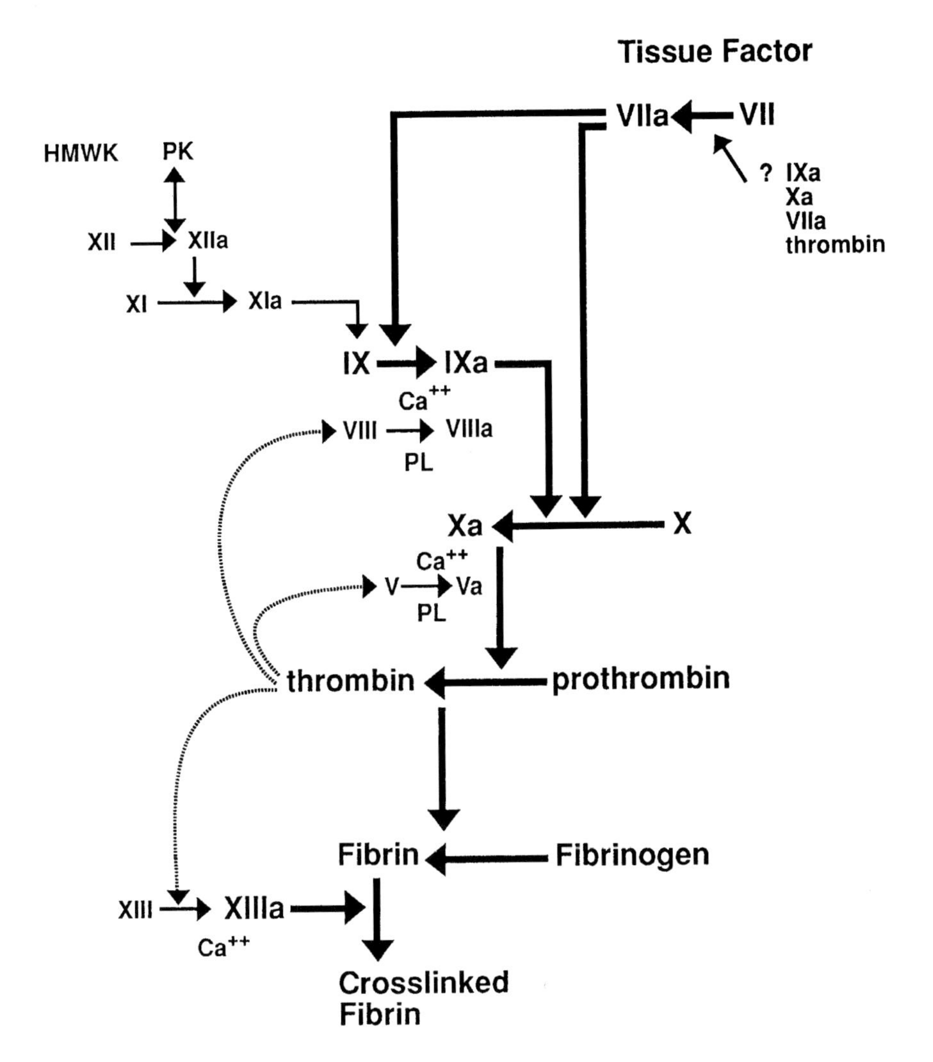

Figure 1.5 Pathways to fibrin generation: recent modifications. HMWK, high-molecular weight kininogen; PK, prekallikrein; PL, phospholipid.

reactions in the intrinsic pathway and might directly activate factor IX (Waaler, 1957; Biggs and Nossel, 1961; Josso et al, 1965; Rapaport et al, 1966). More recently, and working with relatively pure materials, Osterud and Rapaport (1977) showed that the reaction product of tissue factor and factor VII could indeed activate factor IX and thus provide a second mechanism by which the tissue factor pathway could stimulate the production of thrombin (Fig. 1.5).

The relative importance of the tissue factor–factor VII product's action in activating factor IX and thus, indirectly, factor X or of its action in activating factor X directly thus becomes intriguing. In some systems its direct activation of factor X seems faster (Warn-Cramer and Bajaj, 1986; Almus et al, 1989; Komiyama et al, 1990; Rao et al, 1992) but in others its activation of factor IX significantly enhances the activation of factor X (Osterud and Rapaport, 1977; Marlar et al, 1982; Stern et al, 1985; Lawson et al, 1994). Thus it appeared that the tissue factor pathway could enhance thrombin and fibrin formation, not only by direct action on factor X but by short-circuiting activity in the intrinsic path, bypassing the contact system, activating factor IX and further speeding factor X activation, the latter process crucially requiring the presence of factor VIII and being essential for normal haemostasis. This concept goes a considerable way to explaining the contrast between the very severe bleeding in the haemophilias (factor VIII and IX deficiencies) and the relatively trivial bleeding in factor XI deficiency. The biological phenomenon of the bleeding in the haemophilias (factor VIII or IX deficiency) emphasizes the major role for this part of the pathway in normal haemostasis.

The agent that initiates activation of factor VII itself is as yet unknown. A single chain protein, factor VII, like the other procoagulant proteins, is converted to an active enzyme by rupture of an internal bond, in this case arginine 152–Ile. Factor VII conversion is vastly enhanced by its binding to the extracellular N-terminal domain of tissue factor, a single chain membrane glycoprotein that requires association with phospholipid for its function. In equimolar association in the presence of ionic calcium, these agents generate factor VIIa on membranes (Nemerson et al, 1985; Rao et al, 1988; Sakai et al, 1989). Traces of factor Xa, IXa, VIIa itself or thrombin may achieve initial activation of tissue-factor-bound factor VII (Nemerson and Repke, 1985; Rao et al, 1986; Rao and Rapaport, 1988). An interesting observation is the fact that minute quantities of factor VIIa occur in circulating blood but that patients with severe factor IX deficiency show a major reduction in this agent whereas those with factor VIII deficiency do not, suggesting that factor IX plays a role in factor VII activation. However, other possibilities exist (Kazama et al, 1995). Thus, just as in the 1970s and 1980s, we were pursuing the events responsible for initiating activity in the intrinsic pathway, and debating whether contact activation was initiated by autoactivation of factor XII by trace quantities of XIIa or by kallikrein-induced factor XII activation when confronted by a negatively charged surface, so now trace quantities of proteases are sought that may ultimately be responsible for the activation of factor VII when complexed with tissue factor (Rapaport and Rao, 1995). Whether the initiating agent is traces of VIIa, IIa, IXa or Xa is not yet defined.

As in the other steps of the pathway, phospholipid plays a considerable role in enhancing the action of the enzyme factor VIIa. While not essential for the interaction of VIIa and tissue factor, it enhances the binding necessary for factor VII itself to be activated and is required for its activation of its substrates, factor IX and X, partly by providing a binding surface for these substrates.

The tissue factor pathway is only susceptible to neutralization when factor VIIa is active and bound to tissue factor itself. The tissue factor pathway inhibitor (TEPI-1), a Kunitz-type inhibitor, provides some control (Rapaport, 1989, 1991; Broze et al, 1990) and a second similar agent (TFPI-2) has also been recently identified (Sprecher et al, 1994). Heparin releases quantities of TFPI bound to glycosaminoglycans into the circulation (Sandset et al, 1988; Novotny et al, 1991) and heparin also limits clearance of TFPI from the circulation. TFPI binds first to factor Xa and thereafter this complex binds to factors VIIa/TF; the quaternary complex lacks catalytic activity (Rapaport and Rao, 1995; Broze et al, 1988; Warn-Cramer et al, 1988). However, the role of the inhibitor in normal physiology is not yet clear. Platelet factor 4 can also bind to the vitamin K-dependent clotting factors via their Gla domain and inhibit the pathway further (Key et al, 1994). Antithrombin itself clearly exerts a regulatory role on the extrinsic pathway (Rosenberg and Damus, 1973). This agent inhibits active procoagulant proteins, factors IIa, VIIa, IXa, Xa and in addition factor XIa, by complexing with them, a reaction vastly enhanced by the presence of heparin (Kurachi et al, 1976; Kurachi and Davie, 1977; Shigematsu, 1992; Lawson, 1993; Rao et al, 1993).

Control of Thrombin Generation

The first agent clearly identified as a major coagulation inhibitor was antithrombin, originally known as antithrombin III. Its identification came from the study of a family affected by hereditary thrombophilia with an autosomal dominant pattern, now established as being deficient in this protein (Egeberg, 1965). Antithrombin, a 65 kDa protein, functions by targeting thrombin and other activated procoagulants and neutralizing their enzymic activity by complex formation. It can inhibit not only thrombin but also factors XIIa, XIa, IXa and Xa, kallikrein and plasmin. Its function in inhibiting these agents is greatly enhanced by the presence of heparin, which binds to the amino-terminal domain of the molecule rendering the active site, arginine, more available for interaction with the serine of thrombin. The glycosaminoglycans of vascular endothelium presumably act similarly (Marcum et al, 1984). Many mutations on the gene on chromosome 1 controlling this protein have now been identified, some leading to quantitative (type 1) and others to qualitative (type 2) defects. Type 2 defects may affect the reactive site by which the molecule interacts with the activated procoagulants or alternatively with the heparin binding site of the molecule, the thrombophilic potential of the latter being less striking than that of the former (Molho-Sabatier et al, 1989; Lane et al, 1993). Those affecting the active site may transform antithrombin into a substrate for thrombin while others prevent its recognition of its target proteases. A further protein of similar molecular size inhibiting thrombin alone and requiring larger amounts of heparin to function has been identified. This was originally named heparin co-factor II; its action is particularly enhanced by dermatan sulphate and deficiencies have been associated with thrombosis.

An additional system for modifying coagulation or fibrin formation requires two further proteins which are, like some of the procoagulant agents, dependent on vitamin K for their production. These proteins are now known as protein C and protein S. Thrombomodulin, a membrane glycoprotein of endothelial cells, complexes with active thrombin and neutralizes its ability to produce fibrin (Esmon, 1987). The complex product then converts protein C to an active protease, activated protein C (APC; 56 kDa), a single chain protein that destroys by proteolysis the activity of factors Va and VIIIa. This process is markedly enhanced by the presence of the second vitamin K-dependent protein, protein S (69 kDa). This process may thus suppress the generation of further thrombin by a feedback loop. APC also inactivates PAI-1 (see below) so enhancing fibrinolysis. The system thus enhances maintenance of blood fluidity. APC, in turn, is controlled by its own inhibitor, a 57 kDa single chain protein capable of complexing with the activated enzyme. Thrombomodulin has a wide distribution in tissues (Soff et al, 1981). Homozygosity for deletion of thrombomodulin results in death in utero, apparently due to growth retardation in endodermal tissues (Rosenberg, 1995). Heterozygosity is not associated with thrombosis in mice. Deficiencies of protein C and protein S in turn result in thrombotic disorders of varying severity. In humans heterozygosity does enhance the incidence of thrombosis somewhat (Miletich et al, 1987; Bovill et al, 1989; Bertina et al, 1994). Deficiencies of protein C, protein S and antithrombin itself are relatively uncommon and responsible for only a modest proportion of episodes of hereditary thrombophilia. Recently, a further more common hereditary disorder favouring thrombosis has been defined. This is activated protein C resistance, a phenomenon now known to be due to a mutation on the factor V gene that renders factor Va resistant to inactivation by APC (Dahlbeck et al, 1993; Bertina et al, 1994).

The tissue factor pathway inhibitor (TFPI), a recently rediscovered and identified entity (Loeb et al, 1922; Thomas, 1947; Schneider, 1947; Hjort, 1957; Broze, 1987, 1995) is a plasma protein of 38 kDa that inhibits factor Xa directly, complexing with it and in turn inhibiting the action of the factor VIIa/tissue factor complex. In plasma it is bound to lipoproteins, particularly low density lipoproteins (LDL). Its source is probably the endothelium from which it is released into the circulation, a process enhanced by heparin. It possesses three Kunitz type domains. Factor Xa/prothrombin complex inhibition requires the carboxy-terminus of the molecule and the second Kunitz domain which binds to factor Xa. Once this initial complex is formed it binds and inhibits the factor VIIa/tissue factor complex, a reaction in which the first Kunitz domain binds to VIIa. It is suggested that this phenomenon is sufficiently powerful to throw into prominence the requirement of the factor VIII and factor IX pathway in generating factor Xa in the circulation.

α_2-Macroglobulin, α_2-antitrypsin, α_2-antiplasmin, PAI-1 and C1 inactivator are all proteins that will bind or inhibit activated procoagulants in vitro. Their physiological roles in controlling fibrin formation are not established.

A further mechanism modifying thrombin production in vivo is that of clearance of activated coagulant proteins from the circulation. This occurs largely in the liver but there are few clinically relevant quantitative data in this area.

Fibrinolysis

As indicated earlier we are endowed with an efficient system for sealing wounds in our vascular compartment. This leads to the production of a formidable wound seal consisting of fibrin and platelets. Ultimately this requires removal when wound healing is well advanced. Additionally, small quantities of fibrin formed inappropriately within the microvasculature, because of triggering of efficient haemostatic mechanisms, require removal. These processes are achieved by the fibrinolytic mechanism (Fig. 1.6) (Bennett and Ogston, 1995).

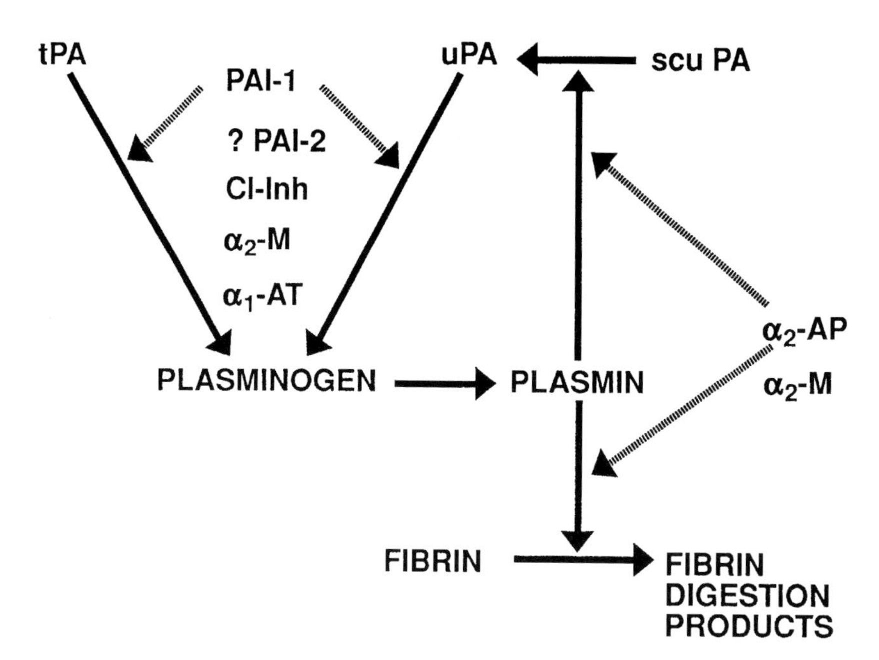

Figure 1.6 The fibrinolytic system. tPA, tissue plasminogen activator; uPA, urokinase; PAI-1, plasminogen activator inhibitor-1; PAI-2, plasminogen activator inhibitor-2; C1-Inh, C1 inhibitor; scu PA, single chain urokinase; α_2-M, α_2-macroglobulin; α_1-AT, α_1-antitrypsin; α_2-AP, α_2-antiplasmin.

Fibrinolysis depends on the production of plasmin, a protease rarely detected in the circulation in an active form. Plasmin is generated from the circulating precursor protein, plasminogen, an inactive glycoprotein of molecular weight 90 kDa that occupies a position in the fibrinolytic system similar to that of prothrombin in coagulation. It is a single chain protein encoded by a gene on chromosome 6, and possesses five "kringle" structures formed by internal disulphate bonds which create loops in the molecule similar to those seen on the prothrombin molecule. These loops contain lysine binding sites, which will be referred to subsequently. It is converted to the active protease, plasmin, by rupture of the arginine 560/valine 561 bond which creates a two chain plasmin molecule. The heavy chain contains the "kringles" the lysine binding sites of which determine its interaction with its major inhibitor, α_2-antiplasmin, or its substrate fibrin. It circulates with an amino-terminal glutamic acid (Glu plasminogen) and a second form with amino-terminal lysine (Lys plasminogen) is generated in the process of plasmin formation. The protease, plasmin, digests not only fibrin but fibrinogen, factors V and VIII and other proteins.

Plasmin formation from plasminogen is achieved by the plasminogen activators, of which two major physiological types exist. The first identified activator was, however, streptokinase, the bacterial product, the first agent used in the now widely employed thrombolytic therapy.

The principal circulating plasminogen activator in man, however, is tissue-type plasminogen activator (tPA) a 70 kDa protein encoded by a gene on chromosome 8 that may exist in single or two chain forms (Rijken and Collen, 1981; Wallen et al, 1982). The active site lies in the light chain while the heavy chain has two "kringle"-like structures similar to those in plasminogen. It converts plasminogen to plasmin as described above and this activity is markedly enhanced in the presence of formed fibrin which not only binds tPA and plasminogen but increases the affinity of tPA for the proenzyme. Fibrin thus brings tPA and plasminogen together, enhancing their interaction, and as plasmin so formed is bound by its lysine binding sites to fibrinogen, it is relatively protected from the inhibitory effect of α_2-antiplasmin (Collen and Lijnen, 1990). The primary source of tPA in the body is the vascular endothelium (Todd, 1959).

In normal individuals tPA and PAI-1 circulate as a complex with a molecular size of 110 kDa (Booth et al, 1987). Stimuli such as exercise result in considerably increased levels of plasminogen activator in the circulation and this represents material released from the endothelium that has not yet complexed with the inhibitor (Booth et al, 1987). However, such free tPA is only detectable briefly. When vast amounts of tPA are released or injected it complexes not only with PAI-1 but also with C1 inhibitor (C1-INH) and α_2-macroglobulin before it is cleared from the circulation (Bennett et al, 1990). Whereas little free tPA activity is normally present in blood because of complexing with PAI-1, the reverse situation occurs in marrow which is rich in free tPA and the tPA/PAI-1 ratio is high (McWilliam et al, 1996).

The first human plasminogen activator identified was urokinase (uPA) from urine (White et al, 1966). It has a molecular size of 54 kDa, is encoded by a gene on chromosome 10 and exists in single chain or two chain forms. The single chain precursor form (scuPA) has been isolated from blood and urine (Wun et al, 1982; Hussain et al, 1983). Minor digestion by plasmin converts it to the enzymatically active two chain form. Unlike tPA, this does not have major fibrin affinity. Traces of urokinase activity can be detected in plasma of patients with hepatic cirrhosis (Booth et al, 1984) and larger quantities in some patients with promyelocytic leukaemia (Bennett et al, 1989).

A second pathway exists which may generate plasminogen activator. This depends on the integrity of the contact activation pathway of the intrinsic system of coagulation. This activator has therefore sometimes been termed the "intrinsic" activator by analogy. Generation of the activator is not possible in blood from patients with Hageman trait, Fletcher trait or Fitzgerald trait and it therefore appears to require the presence of factor XII, prekallikrein, and high-molecular-weight kininogen as well as other less well-defined agents (Ogston et al, 1969). Activated factor XII or kallikrein can activate plasminogen, and kallikrein can convert scuPA to active uPA and this pathway may depend upon these reactions.

Inhibitors of Fibrinolysis

The principal inhibitor of plasminogen activator is known as plasminogen activator inhibitor-1 (PAI-1), a protein of approximately 50 kDa that inhibits both tPA and uPA and has received intense molecular study in recent years (Loskutoff et al, 1989; Booth, 1995). It is synthesized by human endothelial cells in culture (Emeis et al, 1983). It is present in human plasma in small amounts, the agent here having high specific activity; it is also present in an apparently much less active form in platelets but the total quantity in platelets is much greater than that in plasma so the contribution of platelets to the overall inhibitory potential of blood is significant. The two pools of the agent vary independently (Simpson et al, 1991). The ratio of the agent in plasma to tPA is such that most of the tPA normally circulates in a complex with the inhibitor. The agent behaves as an acute-phase reaction, rising after trauma of various sorts, while platelet PAI does not change in these situations (Simpson et al, 1991). It is present in not only plasma and platelets but also in vascular endothelial cells, the muscularis layer of the vessel wall, hepatocytes, megakaryocytes and the neutrophils (Simpson et al, 1991; Haj et al, 1995ab). Although the protein inhibits both tPA and uPA, and tPA–PAI-1 complexes are normally present in human plasma, uPA–PAI-1 complexes are not detected.

A second inhibitor, now known as PAI-2, initially identified in the placenta and in the plasma of pregnant women, is now recognized (Kawano et al, 1968;

Astedt et al, 1987). Not normally present in plasma, it has a molecular size similar to that of PAI-1, though it circulates in two high-molecular-weight forms in the plasma of pregnant women (Booth et al, 1988). Plasma levels rise progressively until the 30th week of pregnancy and remain elevated until term and fall rapidly thereafter (Kruithof et al, 1987). Plasma levels of PAI-1 behave similarly though the decline after delivery is faster. PAI-2 is an intracellular agent and has been detected in several tissues, including monocytes (Kruithof et al, 1986) and malignant promyelocytes (Bennett et al, 1988). Monocyte levels of PAI-2 rise during infection (Haj et al, 1995b). It inhibits uPA more efficiently than tPA. However, its role is as yet unknown.

A third inhibitor, PAI-3, has been detected in human urine which complexes with two chain but not single chain urokinase. It has weak inhibitory activity on two chain tPA and is immunologically similar to protein C inhibitor, requiring heparin for maximal activity. Like PAI-2, its physiological significance is unknown.

Two other agents, α_2-macroglobulin and C1-INH are also known to complex with tPA in vitro and in vivo (Booth et al, 1987; Bennett et al, 1989). These complexes appear to occur only when large quantities of free tPA are circulating and these agents may therefore act as a backup inhibitory pool that is used only when circulating PAI-1 has been exhausted in complexing with tPA.

The principal plasma inhibitor of plasmin itself is α_2-antiplasmin. This single chain 70 kDa protein rapidly forms complexes with any plasmin free in the circulation so that detectable plasmin activity is exceptional (Collen, 1976; Moroi and Aoki, 1976; Mullertz and Clemmensen, 1976). Its complex formation with plasmin is initiated by linking to the lysine binding sites of the "kringles" in the plasmin so that if these sites are occupied by virtue of binding to fibrin itself the inhibitor has greater difficulty in interacting with plasmin (Collen, 1980). Several other serpins such as α_2-macroglobulin and α_1-antitrypsin also inhibit plasmin in vitro. Their role as plasmin inhibitors in vivo is not clear. Clot lysis studies involving plasma alone indicate that α_2-antiplasmin is quantitatively by far the most important inhibitor and only when PAI-1 levels rise considerably does it exercise a significant controlling role on the rate of lysis (Robbie et al, 1993). However, quantitative studies involving platelets and studies on thrombi formed in vivo in humans indicate that concentrations of PAI-1 in such thrombi are vastly in excess of those seen in plasma-derived clots and reach levels at which PAI-1 may significantly control thrombolysis (Robbie et al, 1996a). Considerable quantities of PAI-1 are detectable in arterial walls and the levels are high in atherosclerotic lesions (Robbie et al, 1996b).

Rates of synthesis, release and clearance of fibrinolytic enzymes and inhibitors also exert a major controlling influence over fibrinolysis, but have not been quantified systematically.

Mechanism of Physiological Fibrinolysis

Normally only trace quantities of plasminogen activator are present in the circulation and the amounts of PAI-1 are sufficient to suppress their activity almost completely. However, in the presence of formed fibrin, both plasminogen and tPA are specifically absorbed onto its surface where they are in part protected from the inhibitory role of PAI-1 and α_2-antiplasmin. This concentration of the two active molecules of the fibrinolytic system generates plasmin itself on the surface of fibrin which by virtue of interacting with fibrin via its active and lysine binding sites is not accessible to inhibition by α_2-antiplasmin; thus local deposits may be lysed by relatively small quantities of plasminogen activator and plasminogen while any plasmin entering the general circulation is rapidly neutralized, preventing a generalized proteolytic state.

The Role of the Endothelium

The endothelial cells interact with the haemostatic processes at many points in all the above contributing systems, sometimes exerting positive and sometimes negative influences. Endothelial cells produce von Willebrand factor (vWF), the agent necessary for the platelet link to subendothelial collagen, so when endothelial cell damage occurs this material is locally released to enhance initiation of repair by starting platelet plugging of the wound.

On the inhibitory side of the mechanism, platelets admixed with endothelial cells show vastly different aggregation activity compared with platelets studied alone (Marcus et al, 1980, 1982; Habib et al, 1992). At least three different processes contribute to the interaction of endothelial cells with platelets in ways that reduce platelet accumulation.

Endothelial cells produce prostacyclin from the arachidonic acid pathway metabolites generated initially by platelets themselves, as described above. Prostacyclin has a powerful vasodilator effect and additionally inhibits platelet aggregation locally and thus discourages platelet plug formation or local platelet accumulation and promotes flow in the circulation. Additionally, as described above, endothelial NO production, stimulated by nitric oxide synthetase (NOS), further supports vasodilatation, inhibits platelet adhesion/aggregation reactions and thus discourages platelet-induced vascular obstruction (Moncada et al, 1988; Broekman et al, 1991) by a quite different mechanism. Thirdly, endothelial nucleotidases (Marcus, 1991) hydrolyse aggregating nucleotides opposing platelet accumulation while 13-hydroxoctadecadienoic acid (13-HODE) may further reduce the propensity of platelets to local accumulation (Buchanan and Bastida, 1988).

As far as fibrin formation is concerned, endothelial cells, like other cells, will, if damaged, release tissue factor locally so initiating the coagulation process and the repair of injured tissues while exposed collagen may initiate contact system activation. On the negative side, several endothelial mechanisms are in place to limit unwanted fibrin formation in inappropriate sites. Endothelial cell glycosaminoglycans will enhance the activity of antithrombin and thus limit activity at several stages of the fibrin generating pathway, as discussed elsewhere. The endothelial cell glycoprotein thrombomodulin will complex with and neutralize thrombin and the product produces activated protein C (APC) from protein C (Esmon, 1987, 1989) which, in turn, in the presence of its co-factor, protein S, will inhibit activated factors V and VIII. APC and protein S, in contrast to the four vitamin K-dependent agents described earlier, have an anticoagulant as opposed to a procoagulant effect. They may also enhance fibrinolysis by inhibition of PAI-1 (Sakata et al, 1985). This feedback cycle thus tends to turn off further fibrin generation and provides local control of any tendency to inappropriate intravascular coagulation.

Endothelium generates TFPI, which, as described, slows activity of the tissue factor generated pathways. The role of this agent has not yet been clarified by the study of specific deficiency states, but it seems likely to act as a further control on fibrin generation at the endothelial surface.

In the fibrinolytic system it has long been recognized that the endothelial cells are a primary source of plasminogen activator (Todd, 1959). This material is thus well placed to initiate the lysis of endothelial deposits of fibrin in unwanted locations and the affinity of tPA for fibrin will enhance this function. More recently, however, it has been appreciated that endothelial cells in addition to tPA can produce PAI-1 that, in culture, rapidly complexes with tPA. Thus the endothelial cell is in a position to modify the unbridled activity of its own tPA production.

Endothelial cells further produce P-selectin, a cell adhesion molecule expressed on membranes on the activation of cells. This mediates interaction with, and accumulation of, neutrophils and monocytes. Its absence causes attenuation of fibrin deposition (Palabrica et al, 1992). It is likely that this agent, which is also expressed in platelet membranes, participates in inflammatory responses and in thrombogenesis (Furie and Furie, 1995).

Summary

The three different arms of the haemostatic mechanism – platelet plug formation, fibrin deposition and fibrin lysis – have been outlined in this chapter. Defects in any one of these may result in haemorrhagic disease. However, only when actual wounding occurs would these events occur sequentially. It is important to appreciate that modest activity in one or all may occur in response to the minor challenges of everyday life. Also, in response to more major illness, inflammatory, immune, neoplastic, etc., that do not involve what we would regard as wounds in the classical sense and seem to pose no obvious haemostatic threat, considerable changes in one or more arms of the haemostatic mechanism usually occur. Examples of these are thrombocytosis, the rise in fibrinogen or other procoagulants, or the elevation in fibrinolytic inhibitors occurring in infection, other inflammatory disorders, pregnancy and in some types of malignancy. In general these changes tend to enhance haemostatic security as if our genetic endowment regarded bleeding as the primary danger to guard against when threatened in any way. In this of course it is correct and this review has thus concentrated upon the mechanisms providing haemostatic safety, conferring as they do an advantage to the species. The mechanisms restraining haemostatic processes have also been described as failure of these processes and the changes just outlined that are reactive to other processes contribute to the vascular occlusive disorders, arterial or venous, characterizing the later years of life that are of personal import to individuals and of economic significance to the community rather than a direct threat to continuance of our species.

Acknowledgements

Construction of this manuscript depended crucially on the patience and skill of Miss M. Fletcher. Work in the author's laboratory is supported by grants from the British Heart Foundation, Aberdeen Royal Hospitals NHS Trust Research Committee and Aberdeen University.

References

Almus FE, Rao LVM, Rapaport SI. Functional properties of factor VIIa/tissue factor formed with purified tissue factor and with tissue factor expressed on cultured endothelial cells. *Thrombosis and Haemostasis* 1989; **62:** 1067–1073.

Anson DS, Choo KH, Rees DJG, et al. The gene structure of human anti-haemophilic factor IX. *EMBO Journal* 1984; **3:** 1053–1060.

Astedt B, Leander I, Ny T. The placental-type plasminogen activator inhibitor PAI-2. *Fibrinolysis* 1987: **1**: 203–208.

Aster RH. Studies of the fate of platelets in rats and man. *Blood* 1969; **34:** 117–128.

Bartley TD, Bogenberger J, Hunt P, et al. Identification and cloning of a megakaryocyte growth and development factor that is a ligand for cytokin receptor Mpl. *Cell* 1994; **77:** 117–1124.

Bennett B, Ogston D. Fibrinolytic bleeding syndromes. In: Ratnoff OD, Forbes CD (Eds), *Disorders of Hemostasis*, 3rd edn. Philadelphia: W.B. Saunders, 1996: 327–351.

Bennett B, Booth NA, Croll A, Dawson AA. The bleeding disorder in acute promyelocytic leukaemia: fibrinolysis due to uPA rather than defibrination. *British Journal of Haematology* 1989; **71:** 511–517.

Bennett B, Croll A, Ferguson K, Booth NA. Complexing of tissue plasminogen activation with PAI-1, α_2-macroglobulin and CI Inhibitor. *Blood* 1990; **75:** 671–676.
Bennett JS, Vilaire G, Cines DB. Identification of the fibrinogen receptor on human platelets by photoaffinity labeling. *Journal of Biological Chemistry* 1982; **257:** 8049–8054.
Bertina RM, Koleman BPC, Koster T, et al. Mutation in blood coagulation factor V associated with resistance to activated protein C. *Nature:* 1994; **369:** 64–67.
Bierman HR, Kelly KH, Cordes FL, et al. The release of leukocytes and platelets from the pulmonary circulation by epinephrine. *Blood* 1952; **7:** 683–692.
Biggs R, Nossel HL. Tissue extract and the contact reaction of blood coagulation. *Thrombosis et Diathesis Haemorrhagica* 1961; **6:** 1–14.
Blomback B, Blomback M. The molecular structure of fibrinogen. *Annals of the New York Academy of Sciences* 1972; **202:** 77–97.
Booth NA. The natural inhibitors of fibrinolysis. In: Bloom AL, Forbes CD, Thomas DP, Tuddenham EGD (Eds), *Haemostasis and Thrombosis*. Edinburgh: Churchill Livingstone, 1995: 699–717.
Booth NA, Anderson JA, Bennett B. Plasminogen activators in alcoholic cirrhosis. *Journal of Clinical Pathology* 1984; **37:** 772–777.
Booth NA, Walker E, Maugham R, Bennett B. Plasminogen activator in normal subjects after exercise and venous occlusion: tPA circulates in complex with C1-inhibitor and PAI-1. *Blood* 1987; **69:** 1600–1604.
Booth NA, Reith A, Bennett B. A plasminogen activator inhibitor (PAI-2) circulates in two molecular forms in pregnancy. *Thrombosis and Haemostasis* 1988; **59:** 77–79.
Bouma BN, Griffin JH. Human blood coagulation factor XI. Purification, properties, and mechanisms of activation by activated factor XII. *Journal of Biological Chemistry* 1977; **252:** 6432–6437.
Bovill EG, Bauer KA, Dickerman JD, Calles P, West B. The clinical spectrum of heterozygous protein C deficiency in a large New England Kindred. *Blood* 1989: **73**; 712–717.
Broze GJ Jr, Watten LA, Novotny WF, Higuchi DA, Girard JJ, Miletich JP. The lipoprotein-associated coagulation inhibitor that inhibits the factor VII-tissue factor complex also inhibits factor Xa: insight into its possible mechanism of action. *Blood* 1988; **71:** 335–343.
Broze GJ Jr, Girard TJ, Novotny WF. Regulation of coagulation by a multivalent Kunitz-type inhibitor. *Biochemistry* 1990; **29:** 7539–7545.
Broze GJ, Jr, Miletich JP. Isolation of the tissue factor inhibitor produced by Hep G2 hepatoma cells. Proceedings of the National Academy of Sciences, USA. 1987: **84** 1886–1890.
Broze GJ Jr. Tissue factor pathway inhibitor. *Thrombosis and Haemostasis.* 1995: **74:** 90–93.
Broekman MJ, Eiroa AM, Marcus AJ. Inhibition of human platelet reactivity by endothelium-derived relaxing factor from human umbilical vein endothelial cells in suspension. *Blood* 1991; **78:** 1033–1040.
Buchanan MR, Bastida E. Endothelium and underlying membrane reactivity with platelets, leukocytes and tumor cells: regulation by the lipoxygenase-derived fatty acid metabolites, 13-HODE and HETES. *Medical Hypotheses* 1988; **27:** 317–325.
Budzynski AZ, Olexa SA, Pandya BV. Fibrin polymerization sites in fibrinogen and fibrin fragments. *Annals of the New York Academy of Sciences* 1983; **308:** 301–313.
Chen R, Doolittle RF. Identification of the polypeptide chains involved in the cross-linking of fibrin. *Proceedings of the National Academy of Sciences USA* 1969; **63:** 420–427.
Chen R, Doolittle RF γ–γ cross-linking sites in human and bovine fibrin. *Biochemistry* 1971; **10:** 4486–4491.
Chung DW, Que BG, Rixon MW, Mace M Jr, Davie EW. Characterization of the cDNA and genomic DNA for the b chain of human fibrinogen. *Biochemistry* 1983a; **22:** 3244–3250.
Chung DW, Chan WY, Davie EW. Characterization of the cDNA coding for the c chain of human fibrinogen. *Biochemistry* 1983b; **22:** 3250–3256.
Chung GC, Delaney R, Meck D et al. Partial purification and characterization of the enzyme which converts precursor liver protein to factor X. *Biochimica et Biophysica Acta* 1975; **386:** 556–566.

Cochrane CG, Revack SD, Wuepper KD. Activation of Hageman factor in solid and fluid phases. A critical role of kallikrein. *Journal of Experimental Medicine* 1973; **138:** 1564–1583.
Collen D. Identification and some properties of a new fast reacting plasmin inhibitor in human plasma. *European Journal of Biochemistry* 1976; **69:** 209–216.
Collen D. On the regulation and control of fibrinolysis. *Thrombosis and Haemostasis* 1980; **43:** 77–89.
Collen D, Lijnen HR. Molecular mechanisms of thrombolysis. *Biochemical Pharmacology* 1990; **40:** 177–186.
Coller BS. Disorders of platelets. In: Ratnoff OD, Forbes CD (Eds), *Disorders of Hemostasis*. Orlando: Grune & Stratton, 1984: **73**–176.
Colman RW, Osbahr AJ. New vasoconstrictor bovine peptide-B released during blood coagulation. *Nature* 1967; **214:** 1040–1041.
Colman RW, Bagdesarian A, Telemo RC, et al. Williams trait: human kininogen deficiency with diminished levels of plasminogen proactivator and prekallikrein associated with abnormalities of the Hageman factor-dependent pathways. *Journal of Clinical Investigation* 1975; **56:** 1650–1662.
Crabtree GR, Kant JA. Coordinate accumulation of the mRNAs for the a, b, and c chains of rat fibrinogen following defibrination. *Journal of Biological Chemistry* 1982; **257:** 7277–7279.
Crawford N, Scrutton MC. Biochemistry of blood platelets. In: Bloom AL, Forbes CD, Thomas DP, Tuddenham EGD (Eds), *Haemostasis and Thrombosis*, 3rd edn. Edinburgh: Churchill Livingstone 1994: 89–113.
Davey MG. The survival and destruction of human platelets. *Bibliotheca Haematologica* 1966; **22:** 1–137.
Davie EW, Ratnoff OD. Waterfall sequence for intrinsic blood clotting. *Science* 1964; **145:** 1310–1312.
Degen SJF, MacGillivray RTA, Davie EW. Characterization of the cDNA and gene coding for human prothrombin. *Biochemistry* 1983; **22:** 2087–2097.
Dahlback B, Carlsson M, Svensson PJ Familial thrombophilia due to a previously unrecognised mechanism characterized by poor anticoagulant response to activated protein C. Prediction of a co-factor to activated protein C. *Proceedings of the National academy of Sciences USA* 1993; **90:** 1004–1008.
De Sauvage FJ, Hass PE, Spencer SD, et al. Stimulation of megakaryocytopoiesis and thrombopoiesis by cMpl ligand. *Nature* 1994; **369:** 533–538.
Doolittle RF, Fibrinogen and Fibrin. *Annual Reviews of Biochemistry* 1984; **53:** 195–229.
Eaton D, Rodriguez H, Vehar G. Proteolytic processing of human FVIII. Correlation of specific cleavages by thrombin, FXa and activated protein C with activation and inactivation of factor VIII coagulant activity. *Biochemistry* 1986; **25:** 505–512.
Eaton DL, Hass PE, Riddle L, et al. Characterization of recombinant human factor VIII. *Journal of Biological Chemistry* 1987; **262:** 3285–3290.
Egeberg O. Inherited antithrombin III deficiency causing thrombophilia. *Thrombosis et Diathesis Haemorrhagica* 1965; **13:** 516–530.
Emeis JJ, Van Hinsbergh VWM, Verheijen JH, Wijngaards G. Inhibition of tissue type plasminogen activator by conditioned medium from cultured human and porcine endothelial cells. *Biochemical & Biophysical Research Communications* 1983; **110:** 392–398.
Esmon CT. The regulation of natural anticoagulant pathways. *Science* 1987; **235:** 1348–1352.
Esmon CT. The roles of protein C and thrombomodulin in the regulation of blood coagulation. *Journal of Biological Chemistry* 1989; **264:** 4743–4746.
Esmon CT, Owen Whyte G, Duguid D, Jackson CM. The action of thrombin on blood clotting factor V. Conversion of factor V to a prothrombin-binding protein. *Biochimica et Biophysica Acta* 1973; **310:** 289–294.
Esmon CT, Owen WG, Jackson CM. The conversion of prothrombin to thrombin: a plausible mechanism for prothrombin activation by factor Xa, Phospholipid and calcium ions. *Journal of Biological Chemistry* 1974; **249:** 8045–8047.
Folk JE, Finlayson JS. The ε (γ_1-glutamyl) lysine cross-link and the catalytic role of transglutaminases. *Advances in Protein Chemistry* 1977; **31:** 1–133.
Frazier D, Smith KJ, Cheung W-F, et al. Mapping of monoclonal antibodies to human

factor IX. *Blood* 1989; **74:** 971–977.
Freeman JP, Guillin M-C, Bezeaud A, Jackson CM. Activation of bovine blood coagulation factor V. *Federation Proceedings* 1977; **36:** 675.
Fujikawa K, Coan MH, Legaz ME, Davie EW. The mechanism of activation of bovine factor X (Stuart factor) by intrinsic and extrinsic pathways. *Biochemistry* 1974a; **13:** 5290–5299.
Fujikawa K, Coan MH, Enfield DL, Titani K, Ericsson LH, Davie EW. A comparison of bovine prothrombin, factor IX (Christmas factor) and factor X (Stuart factor). *Proceedings of the National Academy of Sciences USA* 1974b; **71:** 427–430.
Fung MR, Hay CW, MacGillivray RTA. Characterization of an almost full-length cDNA coding for human blood coagulation factor X. *Proceedings of the National Academy of Sciences USA* 1985; **82:** 3591–3595.
Furchgott RF, Zawadzki JV. The obligatory role of endothelial cells in the relaxation of arterial smooth muscle by acetylcholine. *Nature* 1980; **288:** 373–376.
Furie B, Furie BC. The molecular basis of blood coagulation. *Cell* 1988; **53:** 505–518.
Furie B, Furie BC. The molecular basis of platelet and endothelial cell interaction with neutrophils and monocytes: role of P-Selectin and the P Selectin ligand PSGL-1. *Thrombosis and Haemostasis* 1995; **74:** 224–227.
Ginsberg MH, Loftus J, Plow EF. Platelets and the adhesion receptor superfamily. In: Jamieson GA (Ed.), *Platelet Membrane Receptors: Molecular Biology, Immunology, Biochemistry, and Pathology*. New York: Alan R Liss, 1988: 171–195.
Girma J-P, Meyer D, Verweij CL, Pannekoek H, Sixma JJ. Structure – function relationship of human von Willebrand factor (vWF). *Blood* 1987; **70:** 605–611.
Gitschier J, Wood WI, Goralka TM, et al. Characterization of the human factor VIII gene. *Nature* 1984; **312:** 326–330.
Gordon JL. Extracellular ATP: effects, sources and fate. *Biochemical Journal* 1986; **233:** 309–319.
Griffin JH, Beretta G. Molecular mechanisms of surface-dependent activation of Hageman factor. In: Fujii S, Moriya H, Suzuki T (Eds), *Kinins II* New York: Plenum, Press, 1979: 39–51.
Griffin JH Role of surface in surface-dependent activation of Hageman factor (blood coagulation factor XII) *Proceedings of the National Academy of Sciences USA* 1978; **75:** 1998–2002.
Guinto E, Esmon C. Factor Va light chain interaction with phospholipid and factor Xa. *Blood* 1981; **58:** 218.
Habib A, Maclouf J. Comparison of leukotriene Au metabolism into leukotriene C_4 by human platelets and endothelial cells. *Archives Biochemistry & Biophysics* 1992; **298:** 544–552.
Haj MA, Neilly IJ, Robbie LA, Adey G, Bennett B. Influence of white blood cells on the fibrinolytic response to sepsis: studies of septic patients with or without severe leucopenia. *British Journal of Haematology* 1995a; **90:** 541–547.
Haj MA, Robbie LA, Adey G, Bennett B. Inhibitors of plasminogen activation in neutrophils and mononuclear cells from septic patients. *Thrombosis and Haemostasis* 1995b; **74:** 1528–1532.
Hanson SR, Slichter SJ. Platelet kinetics in patients with bone marrow hypoplasia: evidence for a fixed platelet requirement. *Blood* 1985; **66:** 1105–1109.
Harrison P. Platelet alpha-granule fibrinogen. *Platelets* 1992; **3:** 1–10.
Hathaway WE, Belhasen LP, Hathaway HS. Evidence for a new plasma thromboplastin factor. *Blood* 1965; **26:** 521–532.
Heyns AD, Lotter MG, Badenhorst PN, et al. Kinetics, distribution and sites of destruction of indium-III-labelled human platelets. *British Journal of Haematology* 1980; **44:** 269–280.
Heyns AD, Lotter MG, Kotze HF, Pieters H, Wessel SP. Quantification of in vivo distribution of platelets labelled with indium-111-oxine. *Journal of Nuclear Medicine* 1982; **23:** 943–944.
Heyns AD, Badenhorst PN, Lotter MG Pieters H, Wessels P. Kinetics and mobilisation from the spleen of Indium-III -labelled platelets during platelet apheresis *Transfusion* 1985; **25:** 215–218.
Hjort PF. Intermediate reactions in the coagulation of the blood with tissue thromboplastin. Convertin, accelerin, prothrombinase. *Scandinavian Journal of Clinical and Laboratory Investigation* 1957; **9:** (Suppl 27): 1–183.

Hoffman R. Regulation of megakaryocytopoiesis. *Blood* 1989; **74:** 1196–1212.
Holmsen H. Platelet secretion. In: Colman RW, Hirsh J, Marder VJ et al (Eds), *Hemostasis and Thrombosis: Basic Principles and Clinical Practice*, 2nd edn. Philadelphia: Lippincott, 1987; 606–617.
Hougie C, Barrow EM, Graham JB. Stuart Clotting defect. Segregation of an hereditary hemorrhagic state from a heterogeneous group heretofore called 'stable factor' (SPCA, proconvertin, factor VII) deficiency. *Journal of Clinical Investigation* 1957; **36:** 485–496.
Hussain S, Gurevich V, Lipinski B. Purification and characterization of a single chain high molecular weight form of urokinase from human urine. *Archives of Biochemistry & Biophysics* 1983; **220:** 31–38.
Ignarro LJ. Endothelium-derived nitric oxide: actions and properties. *FASEB* 1989; **3:** 31–36.
Ishibashi T, Koziol JA, Burstein SA. Human recombinant erythropoietin promotes differentiation of murine megakaryocytes in vitro. *Journal of Clinical Investigation* 1987; **79:** 286–289.
Jackson CM. Physiology and biochemistry of prothrombin. In: Bloom AL, Forbes CD, Thomas DP, Tuddenham EGD (Eds), *Haemostasis and Thrombosis*, 3rd edn. Edinburgh: Churchill Livingstone, 1995; 397–438.
Jackson CM, Suttie JW. Recent developments in understanding the mechanism of vitamin K and vitamin K-antagonist drug action and the consequence of vitamin K action in blood coagulation. *Progress of Hematology* 1977; **10:** 333–359.
Jackson CM, Esmon CT, Gitel SM, Owen WG, Henriksen RA. The conversion of prothrombin to thrombin: the function of the propiece of prothrombin. In: Hemker HC, Veltkamp JJ (Eds), *Prothrombin and Related Coagulation factors*. Leiden: Leiden University Press, 1974: **59**.
Jackson CM, Esmon CT, Owen WG. The activation of bovine prothrombin. In: Reich E, Rifkin DB, Shaw E (Eds), *Cold Spring Harbor Conferences on Cell Proliferation. Proteases and Biological Control*. New York: Cold Spring Harbor Laboratory, 1975: **95**.
Jaffe EA, Hoyer LW, Nachman RL. Synthesis of antihemophilic factor antigen by cultured human endothelial cells. *Journal of Clinical Investigation* 1973; **52:** 2757–2764.
Josso F, Prou-Wartelle O. Interaction of tissue factor and factor VII at the earliest phase of coagulation. *Thrombosis et Diathisis Haemorrhagica* 1965; Suppl. **17:** 35–44.
Kane WH, Davie EW. Blood coagulation factors V and VIII: structural and functional similarities and their relationship to hemorrhagic and thrombotic disorders. *Blood* 1988; **71:** 539–555.
Kawano T., Morimoto K, Uemura T. Urokinase inhibitor in human placenta. *Nature* 1968; **217:** 253–254.
Kazama Y, Hamamoto T, Foster DC, Kisiel W. Hepsin, a putative membrane-associated serine protease activates human factor VII and initiates a pathway of blood coagulation on the cell surface leading to thrombin. *Journal of Biological Chemistry* 1995; **270:** 66–72.
Key NS, Nelsestuen GL, Slungaard A. Platelet factor 4 (PF4) binds to the gamma-carboxyglutamic acid (GLA) domain of factor X and impairs tissue factor (TF)-mediated coagulation: possible role as physiologic anticoagulant. *Blood* 1994; **84:** 532 (abstract).
Komiyama Y, Pedersen AH, Kisiel W. Proteolytic activation of human factors IX and X by recombinant human factor VIIa: effects of calcium, phospholipids, and tissue factor. *Biochemistry* 1990; **29:** 9418–9425.
Kruithof EKO, Vassali J-D, Schleuning W-D, Mattaliano RJ, Bachmann F. Purification and characterization of a plasminogen activator inhibitor from the histiocytic cell line U-937. *Journal of Biological Chemistry* 1986; **261:** 11207–11213.
Kruithof EKO, Tran-Thang G, Gudinchet A, et al. Fibrinolysis in pregnancy: a study of plasminogen activator inhibitors. *Blood* 1987; **69:** 460–466.
Kurachi K, Davie EW. Activation of human factor XI by factor XIIa. *Biochemistry* 1977; **16:** 5831–5838.
Kurachi K, Davie EW. Isolation and characterization of a cDNA coding for human factor IX. *Proceedings of the National Academy of Sciences USA* 1982; **79:** 6461–6464.
Kurachi K, Fujikawa K, Schmer G, Davie EW. Inhibition of bovine factor IX a and factor Xa by antithrombin III. *Biochemistry* 1976; **15:** 373–377.
Lawson JH, Borenas S, Ribarik, N. Mann KG Complex-dependent inhibition of factor VII by antilhrombin III and heparin. *Journal of Biological Chemistry* 1993; **268:** 767–770.

Lawson JH, Kalafatis M, Stram S, Mann KG. A model for the tissue factor pathway to thrombin. *Journal of Biological Chemistry* 1994; **269:** 23357–23366.
Leytus SP, Chung DW, Kisiel W, Kurachi K, Davie EW. Characterization of a cDNA coding for human factor X. *Proceedings of the National Academy of Sciences USA 1984; 82:* **3699–3702.**
Loeb L, Fleischer MS Tuttle L. The interaction between blood serum and tissue extract in the coagulation of blood. *Journal of Biological Chemistry* 1922: 51: **485–506.**
Lok S, Kauschansky K, Holly RD, et al. Cloning and expression of murine thrombopoietin cDNA and stimulation of platelet production in vivo. *Nature* 1994; **369:** 565–568.
Lorand L, Losowsky MS, Miloszewski KJM. Human factor XIII: fibrin-stabilizing factor. *Hemostasis and Thrombosis* 1980; **5:** 245–290.
Loskutoff DJ, Sawdey M, Mimuro J. Type I plasminogen activator inhibitor. *Progress in Hemostasis and Thrombosis* 1989; **9:** 87–115.
Macfarlane RG. An enzyme cascade in the blood clotting mechanism, and its function as a biochemical amplifier. *Nature* 1964; **202:** 498–499.
MacGillivray RTA, Degen SJF, Chandra T, Woo SLC, Davie EW. Cloning and analysis of a cDNA coding for bovine prothrombin. *Proceedings of the National Academy of Sciences USA* 1980; **77:** 5153–5157.
Magnusson S, Sottrup-Jensen L, Petersen TE, Claeys H. The primary structure of prothrombin. The role of vitamin K in blood coagulation and a thrombin catalysed "negative feed back" control mechanism for limiting the activation of prothrombin. In: Hemker HC, Veltkemp JJ (Eds), *Prothrombin and Related Coagulation Factors.* Leiden: Leiden University Press, 1975: 25–40.
Magnusson S, Petersen TE, Sottrup-Jensen L, Claeys H. Complete primary structure of prothrombin: isolation, structure and reactivity of ten carboxylated glutamic acid residues and regulation of prothrombin activation by thrombin. In: Reich E, Rifkin DB, Shaw E (Eds), *Proteases and Biological Control.* New York: Cold Spring Harbor Laboratory, 1975: 123–149.
Mandle R, Kaplan AP. Hageman factor dependent fibrinolysis. Generation of fibrinolytic activity by interaction of human activated factor XI and plasminogen. *Blood* 1979; **54:** 850–862.
Mandle R, Colman RW, Kaplan AP. Identification of prekallikrein and high molecular weight kininogen as a complex in human plasma. *Proceedings of the National Academy of Sciences USA* 1976; **73:** 4179–4183.
Mann KG, Jenny RJ, Krishnaswamy S. Co-factor proteins in the assembly and expression of blood clotting enzyme complexes. *Annual Review of Biochemistry* 1988; **57:** 915–956.
Marcum JA, Kenney JB, Rosenberg RD. The acceleration of thrombin–antithrombin complex formation in rat hindquarters via naturally occuring heparin-like molecules bound to endothelium. *Journal of Clinical Investigation* 1984; **74:** 341–350.
Marcus AJ. Platelets and their disorders. *In: Ratnoff OD, Forbes CD (Eds), Disorders of Hemostasis 2nd edn. Philadelphia: WB Saunders,* 1991; 75–140.
Marcus AJ, Broekman MJ, Safier LB et al. Formation of leukotrienes and other hydroxy acids during platelet-neutrophil interactions in vitro. *Biochemical Biophysical Research Communications* 1982; **109:** 130–137.
Marcus AJ, Zucker-Franklin D, Safier LB, Ullman HL. Studies on human platelet granules and membranes. *Journal of Clinical Investigation* 1966; **45:** 14–28.
Marcus AJ, Weksler BB, Jaffe EA, Broekman MJ. Synthesis of prostacyclin from platelet-derived endoperoxides by cultured human endothelial cells. *Journal of Clinical Investigation* 1980; **66:** 979–986.
Marlar RA, Kleiss AJ, Griffin JH. An alternative extrinsic pathway of human blood coagulation. *Blood* 1982; **60:** 1353–1358.
McDonald TP, Odell TT, Gosslee DG. Platelet size in relation to platelet age. *Proceedings of the Society for Experimental Biology and Medicine* 1964; **115:** 684–689.
McDonald TP, Cottrell MB, Clift RE, Cullen WC, Lin FK. High doses of recombinant erythropoietin stimulate platelet production in mice. *Experimental Hematology* 1987; **15:** 719–721.
McGee MP, Li LC. Functional difference between intrinsic and extrinsic coagulation pathways. *Journal of Biological Chemistry* 1991; **266:** 8079–8085.

McKee PA, Mattock P, Hill RL. Subunit structure of human fibrinogen, soluble fibrin and cross-linked insoluble fibrin. *Proceedings of the National Academy of Sciences USA* 1970; **66:** 738–744.
McWilliams N, Robbie LA, Barelle CJ *et al.* Evidence for an active fibrinolytic system in normal human bone marrow. *British Journal of Haematology* 1996; **73:** 170–176
Miletich JP, Sherman L, Broze GJ. Absence of thrombosis in subjects with heterozygous protein C deficiency. *New England Journal of Medicine* 1987: **317:** 991–996.
Mohlo-Sabatier P, Aiach M, Gaillard I, et al. Molecular characterization of antithrombin III (AT III) variants using polymerase chain reaction. *Journal of Clinical Investigation* 1989: **84:** 1236–1241.
Moncada S. Biological significance of prostacyclin. *British Journal of Pharmacology* 1982; **76:** 3–31.
Moncada S, Palmer RMJ, Higgs EA. Prostacyclin and endothelium-derived relaxing factor: biological interactions and significance. In: Verstraete M, Vermylen J, Lijnen R (Eds), *Haemostasis and Thrombosis.* Leuven: Leuven University Press, 1987: 597–618.
Moncada S, Radomski MW, Palmer RMJ. Endothelium-derived relaxing factor: identification as nitric oxide and role in the control of vascular tone and platelet function. *Biochemical Pharmacology* 1988; **37:** 2495–2501.
Moncada S, Palmer RMJ, Higgs EA. Biosynthesis of nitric oxide from L-arginine: a pathway for the regulation of cell function and communication. *Biochemical Pharmacology* 1989; **38:** 1709–1715.
Morawitz P. Die chemie der Blutgerinnung *Ergeb Physiol* 1905; **4:** 307–314.
Morawitz P (translated by Hartmann RC, Guenther PF). *The Chemistry of Blood Coagulation.* Springfield, MA: CC Thomas, 1958: 194.
Morita T, Iwanaga S, Suzuki T. The mechanism of activation of bovine prothrombin by an activator isolated from Echis carinatus venom and characterization of new active intermediates. *Journal of Biochemistry* (Tokyo) 1976; **79:** 1089–1108.
Moroi M, Aoki N. Isolation and characterization of the α_2-plasmin inhibitor from human plasma. *Journal of Biological Chemistry* 1976; **251:** 5956–5965.
Mullertz S, Clemmensen J. The primary inhibitor of plasmin in human plasma. *Biochemical Journal* 1976; **159:** 545–553.
Nachman RL, Leung LLK, Kloczewiak M, Hawiger J. Complex formation of platelet membrane glycoproteins IIb and IIIa with the fibrinogen D domain. *Journal of Biological Chemistry* 1984; **259:** 8584–8588.
Nelsestuen GL, Zytkovicz TH, Howard JB. The mode of action of vitamin K. *Journal of Biological Chemistry* 1974; **249:** 6347–6350.
Nemerson Y. Tissue factor and hemostasis. *Blood* 1988; **71:** 1–8.
Nemerson Y, Repke D. Tissue factor accelerates the activation of coagulation factor VII: the role of a bifunctional coagulation co-factor. *Thrombosis Research* 1985; **40:** 351.
Nishimura H. Takeija H, Suehiro K, et al. Characterization of factor IX Fukuoka with substitution of Asn-92 by His in the second epidermal growth factor-like domain. *Thrombosis and Haemostasis* 1991; **65:** 712.
Nishimura H, Takaya H, Miyata T, Suehiro K, Okamura T, Niho Y, Iwanaga S. Factor IX Fukuoka, substitution of Asn-92 by His in the second growth factor-like domain results in defective interaction with factor VIIa. *Journal of Biological Chemistry* 1993; **282:** 24041–24046.
Novotny WF, Brown SG, Miletich JP, Rader DJ, Broze GJ Jr. Plasma antigen levels of the lipoprotein-associated coagulation inhibitor inpatient samples. *Blood* 1991; **78:** 387–393.
Nurden AT. Human platelet membrane glycoproteins. *I*n: Bloom AL, Forbes CD, Thomas DP, Tuddenham EGD (Eds) *Haemostasis and Thrombosis*, 3rd edn. Edinburgh: Churchill Livingstone, 1994: 115–165.
Ogston D, Ogston CM, Ratnoff OD, Forbes CD. Studies on a complex mechanism for the activation of plasminogen by kaolin and chloroform: the participation of Hageman factor and additional co-factors. *Journal of Clinical Investigation* 1969; **48:** 1786–1801.
Osterud B, Rapaport SI. Activation of factor IX by the reaction product of tissue factor and factor VII: additional pathway for initiating blood coagulation. *Proceedings of the National Academy of Sciences USA* 1977; **74:** 5260–5264.

Owen WG, Esmon CT, Jackson CM. The conversion of prothrombin to thrombin. *Journal of Biological Chemistry* 1974; **249:** 594–605.
Palabrica T, Lobb R, Furie BC, Aronovitz M, Benjemin C, Hsu Y-M, Sajer SA, Furie B. Leukocyte accumulation promoted fibrin deposition is mediated in vivo by P-selectin on adherent platelets. *Nature* 1992; **359:** 848–851.
Patek AJ Jr, Taylor FHL. Hemophilia II. Some properties of a substance obtained from normal plasma effective in accelerating the clotting of hemophilic blood. *Journal of Clinical Investigation* 1937; **16:** 113–124.
Phillips DR, Charo IF, Parise LV, Fitzgerald LA. The platelet membrane glycoprotein IIb–IIIa complex. *Blood* 1988; **71:** 831–843.
Quick AJ, Stanley-Brown M, Bancroft FW. A study of the coagulation defect in hemophilia and jaundice. *Americal Journal of Medical Science* 1935; **190:** 501–511.
Radcliffe RD, Nemerson Y. Activation and control of factor VII by activated factor X and thrombin. Isolation and characterization of a single chain form of factor VII. *Journal of Biological Chemistry* 1975; **250:** 388–395.
Randall MD. Vascular activity of the endothelins. *Pharmacology and Therapeutics* 1991; **50:** 73–93.
Rao LVM, Rapaport SI. Activation of factor VII bound to tissue factor: a key early step in the tissue factor pathway of blood coagulation. *Proceedings of the National Academy of Sciences USA* 1988; **85:** 6687–6691.
Rao LVM, Rapaport SI, Bajaj SP. Activation of human factor VII in the initiation of tissue factor-dependent coagulation. *Blood* 1986; **68:** 685–691.
Rao LVM, Robinson T, Hoang AD. Factor VIIa/tissue factor-catalyzed activation of factors IX and X on a cell surface and in suspension: a kinetic study. *Thrombosis and Haemostasis* 1992; **67:** 654–659.
Rao LVM, Rapaport SI, Hoang AD. Binding of factor VIIa to tissue factor permits rapid antithrombin III/heparin inhibition of factor VIIa. *Blood* 1993; **81:** 2600–2607.
Rapaport SI. Inhibition of factor VIIa/tissue factor-induced blood coagulation: with particular emphasis upon a factor Xa-dependent inhibitory mechanism. *Blood* 1989; **73:** 359–365.
Rapaport SI. The extrinsic pathway inhibitor: a regulator of tissue factor-dependent blood coagulation. *Thrombosis and Haemostasis* 1991; **66:** 6–15.
Rapaport SI, Rao VM. The tissue factor pathway: how it has become a 'prima ballerina'. *Thrombosis and Haemostasis* 1995; **74:** 7–17.
Rapaport SI, Schiffman S, Patch MJ, Ames SB. The importance of activation of antihemophilic globulin and Proeccelerin by traces of thrombin in the generation of intrinsic prothrombinase activity. *Blood* 1963; **21:** 221–236.
Rapaport SI, Hjort PF, Patch MJ, Jeremic M. Consumption of serum factors and prothrombin during intravascular clotting in rabbits. *Scandinavian Journal of Haematology* 1966; **3:** 59–75.
Ratnoff OD. Evolution of knowledge about hemostasis. In: Ratnoff OD, Forbes CD (Eds), *Disorders of Hemostasis*. Philadelphia: WB Saunders, 1991: 1–17.
Ratnoff OD, Colopy JE. A familial hemorrhagic trait associated with a deficiency of a clot-promoting fraction of plasma. *Journal of Clinical Investigation* 1955; **34:** 602–613.
Ratnoff OD, Saito H. Surface-mediated reactions. *Current Topics in Hematology* 1979; **2:** 1–57.
Revak SD, Cochrane CG. The relationship of structure and function in human Hageman factor. *Journal of Clinical Investigation* 1976; **57:** 852–860.
Revak SD, Cochrane CG, Griffin JH. The binding and cleavage characteristics of human Hageman factor during contact activation. *Journal of Clinical Investigation* 1977; **59:** 1167–1175.
Revak SK, Cochrane CG, Bouma BN, Griffin JH. Surface and fluid phase activities in two forms of activated Hageman factor produced during contact activation of plasma. *Journal of Experimental Medicine* 1978; **147:** 719–729.
Rijken DC, Collen D. Purification and characterization of the plasminogen activator secreted by human melanoma cells in culture. *Journal of Biological Chemistry* 1981; **256:** 7035–7041.
Rixon MW, Chan WY, Davie EW, Chung DW. Characterization of a cDNA coding for the a chain of human fibrinogen. *Biochemistry* 1983; **22:** 3237–3244.

Robbie LA, Booth NA, Croll AM, Bennett B. The roles of α_2-antiplasmin and plasminogen activator inhibitor 1(PAI-1) in the inhibition of clot lysis. *Thrombosis and Haemostasis* 1993; **70:** 301–306.
Robbie LA, Bennett B, Brown PAJ, Croll AM, Booth NA. Activators and inhibitors of the fibrinolytic system in human thrombi. *Thrombosis and Haemostasis* 1995a; **75:** 127–133.
Robbie LA, Booth NA, Bennett B. Inhibitors of fibrinolysis are elevated in the atherosclerotic plaque. *Arteriosclerosis, Thrombosis and Vascular Biology* 1995b; **16:** 539–545.
Rosenberg RD. The absence of blood clotting regulator thrombomodulin causes embryonic lethality in mice before development of a functional cardiovascular system. *Thrombosis and Haemostasis* 1995; **74:** 52–57.
Rosenberg RD, Damus PS. The purification and mechanism of action of human antithrombin/heparin co-factor. *Journal of Biological Chemistry* 1973; **248:** 6490–6505.
Rosenberg JS, McKenna PW, Rosenberg RD. Inhibition of human factor IXa by human antithrombin. *Journal of Biological Chemistry* 1975; **250:** 8883–8888.
Rosenthal RL, Dreskin OH, Rosenthal N. New hemophilia-like disease caused by deficiency of a third plasma thromboplastin factor. *Proceedings of the Society of Experimental Biology and Medicine* 1953; **82:** 171–174.
Rosing J, van Rijn JL, Bevers EM, van Dieijen G, Comfurius P, Zwaal FN. The role of activated human platelets in prothrombin and factor X activation. *Blood* 1985; **65:** 319–332.
Royle NJ, Irwin DM, Koschinsky ML, MacGillivray RT, Hamerton JL. Human genes encoding prothrombin and ceruloplasmin map to IIpII-q12 and 3q21-24 respectively. *Somatic Cellular and Molecular Genetics* 1987; **13:** 285–292.
Ruoslahti E, Pierschbacher MD. New perspectives in cell adhesion: RGD and integrins. *Science* 1987; **238:** 491–497.
Sadler JE. von Willebrand's disease. *In:* Bloom AL, Forbes CD, Thomas DP, Tuddenham EGD (Eds), *Haemostasis and Thrombosis*. Edinburgh: Churchill Livingstone, 1995: 843–858.
Saito H. The contact phase of blood coagulation. In: Bloom AL, Forbes CD, Thomas DP, Tuddenham EGD (Eds), *Haemostasis and Thrombosis*, 3rd edn. Edinburgh: Churchill Livingstone, 1995: 289–307.
Saito H, Ratnoff OD, Waldmann R, Abraham JP. Fitzgerald trait. Deficiency of a hitherto unrecognised agent, Fitzgerald factor, participating in suface-mediated reactions of clotting, fibrinolysis, generation of kinins and the property of diluted plasma enhancing vascular permeability. *Journal of Clinical Investigation* 1975; **55:** 1082–1089.
Sakai T, Lund-Hansen T, Paborsky L, Pedersen AH, Kisiel W. Binding of human factors VII and VIIa to a human bladder carcinoma cell line (J82): implications for the initiation of the extrinsic pathway of blood coagulation. *Journal of Biological Chemistry* 1989; **264:** 9980–9988.
Sakata Y, Aoki N. Cross-linking of α_2-plasmin inhibitor to fibrin by fibrin-stabilizing factor. *Journal of Clinical Investigation* 1980; **65:** 290–297.
Sakata Y, Curriden S, Lawrence D, Griffin JH, Loskotoff DJ. Activated protein C stimulates the fibrinolytic activity of cultured endothelial cells and decreases antiactivator activity. *Proceedings of the National Academy of Sciences USA* 1985; **82:** 1121–1125.
Samuelsson B, Dahlen S-E, Lindgren JA, Rouzer CA, Serhan CN. Leukotrienes and lipoxins: structures, biosynthesis and biological effects. *Science* 1987; **237:** 1171–1176.
Sandset PM, Abildgaard U, Larsen ML. Heparin induces release of extrinsic coagulation pathway inhibitor (EPI). *Thrombosis Research* 1988; **50:** 803–813.
Schneider CL. The active principle of placental toxin: thromboplastin: its inactivator in blood: antithromboplastin. *American Journal of Physiology* 1947; **149:** 123–129.
Schwartz ML, Pizzo SV, Hill RL, McKee PA. Human factor XIII from plasma and platelets: molecular weights, subunit structure, proteolytic activation and cross-linking of fibrinogen and fibrin. *Journal of Biological Chemistry* 1973; **248:** 1395–1407.
Shattil SJ, Bennett JS. Platelets and their membranes in hemostasis: physiology and pathophysiology. *Annals of Internal Medicine* 1981; **94:** 108–118.
Shigematsu Y, Miyata T, Higashi S, Miki T, Sadler JE, Iwanago S. Expression of human soluble tissue factor in yeast and enzymatic properties of its complex with factor VIIa. *Journal of Biological Chemistry* 1992; **267:** 21329–21337.

Simpson AJ, Booth NA, Moore NR, Bennett B. The platelet and plasma pools of plasminogen activator inhibitor (PAI-1) vary independently in disease. *British Journal of Haematology* 1990; **75:** 543–548.
Simpson AJ, Booth NA, Moore NR, Bennett B. Distribution of plasminogen activator inhibitor (PAI-1) in tissues. *Journal of Clinical Pathology* 1991; **44:** 139–143.
Sixma JJ. Platelet adhesion in health and disease. In: Verstraete M, Vermylen J, Lijnen R (Eds), *Thrombosis and Haemostasis.* Leuven: Leuven University Press, 1987: 127–146.
Sixma JJ, Sakariassen KS, Beeser-Visser NH et al. Adhesion of platelets to human artery subendothelium: Effect of factor VIII-von Willebrand factor (vWF) of various multimeric composition. *Blood* 1984; **63:** 128–139.
Soff G. Jackman RW, Rosenberg RD. Expression of thrombomodulin by smooth muscle cells in culture. *Blood* 1991; **77:** 515–518.
Sporn LA, Chavin SI, Marder VJ, Wagner DD. Biosynthesis of von Willebrand protein by human megakaryocytes. *Journal of Clinical Investigation* 1985; **76:** 1102–1106.
Sprecher CA, Kisiel W, Mathewes S, Foster DC. Molecular cloning, expression, and partial characterization of a second human tissue-factor-pathway inhibitor. *Proceedings of the National Academy of Sciences USA* 1994; **91:** 3353–3357.
Stel HV, Sakariassen KS, de Groot PG, van Mourik JA, Sixma JJ. von Willebrand factor (vWF) in the vessel wall mediates platelet adhesion *Blood* 1985; **65:** 85–90.
Stenflo J, Fernlund P, Egan W, Roepstorff P. Vitamin K-dependent modifications of glutamic acid residues in prothrombin. *Proceedings of the National Academy of Sciences USA* 1974; **71:** 2730–2733.
Stenn K, Blout E. Mechanism of bovine prothrombin activation by an insoluble preparation of bovine factor Xa (thrombokinase). *Biochemistry* 1972; **11:** 4502–4515.
Stern DM, Drillings M, Kisiel W, Nawroth P, Nossel HL, LaGamma KS. Activation of factor IX bound to cultured bovine aortic endothelial cells. *Proceedings of the National Academy of Sciences USA* 1984; **81:** 913–917.
Stern D, Nawroth P, Handley D, Kisiel W. An endothelial cell-dependent pathway of coagulation. *Proceedings of the National Academy of Sciences USA* 1985; **82:** 2523–2527.
Teitel JM, Rosenberg RD. Protection of factor Xa from neutralization by the heparin–antithrombin complex. *Journal of Clinical Investigation* 1983; **71:** 1381–1391.
Telfer TP, Denson KW, Wright DR. A "new" coagulation defect. *British Journal of Haematology* 1956; **2:** 308–316.
Thomas L. Studies on the intravascular-thromboplastic effect of tissue suspensions in mice II. A factor in normal rabbit serum which inhibits the thromboplastic effect of the sedimentable tissue component. *Bulletin of Johns Hopkins Hospital* 1947; **81:** 26–42.
Thompson AR. Structure, function and molecular defects of factor IX. *Blood* 1986; **67:** 565–572.
Thompson CB, Love DG, Quinn PG, Valeri CR. Platelet size does not correlate with platelet age. *Blood* 1983; **62:** 487–494.
Thompson R, Mandle R, Kaplan AP. Association of factor XI and high molecular weight kininogen in human plasma. *Journal of Clinical Investigation* 1977; **60:** 1376–1380.
Todd AS. The histological localization of fibrinolysis activation. *Journal of Pathology and Bacteriology* 1959; **78:** 281–283.
Toole JJ, Knopf JL, Wozney JM, et al. Molecular cloning of a cDNA encoding human antihaemophilic factor. *Nature* 1984; **312:** 342–347.
Tracy PB, Rohrback MS, Mann KG. Functional prothrombinase complex assembly on isolated monocytes and lymphocytes. *Journal of Biological Chemistry* 1983; **258:** 7264–7267.
Turitto VT, Weiss HJ, Zimmerman TS. Factor VIII/von Willebrand factor in subendothelium mediates platelet adhesion. *Blood* 1985; **65:** 823–831.
Vehar G, Davie E. Preparation and properties of bovine FVIII (antihemophilic factor). *Biochemistry* 1980; **19:** 401–410.
Waaler BA. Simultaneous contribution to the formation of thrombin by the intrinsic and extrinsic blood clotting systems. *Scandinavian Journal of Clinical and Laboratory Investigation* 1957; **9:** 322–330.
Wallen P, Bergsdorf N, Ranby M. Purification and identification of two structural variants of porcine tissue plasminogen activator by affinity absorption on fibrin. *Biochimica et Biophysica Acta* 1982; **719:** 318–328.

Walsh PN, Bradford H, Sinha D, Piperna JR, Tuszynski GP. Kinetics of the factor XIa catalyzed activation of human blood coagulation factor IX. *Journal of Clinical Investigation* 1984; **73:** 1392–1399.

Walsh PN Platelet-mediated trigger mechanisms in the contact phase of blood coagulation. *Seminars in Thrombosis and Hemostasis* 1987; **13:** 86–94.

Warn-Cramer BJ, Bajaj SP. Intrinsic versus extrinsic coagulation: kinetic considerations. *Biochemical Journal* 1986; **239:** 757–762.

Warn-Cramer BJ, Rao LVM, Maki SL, Rapaport SI. Modifications of extrinsic pathway inhibitor (EPI) and factor Xa that affect their ability to interact and to inhibit factor VIIa/tissue factor: evidence for a two-step model of inhibition. *Thrombosis and Haemostasis* 1988; **60:** 453–456.

White JG. Platelet ultrastructure. In: Bloom AL, Forbes CD, Thomas DC, Tuddenham EGS (Eds), *Haemostasis and Thrombosis*. Edinburgh: Churchill Livingstone, 1995: 49–87.

White WF, Barlow GH, Mozen MM. The isolation and characterization of plasminogen activator (urokinase) from human urine. *Biochemistry* 1966; **5:** 2160–2169.

Widmer K, Moake JL. Clot reaction: evaluation in dilute suspensions of platelet-rich plasma and gel-separated platelets. *Journal of Laboratory and Clinical Medicine* 1976; **87:** 49–57.

Wiggins RC, Bouma BN, Cochrane CG, Griffin JH. Role of high-molecular-weight kininogen in surface binding and activation of factor XI and prekallikrein. *Proceedings of the National Academy of Sciences USA* 1977; **74:** 4636–4640.

Wion KL, Kelly D, Summerfield JA, Tuddenham EG, Lawn RM. Distribution of factor VIII mRNA and antigen in human liver and other tissues. *Nature* 1985; **317:** 726–729.

Wood WI, Capon DJ, Simonsen CC, et al. Expression of active human factor VIII from recombinant DNA clones. *Nature* 1984; **312:** 330–337.

Wuepper KD, Miller DR, Lacombe MJ. Flaujeac trait. Deficiency of human plasma kininogen. *Journal of Clinical Investigation* 1975; **56:** 1663–1672.

Wuepper KD Prekallikrein deficiency in man. *Journal of Experimental Medicine* 1973; **138:** 1345–1355.

Wun TC, Schleuning WD, Reich E. Isolation and characterization of urokinase for human plasma. *Journal of Biological Chemistry* 1982; **257:** 3276–3281.

Yanagisawa M, Kurihara H, Kimura S, et al. A novel potent vasoconstrictor peptide produced by endothelial cells. *Nature* 1988; **332:** 411–415.

Yoshitake S, Schach BG, Foster DC, Davie EW. Nucleotide sequence of the gene for human factor IX (antihemophilic factor B). *Biochemistry* 1985; **24:** 3736–3750.

2 The Genetics of Blood Coagulation and Haemostasis

FRANCESCO GIANNELLI

Inherited Disorders of Blood Coagulation

The previous chapter has described the proteins involved in blood coagulation and haemostasis, and has shown how their interaction results in the rapid and controlled response to blood vessel injury necessary to maintain the integrity of our closed circulation system. Gene defects that impair the production, structure and function of the above factors may cause defective or abnormal blood coagulation and haemostasis. Defects of most coagulation factors have been reported.

Deficiency of coagulation factor XII (Hageman factor) has been observed (Ratnoff and Colopy, 1955), but rarely causes excessive bleeding. Similarly, deficiency of pre-kallikrein or of kininogen has been found in individuals with anomalies of blood coagulation but no excessive bleeding (Hathaway et al, 1965; Waldmann and Abraham, 1974). Deficiency of factor XI may result in a bleeding diathesis that has so far been reported mainly in Ashkenazi Jews (Biggs et al, 1958). Deficiency of factor VII (Alexander et al, 1951) has been reported in approximately 100 cases of varying severity. Factor X and factor V deficiencies (Owren, 1947; Telfer et al, 1956) are also relatively rare but they are both accompanied by excessive bleeding. Rarer still is prothrombin deficiency (Shapiro et al, 1969). This has been found in patients with mild bleeding tendencies. Fibrinogen abnormalities (Ménaché, 1964) have been described in the literature and they affect different aspects of fibrinogen activity such as fibrinogen release, polymerization and cross-linking. Excessive bleeding may accompany these abnormalities and especially defective fibrinopeptide release, but it is not the inevitable consequence of haematologically detectable fibrinogen defects. Afibrinogenaemia (Rabe and Salomon, 1920) is well known but infrequent. It causes excessive bleeding but this is milder than in severe haemophilia. Deficiency of factor XIII (Duckert et al, 1960) is also rarely encountered. This condition leads to unstable clots and can be associated with a severe tendency to bleed.

The genes for all the above factors are autosomal and the defects therefore show autosomal patterns of inheritance. The most common bleeding disorder, von Willebrand's disease is also autosomal, but those that are associated with greatest morbidity, haemophilias A and B, are X-linked.

Besides the defects of single coagulation factors, one occasionally finds combined deficiency. A well-documented combined deficiency is that of factors V and VIII (Fisher et al, 1988), while a combined deficiency of vitamin K-dependent factors has been tentatively attributed to a congenital disorder of γ-carboxylation (Ekelund et al, 1986).

Defects in factors that exert a negative control on blood coagulation, such as antithrombin III, protein C, and protein S, or resistance to such factors, may lead to excessive blood coagulation: thrombophilia. Recently it has been discovered, in Holland, that a missense mutation of factor V affecting the site of cleavage of activated protein C is a major cause of thrombophilia (Bertina et al, 1994).

This chapter will not consider thrombophilia and the rare haemorrhagic disorders mentioned above any further, but will deal exclusively with the three conditions that are the principal concern of haemophilia centres, namely haemophilia A, haemophilia B and von Willebrand's disease. For the other disorders of blood coagulation, the reader is referred to the reviews by Allaart and Briët (1994) and Rizza (1994).

The Genetics of Haemophilia A and Haemophilia B

The genes for factor VIII and factor IX are both on the long arm of the X chromosome. The former is the most distal of the genes associated with X-linked disease, and lies in band Xq28. The latter occupies a more proximal position, near the boundary between Xq26 and Xq27. Both haemophilias show recessive inheritance. Their relatively high incidence is thus explained by the natural hemizygous state of the male, which allows full expression of recessive mutations.

The characteristic pattern of inheritance of haemophilia, with affected males and unaffected females who transmit the disease, was clearly recognized by Otto in 1803, more than 50 years before Mendel's discovery of the laws of inheritance, and more than 100 years prior to Morgan's definition of sex-linkage (Morgan, 1910). The population genetic features of the two haemophilias are also very similar, and they were defined in the 1930s by Haldane (1935), when haemophilias A and B had not yet been distinguished. Haldane argued that because affected males had a much reduced chance of reproducing, a proportion of the haemophilia genes in the population should be lost at each generation. Taking into account the fact that males carry one-third of the X chromosomes in the population, he calculated that the loss of haemophilia genes in each generation should be equal to $1/3(1-f)I$, where f is the chance that a patient produces offspring relative to that of a normal male, and I is the incidence of the disease. He was then able to show that if such a loss had not been compensated for by new mutations, the observed frequency of haemophilia would imply that at the time of the Norman conquest most Englishmen were haemophiliacs. Since that is absurd, his postulate was proven insofar as this was possible. Recent data have suggested that prior to the introduction of modern replacement therapy, the value of f was 0.5 for both haemophilia A and haemophilia B (Francis and Kasper, 1983; Ferrari and Rizza, 1986). This figure, and Haldane's formula, indicate that the pools of haemophilia A and haemophilia B genes in the population must have been renewed at a rate of 1/6 per generation. It follows that both diseases should be mutationally very heterogeneous, so that unrelated patients should usually carry mutations of independent origin. This, as will be shown later, is consistent with observations, especially for the mutations causing moderate and severe disease, which are subjected to more severe selection. Mild defects may persist longer in the population, and may even attain relatively high population frequencies through genetic drift and founder effects (Ketterling et al, 1991). The mutational heterogeneity predicted by Haldane's theory is a very important genetic feature of both haemophilias, because it creates the greatest challenge to DNA-based carrier and prenatal diagnosis, whilst at the same time providing excellent opportunities to learn about the structural features important to the expression and functions of coagulation factors VIII and IX.

Haldane's theory is also useful in predicting the historic changes that may occur in the incidence of haemophilia. This theory states that, in the absence of external intervention, the mutation rate for either haemophilia A or haemophilia B (μ_A or μ_B) should be equal to the loss of genes resulting from the lower f of affected males, or, to put it more concisely: $\mu_A = 1/3(1-f)\ I_A$ and $\mu_B = 1/3(1-f)I_B$. Since μ_A and μ_B are not expected to change much, it is obvious that treatments increasing f (that is, the probability that a patient will reproduce) should result in an increase in the incidence of the disease, since $I = 3\mu/(1-f)$. Thus if the f of patients with haemophilia B changes from 0.5 to 0.75, the incidence of haemophilia B would be expected to double. In fact, the steady rise in the prevalence of haemophilia observed in recent years may be due partly to the increased life-span of patients, and partly to the change mentioned above. The increase in incidence resulting from the effect of therapy on f could be tempered by the use of prenatal tests for the genetic prevention of the disease. The importance of this factor of course depends on the proportion of parents seeking prenatal tests, and their attitudes to the affected pregnancy. This is influenced by the quality of the tests that can be provided, and by parental perceptions of, and attitudes towards, the quality of life experienced by patients.

A question of considerable biological interest, but also one of some practical relevance, is whether or not the rate of haemophilia mutations in males and females is equal. Haldane, in 1947, was the first to consider this question, and he concluded that the mutation rate in males was 10 times higher than in females. However, indirect estimates of the sex-specific mutation rates suffer from the uncertain values of the patients' effective reproduction (*f*), the effect of ascertainment bias on segregation ratios, and doubtful carrier diagnosis. Thus, in haemophilia A, discordant results have been reported, even if the weight of evidence favours a higher mutation rate in the male (Tuddenham and Giannelli, 1994). In haemophilia B, indirect estimates of the sex-specific mutation rate led to inconclusive results. However, the first direct estimate of such mutations suggested a higher mutation rate in males (Montandon et al, 1992). This is also in keeping with the more recent observations of Ketterling et al (1993).

The Genes for Factor VIII and Factor IX

The factor IX gene

Cloning of the factor IX gene was first reported in 1982 (Choo et al, 1982; Kurachi and Davie, 1982), and the gene was fully characterized and sequenced in the following 3 years (Anson et al, 1984; Yoshitake et al, 1985). This showed that factor IX is encoded by a stretch of DNA approximately 34 kb long, and containing eight exons (Fig. 2.1).

The gene is controlled by a promoter that is being characterized with the help of patients carrying mutations in this part of the gene. Thus several functionally important motifs have been identified. One of these is located in the transcribed region of the gene (residues +1 to +13), and binds members of a well-known family of transcription activating factors: the CCAAT/enhancer binding protein (C/EBP). This is immediately preceded by a second region of functional importance (residues −1 to −15), and then by a region having homology to the binding site for the liver-specific transcription activation factor LF-A1/HNF4 (−15 to −27). This partly overlaps a putative androgen-responsive element (−22 to −36) (Crossley et al, 1992). The precise way in which these and other elements of the factor IX gene promoter exert their activity is not yet understood (Crossley et al, 1992; Picketts et al, 1992; Reijnen et al, 1993).

Transcription of the factor IX gene leads to a mature message of 2802 nt. This includes an untranslated leader of 29 or 50 nt, depending on the true position of the translation start. Three possibilities exist: codon −46, −41 and −39 (the negative signs indicate residues preceding the first amino acid of circulating factor IX). The coding sequence ends with two nonsense codons, and is followed by an untranslated region of 1390 nt, which includes the RNA polyadenylation signal sequence AATAAA 15 nt upstream of the start of the poly A tail of the message. The sequence of the eight exons that form this message encode distinct domains that factor IX shares with large families of proteins.

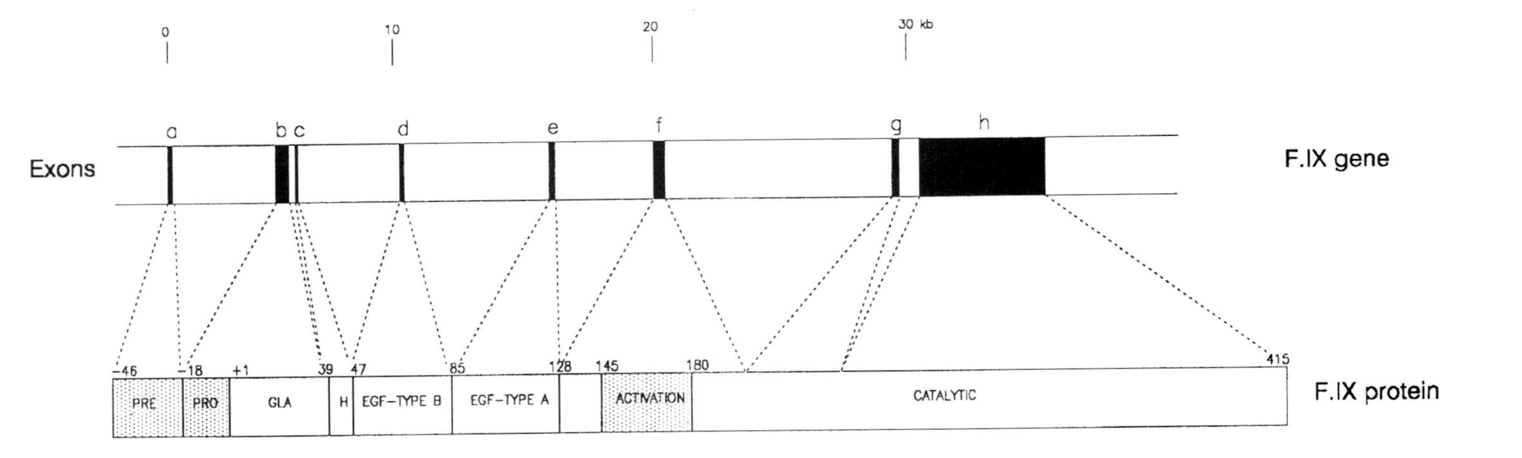

Figure 2.1 The factor IX gene and protein domains. Exons are labelled a–h and shown as filled boxes. Dotted lines between gene and protein indicate protein domains encoded by each exon. Stippled domains are cleaved away during processing and activation of factor IX. The numbers above the protein refer to the residues at the boundaries of relevant domains.

The first exon of the factor IX gene codes for the signal peptide necessary for transport into the endoplasmic reticulum. The second exon codes for the propeptide that acts as a recognition site for the enzyme that γ-carboxylates the first 12 glutamic acid residues of circulating factor IX. The propeptide is cleaved prior to secretion of factor IX, so that the gla region, also encoded by the second exon, is at the amino end of circulating factor IX. The third exon, of only 25 residues, is the smallest exon of the factor IX gene, and encodes a hydrophobic region. The fourth and fifth exons encode two domains homologous to epidermal growth factor (EGF). The first of these EGF domains is of type B, and contains a high-affinity calcium binding site (Handford et al, 1991). The second EGF domain is of type A, and has no calcium binding site. The sixth exon codes for a region comprising the activation peptide (residues 146 to 180) that is cleaved off during the activation of factor IX. The seventh and eighth exons encode the catalytic regions of factor IX. The latter exon is the largest (1936nt) and comprises the long 3′ untranslated tail. The exon/intron organization of the factor IX gene and the domain structure of factor IX are the same as those of factors VII and X, and protein C. The above four genes are therefore thought to derive from the same ancestral gene by duplication (Foster et al, 1985; Leytus et al, 1986; O'Hara et al, 1987).

The factor VIII gene

The factor VIII gene was cloned in 1984 (Gitschier et al, 1984; Toole et al, 1984; Wood et al, 1984), and at that time it was by far the longest known human gene, spanning 186 kb of DNA, and containing 26 exons (Fig. 2.2). The promoter of the gene, which has not yet been functionally characterized, contains a GATAAA sequence 30 bp 5′ of the presumed transcription start that may represent an atypical TATA box. The 26 exons vary considerably in size, from 69 bp (exon 5) to 3106 bp for the exceptionally large exon 14. The exons are separated by introns that also vary considerably in size, from 200 bp (intron 17) to 32.4 kb (intron 22). The latter intron is unusual because it contains an HTF island that is associated with two additional transcripts. One, which is of opposite polarity to the factor VIII transcript, is coded entirely by a 1.8 kb segment of intron 22 and has an open reading frame uninterrupted by introns (Levinson et al, 1990). The second transcript is of the same polarity as the factor VIII transcript and is processed into an mRNA containing exons 23–26 of the factor VIII gene plus a small first exon with eight codons (Levinson et al, 1992). The sequences responsible for these two transcripts have been called genes F8A and F8B, respectively. Interestingly, two additional copies of the sequences that contain gene F8A have been found in the human genome, and they are located 500–600 kb telomeric to the factor VIII gene (Freije and Schlessinger, 1992). The chromosomal orientation of the factor VIII gene has also been determined, and its first exon is the most telomeric.

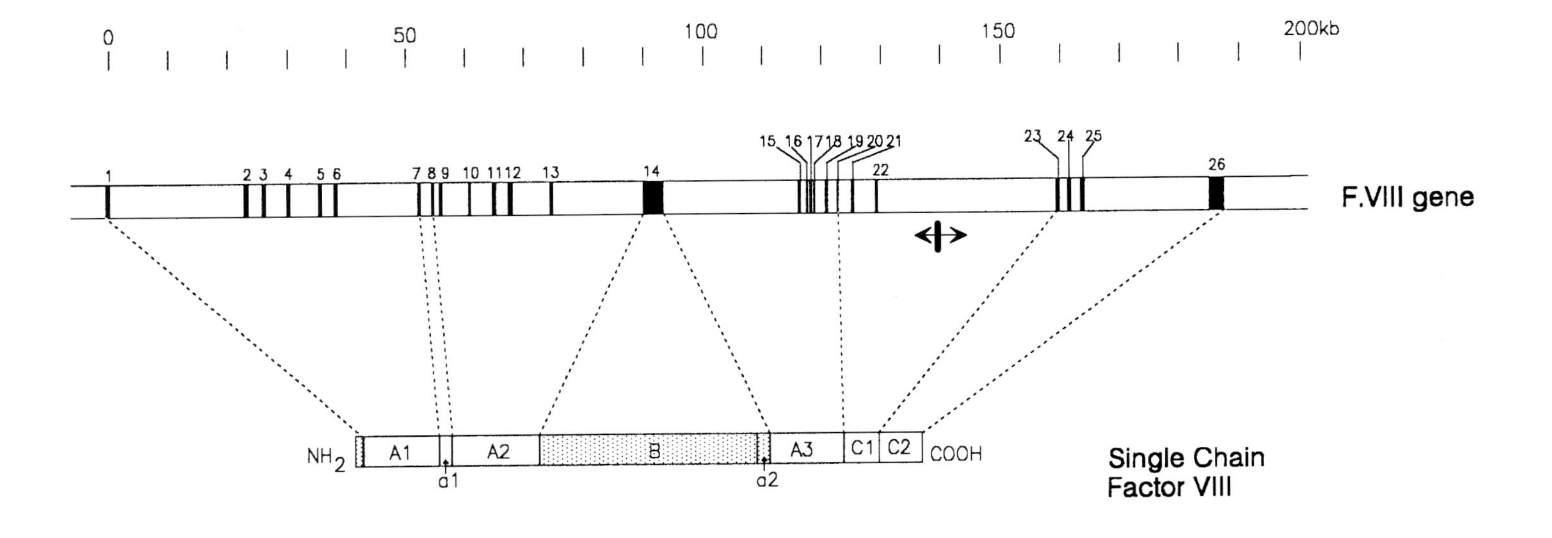

Figure 2.2 The factor VIII gene and protein domains. Exons are labelled 1–26 and shown as filled boxes. The bar and arrows below intron 22 of the gene indicate the position of a CpG island associated with two genes – F8A (left) and F8B (right) – that are transcribed in the direction shown by the arrows. Dotted lines indicate the exons coding for the different protein domains. Stippled domains are excised during processing and activation of factor VIII.

The transcription of the factor VIII gene starts 170, or more rarely 172, bases 5′ of the translation start. This (the first AUG or methionine codon of the message) is followed by an open reading frame comprising 2351 codons, and a 3′ untranslated tail of 1805 nt that includes a TGA stop codon and an AATAAA polyadenylation signal 19 bases from the start of the poly-A segment. The factor VIII mRNA is therefore 9028 nt long, with a coding region of 7053 nt (Gitschier et al, 1984; Toole et al, 1984; Wood et al, 1984). The correspondence between exons and protein domains is not as precise as in factor IX. Exons 1–7 encode the A_1 domain, exon 8 the acidic a_1 peptide, exons 9–13 the A_2 domain, exon 14 the B domain, and small flanking peptides including the a_2 acidic segment, immediately preceding the A_3 domain encoded by exons 15–20, and finally, exons 21–23 and 24–26 specify, at the end of factor VIII, the C_1 and C_2 domains, respectively. Factor V shows homology to factor VIII, but its B domain is unrelated to that of factor VIII, and also the two acidic peptides a_1 and a_2 are not present (Jenny et al, 1987).

Gene Defects in the Haemophilias

The development of rapid and efficient methods for the detection of mutations has allowed marked progress in the understanding of the molecular biology of both haemophilia A and haemophilia B, but further and greater progress has been made in the latter disease.

Haemophilia B mutations

The first haemophilia B mutations were detected by Southern blotting in the course of a specific analysis of patients who had developed antibodies (inhibitors) to therapeutic factor IX, and were gross deletions (Giannelli et al, 1983). Some point mutations were also characterized in the 6 years that followed the cloning of the factor IX gene. This, however, entailed either the analysis of the mutant protein (Noyes et al, 1983), or the cloning and analysis of the gene of each patient investigated. These two procedures are so labour-intensive as seriously to limit the numbers of mutations that could be analysed. The speed of progress accelerated dramatically with the introduction of the polymerase chain reaction (PCR), as this eliminated the need to clone each defective gene, and allowed the direct investigation of the patients' factor IX sequences. The promoter, exons and RNA processing signals that could be considered the essential sequences of the factor IX gene were then isolated by PCR amplification, and either sequenced directly (Bottema et al, 1989; Green et al, 1989) or screened by more rapid procedures that allow reduction of the sequencing effort to mutation-containing regions. The first of these procedures (Montandon et al, 1989) detected mismatches in heteroduplexes formed by amplified test and normal DNA, using two chemicals, osmium tetroxide and hydroxylamine, which specifically and respectively modify mismatched T and C residues (Cotton et al, 1988). This method has the merits of detecting virtually any sequence change, of being able to examine long DNA segments (1.5–1.8 kb), and of indicating the position of the mutation within each segment analysed. A different procedure, called denaturing gel electrophoresis (Myers et al, 1985) was also used in 1989, but simply to examine the region coding for the catalytic domain of factor IX (Attree et al, 1989). This method, based on the detection of differences in the stability of DNA duplexes as they travel through an increasing gradient of denaturant, also has the merit of detecting virtually all sequence changes, but it does not indicate the position of the mutation within each segment analysed, and may examine shorter DNA segments, of 600–700 kb. More recently, other screening procedures have also been used. Popular for its technical simplicity is the method called single-strand conformational polymorphism (SSCP) (Orita et al, 1989). This technique is based on the detection of the effects that mutations have on the conformation of single DNA strands. This method has the disadvantage, however, of detecting only a proportion of mutations (Sheffield et al, 1993), of being less predictable than those mentioned above, of being restricted essentially to DNA segments of 150–300 bp, and of failing to locate the mutation within each segment analysed. The use of methods that are fully effective, together with the analysis of the whole essential sequence of the gene, helps to interpret the functional importance of any observed sequence change (see page 63, 66).

Gross rearrangements of the factor IX gene

These are found in only 2–4% of patients, and are mostly deletions that involve either the whole or part of the factor IX gene. In some patients the deletion is known to include other genes, such as the mcf2 transforming gene or the SOX-3 gene. Patients missing the mcf2 gene do not show features other than haemophilia (Anson et al, 1988), while the patient missing SOX-3 has a particularly large deletion and is mentally retarded (Stevanović et al, 1993).

Several patients with partial deletion of the factor IX gene have been reported, but only one of these showed significant factor IX antigen in circulation (Vidaud et al, 1986). This deletion removes exon d, and should not alter the reading frame of the mRNA. Two large insertions have also been reported, and one appears to result from a new transposition of an Alu repeat (Vidaud et al, 1989).

'Point' mutations of the factor IX gene

These account for the vast majority of haemophilia B families, and a large number of such mutations has been characterized by laboratories around the world. Thus the most recent editions of the world list of haemophilia B mutations contain 806 mutations, comprising 734 single base changes, 54 small deletions, 15 small insertions, and three combined deletion-and-insertion (Giannelli et al, 1993). Twelve of the 806 patients had two, and one had three mutations within the factor IX gene, due to the association of rare neutral changes with the presumptive detrimental mutations. Of the latter, 378 are unique molecular events. The remainder are repeats, chiefly occurring at CpG dinucleotides which are well-known hotspots for transitions (i.e. CpG to TpG or CpA). Some repeatedly observed mutations seem to reveal a founder effect: for example, the transition T→C at nucleotide 31 311 that has been reported 30 times, mostly in the USA (Ketterling et al, 1991).

The small mutational changes mentioned above may cause haemophilia in a variety of ways, and they can accordingly be grouped into those that affect the transcription of the factor IX gene, or the processing of the factor IX mRNA, or the translation of the latter into protein, or, finally, the fine structure of factor IX itself.

The first group of mutations is found in the promoter of the factor IX gene, and the patients carrying them share the intriguing feature of symptoms that improve with age, especially at and after puberty (the so-called 'Leyden phenotype'). To date, 13 different mutations with the Leyden phenotype have been described (Giannelli et al, 1993; Reijnen et al, 1993), and they are all clustered in the –21 to +13 nt region, where +1 is the first nucleotide of the factor IX gene to be transcribed, and negative and positive numbers indicate the distance in nucleotides from the transcription start in the upstream or downstream direction, respectively. One patient with a G→C change at nucleotide –26, in contrast with those above, has not experienced the age-related rise in factor IX. This change affects the weak androgen-responsive element (ARE), overlapping the LF-A1/HFN4 binding site delineated by Crossley et al (1992), and disrupts both sites. All the other mutations disrupt only the above LF-A1/HFN4 site, or a C/EBP site (+1 to +18), or the site for an as yet unidentified factor in the –6 region. It therefore seems probable that the putative ARE of the factor IX gene promoter defined by Crossley et al (1992) is of functional importance, and relevant to the age-related changes in factor IX expression.

RNA processing is expected to be altered in 37 different mutations that disrupt RNA splicing (Giannelli et al, 1993), but unfortunately direct evidence for this effect is difficult to obtain because there is no convenient source of mRNA. All but four of these mutations are within the consensus sequences for acceptor and donor splice sites that may lead to mRNA with exons of abnormal length. The remaining four mutations create a potential acceptor or donor splice site. In addition, a point mutation, identified in a patient with <3% factor IX activity, creates a donor splice site consensus sequence in the 3′ untranslated region. The effect of such a mutation on RNA processing is speculative, but screening of the entire coding region has revealed no other change, and the mutation appears to have occurred independently three times (Vielhaber et al, 1993). Translation of the factor IX message may be altered by frameshifts and nonsense mutations.

Frameshifts result from deletions, insertions or combined deletions and insertions, causing loss or gain of one, two or multiples of one and two bases in the coding sequence. Nonsense mutations are usually caused by single base substitutions that convert a codon for an amino acid into a stop signal for translation. Frameshifts alter the amino acid sequence from the site of mutation onwards, thus usually leading to an abnormal peptide followed by protein truncation. Some frameshifts, however, simply create a nonsense codon at the site of mutation, while others may result in an excessively long protein terminating with an abnormal peptide.

Frameshift and nonsense mutations have been identified throughout the coding sequence of factor IX. With one exception, all patients with such mutations have no detectable factor IX protein, suggesting that either such transcripts are not translated, or the resultant peptide is unstable. The exception is factor $IX_{Lincoln\ Park}$. This mutation is a combined 2 bp deletion (at position 31, 327–8, codon 402) and 8 bp insertion. This creates a frameshift that is predicted to result in the coding of 36 new amino acids, which would result in a mature protein of 438 amino acids (instead of the normal 415). This factor IX is expressed and is fairly stable, since the patient has 9% factor IX:Ag (Rao et al, 1990).

The fine structure of the factor IX protein can be altered by either simple amino acid substitutions (missense mutations) or by single amino acid deletions. The latter are caused by 3 bp deletions affecting the coding sequence, and are relatively rare. So far five such mutations have been identified. Missense mutations instead account for approximately 80% of all small changes causing haemophilia B. So far 234 different amino acid substitutions have been reported. Fifty-three of the factor IX residues show two (or more) different amino acid substitutions, and this very strongly highlights their importance. In fact, substitutions have been detected at most of the residues that could be expected to be important, in spite of the fact that the spectrum of missense mutations causing haemophilia B has not yet been defined completely. The above residues include Asp269 and Ser365 of the catalytic site, seven of the 12 gla residues, Asp47 and Asp64 (involved in Ca^{2+} binding), 21 of the 22 cysteines that form disulphide bridges and the residues adjacent to cleavage sites for signal peptidase, propeptidase, and both factor XI_a and factor VII_a.

The distribution of the amino acid substitutions detected so far is illustrated in Fig. 2.3. These mutations preferentially affect residues conserved in the factor IX homologues. In fact, 122 different substitutions have been found for the 107 residues that are absolutely conserved: 48 for the 73 showing only one conservative substitution; 17 for the 45 with one non-conservative change; and 44 for the 229 less-conserved amino acids. Furthermore, the latter mutations usually affect residues conserved in the factor IX of different mammalian species. The many haemophilia B missense mutations that affect residues conserved in the factor IX homologues suggest that many of the factor IX detrimental mutations are at residues of importance to the overall structure of these complex multidomain serine proteases. Conversely, the mutations that affect residues poorly conserved among the factor IX homologues but highly conserved among the

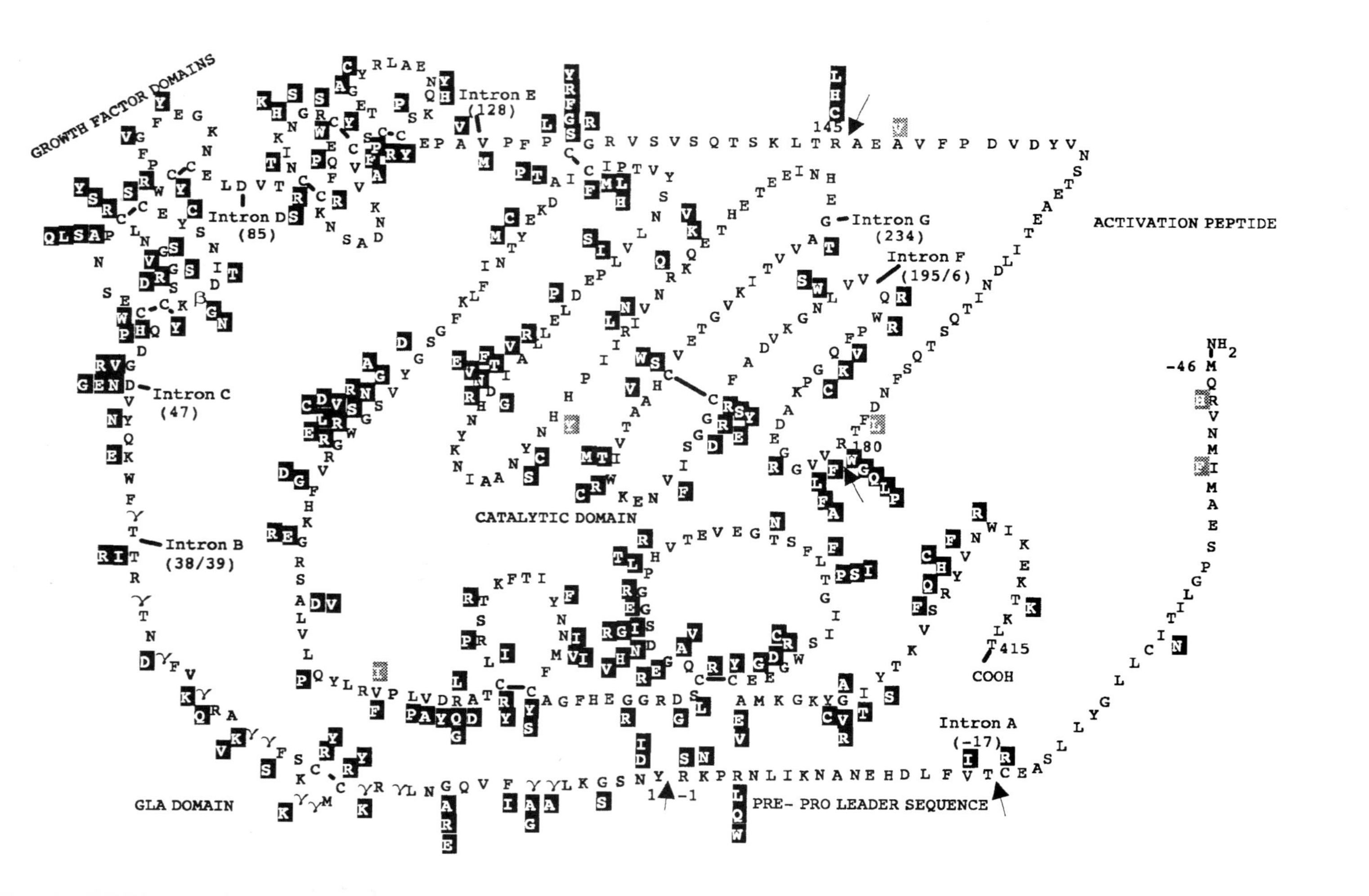
GROWTH FACTOR DOMAINS
ACTIVATION PEPTIDE
CATALYTIC DOMAIN
GLA DOMAIN
PRE- PRO LEADER SEQUENCE
Intron A (-17)
Intron B (38/39)
Intron C (47)
Intron D (85)
Intron E (128)
Intron F (195/6)
Intron G (234)
NH_2
-46
145
180
415
COOH
1
-1

factor IX of different mammalian species may indicate regions important to the specificity of factor IX function. Interesting in this respect is the clustering of mutations observed around Arg333. Several of these involve residues conserved only among the factor IX of different mammalian species (i.e. residues 332–334, 337, 338 and 340), and affect the activity rather than the concentration of circulating factor IX.

The most obvious clustering of missense mutations can be seen in the amino end half of the first EGF domain, the regions containing the cardinal residues of the active site (His221, Asp269, Ser365), and two further segments of the catalytic domain: the peptide comprising residues 305 to 313 and that comprising residues 330 to 340. Also the amino end of the heavy chain of activated factor IX shows a cluster of mutations and this is not surprising, since Val181 interacts with Asp364 of the catalytic centre (Titani and Fujikawa, 1982).

General considerations on the haemophilia B mutations

The functional interpretation of most mutations now found in haemophilia B patients is relatively easy, for the following reasons. A considerable body of information has been gathered in recent years on the factor IX mutations present in haemophilia B patients. There is information on the conservation of each one of the factor IX domains, and there are also some tri-dimensional structural data derived either from the study of factor IX (i.e. the first EGF domain; Baron et al, 1992) or from the study of factor IX homologues (i.e. the gla region of prothrombin; Soriano-Garcia et al, 1992). The main residual problem is represented by splice site mutations affecting poorly conserved elements of the splice consensuses or generating new sites as there is at present no ready access to factor IX mRNA from haemophilia B patients.

From the haematological point of view, patients with haemophilia B may be divided into three groups based on factor IX coagulant and antigen measurements: class I has normal levels of antigen but reduced activity; class II has reduced antigen but greater reduction in activity; and class III has equally reduced antigen and activity. In addition, of course, patients within each of these groups may suffer from mild, moderate or severe disease. Patients in class I are expected to have mutations (mostly missense) that compromise (or abolish) the function of factor IX while not affecting its synthesis, secretion and stability nor suppressing its immunologically detectable epitopes. Functional impairment may result from damage that affects the maturation or activation of factor IX. Examples of this group are the Arg145→His and Arg180→Trp, Arg180→Gly,

Figure 2.3 The reported missense mutations of factor IX. Amino acids are shown with a single letter code. Letters in the black fields indicate mutant residues. Letters in the grey fields show amino acid changes with no detrimental effects.

Arg180→Gln and Arg180→Lys mutations that impair the activation of factor IX; and Arg1→Ser, which preclude cleavage of the propeptide and full γ-carboxylation. This produces a factor IX of abnormal molecular weight that is grossly dysfunctional. Other mutations directly damage the catalytic domain, e.g. Ser365→Arg, or Ser365→Gly and Asp364→His.

Class III phenotypes are associated with a very broad spectrum of mutations because they may result from any change that interferes primarily with the synthesis, secretion or stability of factor IX, or perhaps even with the epitopes that are recognized by the factor IX antigen assays. Thus promoter mutations are expected to result in this phenotype, although usually not in its most severe form. The latter is obligatory for patients with deletions removing the whole gene. Experience so far shows that partial deletions, nonsense mutations, frameshifts and mutations of the GT and AG dinucleotides at the start and end of introns usually cause haemophilia where factor IX activity and antigen are too low to be measured. Whether this is due to problems in synthesis (e.g. instability of mRNA) or in protein stability is not known. Milder type III disease is usually observed when the mutations affect the less conserved features of the splice signals. Probably in this case a proportion of the transcript is correctly spliced.

A problem with factor IX transport and secretion may explain the type III phenotype of a severely affected patient with the missense mutation Ile30→Asn (Green et al, 1993). In this case the introduction of a hydrophilic residue into the hydrophobic core of the prepeptide creates a block of three hydrophilic amino acids (Thr31, Asn30, Cys29) that grossly modifies the usual structure of prepeptides and is therefore likely to prevent transport of the protein into the endoplasmic reticulum.

Other missense mutations may destabilize factor IX or alter its tertiary structure, so that it is rapidly degraded intra- or extracellularly or, perhaps less likely, it is not detected by the factor IX antigen assay and is biologically inactive. These are possible outcomes for mutations altering cysteine residues involved in disulphide bridges and, indeed, a severe type III phenotype is observed in the vast majority of these mutations. However, there are exceptions: the Cys18→Arg mutation causes severe haemophilia with normal levels of factor IX antigen, and both Cys23→Arg and Cys23→Tyr cause a class II phenotype with significant levels of antigen (35% and 19%, respectively). Interestingly, Cys18 and Cys23 contribute to the same disulphide bridge that delimits a minor and well-protected loop of the gla domain (Soriano-Garcia et al, 1992).

Patients with reduced antigen levels but greater reduction in activity (class II) usually have missense mutations, and these are expected to reduce mRNA or protein stability or, possibly, to alter the epitope profile of factor IX, but they obviously have an even greater detrimental effect on factor IX function. An example of this is a patient with 1% factor IX activity, and 12% factor IX antigen, who has an in-frame deletion removing Arg37 from the gla domain of factor IX. This disrupts the amphipathic nature of an α-helix predicted on the basis of information on the crystal structure of the gla region of prothrombin

(Soriano-Garcia et al, 1992). Such a structural change is entirely consistent with an unstable factor IX of low specific activity.

As mentioned earlier, several haemophilia B mutations have been observed repeatedly in unrelated patients, and in many instances such repeats result from independent mutational events. The phenotypic features of patients with these identical mutations appear to be similar enough to suggest that information on the factor IX mutation may serve to predict the severity of the disease. This may be useful in the genetic counselling of families with inadequate clinical information on their affected member(s).

An infrequent but very unfortunate phenotypic feature of haemophilic patients is the development, during the course of treatment, of antibodies against infused factor IX which nullify normal replacement therapy. It was shown for the first time in 1983 that such a complication frequently occurs in patients with gross deletions (Giannelli et al, 1983), and later work has confirmed that patients with gross deletions or functionally equivalent mutations such as nonsense and frameshift mutations are predisposed to this life-threatening complication. It has been proposed that this predisposition is a consequence of the failure to produce a factor IX protein capable, during the maturation of the patient's immune system, of inducing the development of immune tolerance to normal factor IX (Giannelli et al, 1983; Giannelli and Brownlee, 1986).

Haemophilia A mutations

The first haemophilia A mutations were identified in 1985, and comprised both gross deletions and single base substitutions that altered the recognition sequence of the TaqI restriction enzyme (Gitschier et al, 1985). However, since the factor VIII gene is very large, no attempt was made to clone the gene of individual patients, and mutation detection remained limited by the sensitivity of Southern blotting until the introduction of PCR. Nevertheless, TaqI restriction proved relatively efficient at detecting some point mutations, partly because the TaqI recognition sequence, TCGA, contains a CpG dinucleotide that often represents a hotspot for transitions (CpG→TpG or CpA); and partly because the above transitions in the TaqI sites of the factor VIII coding sequence result in nonsense mutations 4.3 times more frequently than expected by chance, and consequently mutations at TaqI sites have a relatively high probability of being so detrimental as to cause haemophilia (Green et al, 1991a).

After the introduction of PCR, and of rapid mutation screening procedures, the size and complexity of the factor VIII gene and the pattern of investigation established in earlier years continued to hinder progress, and much effort was spent in examining limited regions of the factor VIII gene in large series of patients, and thus the spectrum of mutations characterized remained, until recently, grossly biased.

Development of an efficient mutation detection method and discovery of unconventional mutations

The first mutations detected by a procedure that examined all the essential sequences of the factor VIII gene were published in 1991 (Naylor et al, 1991). This procedure relied in part on the amplification of traces of factor VIII mRNA present in peripheral lymphocytes by means of reverse transcription and PCR. Two important advances stem from the use of mRNA: (1) reduction of labour because this molecule presents the coding sequence as a single stretch of 7053nt rather than 26 widely spaced exons; and (2) detection of any mutation causing mRNA abnormalities, irrespective of where they are located within the gene. The detection of haemophilia A mutations by the above method entails the PCR amplification of the putative promoter, the 3106bp exon 14, and the polyadenylation signal region from genomic DNA and reverse transcription plus PCR amplification of the remainder of the coding sequence with nested primers. A total of eight PCR products is thus obtained: two from exon 14, four from the remainder of the coding sequence, and one from each end of the gene. These segments overlap each other, except for that with the polyadenylation signal, and this ensures thorough screening of the whole amplified sequence by the chemical mismatch procedure described earlier (page 50, 51). This allows screening of long DNA segments and identifies and locates any mutation, thus reducing the sequencing reactions needed to characterize fully any sequence change to just one or two. Point mutations affecting the coding sequence are readily confirmed by genomic DNA analysis while gross mRNA changes immediately indicate the segment of genomic DNA to be examined for further characterization of the mutation.

This procedure in 1992 revealed unexpected mutations that are responsible for almost half of all cases of severe haemophilia A, and that had, nevertheless, been missed for 8 years (Naylor et al, 1992, 1993a). This discovery was preceded by the intriguing report that analysis of the promoter, exons, and most exon/intron boundaries of the factor VIII gene, while detecting mutations in most patients with mild and moderate disease, clearly failed in half of severely affected patients (Higuchi et al, 1991a,b). This puzzling result, obtained with a procedure expected to examine almost all essential sequences of the factor VIII gene, generated hypotheses that postulated the existence of remote factor VIII controlling regions or of genes other than factor VIII responsible for haemophilia A. However, the puzzle was solved when examination of factor VIII mRNA showed not only that all patients with haemophilia A had mutations of the factor VIII gene, but also that 45% of the patients with severe disease had an unusual mRNA defect (Naylor et al, 1992). This defect completely prevented amplification of any segment that crossed the boundary between exons 22 and 23, and yet all the coding sequences of the factor VIII gene could be amplified by reactions that avoided the boundary. This assigned the mutations to intron 22, but because the splice signals and the adjacent regions of intron 22 were normal, the mutations clearly affected internal regions of the intron (Naylor et al, 1993a).

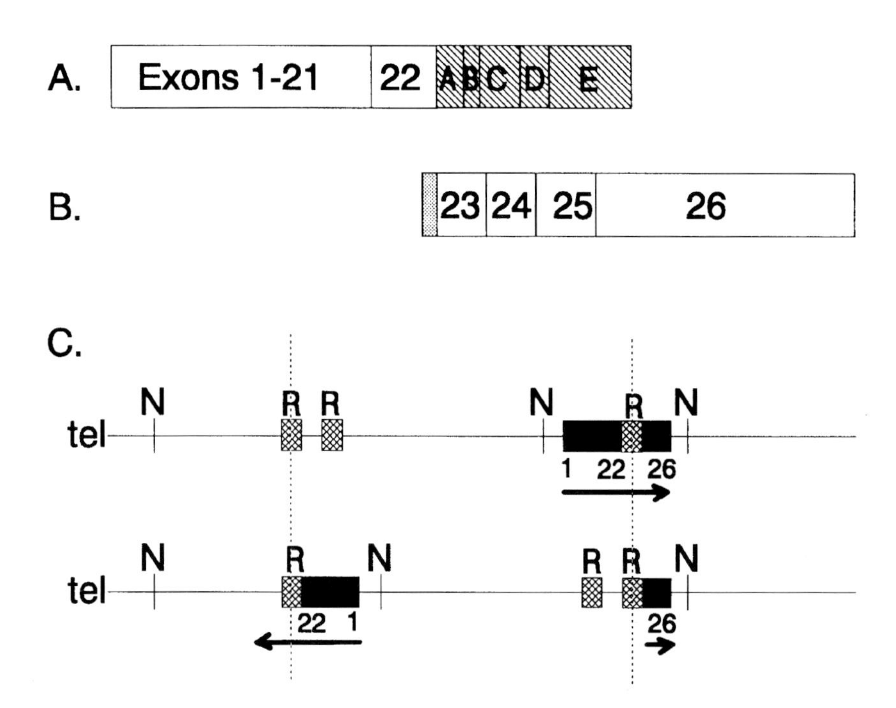

Figure 2.4 mRNA and genomic DNA of severe haemophilia A patients with the inversion involving intron 22. (A) mRNA (not drawn to scale) containing the first 22 exons of the factor VIII gene plus several exons (A–E) from a segment of DNA about 500kb telomeric of the factor VIII gene. (B) mRNA containing exons 23–26 of the factor VIII gene plus an initial exon present in intron 22 of the factor VIII gene. This mRNA is produced by the gene called F8B. (C) (Top) Shows the end of the long arm of the X chromosome in a normal male. The black box is the factor VIII gene. Cross-hatched boxes (R) indicate three copies of the same sequence (one located in intron 22 of the factor VIII gene and two 500–600 kb telomeric to the factor VIII gene). Black arrows show the direction of transcription of mRNA containing factor VIII coding sequences. N, NruI restriction enzyme site used in pulsed field gel analysis; tel, telomere. (Bottom) The end of the long arm of the X chromosome in a patient with the inversion extending from intron 22 to the most telomeric of the repeated sequences. Note how the factor VIII gene is split in intron 22 and exons 1–22 are in inverted orientation. The spacing of the NruI sites is abnormal as detected by pulsed field gel analysis. The dotted lines indicate the inversion boundaries.

The block to amplification across the exon 22–23 boundary was insurmountable, and it therefore seemed probable that the patients' factor VIII mRNA was interrupted 3′ of exon 22, so that exons 23–26 were exclusively expressed as part of the F8B gene controlled by the intron 22 promoter (Fig. 2.4). The successful amplification of the entire F8B message in the patients was in keeping with this idea, and therefore the sequences 3′ of exon 22 were sought in each of the available patients, using a novel strategy for the isolation of the 3′ ends of mRNA (Naylor et al, 1993b). Upon sequencing, these revealed a set of sequence blocks (Fig. 2.4) identifiable as exons on at least three grounds: their precise boundaries, separation by intervening sequences in genomic DNA, and, in one case, the observation of a splice site consensus. The novel exon-like sequences were variably spliced out of or into the patients' abnormal factor VIII message (Naylor et al, 1993b) and were not from intron 22. The possibility that the abnormal sequences had been brought into the patients' intron 22 by insertion or translocation was also excluded, because Southern blotting of the intron 22 sequences from the patients' DNA digested with BamHI, EcoRI or HindIII did not show gross abnormalities. It was therefore postulated that inversions had occurred involving the two telomeric sequences homologous to part of intron 22 (Fig. 2.4), as this would split the factor VIII gene into two fragments but cause minimal disturbance to the restriction map of the intron 22 region (Naylor et al, 1993b). This hypothesis was confirmed using the novel sequences from the patients' mRNA to isolate YAC clones that, when ordered relative to each other and clones containing the factor VIII gene, mapped the novel sequences telomeric of the factor VIII gene and in the region containing the sequences homologous to part of intron 22. Since the first exon of the normal factor VIII gene is telomeric to exon 22, the linear arrangement of sequences in the patients' mRNA clearly indicates inversions (Fig. 2.4). Furthermore, pulse field analysis of the patients' DNA demonstrated that the inversions involved segments of 500–600 kb, i.e. the segments expected if the inversion boundaries were in intron 22 and the telomeric sequences homologous to intron 22 (Naylor et al, 1993b).

Meanwhile, Lakich et al (1993) had thought that the unusual abnormality we had identified in 45% of severely affected patients could be due to recombination between the homologous sequences in intron 22 and those at the two more telomeric locations. If the latter sequences were in opposite orientation to that in intron 22, homologous intra-chromatid recombination would lead to inversions. In the course of testing this hypothesis, they found one restriction enzyme (BclI) that resolved the three homologous sequences as a set of three bands of 21.5, 16 and 14 kb that hybridize to the F8A gene sequences (Fig. 2.5). The 21.5 kb band is contributed by intron 22, while those of 14 and 16 kb contain, respectively, the proximal and distal members of the telomeric pair of repeats. Patients with the intron 22 mutations showed an abnormality of either the 14 kb or 16 kb band, and then invariably of the 21.5 kb band, thus showing that the inversion boundaries on the telomeric side involved either of the two regions containing the telomeric copies of the F8A gene (Lakich et al, 1993). Indeed,

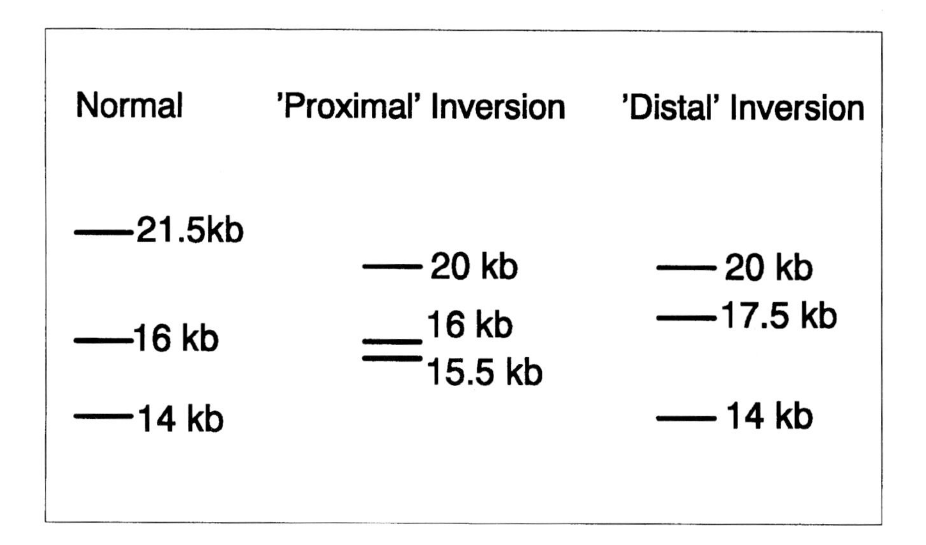

Figure 2.5 BclI Southern blot results. Males with no inversion (normal) are distinguished from those with inversions affecting the telomeric repeat less distant from the factor VIII gene ("proximal") and those with inversions affecting the most telomeric of the repeats ("distal"). A female carrier with one or other of the inversions will show a combination of the normal and either "proximal" or "distal" inversion pattern.

current data indicate that the more distal repeat is preferentially involved (6 : 1) (Lakich et al, 1993; Collins et al, 1994; Goodeve et al, 1994; Ljung, 1994; Naylor et al, unpublished observations)

Patients with any of the above inversions show different haplotypes of the factor VIII gene polymorphisms, thus suggesting that the inversions are as independent in origin as other mutations causing haemophilia A (Lakich et al, 1993; Naylor et al, 1993b). We estimate, therefore, that the rate of mutations leading to inversions is of the order of 4×10^{-6} per gene per gamete per generation. This rate is equivalent to the mutation rate for the whole spectrum of mutations causing haemophilia B, and clearly reveals an unsuspected degree of chromosomal instability (Naylor et al, 1993b).

It is important at this stage to define the structure of the inversion junctions, and to gain further insight into the factors that are responsible for the very high observed inversion rate. Furthermore, these results beg the question of whether the chromosomal instability first discovered in haemophilia A may occur in other regions of the genome, and thus contribute significantly to man's genetic load.

Conventional mutations causing haemophilia A

One-fifth of all haemophilia A mutations is accounted for by the inversions mentioned above, while the remainder consists of changes similar to those observed in haemophilia B, and collectively referred to here as conventional. Recently a summary has been prepared of all such mutations detected in haemophilia A (Tuddenham et al, 1994).

Three to five per cent of haemophilia A patients have gross deletions of the coding sequence, and 75 gross deletions have been reported so far. These may involve the whole or a part of the gene (e.g. a single exon), and do not show obvious preferences for any specific region. Usually deletions result in severe disease, but two have been found in patients with moderate haemophilia: one comprises exon 22 (Youssoufian et al, 1987), and one exons 23 and 24 (Lavergne, 1992: cited by Tuddenham et al, 1994). The mRNA in these cases is expected to maintain the normal reading frame and presumably the deletions simply lead to the loss of the amino acids encoded by the missing exons.

Gross insertions and duplications appear to be quite rare, but two interesting patients have been reported with insertions of the Line repeat sequence in AT-rich regions of exon 14 (Kazazian et al, 1988). These insertions appear to represent recent transpositions, and the sequence representing the probable origin of one of these inserted repeats has been located in chromosome 22 (Dombroski et al, 1991).

Two partial duplications have also been reported: one involving 23 kb of intron 22 inserted between exons 23 and 24, and the other exon 13 (Gitschier, 1988; Murru et al, 1990). The former was found in the mother of a deletion patient, and it was thought to have predisposed the gene to deletion. The latter does not alter the reading frame, and was found in a mildly affected patient.

As in haemophilia B, the vast majority of conventional haemophilia A mutations are small sequence changes, but none so far has been found in the putative promoter of the factor VIII gene (Tuddenham et al, 1994). The above mutations therefore are expected to act by affecting RNA processing (splice site mutations) or mRNA translations (nonsense and frameshifts), or the fine structure of factor VIII (missense and amino acid deletions).

At least eight different splice site mutations have been reported but the mRNA was not examined in most of these. Four mutations affected highly conserved residues of the consensuses (AG at ends of introns), while five involved less conserved elements.

Nonsense mutations have been reported at no fewer than 25 different locations, and several have been observed repeatedly. At 12 of the 25 locations, nonsense codons have arisen by transitions at CpG sites. These mutations are expected to arise frequently, and were therefore deliberately sought by targeted screening of CpG sites by TaqI restriction or by oligonucleotide discriminant hybridization (Gitschier et al, 1985; Pattinson et al, 1990). Nonsense mutations are expected to cause premature termination of translation but recently mRNA analysis has shown that nonsense mutations may sometimes alter RNA processing and cause skipping of the exon containing the nonsense codon (Naylor et al, 1993a), a result that may significantly affect the functional consequences of the mutation. Thus in one patient with a nonsense mutation at codon 1987, the examined mRNA always lacked exon 19, while another with a nonsense codon at position 2116 showed two mRNAs, one of normal structure and one missing the mutant exon 22. The loss of the exon containing the nonsense codon in these two patients should have beneficial effects because in the first patient it results in a factor VIII missing only the amino acids encoded by exon 19, rather than a factor VIII missing those encoded by exons 20 to 26 plus part of exon 19, and in the second patient in the loss of only the residues encoded by exon 22, rather than those encoded by exons 23 to 26 plus part of exon 22.

Frameshift mutations resulting from small deletions or insertions in the coding sequence have been detected so far at, respectively, 31 and 11 different positions.

More subtle changes to the structure of factor VIII are caused by missense mutations and their analysis should gradually help to define the structural features that are important to the transport, processing, stability and function of factor VIII. So far, 145 different missense mutations and two single amino acid deletions have been identified (Table 2.1), but three of the missenses are due to mutations that alter the normal splice consensus (Gly205→Trp, Gln565→Lys and Val2223→Met; see last three lines in Table 2.1), and could therefore also affect mRNA processing. Some of the missense mutations involve sites of known functional importance, such as activation cleavage sites (Arg372→Cys, Arg372→His or Arg372→Pro; Ser373→Leu or Ser373→Pro and Arg1689→Cys or Arg1689→His), and the sulphated tyrosine at position 1680 that is involved in von Willebrand factor binding (Tyr1680→Phe and Tyr1680→Cys). One mutation destroys and two create N-glycosylation sites (Ser584→Ile and Ile566→Thr plus Met1772→Thr). One cysteine involved in a disulphide bridge has been the site of three different amino acid substitutions (Cys329→Tyr, Cys329→Ser, Cys329→Arg) and in total two or more different substitutions have been observed at 20 residues (see Table 2.1).

General considerations on the haemophilia A mutations

A large proportion of the observed factor VIII mutations can undoubtedly be considered detrimental, i.e. gross deletions, insertions, duplications and the inversions involving intron 22. Together these represent a quarter of all haemophilia A mutations. Further mutations that are clearly detrimental are frameshifts, nonsense mutations and alterations of the absolutely conserved elements of the splice site consensuses. A few missense mutations can also readily be recognized as detrimental because they affect regions of known functional importance such as activation cleavage sites and residues important for the factor VIII–von Willebrand binding. The detremintal nature of other missense mutations can be strongly indicated by any of the following three criteria: (1) the change observed

Table 2.1 Missense mutations and single AA deletions in factor VIII gene of haemophilic patients

Line number	Amino acid change	Severity	Line number	Amino acid change	Severity	Line number	Amino acid change	Severity
1	Leu7 → Arg	Severe	50	Tyr473 → Cys	Moderate	99	Met1823 → lle	Moderate
2	Glu11 → Val	Mild	51	lle475 → Thr	Mild	100	Pro1825 → Ser	Moderate
3	Gly22 → Cys	Severe/mild	52	Gly479 → Arg	Moderate/mild	101	Thr1826 → Pro	Mild
4	Gly70 → Asp	Severe	53	Asp525 → Asn	Moderate	102	Ala1834 → Val	Mild
5	Gly73 → Val	Mild	54	Arg527 → Trp	Mild	103	Asp1846 → Asn	Severe
6	Val80 → Asp	Severe	55	Arg531 → Cys	Moderate	104	Asp1846 → Tyr	Severe
7	Val85 → Asp	Mild	56	Arg531 → Gly	Moderate	105	His1848 → Arg	Moderate
8	Lys89 → Thr	Mild	57	Arg531 → His	Mild	106	Pro1854 → Arg	Severe
9	Met91 → Val	Mild	58	Ser535 → Gly		107	Glu1885 → Lys	Severe
10	Leu98 → Arg	Severe	59	Asp542 → Gly	Severe	108	Asn1922 → Asp	Severe/ moderate
11	Gly111 → Arg	Severe	60	Ser558 → Phe	Mild	109	Asn1922 → Ser	Moderate
12	Gln113 → Asp	Severe	61[b]	IIe566 → Thr	Severe/moderate	110	Arg1941 → Gln	Moderate/mild
13	Tyr114 → Cys	Mild	62	Ser577 → Pro		111	Arg1941 → Leu	Moderate
14	Asp116 → Gly	Severe	63[c]	Ser584 → lle		112	Gly1948 → Asp	Moderate
15	Thr118 → lle	Moderate	64	Trp585 → Cys	Severe	113	Gly1960 → Val	Mild/moderate
16	Gly145 → Val	Mild	65	Tyr586 → Ser	Severe	114	His1961 → Tyr	Mild
17	Pro146 → Ser	Severe	66	Arg593 → Cys	Mild	115	Arg1997 → Trp	Moderate/ severe
18	Val162 → Met	Moderate/mild	67	Asn612 → Ser		116	Asn2019 → Ser	Mild
19	Lys166 → Thr	Mild	68	Val634 → Ala	Mild	117	Trp2046 → Arg	Moderate
20	Ser170 → Leu	Moderate	69	Val634 → Met	Severe	118	Ser2069 → Phe	Severe
21	Asp203 → Val	Moderate	70	Ala644 → Val	Mild	119	Asp2074 → Gly	Mild
22	Gly247 → Gln	Severe	71	Phe652 deletion	Severe	120	Phe2101 → Leu	Mild
23	Gly259 → Arg	Severe	72	Phe658 → Leu	Moderate	121	Tyr2105 → Cys	Mild
24	Val266 → Gly	Mild	73	Arg698 → Trp	Mild	122	Arg2116 → Pro	Severe

Table 2.1 *continued*

Line number	Amino acid change	Severity	Line number	Amino acid change	Severity	Line number	Amino acid change	Severity
25	Glu272 → Gly	Moderate	74	Ala704 → Thr	Mild/moderate	123	Ser2119 → Tyr	Moderate
26	Thr275 → lle	Moderate	75	Glu720 → Lys	Mild	124	Arg2150 → His	Mild
27	Asn280 → lle	Mild	76	Glu1038 → Lys	Moderate	125	Pro2153 → Gln	Moderate
28	Arg282 → His	Severe	77	Asn1441 → Lys	Moderate	126	Thr2154 → lle	Mild
29	Arg282 → Leu	Severe	78	Leu1462 → Pro		127	Arg2159 → Cys	Mild
30	Ser289 → Leu	Mild	79	Val1634 → Ala	Moderate	128	Arg2159 → Leu	Mild
31	Phe293 → Ser	Mild	80	Val1634 → Met	Severe	129	Arg2159 → His	Mild
32	Thr295 → Ala	Mild	81[d]	Tyr1680 → Phe	Mild	130	Arg2163 → His	Moderate
33	Leu308 → Pro	Severe	82[d]	Tyr1680 → Cys	Severe	131	Arg2163 → Cys	Moderate
34	Val326 → Leu	Severe/moderate	83[a]	Arg1689 → Cys	Moderate/severe	132	Leu2166 → Ser	Severe
35	Cys329 → Arg	Severe	84	Arg1689 → His	Mild	133	Ala2192 → Pro	Moderate
36	Cys329 → Tyr	Severe	85	Arg1696 → Gly	Mild	134	Pro2205 deletion	Moderate
37	Cys329 → Ser	Moderate	86	Arg1698 → Cys	Severe	135	Arg2209 → Leu	Moderate
38[a]	Arg372 → Cys	Moderate	87	Glu1704 → Lys	Severe	136	Arg2209 → Gln	Severe/mild
39[a]	Arg372 → His	Moderate/mild	88	Tyr1709 → Cys	Moderate	137	Arg2209 → Gly	Severe
40[a]	Arg372 → Pro	Severe	89	Gly1750 → Arg	Mild	138	Trp2229 → Cys	Moderate
41	Ser373 → Leu	Mild	90	Leu1756 → Val	Moderate	139	Trp2246 → Arg	Moderate
42	Ser373 → Pro	Mild	91	Leu1756 → Phe	Mild	140	Pro2300 → Leu	Mild
43	lle386 → Ser	Severe	92	Gly1760 → Glu	Severe	141	Arg2304 → Cys	Mild
44	Glu390 → Gly	Moderate/severe	93[b]	Met1772 → Thr	Severe	142	Arg2304 → His	Mild
45	Leu412 → Phe	Mild/moderate	94	Arg1781 → His	Mild/moderate	143	Arg2307 → Leu	Severe/mild
46	Lys425 → Arg	Severe	95	Arg1781 → Cys	Mild	144	Arg2307 → Gln	Moderate/mild
47	Tyr431 → Asn	Moderate	96	Arg1781 → Gly	Mild	145	Gly205 → Trp	Moderate[e]
48	Ala469 → Gly	Moderate	97	Ser1784 → Tyr	Severe	146	Gln565 → Lys	Moderate[e]
49	Tyr473 → His	Mild	98	Leu1789 → Phe	Mild	147[e]	Val2223 → Met	

[a]Activation cleavage site; [b]Generates new glycosylation site; [c]Causes loss of glycosylation site; [d]Sulphated residue involved in von Willebrand factor binding; [e]Mutations also altering splice site consensuses

in a patient is the only one affecting his gene; (2) the mutation is of recent origin; (3) the mutation has occurred independently in two or more families. In order to apply the first of the above criteria, it is necessary to use a mutation detection method that screens all the essential sequences of the gene with virtually 100% efficiency, such as the method of Naylor et al (1991). The second criterion relies on family studies, and the availability of ascendant relatives, and the third on differences between the patients' factor VIII markers. Weaker inferences can be based on the evolutionary conservation of the residue involved in the mutation, or on the difference between the mutant and wild-type residue. In fact, factor VIII has few homologues, and very little is known about its tridimensional structure or the functional importance of its individual domains. Site-directed mutagenesis and expression of factor VIII in cultured cells has been used to confirm the importance of factor VIII residues suspected to be functionally important (Eaton et al, 1986; Pittman and Kaufman, 1988, 1989), but this method does not provide a general approach for determining the detrimental nature of factor VIII mutations. In fact the vast majority of haemophilia A mutations result in deficits of factor VIII protein in circulation and the factors that determine the concentration of factor VIII in circulation cannot be reproduced in cell culture systems. Residues that in patients are affected by two or more missense mutations may indicate residues of clear structural and functional importance.

Analysis of the mRNA is important for the functional interpretation of mutations. Of course any mutation altering splice sites and especially those affecting poorly conserved elements of the splice site consensus should be examined at the mRNA level. This analysis is also essential for mutations likely to create a new splice site. Gross structural changes such as partial deletions and duplications or insertions could also affect splicing in ways that cannot be predicted by DNA analysis, and direct examination of the mRNA is appropriate. Furthermore, as mentioned above, even a single base pair substitution causing a nonsense codon may result in exon skipping (Naylor et al, 1993a).

With regard to the correlation between phenotype and genotype, patients with mild and moderate disease usually carry missense mutations, but the converse is not necessarily true and several missense mutations have been found in patients with severe disease (Higuchi et al, 1991b; Naylor et al, 1993a; Tuddenham et al, 1994). Sometimes marked differences in severity have been reported between patients with the same mutation (see Table 2.1 and Tuddenham et al, 1994), but it is difficult at present to assess how much this is due to variations in haematological assays, problems with the characterization of mutations such as failing to detect a second change because of incomplete screening of the essential sequences of the gene, or true biological variation. The latter would seem most probable if differences were observed among relatives examined by the same laboratory, and in this case perhaps variations in the proteins that interact with factor VIII – such as, for example, von Willebrand factor – could be responsible. Haemophilia A shows a greater proportion of severely affected patients than haemophilia B. The fact that one-fifth of all haemophilia A cases are due to inversions that disrupt the factor VIII gene may, at least in part, explain this difference.

One of the most worrying phenotypic features of haemophilia A patients is the development of antibodies against therapeutic factor VIII (inhibitors). Mutation analysis has clearly indicated that the individual predisposition to develop such a disastrous complication is strongly influenced by the nature of the patient's mutation. Thus 53 of 57 patients with inhibitors show a gross deletion, nonsense or frameshift mutations and only four had missense mutations. The former represent 35% of the patients with a deletion, nonsense or frameshift mutation whose inhibitor status is known, while the latter represent 1.7% of the patients with missense mutations and known inhibitor status (Tuddenham et al, 1994).

The correlation between the individual's mutation and his predisposition to the inhibitor complication can best be explained by the hypothesis that failure to produce a coagulant factor resembling the normal one does not allow the natural development of immune tolerance to the latter. It is interesting to consider the frequency of inhibitors among groups of patients with different nonsense mutations. Tuddenham et al (1994) have noted that this seems to vary. Thus none of the six known patients with a nonsense mutation at codon 2116 has inhibitors, whilst 11 of the 21 with nonsense mutations at codons 1941, 2147 and 2209 have the complication. It is at least conceivable that this difference may be due to the fact, mentioned earlier, that patients with an Arg2116→Stop mutation produce mRNA where exon skipping eliminates the nonsense codon. This leads to the synthesis of factor VIII missing only the amino acids encoded by exon 22. Since a patient with a deletion affecting only exon 22 has moderate disease and 2–5% factor VIII antigen in circulation (Youssoufian et al, 1987), it seems that factor VIII missing the amino acids encoded by exon 22 is partially stable and functional. Such a factor VIII could allow development of immune tolerance toward factor VIII during the maturation of the patient's immune system.

Carrier Detection, Prenatal Diagnosis and Genetic Counselling in the Haemophilias

The problem and its initial solution

The X-linked recessive nature of both haemophilias, and the extreme rarity of matings between affected males and carrier females ensures that affected males generally produce only normal sons and carrier daughters, while carrier females have equal chances (1/2) of producing affected or normal sons and carrier or normal daughters. Nevertheless, affected females are occasionally observed, and some have clearly been shown to be manifesting heterozygotes (Kling et al, 1991). One possible explanation for this phenomenon is the abrogation of the random pattern of X-inactivation in early female embryos so that systematic inactivation of either the maternally or paternally derived X chromosome occurs. This is usually brought about by structural aberrations of one X chromosome. Some bias in the X chromosome inactivation of coagulant factor synthesizing cells may also occur by chance. This causes a very broad spectrum of factor VIII or factor IX levels in heterozygotes. Consequently, haematological data are equivocal about the carrier status, except when the assays give very low values, or when coagulant activity is much more reduced than the protein concentration in the relatives of patients that clearly show the same kind of discrepancy between the factor IX or factor VIII coagulant and antigen assays. Much work was done prior to the cloning of the factor IX and factor VIII genes to optimize assessment of carrier status by haematologic tests and pedigree analysis, but even with optimal procedures error rates were greater than 15%, and consisted mainly of false-negative diagnoses (Barrow et al, 1982).

Carrier diagnosis is an essential component of the genetic counselling for haemophilia. Any female blood relation of a haemophilic patient is at risk of being a carrier, and a patient may typically be expected to have five or six such female relatives. In the UK there could therefore be approximately 30 000 women who would benefit from carrier testing for haemophilia A, and 5000 for haemophilia B. The expected carrier frequencies for haemophilia A and haemophilia B are approximately 1/2500 and 1/15 000, respectively, and such carriers may wish to have their male fetuses tested for the disease.

In the late 1970s, prenatal diagnosis for both haemophilia A and haemophilia B became available. This was based on haematological assays, and required fetoscopy to obtain a fetal blood sample at 18–20 weeks of pregnancy. The procedure can only be performed in a very few experienced centres, and has shown a low level of acceptability because it is invasive and is applied at an advanced stage of pregnancy. Nevertheless, in good hands definite diagnoses were obtained at apparently no risk to the mother, but at a definite (though small) risk to the fetus. Thus in the UK the operative loss and abortion rate was 2.4%, and the pre-term delivery rate 15% (Mibashan et al, 1986).

Progress in the DNA era

The cloning of the factor IX and factor VIII genes heralded substantive advances in carrier detection and prenatal diagnosis, and consequently also in the genetic counselling of the haemophilias. But if diagnosis based on haematologic tests had been hampered by the vagaries of X chromosome inactivation in females, and the technical problems of obtaining adequate fetal blood samples, DNA-based diagnosis had to face the problems derived from the very high mutational heterogeneity of haemophilias A and B. The solution of this problem has required targeted efforts that have led to the development of a fully effective strategy for haemophilia B, and to the creation of the technical conditions required for the implementation of ideal strategies also in haemophilia A. Such progress entailed the following phases: detection of gene-specific polymorphic markers and their application to indirect carrier and prenatal tests; development of rapid procedures for the detection of gene mutations and their application to direct carrier and prenatal tests; and formulation and implementation of a strategy to maximize the benefits of diagnosis based on the direct detection of the gene defect.

Haemophilia B

Until the development of rapid methods for the detection of mutations, carrier and prenatal tests based on the direct identification of the gene defect were limited to conditions where a few mutations accounted for all or most of the individuals at risk in the population. This was not expected to be the case in haemophilia B, and therefore polymorphic variations were sought within the factor IX gene to help with carrier and prenatal tests. An indirect strategy could then be used. This is based on the principle that polymorphic DNA markers very closely linked to a disease-causing mutation may help to follow the transmission of the latter within individual families (Fig. 2.6). This approach, which was first applied in 1984 (Camerino et al, 1984; Giannelli et al, 1984), can provide definitive carrier diagnosis and first-trimester prenatal diagnosis based on the analysis of DNA extracted from chorion villus samples taken at 10 weeks of pregnancy: a considerable advantage over fetoscopy and blood sampling at 18–20 weeks of gestation. However, this indirect procedure has several drawbacks and inevitably fails in a large proportion of cases. The drawbacks include:

1. The necessity of examining a complete family group for each diagnosis. This group typically includes the proband, one affected male relative to establish the association of markers with the defective gene, the mother, and, for carrier diagnosis, often the father of the proband also.
2. The requirement that the proband's mother should be heterogeneous for a marker.
3. The need for paternity testing when investigation of the proband's father is required.
4. The failure to provide information on the nature of the detrimental mutation and thus to advance knowledge of the molecular biology of the disease.
5. The risk of recombination between the marker(s) and the disease-causing mutation, which could lead to erroneous diagnosis. However, in haemophilia B the probability of such an error is small, if only factor IX-specific markers are used.
6. The large proportion of families where the procedure does fail. Failure may occur because of: (a) homozygosity for all markers in the proband's mother; (b) lack of samples from essential relatives; and (c) lack of positive family history. Analysis of the UK population has shown that (a) accounts

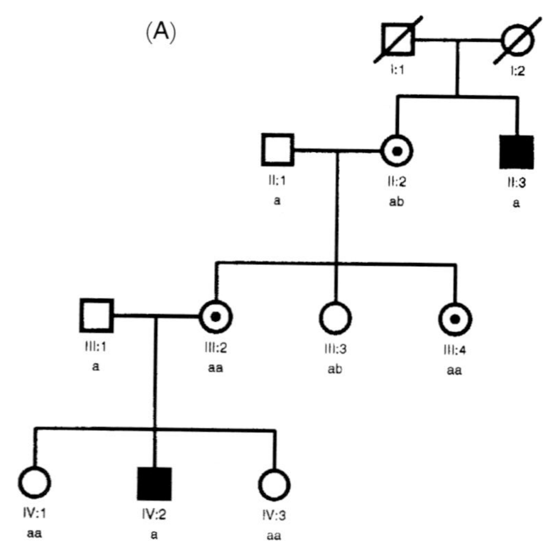

(A)
I:1
I:2
II:1
a
II:2
ab
II:3
a
III:1
a
III:2
aa
III:3
ab
III:4
aa
IV:1
aa
IV:2
a
IV:3
aa

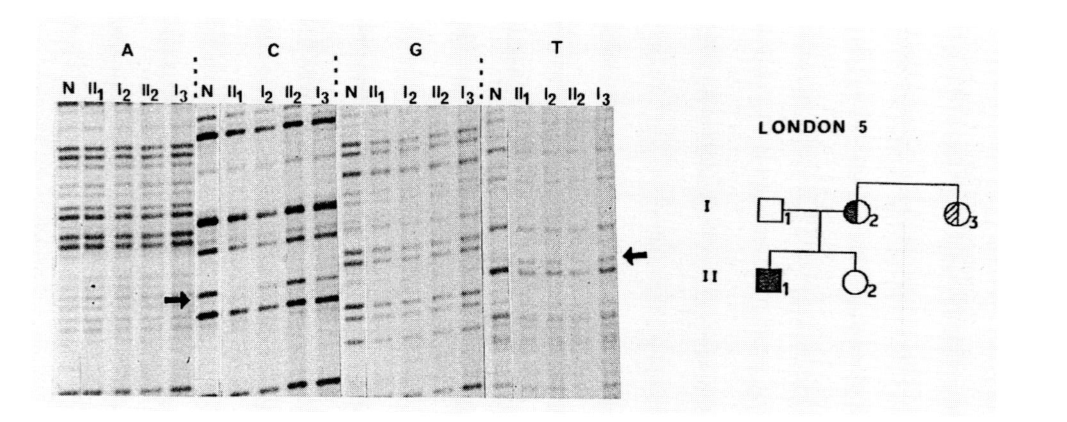

(B)
A
C
G
T
N
II1
I2
II2
I3
LONDON 5
I
II
1
2
3

for diagnostic failures in 11% of families; (b) in 6%, while (c) affects 50% of families (Saad et al, 1994). In the last families, it is sometimes possible to exclude carrier status in female relatives, and the disease in fetuses at risk, but never to provide positive diagnoses.

In order to overcome the above limitations and approach 100% success in carrier and prenatal diagnosis, the direct detection of gene defects was advocated (Giannelli, 1987). This was achieved in 1989, as rapid methods of mutation detection were developed (Bottema et al, 1989; Green et al, 1989; Montandon et al, 1989). Nevertheless, in order to switch completely and definitively from indirect to direct diagnostic procedures, it was necessary to develop a strategy to maximize the benefits that may derive from the direct approach. In 1989, therefore, Giannelli proposed the creation of a UK resource that would enable any individual at risk to obtain carrier or prenatal tests in only a few days, simply by offering a sample of cells and information on their family. This resource would consist of pedigree, haematological and mutation data to be obtained by examining an index person in each affected family.

The considerations that led to this strategy, now being implemented with the collaboration of the UK haemophilia centres, are the following.

Once the mutation in an index person has been characterized, carrier and prenatal diagnoses on any of his blood relatives for generation after generation can be based solely on the analysis of the region of the gene that is abnormal in the index patient, thus allowing rapid, economic and yet definite and accurate diagnostic tests. The preliminary study of mutations in the index individuals not only rapidly advances the understanding of the disease but also ensures a

---

Figure 2.6 Indirect and direct carrier diagnosis in haemophilia B. (A) The pedigree shows how an RFLP marker (*a*, *b*) can be used to determine that III:4 is a carrier of haemophilia B. II:2 is obviously an obligate carrier and her factor IX gene with the *a* marker is the mutant allele because this is present in the affected males II:3 and IV:2. III:4 has obviously inherited the mutant gene from the mother. By contrast III:3 appears to have inherited the normal maternal allele and therefore should not be a carrier. This conclusion, however, is conditional to positive paternity tests. Please note that the same marker cannot help in testing the carrier state of IV:1 and IV:3 because their mother (III:2) is homozygous for the marker. (B) Direct diagnosis. Arrows in a sequencing gel point to C→T transition in patient II_1 (see pedigree on right). This mutation is demonstrated by the lack of a band in section C, track II_1 accompanied by an abnormal band in the same position of section T, track II_1. In section T, tracks I_2 and I_3 show an abnormal band while II_2 has a pattern identical to the normal control (track N). This indicates that I_2 and I_3 are carriers and II_2 is not. I_2 and I_3 have a normal band in section C (arrow), since they have one normal factor IX gene. Please note that carrier diagnoses are not dependent on pedigree structure and can be achieved in the families of isolated patients such as that shown here.

sound theoretical basis for the provision of diagnostic services, because it thoroughly tests the technical procedures, it yields data to help assess the functional consequences of any sequence change, and it shows correlations between mutations and phenotypes that may offer valuable prognostic information. Finally, this work should lead to such interaction between clinicians and molecular geneticists as to ensure optimal transfer of information and clinicians' access to state-of-the-art technology. After a pilot study on a sample of the Swedish population, the strategy was applied to the UK population (Green et al, 1991b; Giannelli et al, 1992), where it appears to fulfil all its promise (Saad et al, 1994). National registers of haemophilia B mutations are also being constructed in Sweden (Ljung, personal communication) and New Zealand (van der Water et al, 1992).

At present it is therefore possible to offer exact carrier and prenatal diagnoses to almost all families with haemophilia B. The last remaining problem is our ignorance of the incidence of gonadal mosaicism for the haemophilia B mutations. Gonadal mosaicism affects the recurrence risk of the sporadic patients' mothers who test, on somatic cells, as homozygous normal. Since it may be expected that at least a proportion of gonadal mosaics may also show mosaicism in their soma, it is useful to employ carrier detection methods that can detect the mutant gene even when this represents a minor proportion of the factor IX alleles. The mismatch detection method we use (Montandon et al, 1989) seems able to detect mutant alleles representing only 5–10% of the total (Montandon and Green, unpublished observations). However, in order to provide more precise counselling, estimates of the incidence of ovarian mosaicism must be obtained. This requires systematic family studies in large populations, since ovarian mosaicism is revealed every time two children inherit a defective factor IX gene from a mother with homozygous normal somatic cells.

Haemophilia A

Delay in the development of rapid procedures for the detection of haemophilia A mutations has so far caused carrier tests and prenatal diagnoses to rely essentially on the indirect method. The first factor VIII intragenic polymorphisms were detected in 1985, but these and other markers detected up to 1991 were only moderately informative, since only 70% of carrier females could be expected to be heterozygous for at least one marker (Tuddenham, 1989; Lalloz et al, 1991). In order to increase the proportion of successful diagnostic tests, therefore, two extragenic markers were used: DXS15 and DXS52. These showed significant recombination with the factor VIII gene, and therefore did not allow definite diagnoses. The value of the results obtained with these markers was very much dependent on the distance of the blood relationship between the proband and the affected relative used to determine which markers were associated with the detrimental mutation segregating in the family. Nevertheless, by applying correct mathematical procedures, the results obtained with these markers could be used to offer reasonable estimates of the proband's probability of being a carrier, or of having conceived an affected boy. In 1991, an intragenic polymorphism resulting from variable numbers of tandem repeats (VNTRs) was discovered in intron 13 (Lalloz et al, 1991). This greatly increased the informativeness of the intragenic markers and overcame the need to use DXS15 and DXS52. However, the indirect polymorphism-based approach in haemophilia A has the same shortcomings mentioned for haemophilia B (see page 69–71), and it will in future be phased out in favour of diagnoses based on the direct detection of the gene defect. These became feasible in 1991, because of the development by Naylor et al (1991) of a rapid method for the characterization of haemophilia A mutations (see page 58). However, the non-conventional mutations causing 45% of severe haemophilia (Naylor et al, 1992, 1993a) represented a problem because the carriers of these mutations could not be identified by mRNA analysis. Ironically, these mutations have now become the easiest to detect, because a Southern blot of DNA cut with BclI and hybridized to a probe from intron 22 of the factor VIII gene (gene F8A) usually detects three bands, of which two are abnormal in the patients (Lakich et al, 1993). These abnormal bands are also present in carriers where they coexist with a full set of normal segments. We can therefore expect that henceforward progress in the genetic counselling of haemophilia A will be fast, and will eventually follow the model of haemophilia B.

Genetics of von Willebrand's Disease

In 1926 von Willebrand described a severe bleeding disorder in a family from Föglö, an island between Finland and Sweden. The condition appeared distinct from haemophilia on both clinical and genetic grounds, as inheritance was clearly autosomal. Indeed, von Willebrand suggested an autosomal dominant inheritance, although marked differences in the severity of the disease could be seen between the parents and some of their affected offspring in the first family he reported.

Subsequent research has shown that von Willebrand's disease is very heterogeneous, both with regard to clinical and biochemical features (Holmberg and Nilsson, 1972) and to familial transmission. Thus pedigrees are found with a clear recessive pattern of inheritance, while others display a dominant pattern, often with variation in both penetrance (the probability that a person carrying the defective gene will manifest the disease) and expressivity (the severity of the phenotypic effect of the defective gene).

Much uncertainly also exists about the incidence of the disease, as inherited abnormalities of von Willebrand factor are observed in 1 in 125 individuals (Rodighiero et al, 1987), while clinically significant von Willebrand's disease affects 1 in 8000 people (Holmberg and Nilsson, 1985) and only 1 in 700 000 has the severe autosomal recessive form.

In order to construct a logical framework to understand the genetics of von Willebrand's disease, it is necessary to consider at least some of the features of von Willebrand factor. As detailed in the previous chapter, von Willebrand factor is synthesized in the vascular endothelial cells and megakaryocytes as a primary polypeptide of 2813 amino acids which undergoes complex changes. Of particular importance is the interaction of the pro-vWF subunits to form dimers and then multimers that are processed into mature species with different numbers of subunits. The normal biological function of von Willebrand factor is due to the longer multimers and it involves the interaction with many other factors such as the platelet GPIb–IX complex of nonactivated platelets, the GPIIb–IIIa complex of activated platelets, macromolecules of the subendothelial matrix, and factor VIII (Ruggeri and Ware, 1992). The phenotypic effects of a mutation causing von Willebrand's disease therefore depends both on the interactions of von Willebrand factor subunits with each other and the interaction of von Willebrand factor multimers with other molecules. It is therefore logical to assume that a mutation that results essentially in a reduction or ablation of subunit production from the defective gene may have phenotypic effects different from those of mutations causing the production of abnormal subunits. In fact a person with one completely silent and one normal allele will produce half the normal amount of von Willebrand factor but this factor will have a perfectly normal structure. This situation, not surprisingly, appears to be associated with a normal phenotype (Ngo et al, 1988) and therefore mutations of this type may be expected to show recessive inheritance.

By contrast, a person heterozygous for a mutation causing the production of an abnormal subunit in normal amounts will produce at best only a trace of von Willebrand factor with a perfectly normal structure since the bulk of the multimers will be formed of a mixture of normal and abnormal subunits. If such von Willebrand factor is sufficiently dysfunctional, von Willebrand's disease will result, and this will show dominant inheritance. A great variety of functional consequences may result from the interactions of mutant and normal von Willebrand factor subunits, depending on the domain affected by the mutation and the amount of the mutant subunit available for interaction with the normal one. Furthermore, because several protein polymorphisms for von Willebrand factor are known, the range of phenotypic variation can be increased by additive, subtractive, synergistic and antagonistic interactions between all sequence variations affecting the von Willebrand factor subunits. This could, at least in part, account for variations in penetrance and expressivity.

The phenotypic consequences of von Willebrand factor mutations depend on the function they impair. Thus mutations that affect the binding of von Willebrand factor to factor VIII cause von Willebrand's disease that appears to be an autosomal recessive form of haemophilia A, because the dominant symptoms are caused by the low levels of factor VIII in plasma and only individuals with mutations that impair factor VIII binding in both of their von Willebrand factor genes have factor VIII deficits severe enough to cause disease. It is obvious that any variation in the factors that interact with von Willebrand factor may also modulate the ultimate phenotypic effect of von Willebrand factor gene mutations and thus account for variations in penetrance and expressivity.

Clear understanding of the genetics of von Willebrand's disease will eventually come from the detailed study of the structural features of von Willebrand factor (vWF) genes in individuals with different forms of the disease as well as families with different patterns of inheritance and variation in penetrance and expressivity. At present our understanding is too poor to present a coherent picture of the population genetics of the disease. On the basis of the prevalence of the different types of von Willebrand's disease or von Willebrand factor defects mentioned above, one may come to the following tentative conclusions. The mutations that cause severe autosomal recessive disease may have a population frequency of 0.0012 while those that cause dominant von Willebrand's disease seem 20-fold rarer, with a frequency of 0.000062; it is difficult to know what is the frequency of mutations causing laboratory evidence of von Willebrand factor defects without clinically obvious von Willebrand's Disease.

The von Willebrand factor Gene

The von Willebrand factor gene (Fig. 2.7) is located near the tip of the short arm of chromosome 12 (band 12p12-ter); it is 180 kb long and contains 52 exons (Mancuso et al, 1989). Its promoter contains a typical TATA box 30bp upstream of the transcription start but is not yet functionally well characterized. The exons vary in size from 40 (exon 50) to 1379bp (exon 28), while the introns vary fron 97 bp (intron 29) to 20 kb (intron 6). The first exon of the gene codes for the 250nt long non-coding 5′ leader of the mRNA and the second exon for most of the prepeptide. Exons 3–10 code for the D_1 and exons 11–17 for the D_2 domains of the propeptide. Exons 18, 19 and part of 20 code for the D1 segment at the amino end of the mature von Willebrand factor monomeric unit. The remainder of exon 20 plus exons 21–27 and part of 28 code for the D_3 domain. The large exon 28 also codes for the A_1 and A_2, as well as the start of the A_3, domains. The latter also spans exons 29–32. There follows a stretch of 74 amino acids encoded by exons 33 and 34. The following five exons (35–39) encode the D_4 domain while individual exons code for the short B_1 and B_2 regions. Exon 42 encodes the B_3 domain and the start of the C_1 domain that extends to comprise exons 43 and 44. The following four exons (45–48) encode the C_2 domain, while the remainder (exons 49–52) specify the last 151 amino acids of the protein and the short non-coding 3′ tail of the mRNA. The latter contains a stop codon and the AATAAA polyadenylation signal that is located 19 bp upstream of the poly A addition site.

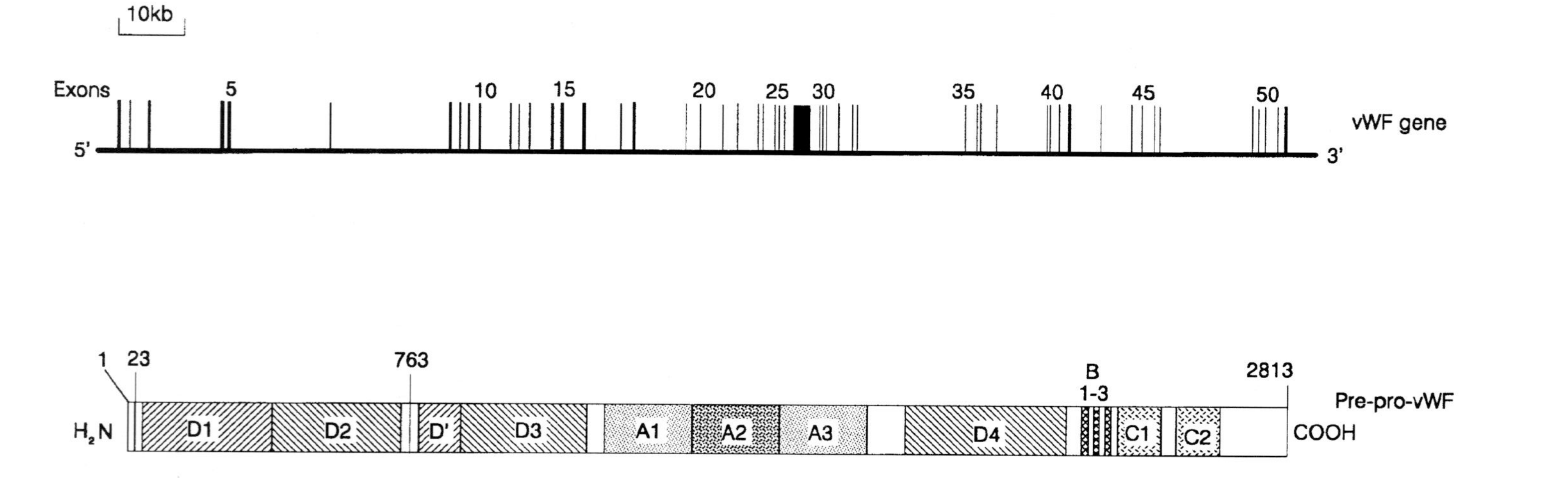

Figure 2.7 The von Willebrand factor (vWF) gene and von Willebrand factor (vWF) domains. The 52 exons of the gene are indicated by vertical lines. The domain organization of the protein shows the repeated domain structure and the amino acid positions delimiting the prepeptide, propeptide and mature monomer of vWF.

A copy of part of the von Willebrand factor gene containing exons 23–34 is found in chromosome 22 (band 22q11–q13). This non-functional entity or pseudogene has diverged from the active gene by only 3.1% and may therefore owe its existence to a recent event (<20–30 million years ago). The von Willebrand factor gene produces an mRNA of approximately 9 kb consisting of a long non-coding 5′ leader of 250nt, an open reading frame of 8439nt, a stop codon and a 3′ non-coding tail of 134nt (Ginsburg et al, 1985; Lynch et al, 1985; Sadler et al, 1985; Verveij et al, 1985).

Thirty-three polymorphisms have been reported in the von Willebrand factor gene (Sadler and Ginsburg, 1993) and 21 have been characterized at the sequence level. Sixteen of the polymorphisms are within exons and approximately half of these affect the amino acid sequence of von Willebrand factor. A very informative polymorphic system is due to a tetranucleotide repeat about 600 bp long in intron 40. Ninety-eight different alleles have been found at this site, which shows 98% heterozygosity.

Gene Defects in von Willebrand's disease

The first von Willebrand factor gene mutations to be characterized were gross deletions detected by Southern blotting (Shelton-Inloes et al, 1987), and later PCR amplification and sequencing was used to detect smaller changes such as single base substitutions (Ginsburg et al, 1989). Protein information in some forms of von Willebrand's disease and functional studies of von Willebrand factor have indicated potential mutation targets and directed efforts in mutation studies. Furthermore the size of the gene, the large number of exons, the abundance of polymorphisms and the presence in each individual of two alleles and attendant pseudogenes has discouraged attempts to screen all essential regions of the von Willebrand factor gene. Thus mutations analysis in von Willebrand's disease is following a course different from current haemophilia research. One exon of the von Willebrand factor gene, the large exon 28 that codes for important functional domains, has been a favourite target of mutation studies. As a consequence of this selective pattern of mutation analysis, most of the patients whose point mutations have been characterized belong to specific subtypes of von Willebrand's disease that show qualitative changes of von Willebrand factor (Ginsburg and Sadler, 1993). In this case the causative role of any observed mutation can be established by expressing in vitro genes with these mutations in order to test whether they produce von Willebrand factor with features corresponding to those of the patients' von Willebrand factor. Unfortunately, the above procedure could not easily establish the causative role of mutations that result in quantitative changes of von Willebrand factor because the conditions that determine the level of expression, stability and possibly secretion of von Willebrand factor may substantially differ between patients' and mammalian cells in culture.

So far, in no case has the whole essential sequence of the von Willebrand factor gene been examined, and therefore we are completely ignorant of the effects that different sequence changes in the same or different monomeric subunits of von Willebrand factor may have on its structure and function. Much work is therefore still needed to understand the role of mutations on the function of von Willebrand factor and the aetiology of von Willebrand's disease. Nevertheless some very interesting insights have been obtained. A brief summary of these findings is presented below.

Type I von Willebrand's disease

This is the most common form of von Willebrand's disease and shows autosomal dominant inheritance. It is accompanied by decreases in von Willebrand factor antigen, ristocetin co-factor activity and factor VIII activity, but normal von Willebrand factor multimer structure. These phenotypic features suggest mutations that cause quantitative defects of von Willebrand factor but none of the changes associated with this form of von Willebrand's disease has yet been identified (Ginsburg and Sadler, 1993).

Type III von Willebrand's disease

This autosomal recessive form of severe von Willebrand's disease shows gross quantitative deficits of von Willebrand factor and some of the causative mutations have been characterized. These include six nonsense mutations and five gene deletions that in four cases involve the whole gene (Zhang et al, 1992; Ginsburg and Sadler, 1993). A frameshift due to a single base deletion has been found to be common in Swedish patients. As these types of mutations are expected to be amorphic (i.e. to lead to no stable gene product), they fit the tentative explanation of the inheritance of von Willebrand's disease presented above.

Following treatment with preparations of von Willebrand factor, development of inhibitors has been observed in patients homozygous for gross deletions. This is analogous to the situation encountered in haemophilias A and B.

Type IIA von Willebrand's disease

This form of the disease shows autosomal dominant inheritance, decreased von Willebrand factor ristocetin co-factor activity and absence of large von Willebrand factor multimers in plasma accompanied by increase of a satellite band migrating below each multimer in electrophoretic studies. The characterization of a 176 kDa C-terminal proteolytic von Willebrand factor fragment increased in the plasma of patients with this form of the disease directed attention to the A_2 domain of von Willebrand factor and so far most of the mutations associated with this form of the disease have been found in a 134 amino acid segment (residues 742–875) encoded by part of exon 28. Two subtypes of the disease have been distinguished: one where secretion of the von Willebrand factor appears to be diminished and one where platelets, in contrast to plasma, show a normal pattern of multimers. In the latter form the loss of high molecular weight multimers from plasma has been tentatively attributed to a sensitivity to plasma proteases. The mutations characterized in the first group include Arg844→Asp, Gly742→Arg, Ser743→Leu, and those in the second group Arg834→Trp, Gly742→Glu (Ginsburg and Sadler, 1993). Recurrence of transitions affecting CpG sites has been observed in patients with von Willebrand's disease, in keeping with observations in other genes.

Type IIB von Willebrand's disease

This form of the disease shows autosomal dominant inheritance, loss of the largest von Willebrand factor multimers from plasma and marked increase of the von Willebrand factor affinity for platelet glycoprotein 1b (GP1b). This property is most marked in the largest multimers that spontaneously bind to platelets and are thus cleared from the circulation. Most of the mutations associated with this form of the disease cluster within a short segment of the A_1 domain (residues 540–578) also encoded by exon 28 (Ginsburg and Sadler, 1993). This segment is located within the putative GP1b binding region of von Willebrand factor. This group of gain of function mutations includes His505→Asp, Arg543→Trp, Arg545→Cys, Trp550→Cys, Val551→Leu, Val553→Met, Pro574→Leu and Arg578→Gln.

von Willebrand's Disease with decreased factor VIII affinity

This form of von Willebrand's disease results in an autosomal recessive form of haemophilia with markedly decreased factor VIII levels and a clinical picture of mild to moderate haemophilia. Five mutations in the amino end segment of von Willebrand factor have been found associated with this disease and have been shown to cause reduced affinity of von Willebrand factor for factor VIII. These mutations are Arg19→Trp, His54→Gln, Thr28→Met, Arg53→Trp and Arg91→Gln. It is interesting, however, that Arg89→Gln is a polymorphic change that does not affect factor VIII binding (Ginsburg and Sadler, 1993). This suggests rather specific conformational requirements for factor VIII binding.

Other mutations

These have been found in individual patients (Ginsburg and Sadler, 1993). A gross deletion (exons 26–34) that may not affect the reading frame of the mRNA has been found in a type II von Willebrand's disease possibly suggesting that the deleted protein monomer interfered with the multimer assembly. An amino acid substitution, Gly561→Ser, was found in a patient showing a contrast between ristocetin and botrocetin co-factor activity, the former being absent and the latter normal.

Mutations in loci other than von Willebrand factor

Such mutations may result in syndromes that mimic von Willebrand's disease and are therefore called pseudo-von Willebrand's disease. For example, mutations of the GP1b α chain have been found in platelet-type von Willebrand's disease (Miller et al, 1991).

Genetic Counselling in von Willebrand's Disease

In contast to the haemophilias, where genetic counselling is a very important component of clinical care, in von Willebrand's disease genetic counselling plays a minor role because most patients have a relatively mild disease that can be very adequately controlled. The most severely affected patients are those with type III von Willebrand's disease, which shows autosomal recessive inheritance. In this case the parents of one affected child have a 1 : 4 chance of a second affected offspring and prenatal diagnosis may be required. This may be based on analysis of the segregation of the von Willebrand factor polymorphic markers or on direct detection of the gene defects if these have been previously identified in the patient and his/her parents. As mentioned earlier, several DNA polymorphisms exist in the von Willebrand factor gene and can be used for indirect diagnosis by PCR-based procedures. However, in this case it is important to know that the disease is truly due to defects of the von Willebrand factor gene rather than to defects of genes for factors interacting with von Willebrand factor, as is the case in pseudo-vWD.

In the recessive forms of von Willebrand's disease, diagnostic tests for genetic counselling are usually necessary only for the sibship of the affected individual because other collateral or descendant relatives are at a very low risk of producing affected children unless they marry within their family. In the dominant forms of von Willebrand's disease, each affected has a 1 : 2 chance of producing an affected child. However, severity of the disease may vary from individual to individual within the same family.

Conclusions

Advances in molecular genetics have allowed much progress on the haemophilias. Inferences on the population genetics of the haemophilia made by Haldane before the discovery that two forms of haemophilia exist have been confirmed and the molecular genetics of both diseases has been clarified. Fully efficient DNA-based strategies for the genetic counselling of haemophilia B are now in place and steps have been taken toward the extension of such strategies to haemophilia A. The analysis of mutations in haemophilia A has revealed an unexpected chromosomal instability that results in gross inversions disrupting the factor VIII gene in one-fifth of all haemophilia A patients and almost half of those severely affected.

In von Willebrand's disease the analysis of mutations is supplementing the insight into the molecular biology of the disease and the function of von Willebrand factor that has been obtained by protein studies. Much, however, remains to be discovered about the mutations and the molecular genetics of von Willebrand's disease. Advances in this field are necessary to understand the population genetics of von Willebrand's disease. An interesting challenge for the future is the investigation of how different changes in the von Willebrand factor monomers may interact to modify the structure and function of von Willebrand factor.

References

Alexander B, Goldstein R, Landwehr G, Cook CD. Congenital SPCA deficiency. A new hitherto unrecognised defect with hemorrhage rectified by serum and serum fractions. *Journal of Clinical Investigation* 1951; **30:** 596.

Allaart CF, Briët E. Familial venous thrombophilia. In: Bloom AL, Forbes CD, Thomas DP, Tuddenham EGD (Eds), *Haemostasis and Thrombosis* 3rd edn. Edinburgh: Churchill Livingstone, 1994.

Anson DS, Choo KH, Rees DJG, et al. The gene structure of human anti-haemophilic factor IX. *EMBO Journal* 1984; **3:** 1053.

Anson DS, Blake DJ, Winship PR, Birnbaum D, Brownlee GG. Nullisomic deletion of the mcf2 transforming gene in two haemophilia B patients. *EMBO Journal* 1988; **7:** 2795.

Attree O, Vidaud D, Vidaud M, Amselem S, Lavergne JM, Goosens M. Mutations in the catalytic domain of human coagulation factor IX: rapid characterisation by direct genomic sequencing of DNA fragments displaying an altered melting behaviour. *Genomics* 1989; **4:** 266.

Baron M, Norman DG, Harvey TS, Handford, PA. The three-dimensional structure of the first EGF-like module of human factor IX: comparison with EGF and TGF-α. *Protein Science* 1992; **1:** 81.

Barrow ES, Miller CH, Reisner HM, Graham JB. Genetic counselling in haemophilia by discriminant analysis 1975–1980. *Journal of Medical Genetics* 1982; **19:** 26.

Bertina RM, Koeleman BPC, Koster T, et al. Poor anticoagulant response to activated protein C is associated with a single base pair transition in the gene for blood coagulation factor V. *Nature* 1994; **369:** 64–67.

Biggs R, Sharp AA, Margolis J, Hardisty RM, Stewart J, Davidson WM. Defects in the early stages of blood coagulation: a report of four cases. *British Journal of Haematology* 1958; **4:** 177.

Bottema CDK, Ketterling RP, Cho HI, Sommer SS. Hemophilia B in a male with a four-base insertion that arose in the germline of his mother. *Nucleic Acids Research* 1989; **17:** 10139.

Camerino G, Grzeschik KH, Jaye M, et al. Regional localisation on the human X chromosome and polymorphism of the coagulation factor IX gene (haemophilia B locus). *Proceedings of the National Academy of Sciences USA* 1984; **81:** 498.

Choo KH, Gould KG, Rees DJG, Brownlee GG. Molecular cloning of the gene for human anti-haemophilic factor IX. *Nature* 1982; **299:** 178.

Collins PW, Jenkins PV, Goldman E, Lee CA, Pasi KJ. Intron 22 inversions and haemophilia. *Lancet* 1994; **343:** 791.

Cotton RGH, Rodrigues NR, Campbell RD. Reactivity of cytosine and thymine in single-base-pair mismatches with hydroxylamine and osmium tetroxide and its application to the study of mutations. *Proceedings of the National Academy of Sciences USA* 1988; **85:** 4397.

Crossley M, Ludwig M, Stowell KM, De Vos P, Olek K, Brownlee GG. Recovery from haemophilia B Leyden: an androgen-responsive element in the factor IX promoter. *Science* 1992; **257:** 377.

Dombroski BA, Mathias SL, Nanthakumar E, Scott AF, Kazazian HH Jr. Isolation of an active human transposable element. *Science* 1991; **254:** 1805.

Duckert F, Jung E, Schmerling DH. Hitherto undescribed congenital haemorrhagic diathesis probably due to fibrin stabilising factor deficiency. *Thrombosis et Diathesis Haemorrhagica* 1960; **5:** 179.

Eaton D, Rodriguez H, Vehar GA. Proteolytic processing of factor VIII: correlation of specific cleavages by thrombin, factor Xa and activated protein C with activation and inactivation of factor VIII:C coagulant activity. *Biochemistry* 1986; **25:** 505.

Ekelund H, Lindeberg L, Wranne L. Combined deficiency of coagulation factors II, VII, IX and X: a case of probable congenital origin. *Pediatric Hematology and Oncology* 1986; **3:** 187.

Ferrari N, Rizza CR. Estimation of genetic risks of carriership for possible carriers of Christmas disease (haemophilia B). *Brazilian Journal of Genetics* 1986; **9:** 87.

Fisher RR, Giddings JC, Roisenberg I. Hereditary combined deficiency of clotting factors V and VIII with involvement of von Willebrand factor. *Clinical and Laboratory Haematolosy* 1988; **10:** 53.

Foster DC, Yoshitake S, Davie EW. The nucleotide sequences of the gene for human protein C. *Proceedings of the National Academy of Sciences USA* 1985; **82:** 4673.

Francis RB, Kasper CK Reproduction in haemophilia. *Journal of the American Medical Association* 1983; **250:** 3192.

Freije D, Schlessinger D. A 1.6 Mb contig of yeast artificial chromosomes around the human factor VIII gene reveals three regions homologous to probes for the DXS115 locus and two from the DXYS64 locus. *American Journal of Human Genetics* 1992; **51:** 66.

Giannelli F. The identification of haemophilia B mutations. In: Peeters H (Ed.), *Protides of the Biological Fluids. Proceedings of the 25th Colloquium*, Oxford: Pergamon Press, 1987.

Giannelli F. Factor IX. In: Tuddenham EGD (Ed.), *The Molecular Biology of Coagulation*. New York, London: Baillière Tindall, 1989.

Giannelli F, Brownlee GG. Cause of the "inhibitor" phenotype in the haemophilias. *Nature* 1986; **320:** 196.

Giannelli F, Choo KH, Rees DJG, Boyd Y, Rizza CR. Gene deletions in patients with haemophilia B and anti factor IX antibodies. *Nature* 1983; **303:** 181.

Giannelli F, Anson DS, Choo KH, et al. Characterisation and use of an intragenic polymorphic marker for detection of carriers of haemophilia B (factor IX deficiency). *Lancet* 1984; **i:** 239.

Giannelli F, Green PM, High KA, et al. Haemophilia B: database of point mutations and short additions and deletions – third edition. *Nucleic Acids Research* 1992; **20:** Suppl 2027.

Giannelli F, Green PM, High KA, et al. Haemophilia B: database of point mutations and short additions and deletions – fourth edition, 1993. *Nucleic Acids Research* 1993; **21:** 3075.

Ginsburg D, Sadler JE. Von Willebrand disease : a database of point mutations, insertions and deletions. *Thrombosis and Haemostasis* 1993; **69:** 177.
Ginsburg D, Handin RI, Bonthrow DT, et al. Human von Willebrand factor (vWF): isolation of complementary DNA (cDNA) clones and chromosome localisation. *Science* 1985; **228:** 1401.
Ginsburg D, Konkle BA, Gill JC, et al. Molecular basis of human von Willebrand disease: analysis of platelet von Willebrand factor mRNA. *Proceedings of the National Academy of Sciences USA* 1989; **86:** 3723.
Gitschier J. Maternal duplication associated with gene deletion in sporadic haemophilia. *American Journal of Human Genetics* 1988; **43:** 274.
Gitschier J, Wood WI, Goralka TM, et al. Characterization of the human factor VIII gene. *Nature* 1984; **312:** 326.
Gitschier J, Wood WI, Tuddenham EGD, et al. Detection and sequence of mutations in the factor VIII gene of haemophiliacs. *Nature* 1985; **315:** 427.
Goodeve AC, Preston FE, Peake IR. Factor VIII gene rearrangements in patients with severe haemophilia A. *Lancet* 1994; **343:** 329.
Green PM, Bentley DR, Mibashan RS, Nilsson IM, Giannelli F. Molecular pathology of haemophilia B. *EMBO Journal* 1989; **8:** 1067.
Green PM, Montandon AJ, Bentley DR, Giannelli F. Genetics and molecular biology of haemophilia A and B. *Blood Coagulation and Fibrinolysis* 1991a; **2:** 539.
Green PM, Montandon AJ, Ljung R, et al. Haemophilia B mutations in a complete Swedish population sample. A test of new strategy for the genetic counselling of diseases with high mutational heterogeneity. *British Journal of Haematology* 1991b; **78:** 390.
Green PM, Mitchell VE, McGraw A, Goldman E, Giannelli F. Haemophilia B caused by a missense mutation in the prepetide sequence of factor IX. *Human Mutations* 1993; **2:** 103.
Haldane JBS. The rate of spontaneous mutation of a human gene. *Journal of Genetics* 1935; **31:** 317.
Haldane JBS. The mutation of the gene for haemophilia and its segregation ratios in males and females. *Annals of Eugenics* 1947; **13:** 262.
Handford PA, Mayhew M, Baron M, Winship PR, Campbell ID, Brownlee GG. Key residues involved in calcium-binding motifs in EGF-like domains. *Nature* 1991; **351:** 164.
Hathaway WE, Belhasen LP, Hathaway HS. Evidence for a new plasma thromboplastin factor. I. Case report, coagulation studies and physicochemical properties. *Blood* 1965; **26:** 521.
Higuchi M, Antonarakis SE, Kasch L, et al. Towards complete characterization of mild-to-moderate hemophilia A: detection of the molecular defect in 25 of 29 patients by denaturing gradient gel electrophoresis. *Proceedings of the National Academy of Sciences USA* 1991a; **88:** 8307.
Higuchi M, Kazazian HH, Kasch L, et al. Molecular characterization of some hemophilia A suggests that about half the mutations are not within the coding regions and splice junctions of the factor VIII gene. *Proceedings of the National Academy of Sciences USA* 1991b; **88:** 7405.
Holmberg L, Nilsson IM. Genetic variants of von Willebrand's disease. *British Medical Journal* 1972; **3:** 317.
Holmberg L, Nilsson IM. von Willebrand's disease. *Clinical Haematology* 1985; **14:** 461.
Jenny RJ, Pittman DD, Toole JJ, et al. Complete cDNA and derived amino acid sequence of human factor V. *Proceedings of the National Academy of Sciences USA* 1987; **84:** 4846.
Kazazian HH, Wong C, Youssoufian H, et al. Haemophilia A resulting from de novo insertion of L1 sequences represents a novel mechanism for mutation in man. *Nature* 1988; **332:** 164.
Ketterling RP, Bottema CDK, Phillips JA, Sommer SS. Evidence that descendants of three founders constitute about 25% of hemophilia B in the United States. *Genomics* 1991; **10:** 1093.
Ketterling RP, Ricke DO, Wurster MW, Sommer SS. Deletions with inversions: report of a mutation and review of the literature. *Human Mutations* 1993; **2:** 53.
Kling S, Coffey AJ, Ljung R, et al. Moderate haemophilia B in a female carrier caused by preferential inactivation of the paternal X chromosome. *European Journal of Haematology* 1991; **47:** 257.

Kurachi K, Davie EW. Isolation and characterisation of a cDNA coding for human factor IX. *Proceedings of the National Academy of Sciences USA* 1982; **79:** 6461.
Lakich D, Kazazian HH, Antonarakis SE, Gitschier J. Inversions disrupting the factor VIII gene as a common cause of severe hemophilia A. *Nature and Genetics* 1993; **5:** 236.
Lalloz MR, McVey JH, Pattinson JK, Tuddenham EGD. Haemophilia A diagnosis by analysis of a hypervariable dinucleotide repeat within the factor VIII gene. *Lancet* 1991; **338:** 207.
Levinson B, Kenwrick S, Lakish D, Hammonds G Jr, Gitschier J. A transcribed gene in an intron of the human factor VIII gene. *Genomics* 1990; **7:** 1.
Levinson B, Kenwrick S, Gamel P, Fisher K, Gitschier J. Evidence for a third transcript from the human factor VIII gene. *Genomics* 1992; **14:** 585.
Leytus SP, Foster DC, Kurachi K, Davie EW. Gene for human factor X: a blood coagulation factor whose gene organisation is essentially identical with that of factor IX and protein C. *Biochemistry* 1986; **25:** 5098.
Ljung RCR. Intron 22 inversions and haemophilia. *Lancet* 1994; **343:** 791.
Lynch DC, Zimmerman TS, Collins CJ, et al. Molecular cloning of cDNA for human von Willebrand factor. Authentication by a new method. *Cell* 1985; **41:** 49.
Mancuso DJ, Tuley EA, Westfield LA, et al. Structure of the gene for human von Willebrand factor. *Journal of Biological Chemistry* 1989; **264:** 19514.
Ménaché D. Constitutional and familial abnormal fibrinogen. *Thrombosis et Diathesis Haemorrhagica* 1964; **13:** 173.
Mibashan RS, Giannelli F, Pembrey ME, Rodeck CH. The antenatal diagnosis of clotting disorders. In: Brown MJ (Ed.), *Advanced Medicine 21*, Edinburgh: Churchill Livingstone, 1986.
Miller JL, Cunningham D, Lyle VA, Finch CN. Mutation in the gene encoding the α chain of platelet glycoprotein 1b in platelet-type von Willebrand's disease. *Proceedings of the National Academy of Sciences USA* 1991; **88:** 4761.
Montandon AJ, Green PM, Giannelli F, Bentley DR. Direct detection of point mutations by mismatch analysis: application to haemophilia B. *Nucleic Acids Research* 1989; **17:** 3347.
Montandon AJ, Green PM, Bentley DR, et al. Direct estimate of the haemophilia B (factor IX deficiency) mutation rate and of the ratio of the sex-specific mutation rates in Sweden. *Human Genetics* 1992; **89:** 319.
Morgan TH. Sex-linked inheritance in *Drosophilia. Science* 1910; **32:** 120.
Murru S, Casula L, Pecorara M, Mori P, Cao A, Pirastu M. Illegitimate recombination produced by a duplication within the factor VIII gene in a patient with mild haemophilia A. *Genomics* 1990; **7:** 115.
Myers RM, Fisher SG, Lerman LS, Maniatis T. Nearly all single base substitutions in DNA fragments joined to a GC-clamp can be detected by denaturing gradient gel electrophoresis. *Nucleic Acids Research* 1985; **13:** 3131.
Naylor JA, Green PM, Montandon AJ, Rizza CR, Giannelli F. Detection of three novel mutations in two haemophilia A patients by rapidly screening whole essential regions of the factor VIII gene. *Lancet* 1991; **337:** 635.
Naylor JA, Green PM, Rizza CR, Giannelli F. Factor VIII gene explains all cases of haemophilia A. *Lancet* 1992; **340:** 1066.
Naylor JA, Green PM, Rizza CR, Giannelli F. Analysis of factor VIII mRNA reveals defects in every one of 28 haemophilia A patients. *Human Molecular Genetics* 1993a; **2:** 11.
Naylor J, Brinke A, Hassock S, Green PM, Giannelli F. Characteristic mRNA abnormality found in half the patients with severe haemophilia A is due to large DNA inversions. *Human Molecular Genetics* 1993b; **2:** 1773.
Ngo KY, Glotz T, Koziol JA, et al. Homozygous and heterozygous deletions of the von Willebrand factor gene in patients and carriers of severe von Willebrand's disease. *Proceedings of the National Academy of Sciences USA* 1988; **85:** 2753.
Noyes CM, Griffith MJ, Roberts HR, Lundblad RL. Identification of the molecular defect in factor IX Chapel Hill: substitution of histidine for arginine at position 145. *Proceedings of the National Academy of Sciences USA* 1983; **80:** 4200.
O'Hara PJ, Grant FJ, Haldman BA, et al. Nucleotide sequence of the gene coding for human factor VII, a vitamin K-dependent protein participating in blood coagulation. *Proceedings of the National Academy of Sciences USA* 1987; **84:** 5158.

Orita M, Suzuki Y, Sekiya T, Hayashi K. Rapid and sensitive detection of point mutations and DNA polymorphisms using the polymerase chain reaction. *Genomics* 1989; **5:** 874.
Otto JC. An account of an haemorrhagic disposition existing in certain families. *Medical Repository* 1803; **6:** 1.
Owren PA. The coagulation of blood. Investigations on a new clotting factor. *Acta Medical Scandinavica* 1947; Suppl 194.
Pattinson JK, Millar JH, McVey JH, et al. The molecular genetic analysis of hemophilia A: a directed search strategy for the detection of point mutations in the human factor VIII gene. *Blood* 1990; **76:** 2242.
Picketts DJ, D'Souza C, Bridge PJ, Lillicrap D. An A to T transversion at position –5 of the factor IX promoter results in hemophilia B. *Genomics* 1992; **12:** 161.
Pittman DD, Kaufman RJ. Proteolytic requirements for thrombin activation of anti-hemophilic factor (factor VIII). *Proceedings of the National Academy of Sciences USA* 1988; **85:** 2429.
Pittman DD, Kaufman RJ. Structure–function relationships of factor VIII elucidated through recombinant DNA technology. *Thrombosis and Haemostasis* 1989; **61:** 161.
Rabe F, Salomon E. Ueber Faserstoffmangel im Blute bei einem Falle von Haemophilie. *Deutsches Archiv fur Klinische Medizin* 1920; **132:** 240.
Rao KJ, Lyman G, Hamsabhushanam K, Scott JP, Jagadeeswaran P. Human factor IX (Lincoln Park): a molecular characterization. *Molecular and Cellular Probes* 1990; **4:** 335.
Ratnoff OD, Colopy JH. A familial hemorrhagic trait associated with a deficiency of clot promoting fraction of plasma. *Journal of Clinical Investigations* 1955; **34:** 601.
Reijnen MJ, Peerlinck K, Maasdam D, Bertina RM, Reitsma PH. Hemophilia B Leyden: substitution of thymine for guanine at position –21 results in a disruption of a hepatocyte nuclear factor 4 binding site in the factor IX promoter. *Blood* 1993; **82:** 151.
Rizza CR. Haemophilia and related inherited coagulation defects. In: Bloom AL, Forbes CD, Thomas DP, Tuddenham EGD (Eds), *Haemostasis and Thrombosis*, 3rd Edn. Edinburgh: Churchill Livingstone, 1994.
Rodighiero F, Castaman G, Dini E. Epidemiological investigation of the prevalence of von Willebrand's disease. *Blood* 1987; **69:** 454.
Ruggeri ZM, Ware J. The structure and function of von Willebrand factor. *Thrombosis and Haemostasis* 1992; **67:** 594.
Saad S, Rowley G, Tagliavacca L, Green PM, Giannelli F. UK Haemophilia Centres. First report on UK database of haemophilia B mutations and pedigrees. *Thrombosis and Haemostasis* 1994; **71:** 563–5.
Sadler JE, Ginsburg D. A database of polymorphisms in the von Willebrand factor gene and pseudogene. *Thrombosis and Haemostasis* 1993; **69:** 185.
Sadler JE, Shelton-Inloes BB, Sorace JM, Harlan JM, Titani K, Davie EW. Cloning and characterization of two cDNAs coding for human von Willebrand factor. *Proceedings of the National Academy of Sciences USA* 1985; **82:** 6394.
Shapiro SS, Martinez J, Holburn RR. Congenital dysprothrombinemia: an inherited structural disorder of human prothrombin. *Journal of Clinical Investigation* 1969; **48:** 2251.
Sheffield VC, Beck JS, Kwitek AE, Sandstrom DW, Stone EM. The sensitivity of single-strand conformation polymorphism analysis for the detection of single base substitutions. *Genomics* 1993; **16:** 325.
Shelton-Inloes BB, Chebab FF, Mannucci PM, Federici AB, Sadler JE. Gene deletions correlate with the development of alloantibodies in von Willebrand's disease. *Journal of Clinical Investigation* 1987; **79:** 1459.
Soriano-Garcia M, Padmanabhan K, de Vos AM, Tulinsky A. The Ca^{++} ion and membrane binding structure of the gla domain of Ca-prothrombin fragment I. *Biochemistry* 1992; **31:** 2554.
Stevanović M, Lovell-Badge R, Collignon J, Goodfellow P. *SOX3* is an X-linked gene related to *SRY*. *Human Molecular Genetics* 1993; **2:** 2013.
Telfer TP, Denson KW, Wright DR. A "new" coagulation defect. *British Journal of Haematology* 1956; **2:** 308.
Titani K, Fujikawa K. The structural aspects of vitamin K-dependant blood coagulation factors. *Acta Haematologica Japonica* 1982; **45:** 807.

Toole JJ, Knopf JL, Wozney JM, et al. Molecular cloning of a cDNA encoding human antihaemophilic factor. *Nature* 1984; **312:** 342.
Tuddenham EGD. Factor VIII and haemophilia A. In: Tuddenham EGD (Ed.), *The Molecular Biology of Coagulation, Baillière's Clinical Haematology, Volume 2*. London: Baillière Tindall, 1989.
Tuddenham EGD, Giannelli F. Molecular genetics of haemophilia A and B. In: Bloom AL, Forbes CD, Thomas DP, Tuddenham EGD (Eds), *Haemostasis and Thrombosis, 3rd edn*. Edinburgh: Churchill Livingstone, 1994.
Tuddenham EGD, Cooper DN, Gitschier J, et al. Haemophilia A: database of nucleotide substitutions, deletions and rearrangements of the factor VIII gene. *Nucleic Acids Research* 1994; **22:** 4851–4868.
van de Water NS, Berry EW, Ockelford PA, Browett PJ. Molecular analysis of the factor IX gene in haemophilia B. In: *ISH 24th Congress Abstracts*. Oxford: Blackwell Scientific Publications, 1992.
Verveij CL, DeVries CJM, Distel B, et al. Construction of cDNA coding for human von Willebrand factor using antibody probes for colony-screening and mapping of the chromosomal gene. *Nucleic Acids Research* 1985; **13:** 4699.
Vidaud M, Chabret C, Gazengel C, Grunebaum L, Cazenave JP, Goossens M. A de novo intragenic deletion of the potential EGF domain of the factor IX gene in a family with severe haemophilia B. *Blood* 1986; **68:** 961.
Vidaud M, Vidaud D, Siguret V, Lavergne JM, Goossens M. Mutational insertion on an Alu sequence causes haemophilia B. *American Journal of Human Genetics* 1989; **45:** A226.
Vielhaber E, Jacobson DP, Ketterling RP, Liu JZ, Sommer SS. A mutation in the 3′ untranslated region of the factor IX gene in four families with hemophilia B. *Human Molecular Genetics* 1993; **2:** 1309.
von Willebrand EA. Hereditär pseudohemofili. *Finska Läkaresällskapets Handungar* 1926; **67:** 7.
Waldmann R, Abraham JP. Fitzgerald factor: a heretofore unrecognised coagulation factor. *Blood* 1974; **44:** 934.
Wood WI, Capon DJ, Simonsen CC, et al. Expression of active human factor VIII from recombinant DNA clones. *Nature* 1984; **312:** 330.
Yoshitake S, Schach BG, Foster DC, Davie EW, Kurachi K. Nucleotide sequence of the gene for human factor IX (antihemophilic factor B). *Biochemistry* 1985; **24:** 3736.
Youssoufian H, Antonarakis SE, Aronis S, Tsiftis G, Phillips DG, Kazazian HH Jr. Characterization of five partial deletions of the factor VIII gene. *Proceedings of the National Academy of Sciences USA* 1987; **84:** 3772.
Zhang ZP, Falk G, Blombäck M, Euberg N, Anvret M. A single cytosine deletion in exon 18 of the von Willebrand factor gene is the most common mutation in Swedish vWD type III patients. *Human Molecular Genetics* 1992; **1:** 767.

Clinical Features and Diagnosis of Haemophilia, Christmas Disease and von Willebrand's Disease

3

CHARLES R. RIZZA

Haemophilia A is the most common of the severe, inherited bleeding disorders. It affects males and is transmitted by women who are apparently normal. The condition is present from birth, is lifelong and is characterized by recurrent and persistent episodes of bleeding involving mainly the deep tissues of muscles and joints. In many instances the patient cannot recall any injury as a cause of bleeding. Superficial cuts and scratches, unless they are deep, usually stop bleeding in the normal time. Bleeding is due to the absence of factor VIII which is essential for normal haemostasis and for blood to clot normally. Haemophilia B, or Christmas disease, which has similar clinical features and the same mode of inheritance, is caused by a deficiency of factor IX, one of the vitamin K-dependent clotting factors manufactured in the liver.

History of Haemophilia

The earliest references to what may have been haemophilia are to be found in Jewish writings of the 2nd century AD. In the Tractat Jebamoth the experiences of four sisters who lived in Zipporah are described. The first had her child circumcised and he died; likewise the sons of the second and third sisters died following circumcision. The fourth sister went to Rabbi Ben Gamaliel who ordered that her child was not to be circumcised. Although bleeding is not specifically mentioned (the term "looseness of the blood" is used), this would seem the most likely complication of the procedure. Similar rulings were made if two sons of a boy's maternal aunt had died following circumcision. Maimonides in the 12th century also ordered that a boy was not to be circumcised if his two brothers by the same mother but different father had died after the operation. In the 10th century the Moorish surgeon Khalaf ibn Abbas (known also as Albucasis or Alsaharavius) described how men in certain villages bled to death from minor wounds. Similarly, the boys sometimes bled to death if their gums were rubbed too vigorously. Presumably this was done to encourage eruption of the teeth. During the following centuries there were numerous reports of severe bleeding affecting men. It is difficult to know how many of these were cases of haemophilia.

In 1803 Dr John C. Otto, a physician working in Philadelphia published "An account of an haemorrhagic disposition existing in certain families" in which he described the bleeding symptoms in the male relatives of a woman named Smith who had settled near Plymouth, New Hampshire around about 1725. Otto noted that "males only are affected and all are not liable to it. Though females are free they are capable of transmitting it to their children". Those who suffered from the condition were known as "bleeders". Although it seems possible that Otto had no first-hand experience of the condition and was describing what had been reported to him by other doctors and "gentleman of character", his account was instrumental in raising general interest in the condition. Several individual cases were reported from America and Europe during the next few years but it is not certain how many of those were truly cases of haemophilia. In 1820 Nasse, who was Professor of Medicine in Bonn, published two papers in which most of the known cases were reviewed. From his observations he was able to say that only males suffered from the disease and that the disease was transmitted by apparently normal females. This mode of inheritance came to be known as Nasse's law although it has been described clearly by several authors before Nasse. During the remainder of the 19th century haemophilia continued to attract a good deal of attention. This was no doubt due in part to the appearance of haemophilia in the family of Queen Victoria and its transmission to several European royal families. Grandidier spent a large part of his life collecting information on haemophilia and published in 1855 a vast amount of data, much of it collected rather uncritically from abstracts in journals and year books. In 1872 Wickham Legg published his scholarly and authoritative *Treatise on Haemophilia* and this was followed in 1879 by Immerman's very full and careful handling of the subject.

In 1911 Bulloch and Fildes published their classical monograph on haemophilia. In this massive work they reviewed all the previous literature dealing with haemorrhagic disorders and presented clinical accounts and pedigrees of cases which they thought represented haemophilia. Their work is a landmark in the study of haemophilia notwithstanding the fact that their definition of haemophilia has had to be modified over the years as new knowledge became available; for example, Bulloch and Fildes were not willing to accept the diagnosis in a family in which there was transmission by the male line even if this was grandfather to grandson. They were also suspicious of the diagnosis in the absence of a previous family history. It is now known that a haemophiliac can transmit the condition to his grandsons through his daughters who are all obligatory carriers. Moreover, it is now known that approximately 30–40% of haemophiliacs have no previous family history. That Bulloch and Fildes could not be convinced of grandfather to grandson transmission probably in part reflects the high mortality in young haemophiliacs before they could reproduce.

Liston (1839) was probably the first to recognize that slow clotting of the blood was the cause of the clinical symptoms of haemophilia when he noted that there seemed to be a "want of coagulability". This became generally recognized when Wright (1893) introduced his method for measuring the blood clotting time. Weil (1906) was one of the first to show that the addition of normal blood to haemophilic blood in vitro or in vivo shortened the clotting of the latter. Subsequently, Addis (1911) in a series of careful experiments showed that the addition of as little as 20% of normal plasma to haemophilic plasma shortened the clotting time. Moreover he showed that a crude globulin fraction prepared from normal plasma by acid precipitation was effective at a concentration of 1 part in 200 in correcting the haemophilic defect. Addis believed that his globulin fraction, from which he had removed the fibrinogen, consisted only of prothrombin and concluded that haemophilia was due to a prothrombin defect. This interpretation was soon shown to be incorrect and 25 years were to pass before Patek and Stetson (1936) and Patek and Taylor (1937) repeated Addis' experiments and demonstrated that normal plasma contained a globulin substance that corrected the haemophilic clotting defect. This came to be known as antihaemophilic globulin or antihaemophilic factor and later was assigned the name factor VIII by the International Committee on Blood Clotting Factors (Wright 1962).

With advances in knowledge of blood clotting and with improvement in laboratory techniques, it became apparent in the 1940s that haemophilia was not a homogeneous disorder. Several workers found that occasionally blood from a known case of haemophilia would correct the clotting defect in another case also thought to be haemophiliac (Castex et al, 1944; Pavlovsky, 1947). These observations suggested not only that the two samples of blood which corrected each other were deficient in different factors but also that a deficiency of two quite different clotting factors could produce the same clinical features. This was found to be the case when Aggeler et al (1952) reported a patient who was supposed to have haemophilia but was found to have a deficiency of a serum factor. Unlike antihaemophilic factor, this factor was present in normal serum and could be adsorbed by adsorbents such as barium sulphate.

Later in the same year Biggs and her colleagues (1952) described seven cases with clinical features of haemophilia, four of whom also showed sex-linked inheritance. These patients lacked a serum factor required for normal thromboplastin generation. Aggeler and associates called the missing factor plasma thromboplastin component (PTC) whereas Biggs and her colleagues called it Christmas factor after the surname of one of the patients studied by them. This factor is now known as factor IX and the deficiency state is known as haemophilia B or Christmas disease.

Prevalence

Haemophilia, at one time thought to be a disease of Anglo-Saxon races, has been described in most other races. The condition has also been described and studied in several animal species such as the dog, cat and horse. Studies carried out in large dog colonies have provided reliable information on inheritance as well as on the pathology of the joint changes. The prevalence in humans is difficult to assess accurately because of lack of information but where such data are available, they show a prevalence of 80–110 per million. In the UK there are approximately 5500 patients with all grades of haemophilia A, giving a prevalence of 90 per million of population. There may be many mildly affected individuals who have escaped major injury or surgery and so have escaped diagnosis. This is particularly likely if there is no previous history of bleeding in other family members. If only severely affected individuals are considered, the prevalence is approximately 40 per million of population. This is equivalent to 80 severely affected patients per million males. The prevalence of haemophilia B in the UK is approximately one-fifth of that of haemophilia A. Since 1969, when data began to be collected annually, there has been a steady increase in the number of registered haemophiliacs in the UK, in spite of the increased death rate in haemophiliacs brought about by AIDS.

Inheritance

Haemophilia and Christmas disease are both inherited as sex-linked disorders. The mode of inheritance is illustrated in Fig. 3.1. It should be noted that all daughters of affected males are obligatory carriers whereas all sons are normal. The children of a carrier woman have an equal chance of being normal or affected if males, normal or carriers if females. The marriage of an affected male with a carrier female has on rare occasions taken place and has resulted in affected (homozygous) females with all symptoms of haemophilia including haemarthroses and bleeding into muscles. The family described by Treves in 1886 and studied again in later years by Handley and Nussbrecher (1935), Merskey (1951) and Kernoff and Rizza (1973) contains an example of such a marriage.

Approximately 40% of haemophiliacs have no family history (Kerr, 1965). This may reflect a recent mutation in the gene controlling factor VIII production or the fact that so few males have been born in previous generations that the condition has not shown itself clinically but has been passing silently down through female members.

In families with a history of haemophilia it is usually found that the severity of the disease is the same in the different affected members. If a member of a mildly affected family is found to be clinically severely affected, tests should be done to see if he has developed antibodies to factor VIII.

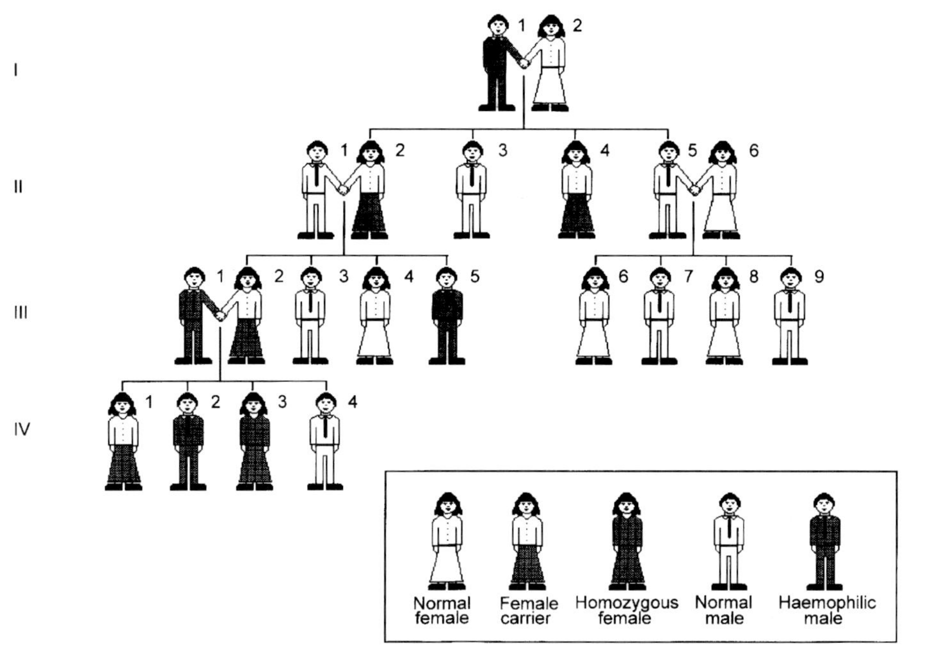

Figure 3.1 Mode of transmission of haemophilia A and Christmas disease (haemophilia B) showing: I1, transmission of gene by affected male; II2, transmission of gene by carrier female; III1 and III2, transmission of gene by affected male marrying carrier female.

Nature of the Defect in Haemophilia and Christmas Disease

The prolonged bleeding seen in a patient with haemophilia and Christmas disease is due to deficiency of factor VIII and factor IX, respectively. Both factors play an important role in the intrinsic mechanism of blood coagulation leading to conversion of fibrinogen to fibrin. Factor VIII acts as a co-factor with phospholipid, calcium ions and factor IXa in the activation of factor X. In the case of factor IX it undergoes cleavage during clotting to yield a powerful serine protease which, in the presence of factor VIIIa, phospholipid and calcium ions, activates factor X.

The details of the blood coagulation process and the part played by factor VIII and factor IX are discussed in detail in Chapter 1. The nature of the genetic defect and the gene mutations associated with failure of production of these two clotting factors is dealt with in Chapter 2.

Clinical features

The clinical features of haemophilia A and Christmas disease are identical and the following description refers to both conditions although haemophilia A may be the condition specifically mentioned. The treatment of both conditions, however, is different, as will be seen in the chapters dealing with management.

The following account describes the signs and symptoms as they are seen in the untreated patient. The natural course of both haemophilia A and haemophilia B has been greatly changed by the immense progress made in transfusion therapy, in particular by the development of potent, safe factor concentrates. Because of this the more severe complications of haemophilic bleeding are becoming less common, at least in the developed countries.

The haemophilic defect is present at birth and factor assays carried out on samples of cord blood from severely affected boys confirm this. Curiously, in spite of the severe factor deficiency, bleeding during the neonatal period is uncommon. Bruising, intracranial haemorrhages and gastrointestinal bleeding characteristic of haemorrhagic disease of the newborn caused by vitamin K deficiency are rarely seen. Prolonged bleeding following separation of the umbilical cord is rarely a problem unless the stump becomes infected. Commonly there are no bleeding symptoms until several months after birth unless the child undergoes circumcision or some other surgical procedure. In a retrospective analysis of data on 56 children to investigate at which age the diagnosis was made, Conway and Hilgartner (1994) found that 35 of the children were diagnosed during the first month of life. In 12 cases this was as a consequence of bleeding following some medical procedure such as heel stab (2) or circumcision (10). In six cases, spontaneous bleeding led to the diagnosis.

The time of onset of first bleeding in a patient is determined by the severity of the condition and this in turn is inversely related to the level of factor VIII or factor IX as determined by in vitro assays of biological clotting activity. Levels of factors VIII and IX in plasma are usually expressed as a percentage of average normal levels or as iu/dl. By definition, average normal plasma contains 100 iu/dl. The range of factor VIII levels in the normal population is wide, being 50–200 iu/dl (Preston and Barr, 1964). The range of levels of factor IX is narrower. Severely affected individuals have factor levels of less than 1 iu/dl, bleed spontaneously and suffer joint and muscle haemorrhages. Patients who are moderately affected generally have factor levels between 1 and 5 iu/dl. Such individuals are less likely to bleed spontaneously but bleed excessively after quite minor surgery and other minor trauma.

People with levels between 5 and 40 iu/dl rarely bleed spontaneously but can bleed severely following surgery or serious accidents. Occasionally patients are encountered in whom this correlation between factor level and severity of symptoms is not seen. For example, we have seen a patient with a level of 8 iu/dl who bled spontaneously into his joints and had evidence of chronic arthropathy; another patient with a factor VIII level of <1 iu/dl has reached adolescence without having experienced any joint bleeding. Patients such as these are relatively uncommon but are very interesting and raise the question as to whether or not the assay methods used are in some way showing varying degrees of sensitivity to different forms of factor VIII. Other factors that may account for the discrepancy between factor level and clinical severity include such things as the boy's level of physical coordination, whether or not he participates in potentially damaging sporting activities and whether he is accident prone. In addition, the boy's anatomical make-up, bone and joint alignment and gait may be an important factor with regard to abnormal stresses on joints and predisposition to joint bleeding.

The first manifestations of haemophilia usually appear in early childhood when the child begins to explore his surroundings. Prolonged bleeding from the mouth is one of the most common early features. With the eruption of the lower incisor teeth at the age of 6–9 months, the child may bite his tongue or lip. Bleeding from the frenulum of the upper or lower lip is relatively common and probably arises from injuries caused by the child chewing on a toy or exploring objects with his mouth. Bleeding from the mouth may persist for weeks if not treated by factor replacement. Typically, bleeding is not profuse, may last for only a few minutes at a time and the volume of blood lost at any one time may seem small and cause little alarm to the parents, especially if there is no family history of haemophilia. As a consequence the child may become severely anaemic and ill before medical treatment is sought. In families with a history of haemophilia the significance of mouth bleeding is usually well recognized and alerts the parents to the likely diagnosis and the need for treatment.

As the boy becomes more mobile and begins to crawl he may strike his head against the legs of tables and chairs causing bruising of the forehead. Sometimes these bruises can be very large and may take many weeks to diminish in size even with adequate factor replacement. The temptation to incise these haematomas should be resisted unless the overlying skin is becoming devitalized and there is a danger of its breaking down.

When the child is learning to walk he will often fall down, characteristically into the sitting position, and may, if he lands on a hard object, such as a toy, develop a haematoma of the buttocks. These haematomas can be extremely tense causing great pain and distress to the child and may extend into the perineum and scrotum.

Bruising may affect any part of the body and is characteristically lumpy and tender. The extensor aspects of the forearms, the shins and the rib margins are common sites of bruising in the young child. Sometimes bruising is so marked that the question of "baby battering" is raised. This is particularly likely if there is no history of haemophilia in the family. This must be one of the few situations where parents may be relieved when a diagnosis of haemophilia is made.

Bleeding into joints

Haemarthroses and the consequent joint deformities are the characteristic lesions of severe haemophilia A and B. Mildly affected haemophiliacs with factor levels greater than 2–3% of normal rarely bleed into joints spontaneously and rarely have crippling joint deformities. Bleeding often occurs without any trauma that can be recalled and this has led to such haemorrhages being called "spontaneous". Careful questioning, however, may elicit a history of injury, often very minor and often sustained 24–48 hours before the onset of bleeding.

Bleeding into joints usually starts at the age of 2–3 years and continues at frequent intervals, sometimes every 1–2 weeks, throughout the patient's life. To begin with, the ankles seem to be the most commonly affected joint but later the knees take precedence followed by the ankles and elbows. Other joints such as the wrists, shoulders and finger joints are less frequently affected.

In the untreated or poorly treated haemophiliac, repeated bleeding into joints leads to thickening and increased vascularity of the synovial membrane, which predisposes to further bleeding. The synovial membrane and joint cartilage become pigmented with the breakdown products of blood and as the condition progresses there is loss of cartilage, loss of joint space, cystic changes in the subchondral bone and osteoporosis. Eventually the anatomy of the joint surfaces become severely disturbed, the joint lining and surrounding soft tissues become fibrosed and normal joint function is severely impaired (see Chapter 7).

Bleeding into muscles

Muscle haemorrhages are common in severe haemophilia and may occur without any injury that the patient can recall. This may in part be due to the fact that bleeding may not appear until several days after an injury so that the patient does not connect the two. Bleeding can occur into almost any muscle group in the body. Large muscle bleeds may result in hypovolaemia, shock and anaemia.

Particularly commonly affected are the flexor muscles of the limbs, the iliacus muscles and the psoas muscles. Besides causing pain, swelling and loss of function, muscle haemorrhages may press on important blood vessels and nerves putting the viability of the whole limb at risk. Bleeding into the iliacus muscle often causes femoral nerve palsy with loss of sensation down the front of the thigh, quadriceps weakness and loss of the patellar reflex. Bleeding into the calf muscle may cause shortening of the achilles tendon and equinus deformity of the ankle.

If muscle haematomas are not treated adequately they may progress over a period of months or years to form blood cysts. These, once established, develop thick fibrous walls and contain broken down clots and muscle. They tend to re-bleed and so become gradually larger causing pressure necrosis of local soft tissues and, not infrequently, resorption and fracture of bones. Ultimately they may cause necrosis of the overlying skin and rupture. When this happens the risk of infection is great and mortality is high. The management of haemophilic cysts is dealt with in detail in Chapter 7.

Haematuria

Bleeding from the renal tract is relatively common in haemophiliacs and in one survey over a 5-year period, was seen to occur in 60% of haemophilic boys (Stuart et al, 1966). It is rare before the ages of 12 or 13 years. Most episodes of haematuria occur without a history of trauma, are usually of short duration and stop spontaneously without causing the patient any pain or discomfort. The amount of blood loss is usually small and is rarely enough to cause anaemia. Even in the days before transfusion therapy, haematuria rarely caused death (Legg, 1872).

The early morning concentrated urine sample tends to be the most heavily discoloured with blood and as the day progresses the urine appears to lighten in colour. Heavy large clots may be passed and may cause severe pain in the abdomen and back as they pass down the ureter. The pain may be so severe as to require treatment with pethidine or morphine. Accumulation of clots in the bladder may cause bladder obstruction with severe distension and lower abdominal pain. It is interesting to note that even in untreated patients, blood present in the urine may clot. This may be due to the presence of thromboplastin in the urine. The giving of clotting factor concentrates is likely to produce large firm clots in the urinary tract and it is therefore advisable before administering concentrates to encourage the patient to drink plenty of water to produce a good diuresis and so bring about dilution of the blood in the urine. Antifibrinolytic drugs should not be used in the treatment of haematuria as this may lead to insoluble clots and renal obstruction (Barkhan, 1964).

It is felt by some who have a long experience of treating haemophiliacs that the incidence of haematuria has decreased in recent years. This has been attributed to the widespread use of home therapy and prophylaxis. Another possible explanation is the great reduction in the use of aspirin and aspirin-containing drugs since it became known that these drugs impair platelet function.

There have been several studies of the long-term effect of haematuria on renal function. In one study (Prentice et al, 1971), intravenous pyelography revealed a filling defect in the renal tract in 38% of patients studied who had had no recent haematuria. These filling defects were attributed to old clots. In addition 10% of patients studied showed dilatation of the pelvis, calyx or ureter of the kidney, suggesting some obstruction to outflow. They also found that 30% of patients studied had abnormal creatinine clearance. In more recent studies, however, renal function seemed to be well preserved (Small et al, 1982; Roberts et al, 1983).

Haematuria is such a common feature of haemophilia that most episodes are not investigated apart from carrying out urine culture to exclude infection as a cause. However, should the character of a patient's haematuria change, e.g.

become more frequent, be associated with unusual pain or with heavy clots, it is wise to look for some underlying pathology in the kidneys or bladder.

Intracranial bleeding

Before the appearance of HIV infection, intracranial bleeding was the most common cause of death in haemophiliacs, accounting for approximately 25% of deaths (Rizza and Spooner, 1983). Bleeding may be subdural, subarachnoid or into the substance of the brain, may follow minor injury or may appear spontaneously. In a review of the literature from 1960 to 1974 and including cases from her own institution, van Trotsenburg found 46 patients who had suffered intracranial bleeding. Thirty patients gave a history of preceding injury, 32 were less than 20 years of age and 15 of the patients died. Because of the high mortality associated with intracranial bleeding in haemophiliacs, it is our policy to admit to hospital patients who have suffered head injury. This is particularly important if the patient was unconscious after the injury, was dazed or vomited. The patient is given large doses of factor concentrate to maintain the factor level at approximately 100 iu/dl and is observed closely for signs and symptoms of intracranial bleeding. If there is a suspicion that bleeding has taken place, it is important to carry out computed tomographic (CT) scanning as soon as possible to localize the site of bleeding and allow surgical intervention if this is thought necessary. Parents of young haemophiliacs should be warned of the dangers of intracranial bleeding and should be encouraged to seek help and advice if the child injures his head, especially if the injury was sufficient to cause an external haematoma or to break the skin.

Intracranial haemorrhage in childhood, although very uncommon, may follow quite trivial injury to the head and before the availability of scanning and other sensitive techniques may have been mistaken for meningitis.

Gastrointestinal bleeding

Bleeding from the gastrointestinal tract is not uncommon in haemophilia and is sometimes associated with peptic ulceration. In a significant number of patients, however, no lesion can be demonstrated on X-ray examination. In one study (Forbes et al, 1973), peptic ulceration was found by barium meal examination or endoscopy in 13% of the adult haemophilic population surveyed. This incidence was higher than that in a comparable non-haemophilic population and these authors speculated that this might be due to the continuous stress suffered by haemophiliacs.

Aspirin and related drugs are known to impair platelet function and this, along with their local irritant effect on the gastric mucosa, makes them potent causes of gastrointestinal bleeding. The passage of bright red blood in the stool, especially in the older patient, requires investigation unless it is clearly due to haemorrhoids.

Many haemophiliacs have been infected with the hepatitis C virus and significant numbers are now showing evidence of progressive liver disease. It is therefore important to keep in mind the possibility of oesophageal varices when investigating haematemesis in a haemophiliac.

Other types of bleeding

Epistaxis is common in haemophilia and is usually associated with a blow to the nose. Congestion of the nasal mucosa either by upper respiratory tract infection or by pollen allergy can also cause bleeding. Another common cause of bleeding is nose-picking, especially in children. Bleeding from the nose can be severe, difficult to control and very frightening for the patient and his relatives. If nasal packing is required it should be done gently, preferably by someone with experience and the pack should be removed as soon as possible so as to avoid local infection and irritation and further bleeding.

As mentioned earlier, bleeding from the mucous membrane of the mouth is common in early childhood and is usually due to injury to the mucosa. Because of moistness of the mucous membranes and its constant movement in swallowing, talking, crying and eating, clots formed in the mouth are easily disturbed, causing recurrence of bleeding, and over a period of several days a reddish-grey, berry-like excrescence of fibrin forms. The frenulum of the upper lip is a common site for this to occur.

Bleeding from a bitten tongue is also occasionally seen. This is potentially serious, as the tongue may swell very rapidly and cause obstruction to the airway. Prompt treatment by factor replacement is essential. Similarly, bleeding into the floor of the mouth causing respiratory obstruction can be a hazard of inferior dental block administered during dental treatment.

The eruption of deciduous teeth usually takes place without gum bleeding. Similarly if these teeth are allowed to fall out naturally, bleeding is rarely a problem. If, however, attempts are made to pull them out when they are only slightly loose, prolonged bleeding may ensue. Dental extraction, like tonsillectomy, is a sensitive indicator of haemostatic efficiency and in the days before there was any effective transfusion therapy these procedures were not an uncommon cause of death (Birch, 1937). Haemophiliacs should be encouraged to pay particular attention to oral hygiene so as to reduce the risk of dental caries and the need for dental extraction.

Superficial cuts and scratches and skin punctures usually stop bleeding in the normal time. Deeper cuts may also stop bleeding normally in the first instance but have a tendency to start bleeding several hours or even days later, especially if the wound is disturbed, becomes infected or if adequate factor replacement is not given. Control of this secondary haemorrhage can sometimes be difficult, especially if the wound is infected. Wounds that have been sutured without adequate factor replacement may continue to bleed. This results in a buildup of pressure in the wound with widespread tracking of blood into surrounding tissues and eventual breakdown of the wound. Tight stitching of a bleeding wound will not by itself control haemorrhage. Factor replacement must also be given.

Venepuncture can be carried out safely in haemophiliacs providing that one does not persist in trying to enter a vein that has already been damaged. Most venepuncture haematomas can be avoided if the operator remembers to remove the tourniquet before withdrawing the needle and sees to it that pressure is applied to the puncture site for 3–4 minutes with the arm held straight and elevated above the head. Vaccination and immunization can be carried out safely in severely affected patients providing the procedure is carried out gently, using a small-gauge needle subcutaneously. Gentle pressure should be applied to the puncture site for several minutes after the injection.

Any form of surgery, even in mildly affected patients, is likely to be followed by prolonged bleeding, haematoma formation and infection unless adequate factor replacement is given before surgery and for several days afterwards until wound healing is well advanced. The mildly affected haemophiliac is particularly prone to get into trouble. This is usually because his medical attendants and he himself may think that because he leads a normal and active life with few bleeding problems, surgery will be safe. This is not the case. Mildly affected patients can bleed severely after surgery and often require as much factor VIII to control bleeding as severely affected patients.

The clinical features described above are those seen in the untreated haemophiliac. A very graphic account of the lot of the haemophiliac before the advent of effective treatment has been given by Kerr (1963). Thanks to the wide availability of factor concentrates, at least in developed countries, the natural history of haemophilia has changed dramatically. Death from exsanguination, formerly the most common cause of death, is now rarely seen and life expectancy before the appearance of HIV was approaching that of the non-haemophilic male (Rizza and Spooner, 1983; Larsson, 1985; Jones and Ratnoff 1991).

Psychological and Socio-economic Problems

Haemophilia, being a familial disease, has a major effect on the lives of all members of the family besides the patient. The mother usually feels guilt at having passed on the disease and this guilt may extend back to include the grandmother or grandfather. The appearance of HIV in recent years has made matters worse as many mothers or fathers feel that they may have been responsible for infecting their son during administration of home therapy. Sometimes the father of the haemophiliac is resentful at not having a son who can participate with him in rough sporting activities and may blame his wife for this. The unaffected children in the family often feel neglected as the affected child is usually the focus of attention and anxiety of the family, neighbours and friends and as a consequence the normal siblings may suffer psychological disturbance. The sisters and other female relatives have the added anxiety that they may be carriers of the condition. It is possible, in more than 90% of cases, to define the carrier status of these women by means of linkage analysis identifying and tracking DNA polymorphisms. Care must be taken, however, to see that a child is not caused added anxiety by having her carrier status discussed and carrier testing offered at an age when she is not able emotionally to come to terms with the procedure or the results.

For the haemophiliac, the repeated, painful, unpredictable haemorrhages cause serious disruption of his education, work and social activities. Overprotection by his parents may lead to overdependency and this, along with his joint deformities, may make him unable to go out into the world and compete. Fortunately this picture is being seen less and less. Some young haemophiliacs react to their condition by setting out to prove that they are as good, if not better, than their friends in pursuing dangerous sporting activities and hobbies. The majority, however, are well adjusted to their haemophilia, and in spite of many problems, lead full and useful lives contributing to their community and providing for their families. There is no doubt that the freedom offered by home therapy was of great psychological benefit to the haemophiliac and also to his family. Sadly, the appearance of HIV as well as hepatitis C has brought new anxieties, anxieties quite unlike those well-understood anxieties provoked by bleeding.

Clinical and Laboratory Diagnosis of Haemophilia and Christmas Disease

Accurate diagnosis of haemophilia and Christmas disease rests on a carefully taken clinical history and clinical examination. Having decided on the basis of these enquiries that the patient is suffering from a significant haemorrhagic condition, the next step is to define the nature of the defect accurately by means of laboratory tests and specific assays for the various clotting factors. In severely affected patients the diagnosis is generally easy. In mildly affected patients the diagnosis may prove to be more difficult, especially if the patient has not previously been exposed to surgery or accidental injury.

Clinical history

The importance of taking a detailed clinical history cannot be overstressed. Indeed, a well-taken clinical history is probably the best "screening test" available. Normal laboratory results on a patient with a clear-cut history of bleeding should be viewed with suspicion and the patient should not be subjected to major surgery without further testing and discussion about the need for the surgery and the potential risks and benefits of the procedure.

Enquiry should be made about easy or excessive bruising, the site of bruising, whether they are spontaneous or only follow injury and whether they are lumpy, persistent and painful. Most active children have small bruises from time to time over bony areas such as the front of the shin, over the elbows and over the iliac crest. Such bruises are usually small, not more that 2–3 cm across, rarely lumpy and not particularly painful. In the haemophiliac the bruising is usually tender, sometimes spreads to a considerable size and is out of proportion to the injury causing it. A history of bleeding into joints or muscles is particularly relevant with regard to haemophilia and Christmas disease, especially if they appear spontaneously or following only minimal injury. The patient should be questioned about prolonged bleeding from superficial injuries. A history of prolonged bleeding from small cuts in the mucous membranes of the mouth or tongue in a male child should make the doctor think of haemophilia or Christmas disease. The patient should be questioned closely about bleeding following any form of surgery including dental extraction and whether blood transfusion or a course of iron therapy was ever required after the surgery. Tonsillectomy is a particularly severe challenge to haemostasis and usually results in excessive bleeding, even in patients with only a mild deficiency of factor VIII or factor IX. If the patient did not bleed excessively after tonsillectomy, it is unlikely that he is suffering from any inherited coagulation defect, severe or mild.

The family history may be very helpful and it is important to draw a pedigree chart and to ask about bleeding in other family members. Particular attention should be paid to any history of bleeding in male members on the maternal side of the family. Physical examination is important to assess the extent and severity of any current bleeding. In addition, in the older severely affected haemophiliac, the typical joint deformities of chronic haemarthrosis will usually be found. It is unusual to find such changes in a young child although there may be evidence of multiple bruising, old and new.

Laboratory tests

Factor VIII and factor IX are necessary for blood coagulation via the intrinsic system. As a consequence, only tests that reflect the integrity of the internal pathway are abnormal in haemophilia and Christmas disease. Hence, in both conditions, providing they are uncomplicated by liver disease, the prothrombin time is normal, as is the platelet count and the bleeding time. In contrast the whole blood clotting time, prothrombin consumption test and activated partial thromboplastin time (APTT) are abnormal in severely affected patients but may be near normal or normal in mildly affected patients.

To make a specific diagnosis it is necessary to assay the level of factor VIII or factor IX in a sample of fresh citrated plasma obtained from the patient by clean venepuncture. Faulty or difficult venepuncture may produce a sample of blood that is partially clotted and will yield spurious and useless results. Since this is most likely to occur when dealing with children, it is essential that the person doing the venepuncture is experienced in venepuncturing children. This is important not only because of the need to obtain a satisfactory sample, but also to spare the child distress and give him confidence in doctors, especially if he is found to be affected and is going to require many venepunctures for purposes of treatment in the future.

The assay method most widely used is the one-stage assay, which is based on the ability of the patient's plasma to correct the prolonged clotting of known haemophilic plasma in a modified APTT. This assay requires plasma from a severely affected haemophiliac free from HIV, hepatitis B or other infection. Artificial factor VIII-deficient plasma samples prepared from normal plasma by immunoabsorption procedures are available (Takasi et al, 1987). At present there is no artificial factor IX-deficient substrate available.

Factors VIII and IX may also be assayed using a two-stage method based on the thromboplastin generation test (TGT). The two-stage assay has been shown to be more precise than the one-stage method (Kirkwood et al, 1977) and does not require haemophilic plasma as a substrate, but it is a more complicated assay requiring specially prepared serum, phospholipid and factor V reagents.

In the above assay methods the end-point of the assay is the formation of a fibrin clot. These methods can be modified so that the end-point is a change in colour of a chromogenic substrate which is detected in a spectrophotometer (Rosen, 1984; Blomback and Egberg, 1987). At present these methods are not widely used in clinical laboratories although they are frequently used in research laboratories or plasma fractionation laboratories.

The importance of accurately calibrated standards for the assay of clotting factors is now well recognized and many countries now provide freeze-dried plasma which can be used as a working standard or to calibrate "in-house" standards. This important topic is reviewed in Chapter 4.

Haemophilia B (Christmas Disease)

Haemophilia B is a life-long bleeding disorder that affects males and shows the same clinical features and inheritance pattern as haemophilia A. It is due to deficiency of factor IX, one of the vitamin K-dependent clotting factors, and the severity of bleeding symptoms is inversely related to the concentration of factor IX in the blood. In 1956 Fantl et al showed that the plasma of one of their patients contained material that was capable of neutralizing a factor IX antibody that had developed in another patient. Similar results were obtained by others using a variety of techniques, (Roberts et al, 1968; Thompson, 1977; Holmberg et al, 1980), and it became clear that there were several variants of haemophilia B. One of the most interesting variants is haemophilia B Leiden in which there is a reduced level of factor IX during childhood but as the boy passes through puberty the level of factor IX rises progressively towards normal (Veltkamp et al, 1970; Briet et al, 1982). Analysis of the DNA of these patients has revealed mutations in the promoter region of the factor IX gene (Reitsma et al, 1988; Crossley et al, 1989). These findings, along with other aspects of the molecular genetics of haemophilia B and its variants, are discussed in detail in Chapter 2.

Prevalence

The prevalence of haemophilia B is less than that of haemophilia A, being about 18 per million in the UK. In some areas, however, because of geographical isolation or for religious reasons, the prevalence may be greater, e.g. in the Tenna valley in Switzerland (Duckert and Koller, 1975) and amongst the Amish in the USA (Wall et al, 1967).

Diagnosis

The severity of bleeding in haemophilia B is related to the level of factor IX in the blood. At one time it was thought that haemophilia B was a less severe condition than haemophilia A but this is now known not to be the case as patients with haemophilia B suffer the same severe bleeding episodes and crippling arthropathy as patients with haemophilia A. Diagnosis rests on a carefully taken personal and family history and appropriate laboratory tests. In severely affected patients the whole blood clotting time, APTT and prothrombin consumption test are abnormal. The bleeding time and platelet count are normal, as is the prothrombin time except in patients with the haemophilia Bm variant who have an abnormal prothrombin time when tested with bovine thromboplastin. Factor IX can be assayed using a one-stage method based on the APTT or by a two-stage method based on the thromboplastin generation test. The one-stage method is the more widely used as it is easier to carry out. As with the assay of factor VIII, suitable, carefully calibrated standards must be used if reliable and reproducible results are to be obtained.

Inhibitors to factors VIII and IX

Factor VIII or factor IX inhibitors are antibodies that may develop in haemophiliacs as a result of transfusion therapy and, after AIDS and hepatitis, constitute the most important complication of treatment. Their presence makes control of haemorrhage extremely difficult. The antibodies are immunoglobulins of the IgG class showing restricted heterogeneity. In the case of factor VIII antibody, usually only a single light chain is present (kappa or lambda) with a predominance of type 4 gamma heavy chain. Fewer factor IX antibodies have been studied in detail but the evidence available suggests they are more heterogeneous than factor

VIII antibodies. Factor VIII antibodies are both temperature and time-dependent in their reaction with factor VIII and may show simple or complex reaction kinetics (Biggs et al, 1972a,b; Gawryl and Hoyer, 1982). The antibody may be assayed using the "Bethesda method" (Kasper et al, 1975) or the "New Oxford method" (Rizza and Biggs, 1973).

The prevalence of factor VIII antibody is of the order of 15–25% in severely affected patients. More than 90% of antibodies arise in patients whose factor VIII level is less than 3 iu/dl and generally occur early in the patient's treatment history, usually after a median time of 9–11 days of treatment (Lusher et al, 1993). The possible relationship between the purity of the concentrate and the development of antibodies is currently being studied.

Factor IX antibodies are less common than factor VIII antibodies and prevalence rates vary between 1 and 5%. The antibody is almost instantaneous in its reaction with factor IX and can be assayed roughly using a titring method based on the principles of the Bethesda assay for factor VIII antibodies.

A detailed account of inhibitors and their management is given in Chapter 11. Whether or not a patient develops antibodies to factor VIII or factor IX may be influenced by the nature of the gene mutation causing his haemophilia. Gross gene deletions, nonsense and frameshift mutations are associated with a high incidence of antibody formation (see Chapter 2).

Von Willebrand's Disease

Von Willebrand's disease is a familial bleeding disorder which affects males and females. It was first described in 1926 by A.E. von Willebrand among inhabitants of Foglo, an island in the Aaland archipelago off the west coast of Finland (von Willebrand, 1926). Von Willebrand called the condition "pseudo-haemophilia" and commented that it differed from haemophilia in several respects namely:

1. Inheritance was autosomal dominant and not sex-linked recessive as in haemophilia. Also both sexes were affected equally.
2. Bleeding was usually from mucous membranes and skin. Haemarthroses were rare.
3. The bleeding time as assessed from skin puncture was prolonged whereas in haemophilia it is normal.

From his observations he concluded that bleeding was due to a qualitative platelet defect. Others believed that there was a defect in the capillaries (Macfarlane, 1941; Blackburn, 1961). It is now known that platelet function is certainly abnormal in von Willebrand's disease but that this is due to a defect in their plasma environment.

Progress in the understanding of the pathophysiology probably began when Alexander and Goldstein (1953) reported a deficiency of factor VIII in association with a prolonged bleeding time in patients suffering from an autosomally inherited bleeding disorder. Further studies in patients with von Willebrand's disease showed that infusions of normal plasma, plasma fractions, normal serum and haemophilic plasma brought about a prolonged rise in the level of factor VIII in the patient's blood. The increase of factor VIII was often greater than what would have been anticipated from the amount of factor VIII transfused. This, of course, was most striking in those experiments where haemophilic plasma was transfused (Nilsson et al, 1957; Biggs and Matthews, 1963; Cornu et al, 1963). Other studies revealed that there was impaired adhesion of platelets to wounds (Borchgrevink, 1960) and to exposed sub-endothelial connective tissue (Tschopp et al, 1974), and that platelets of patients with von Willebrand's disease showed diminished retention when their blood was passed down a column of glass beads (Salzman, 1963). Further evidence for a deficiency of platelet-related activities was obtained when it was shown that the antibiotic ristocetin, which caused aggregation of platelets in normal platelet-rich plasma, failed to do so in platelet-rich plasma from patients with von Willebrand's disease (Howard and Firkin, 1971). In the same year Zimmerman et al (1971a,b) demonstrated a deficiency of what is now called von Willebrand's factor antigen (vWFAg) by means of a Laurell immunoassay employing a rabbit antibody raised against human factor VIII concentrates. The biochemical nature of procoagulant factor VIII and vWFAg has been intensively studied over the past 25 years and it is now generally agreed that the smaller procoagulant molecule is non-covalently linked to the large vWFAg molecule, which serves to protect or stabilize the smaller coagulant molecule and to act as a carrier. The vWFAg itself comprises a series of multimers of large molecular weight ($1-15 \times 10^6$). It is the larger multimers that seem to be important in promoting platelet adhesion and haemostasis. This activity of vWFAg has been called von Willebrand factor. There have been numerous studies in recent years of the gene defects that cause von Willebrand's disease. These are dealt with in detail in Chapter 2.

Prevalence

Von Willebrand's disease is probably the most common inherited bleeding disorder if all forms of the disease are considered. Unfortunately, because of the wide range of clinical and laboratory features encountered in the condition, it is difficult to arrive at a precise figure for prevalence. Estimates of 30–40 per million and 70 per million have been made for the UK (Bloom, 1980) and Switzerland (Bachman, 1980), respectively. The reported prevalence in Sweden is 125 per million with most being mildly affected. The severe condition affected approximately 3 per million (Holmberg and Nilsson, 1985). The prevalence in the USA is approximately 1.5 per million (Weiss et al, 1982a).

Varieties of von Willebrand's disease

Von Willebrand's disease can be classified broadly into three types: type I, type II and type III. Types I and II both comprise several subgroups. In type I disease there is a quantitative deficiency of the factor VIII complex with factor VIII coagulant activity, vWFAg and von Willebrand factor all being reduced to roughly the same extent. In type II there are qualitative abnormalities affecting mainly the multimeric structure of vWFAg and in type III disease, which is inherited in an autosomal recessive fashion, vWFAg and all its associated activities are very low or completely absent.

Type I or classical von Willebrand's disease shows autosomal dominant inheritance with variable but usually mild bleeding symptoms in the heterozygous patient. It is the most common form of the disease and in one survey accounted for about 70% of the cases (Hoyer et al, 1983). The condition is characterized by a prolongation of the bleeding time and a concordant reduction of all activities of the factor VIII complex, namely factor VIII coagulant activity, vWFAg and von Willebrand factor. Crossed immunoelectrophoresis of vWFAg shows normal mobility and more detailed studies of vWFAg by multimer analysis shows a normal pattern. These findings are consistent with a quantitative deficiency of normal multimers.

Several subtypes of type I von Willebrand's disease have been reported based on the relative levels and multimeric structure of vWFAg in plasma and platelets and on response to 1-deamino-8-D-arginine vasopressin (DDAVP). Some of those cases with abnormal multimeric structure and function probably fit better into the type II category.

Type II von Willebrand's disease is characterized by a disproportionate reduction of von Willebrand factor compared with factor VIII clotting activity and vWFAg. The level of von Willebrand factor as measured by ristocetin co-factor assay is often very low and the bleeding time is prolonged. Several subtypes have been described. In type IIA crossed immunoelectrophoresis shows a relative lack of the high molecular weight slow-moving multimers of vWFAg and this is confirmed on multimer analysis, which in addition shows that the normal triplet pattern of the multimers is disturbed. The patient's platelets are deficient in the high molecular weight multimers and show reduced aggregation when ristocetin is added to platelet-rich plasma. Administration of DDAVP to the patient brings about an increase in the concentration of only smaller multimers with only partial correction of the bleeding time.

Type IIB von Willebrand's disease is relatively uncommon, accounting for approximately 20% of type II cases. Levels of vWFAg and von Willebrand factor are normal or only moderately reduced and the analysis of vWFAg multimers shows loss of the high molecular weight components in the plasma but a normal pattern in platelets. A characteristic feature of this variant is that the patient's platelets in platelet-rich plasma show increased sensitivity to ristocetin and are aggregated by low concentrations of ristocetin, which has no effect on normal platelet-rich plasma. It is thought that these patients synthesize an abnormal von Willebrand factor that is able to bind directly to platelets thereby bringing about their aggregation and removal from the circulation. This probably explains the variable thrombocytopenia seen in some patients. Thrombocytopenia may be made worse by surgery, pregnancy or exercise, all of which raise the level of von Willebrand factor. Thrombocytopenia may also follow the administration of DDAVP (Holmberg et al, 1983; Saba et al, 1985; Hultin and Sussman, 1990).

The condition known as "pseudo-von Willebrand's disease" or "platelet von Willebrand's disease" (Takahashi, 1980; Weiss et al, 1982b) has clinical and laboratory features very like those seen in type II von Willebrand's disease. There is a reduction of the larger multimers of vWFAg in plasma but not in platelets and the platelets show increased sensitivity to ristocetin. The underlying pathology is thought to lie in the platelets, which have an increased affinity for the larger multimers of normal vWFAg and undergo aggregation and removal from the circulation along with the attached multimers. This has clinical implications as administration of cryoprecipitate or DDAVP to these patients may cause thrombocytopenia.

Several other variants of type II have been described. Most are autosomal dominant in inheritance and in most cases the reports relate to single families or to only a few families. These variants include type IIC (Armitage and Rizza, 1979; Ruggeri et al, 1982; Mazurier et al, 1986), type IID (Kinoshita et al, 1984), type IIE (Zimmerman et al, 1986), type IIF (Mannucci et al, 1986), type IIG (Gralnick et al, 1987), type IIH (Federici et al, 1989) and type II-I (Castaman et al, 1992). The diagnosis of these variants rests on detailed analysis of the patterns of the von Willebrand factor multimers.

Another unusual type of von Willebrand's disease is von Willebrand's disease "Normandy" named after the birthplace of one of the early patients (Nishino et al, 1989; Mazurier et al, 1990). This condition is characterized by a moderate reduction of factor VIII clotting activity, normal levels of vWFAg and ristocetin co-factor activity and a normal von Willebrand factor multimer pattern. The clinical features resemble those of haemophilia A but the inheritance is autosomal recessive. The underlying defect is a mutation affecting the factor VIII binding site of the von Willebrand factor molecule leading to poor binding of factor VIII to von Willebrand factor. The unbound factor VIII is unstable in the circulation hence the secondary deficiency of factor VIII.

Type III von Willebrand's disease is characterized by autosomal recessive inheritance, very low or undetectable levels of von Willebrand factor, low levels of factor VIII and a greatly prolonged bleeding time. Bleeding symptoms are often severe and, in addition to the bleeding from mucous membranes so typical of von Willebrand's disease, may include haemophilic-type bleeding such as haemarthroses and muscle haematomas. The parents and first-degree relatives of affected individuals are usually symptom-free with a normal or only slight reduction in the level of von Willebrand factor. The incidence of parental consanguinity may be high (Shoa'i et al, 1977).

A simpler scheme of classification (Sadler, 1994) has recently been accepted by the International Society for Thrombosis and Haemostasis. In this scheme, quantitative deficiencies of von Willebrand factor are divided into type 1 (partial deficiency) and type 3 (severe deficiency). Qualitative defects (type 2) are divided into four sub-categories:

- Type 2A shows a reduction in platelet-related function of von Willebrand factor along with a loss of high molecular weight multimers.
- Type 2B shows increased affinity of von Willebrand factor for platelet glycoprotein 1b.
- Type 2M shows decreased platelet-related function of von Willebrand factor but no loss of high molecular weight multimers.
- Type 2N shows decreased affinity of von Willebrand factor for factor VIII.

Clinical features

In the more common heterozygous form of the disease, bleeding symptoms are usually mild to moderate in severity. Easy bruising and excessive bleeding from cuts and scratches are common as well as bleeding from the mucous membranes of the nose, mouth and gastrointestinal tract. In women, menorrhagia may be the chief complaint. Postpartum haemorrhage can be severe and may not occur until 7–10 days after delivery by which time the increased level of the factor VIII complex seen in pregnancy will have returned to the low pre-pregnancy level. Excessive bleeding may occur after surgery, especially if this involves mucous membranes. Typically bleeding starts immediately after the surgery and in this respect is different from haemophilic bleeding, which is usually delayed for several hours, or even days. Bleeding symptoms vary greatly between families and within families and may even vary in the same patient at different times.

Patients with homozygous von Willebrand's disease are severely affected and, in addition to bleeding from mucous membranes, often experience haemophilia-like bleeding, including haemarthroses, muscle haemorrhage and retroperitoneal bleeding.

Diagnosis

Diagnosis of von Willebrand's disease, especially the homozygous form, can usually be made on the basis of the patient's clinical history, family history and results of laboratory tests. Some problems may be encountered in the milder forms of the disease where the clinical features and laboratory tests may be variable and there may be difficulty in distinguishing the condition from mild haemophilia. The distinction between the two conditions is important from the point of view of both genetic counselling and of treatment. It is also very important to try to distinguish between mild von Willebrand's disease and normal and a good deal of thought should be given to the possible consequences for the

Table 3.1 Classification and laboratory findings in the major types of von Willebrand's disease

Type	Bleeding Time	Factor VIII	vWFAg	vWF	Multimer pattern
I	Normal or prolonged	Reduced	Reduced	Reduced	All present but reduced in amount
IIa	Prolonged	Normal or reduced	Normal or reduced	Reduced	Large and intermediate forms absent
IIb	Prolonged	Normal or reduced	Normal or reduced	Normal* or reduced	Large multimers absent
IIc	Prolonged	Normal or reduced	Normal or reduced	Normal or reduced	Large multimers absent but prominent smaller forms or larger and intermediate present with prominent small forms
II 'Normandy'	Normal	Reduced	Normal	Normal	Normal
III	Prolonged	Reduced	None detected	None detected	None detected

*Platelets in platelet-rich plasma aggregated by low concentrations of ristocetin.

patient of having this diagnosis made. With a diagnosis of von Willebrand's disease, not only may he find difficulty in getting life insurance or a mortgage but he may find certain occupations such as the armed forces or civil aviation closed to him. If, therefore, having carefully reviewed the clinical history, it is felt that the diagnosis is likely to be more of a disadvantage to the patient than his borderline symptoms, it is wise not to attach a diagnosis of von Willebrand's disease.

Laboratory tests

In a typical case the skin bleeding time, performed by a template method or by the Ivy method, is prolonged and the levels of factor VIII procoagulant activity and vWFAg are reduced. There is also a reduction in von Willebrand factor as assessed by the ability of the patient's plasma to support aggregation of washed, fixed, normal platelets in the presence of ristocetin. Two-dimensional immunoelectrophoresis of vWFAg can be useful and may demonstrate altered mobility of vWFAg or alteration in the proportions of multimers present. A more detailed picture of the multimeric structure of vWFAg can be obtained by means of SDS agarose electrophoresis. The typical laboratory findings in the different variants of von Willebrand's disease are shown in Table 3.1.

The bleeding symptoms seen in von Willebrand's disease are very similar to those seen in platelet disorders. It is therefore important to exclude primary platelet disorders and the possibility of ingestion of aspirin or other antiplatelet drugs. Studies of platelet aggregation in the presence of ADP, arachidonate, thrombin and collagen are of value here. Bernard-Soulier syndrome may be distinguished by the presence of giant platelets and failure of platelets to aggregate on addition of ristocetin or bovine factor VIII, even when normal plasma is added to the test system.

References

Addis T. The pathogenesis of hereditary haemophilia. *Journal of Pathology and Bacteriology* 1911; **15:** 427–452.

Aggeler PM, White SG, Glendening MB, Page EW, Leake TB, Bates G. Plasma thromboplastin component (PTC) deficiency: a new disease resembling hemophilia. *Proceedings of the Society for Experimental Biology and Medicine* 1952; **79:** 692–694.

Alexander B, Goldstein R. Dual hemostatic defect in pseudohemophilia. *Journal of Clinical Investigation* 1953; **32:** 551.

Alzaharavius al Tasrif (10th century) Translation 1519 by Paul Ricius. *Liber theoreticae necnon practicae Alsaharavii.* Tract. XXXI Sect. ii. Cap. XV folio CXLV. Published Augsburg. Cited by Legg JW. In: *A Treatise on Haemophilia.* London: HK Lewis.

Armitage H, Rizza CR. Two populations of factor VIII-related antigen in a family with von Willebrand's disease. *British Journal of Haematology* 1979; **41:** 279–289.

Bachman F. Diagnostic approach to mild bleeding disorders. *Seminars in Hematology* 1980; **17:** 292–305.

Barkhan P. Haematuria in a haemophilic treated with E-aminocaproic acid. *Lancet* 1964; **ii**, 1061.

Biggs R, Matthews JM. The treatment of haemorrhage in von Willebrand's disease and the blood level of factor VIII (AHF). *British Journal of Haematology* 1963; **9:** 203–214.

Biggs R, Douglas AS, Macfarlane RG, et al. Christmas disease: a condition previously mistaken for haemophilia. *British Medical Journal* 1952; **2:** 1378–82.

Biggs R, Austen DEG, Denson KWE, Rizza CR, Borrett R. The mode of action of antibodies which destroy factor VIII. I. Antibodies which have second order concentration graphs. *British Journal of Haematology* 1972a; **23:** 125–135.

Biggs R, Austen, DEG, Denson KWE, Borrett R, Rizza CR. The mode of action of antibodies which destroy factor VIII. II. Antibodies which give complex concentration graphs. *British Journal of Haematology* 1972b; **23:** 137–155.

Birch C La F. *Hemophilia: Clinical and Genetic Aspects*. Urbana: University of Illinois, 1937.

Blackburn EK. Primary capillary haemorrhage (including von Willebrand's disease). *British Journal of Haematology* 1961; **7:** 239–249.

Blomback M, Egberg N. Chromogenic peptide substrates in the laboratory diagnosis of clotting disorders. In: Bloom AL, Thomas DP (Eds), *Haemostasis and Thrombosis*, London: Churchill Livingstone, 1987: 967–981.

Bloom AL. The von Willebrand syndrome. *Seminars in Haematology*, 1980; **17:** 215–227.

Borchgrevink, CF. A method for measuring platelet adhesiveness in vivo. *Acta Medica Scandinavica* 1960; **168:** 157–164.

Briet E, Bertina RM, van Tilburg NH, Veltkamp JJ. Hemophilia B Leyden. A sex-linked hereditary disorder that improves after puberty. *New England Journal of Medicine* 1982; **306:** 788–790.

Bulloch W, Fildes P. *Treasury of Human Inheritance*, Parts V and VI, Section XIVa, Haemophilia. London: Dulau, 1911.

Castaman G, Rodeghiero F, Lattuada A, Mannucci PM. A new variant of von Willebrand disease (type II-I) with a normal degree of proteolytic cleavage of von Willebrand factor. *Thrombosis Research* 1992; **65:** 343–351.

Castex MR, Pavlovsky A, Simonetti. Contribucion al estudis de la fisiopatogenia de la hemofilia. *Medicina (Buenos Aires)* 1944; **5:** 16.

Conway JH, Hilgartner MW. Initial presentations of pediatric hemophiliacs. *Archives of Pediatric and Adolescent Medicine* 1994; **148:** 589–94.

Cornu P, Larrieu MJ, Caen J, Bernard J. Transfusion studies in von Willebrand's disease; effect on bleeding time and factor VIII assay. *British Journal of Haematology* 1963; 9: **189–203.**

Crossley PM, Winship PR, Black A, Rizza CR, Brownlee GG. Unusual case of haemophilia B (letter). *Lancet*, 1989; **1:** 960.

Duckert F, Koller F. The old Swiss haemophilia families of Tenna and Wald. In: Duckert F, Koller F, Brinkhous KM, Hemker HC (Eds), *Handbook of Hemophilia*. Amsterdam: Excerpta Medica, 1975; 21–29.

Fantl P, Sawers RJ, Marr AG. Investigation of a haemorrhagic disease due to beta-prothromboplastin deficiency complicated by a specific inhibitor of thromboplastin formation. *Australasian Annals of Medicine* 1956; **5:** 163–176.

Federici AB, Mannucci PM, Lombardi R, et al. Type IIH von Willebrand disease: a new structural abnormality of plasma and platelet von Willebrand factor in a patient with prolonged bleeding time and borderline levels of ristocetin cofactor activity. *American Journal of Hematology* 1989; **32:** 287–293.

Forbes CD, Barr RD, Prentice CRM, Douglas AS. Gastrointestinal bleeding in haemophilia. *Quarterly Journal of Medicine* 1973; **42:** 503–511.

Gawryl MS, Hoyer LW. Inactivation of factor VIII coagulant activity by two different types of human antibodies. *Blood*, 1982; **60:** 1103.

Gralnick HR, Williams SB, McKeown LP, Maisonneuve P, Jenneau C, Sultan Y. A variant of type II von Willebrand disease with an abnormal triplet structure and discordant effects of protease inhibitors on plasma and platelet von Willebrand factor structure. *American Journal of Hematology*, 1987; **24:** 259–266.

Grandidier L. (1855). *Die Hamophilie, order die Bluterkrankheit*. Leipzig: Otto Wigand.

Handley RS, Nussbrecher AM. Hereditary pseudohaemophilia. *Quarterly Journal of Medicine* 1935; **4:** 165–178.
Holmberg L, Nilsson IM. Von Willebrand disease. In: Ruggeri ZM (Ed.), *Clinics in Hematology Coagulation Disorders*. London: WB Saunders Company 1985: p.476.
Holmberg L, Gustavii B, Cordesius E, et al. Prenatal diagnosis of hemophilia B by an immunoradiometric assay of factor IX. *Blood* 1980; **56:** 397–401.
Holmberg L, Nilsson IM, Borge L, Gunnanson M, Sjorin E. Platelet aggregation induced by 1-desamino-8-D-arginine vasopressin (DDAVP) in Type IIB von Willebrand's disease. *New England Journal of Medicine* 1983; **309:** 816–821.
Howard MA, Firkin BG. Ristocetin – a new tool in the investigation of platelet aggregation. *Thrombosis et Diathesis Haemorrhagica* 1971; **26:** 362–369.
Hoyer LW, Rizza CR, Tuddenham EG, Carta CA, Armitage H, Rotblat F. von Willebrand multimer patterns in von Willebrand's disease. *British Journal of Haematology* 1983; **55:** 493–507.
Hultin MB, Sussman LN. Postoperative thrombocytopenia in type IIB von Willebrand disease. *American Journal of Hematology* 1990; **33:** 64–68.
Immermann H. "Hamophilie" In: *Ziemssen's Handbuch der speciellen Pathologie und Therapie.* 1879.
Jones PK, Ratnoff OD. The changing prognosis of classic hemophilia (factor VIII "deficiency"). *Annals of Internal Medicine* 1991; **114:** 641–648.
Kasper CK, Aledort LM, Counts RB, et al. A more uniform measurement of factor VIII inhibitors. *Thrombosis et Diathesis Haemorrhagica*, 1975; **34:** 875–876.
Kernoff PBA, Rizza CR. Factor VIII-related antigen in female haemophilia. (letter). *Lancet* 1973; **2:** 734.
Kerr CB. The fortunes of haemophiliacs in the nineteenth century. *Medical History* 1963; **7:** 359–370.
Kerr CB. Genetics of human blood coagulation. *Journal of Medical Genetics* 1965; **2:** 221–308.
Kinoshita S, Harrison J, Lazerson J, Abildgaard CF. A new variant of dominant type II von Willebrand's disease with aberrant multimeric pattern of factor VIII-related antigen (type IID). *Blood* 1984; **63:** 1369–1371.
Kirkwood TBL, Rizza CR, Snape TJ, Rhymes IL, Austen DEG. Identification of sources of inter-laboratory variation in factor VIII assay. *British Journal of Haematology* 1977; **37:** 559–568.
Larsson SA. Life expectation of Swedish haemophiliacs, 1831–1980. *British Journal of Haematology* 1985; **59:** 593–602.
Legg JW. *A Treatise on Haemophilia, Sometimes Called the Hereditary Haemorrhagic Diathesis.* London: HK. Lewis, 1872.
Liston R. Haemorrhagic Idiosyncrasy. *Lancet* 1839; **ii:** 136–138.
Lusher JM, Arkin S, Abildgaard CF, Schwartz RS. and the Kogenate study group. Recombinant factor VIII for the treatment of previously untreated patients with hemophilia A. *New England Journal of Medicine* 1993; **328:** 453–459.
Macfarlane RG. Critical review: The mechanism of haemostasis. *Quarterly Journal of Medicine* 1941; **10:** 1.
Mannucci PM, Lombardi R, Federici AB, Dent JA, Zimmerman TS, Ruggeri ZM. A new variant of type II von Willebrand disease with aberrant multimeric structure of plasma but not platelet von Willebrand factor (type IIF). *Blood*, 1986; **68:** 269–274.
Mazurier C, Mannucci PM, Parquet-Gernez A, Goudemand M, Meyer D. Investigation of a case of subtype IIC von Willebrand disease: Characterization of the variability of this subtype. *American Journal of Hematology* 1986; **22:** 301–311.
Mazurier C, Gaucher C, Jorieux S, Parquet-Gernez A, Goudemand M. Evidence for a von Willebrand factor defect in factor VIII binding in three members of a family previously misdiagnosed mild haemophilia A and haemophilia A carriers. Consequences for therapy and genetic counselling. *British Journal of Haematology* 1990; **76:** 372–379.
Merskey C. The occurrence of haemophilia in the human female. *Quarterly Journal of Medicine* 1951; **20:** 299–312.
Nasse CF. Von einer erblichen Neigung zu todtlichen Blutungen. In *Archiv fur medizinische Erfahrung im Gebiete der praktischen Medizin und Staatsartzneikunde*. Berlin: 1820; p. 385.
Nilsson IM, Blomback M, Jorpes EJ, Blomback B, Johansson SA. von Willebrand's disease and its correction with human fraction I-O. *Acta Medica Scandinavica* 1957; **159:** 179–188.

Nishino M, Girma, J-P, Rothschild C, Fressinaud E, Meyer D. New variant of von Willebrand disease with defective binding to factor VIII. *Blood* 1989; **74:** 1591–1599.
Otto JC. An account of an haemorrhagic disposition existing in certain families. *The Medical Repository* 1803; **6:** 1–4.
Patek AJ Jr, Stetson RP. Hemophilia I. The abnormal coagulation of the blood and its relation to the blood platelets. *Journal of Clinical Investigation* 1936; **15:** 531–542.
Patek AJ, Taylor FHL. Hemophilia. II. Some properties of a substance obtained from normal human plasma effective in accelerating the coagulation of hemophilic blood. *Journal of Clinical Investigation* 1937; **16:** 113–124.
Pavlovsky A. Contribution to the pahogenesis of hemophilia. *Blood* 1947; **2:** 185–191.
Prentice CRM, Lindsay R, Barr RD, et al. Renal complications in haemophilia and Christmas disease. *Quarterly Journal of Medicine* 1971; **40:** 47–61.
Preston AE, Barr A. The plasma level of factor VIII in the normal population. *British Journal of Haematology*, 1964; **10:** 238–245.
Reitsma PH, Mandalaki T, Kasper CK, Bertina RM, Briet E. Two novel point mutations correlate with an altered developmental expression of blood coagulation factor IX (hemophilia B Leyden phenotype). *Blood* 1989; **73:** 743–746.
Rizza CR, Biggs R. The treatment of patients who have factor VIII antibodies. *British Journal of Haematology* 1973; **24:** 65–82.
Rizza CR, Spooner RJD. Treatment of and related disorders in Britain and Northern Ireland during 1976–1980: report on behalf of the directors of haemophilia centres in the United Kingdom. *British Medical Journal* 1983; **286:** 929–933.
Roberts GM, Evans KT, Bloom AL, Al-Gailani F. Renal papillary necrosis in haemophilia and Christmas disease. *Clinical Radiology* 1983; **34:** 201–206.
Roberts HR, Grizzle JE, McLester WD, Penick GD. Genetic variants of hemophilia B: detection by means of a specific inhibitor. *Journal of Clinical Investigation* 1968; **47:** 360–365.
Rosen S. Assay of factor VIII C with a chromogenic substrate. *Scandinavian Journal of Haematology* 1984; **33:** (suppl 40) 139–145.
Ruggeri ZM, Nilsson IM, Lombardi R, Holmberg L, Zimmerman TS. Aberrant multimeric structure of von Willebrand factor in a new variant of von Willebrand's disease (type IIC). *Journal of Clinical Investigation* 1982; **70:** 1124–1127.
Saba HI, Saba SR, Dent J, Ruggeri ZM, Zimmerman TS. Type IIB Tampa: a variant of von Willebrand disease with chronic thrombocytopenia, circulating platelet aggregates and spontaneous platelet aggregation. *Blood* 1985; **66:** 282–286.
Sadler JE. A revised classification of von Willebrand's disease. For the Subcommittee on Von Willebrand factor of the Scientific and Standardization Committee of the International Society on Thrombosis and Haemostasis. *Thrombosis and Haemostasis* 1994; **71:** 520–525.
Salzman EW Measurement of platelet adhesiveness. A simple in vitro technique demonstrating an abnormality in von Willebrand's disease. *Journal of Laboratory and Clinical Medicine* 1963; **62:** 724–735.
Shoa'i I, Lavergne J-M, Ardaillou N, Obert B, Ala F, Meyer D. Heterogeneity of von Willebrand's disease: study of 40 Iranian families. *British Journal of Haematology* 1977; **37:** 67–83.
Small, M, Rose, PE, McMillan, N, et al. Haemophilia and the kidney: assessment after 11-year follow up. *British Medical Journal* 1982; **285:** 1609–1611.
Stuart J, Davies SH, Cumming RA, Girdwood, RH, Darg, A. Haemorrhagic episodes in haemophilia: a 5-year prospective study. *British Medical Journal* 1966; **2:** 1642–1662.
Takahashi H. Studies on the pathophysiology and treatment of von Willebrand's disease. IV. Mechanism of increased ristocetin-induced platelet aggregation in von Willebrand's disease. *Thrombosis Research* 1980; **19:** 857–867.
Takase T, Rotblat F, Goodall A, et al. Production of factor VIII deficient plasma by immunodepletion using three monoclonal antibodies. *British Journal of Haematology* 1987; **66:** 497–502.
Thompson AR. Factor IX antigen by radioimmunoassay. Abnormal factor IX protein in patients on warfarin therapy and with hemophilia B. *Journal of Clinical Investigation* 1977; **59:** 900–910.
Tractate Yevamoth 64b. In the *Babylonian Talmud*, edition of Otzar Hasefarim. New York, 1957.
Treves F. A case of haemophilia: pedigree through five generations. Lancet 1886; **ii:** 533–4.

Tschopp TP, Weiss HJ, Baumgartner HR. Decreased adhesion of platelets to subendothelium in von Willebrand's disease. *Journal of Laboratory and Clinical Medicine* 1974; **83:** 296–300.
Van Trotsenburg L. Neurological complications of hemophilia. In *Handbook of Hemophilia*. Brinkhous KM, Hemker HC (eds). Amsterdam: Excerpta Medica. 1995, pp. 389–404.
Veltkamp JJ, Meilof J, Remmelts, HG, van der Vlerke D, Loeliger, EA. Another genetic variant of haemophilia B: haemophilia B Leyden. *Scandinavian Journal of Haematology* 1970; **7:** 82–90.
Wall RL, McConnell JL, Moore D, MacPherson CR, Marson A. Christmas disease colour blindness and blood group Xga. *American Journal of Medicine* 1967; **43:** 214–226.
Weil MPE. Etude du Sang chez les Hemophiles. *Bulletins et Memoires de la Societe Medicale des Hopitaux de Paris*. 1906; **23:** 1001–1018.
Weiss HJ, Ball AP, Mannucci PM. Incidence of severe von Willebrand's disease. *New England Journal of Medicine* 1982a; **307:** 127.
Weiss HJ, Meyer D, Rabinowitz R, et al. Pseudo-von Willebrand's disease. An intrinsic platelet defect with aggregation by unmodified human factor VIII/von Willebrand factor and enhanced adsorption of its high molecular weight multimers. *New England Journal of Medicine* 1982b; **306:** 326–333.
Willebrand von EA. Hereditare pseudohemofili. *Finska Lakaresallskapets Handlingar* 1926; **67:** 7–12.
Wright AE. On a method of determining the condition of blood coagulability for clinical and experimental purposes and on the effect of the administration of calcium salts in haemophilia and actual or threatened haemorrhage. *British Medical Journal* 1893; **2** 223–5.
Wright IS. The nomenclature of blood clotting factors. *Thrombosis et Diathesis Haemorrhagica* 1962; **7:** 381–388.
Zimmerman TS, Ratnoff OD, Littell AS. Detection of carriers of classic hemophilia using an immunologic assay for antihemophilic factor (factor VIII). *Journal of Clinical Investigation* 1971a; **50:** 255–258.
Zimmerman, TS, Ratnoff OD, Powell AE. Immunologic differentiation of classic hemophilia (factor VIII deficiency) and von Willebrand's disease with observations on combined deficiencies of antihemophilic factor and proaccelerin and on acquired circulating anticoagulant against antihemophilic factor. *Journal of Clinical Investigation* 1971b; **50:** 244–254.
Zimmerman, TS, Dent, JA, Ruggeri, ZM, Nannini LH. Subunit composition of plasma von Willebrand factor. Cleavage is present in normal individuals, increased in IIA and IIB von Willebrand disease but minimal in variants with aberrant structure of individual oligomers (types IIC, IID, and IIE) *Journal of Clinical Investigation* 1986; **77:** 947–951.

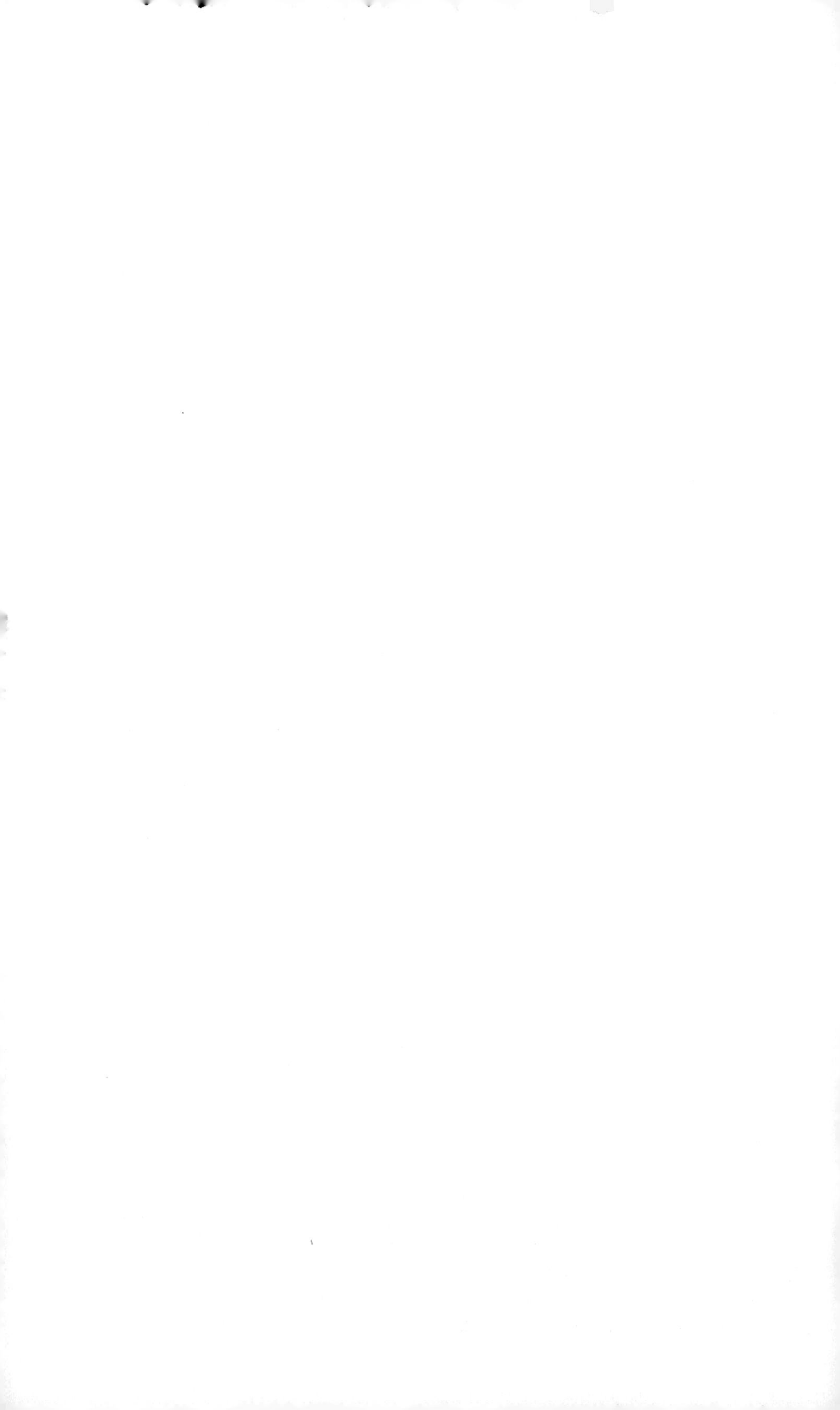

Standards and Quality Control in the Blood Coagulation Laboratory

4

TREVOR W. BARROWCLIFFE AND
KATHY B. MATTHEWS

Introduction

The overall aim of standardization and quality control is to ensure that measurements of a particular clotting factor give the same result when carried out at different times in the same laboratory, in different laboratories and by different methods. There are many factors that are important in ensuring reproducibility of coagulation assays, but two of the most critical are the provision of appropriate reference standards and procedures for quality control, both internal and external. In this chapter these two important aspects will be described, with particular reference to factors VIII and IX and von Willebrand factor (vWF).

Units of Activity

The units of activity used to standardize coagulation assays have been measured in three ways.

"Absolute" units

Here the unit is defined as the activity measured under certain well-defined assay conditions. This was used for instance to define the NIH unit for thrombin, being the amount of thrombin that would clot a standardized solution of fibrinogen in 15 seconds. Fibrinogen itself can be measured in milligrams using a suitably defined method and several purified clotting enzymes can be measured in molar terms using chromogenic substrates. Although such measurements may be suitable for purified materials, they are rarely applicable to plasma or impure concentrates and they have the disadvantage of requiring precise fulfilment of a specified set of reaction conditions.

For most coagulation measurements, adequate standardization can only be achieved by comparison of the unknown sample against a standard of defined activity, assayed under the same conditions. Variations in the system from assay to assay and from one laboratory to another affect both the standard and test sample, so that the final measurement should be largely independent of such variations.

Normal plasma units

Because assays for most coagulation factors were developed before they had been purified, the first standard to be established consisted simply of normal plasma, the unit of activity being defined as that amount in 1 ml of "average normal plasma". One advantage of this system of units is that the severity of a clotting factor deficiency in a patient can be easily related to normal on a percentage scale, calling the normal 100%. Another important advantage is that the denaturation that tends to occur on purification is avoided and, because most assays of clotting factors are carried out on plasma, normal plasma is an appropriate standard on the basis of a general preference for assaying "like against like" in bioassays. The main disadvantage of normal plasma as a standard is the very wide range of levels of clotting factors in the "normal" population, due to differences associated with age, sex, race and blood group, as well as intrinsic biological variability and the influence of drugs, such as oral contraceptives. The combined effects of these differences can result in appreciable variations in the clotting factor content of multidonor pools: it is not uncommon in many laboratories to find 20% differences in the factor VIII content of successive pools of plasma, and pools from different laboratories may differ even more widely. For instance, in an international collaborative study, the factor VIII content of 21 pools of 15 or more donors ranged from 63% to 135% (Barrowcliffe et al, 1983). A further problem is that successive pools can only be assayed against the previous pool and, because of the poor stability of some clotting factors, especially factors V and VIII, this can result in a "drift" of the value of the unit over a period of time. The only satisfactory solution to these problems is the provision of stable reference standards against which successive batches of working standard can be compared.

Reference standards

In most areas of biological measurement, greatest uniformity has been achieved through the establishment of stable reference standards. The general principle of defining a unit of biological activity as the activity in a specified amount of single reference substance was first established for insulin (Dale, 1925, Unpublished Letter). It has since been applied to many other biological substances and in the last 25 years International Reference Standards have been established for most of the major clotting factors and inhibitors.

Characteristics of Reference Standards

In general, reference standards should have four main characteristics.

An agreed potency

The potency of a local standard may be "agreed" by arbitrarily assigning a figure of 100% to a pool of normal plasmas. This may be adequate in one laboratory, but the potency of different laboratories' local standards can only be related to each other by comparison against national and international standards. One of the main features of national and international standards is that their potency is established after a collaborative study, by agreement with the participants.

Stability

Some clotting factors, notably factors V and VIII, are quite labile in plasma and this can cause uncertainty in the use of normal plasma pools as local standards. For any standards that are going to be used over a lengthy period, their stability needs to be checked by repeat assay against a reference standard. For long-term reference standards themselves, their stability has to be checked by accelerated degradation studies of their degradation rate at different temperatures.

All samples should be identical

For frozen materials, this is easy to achieve by freezing all samples together as a batch but, for freeze-dried standards, it is also necessary to check the accuracy of filling.

Like versus like

In addition to these three aspects, the other important point about a standard is that it should be, as far as possible, closely similar in composition to the test samples being assayed against it. This principle of assaying "like against like" is most important in biological standardization, and the discrepancies that arise between laboratories and between assay methods (see following sections) can mostly be traced to the assay against one another of dissimilar materials.

Preparation of International Standards

To avoid confusion caused by a multiplicity of standards, a single primary reference preparation is established as the International Standard (IS) against which all other standards are calibrated, though for some clotting factors it has been found necessary to establish two International Standards, one for concentrates and one for plasma (see later). The main feature of such International Standards is that they are calibrated by many laboratories around the world; the donor population is thus much wider than can be achieved in a single laboratory, and results from all the laboratories with a variety of assay methods are distilled into a single agreed figure, which then defines the international unit for that clotting factor.

In setting up reference standards for coagulation, use has been made of the general principles of biological standardization which have been developed over many years for other substances. The basic processes in establishing such a reference standard are described as follows.

Ampouling of one or more candidate reference preparations. An accuracy of filling of less than 1% is considered desirable for international and national standards and the steps taken to achieve this have been described in detail by Campbell (1974).

Preliminary testing of proposed standards against the current standard and comparison with test substances likely to be assayed against the proposed standard. This is a basic check on whether the proposed reference substance has adequate activity and gives valid assays against the materials with which it is going to be compared.

Testing stability of proposed standards. To act as a long-term reference preparation, the proposed standard should display no significant losses in potency when stored under its normal conditions (usually –20 °C) for up to 10 years and should also be able to withstand short periods at higher temperatures, so that it can be mailed at ambient temperatures without losses of activity. The general principle used in producing stable biological standards is that of removal, as far as possible, of the main agents of chemical change, i.e. water, oxygen, heat and light. Thus most standards are freeze-dried and the drying process has been developed both to ensure minimum losses of biological activity and to reduce moisture levels as much as possible, i.e. less than 1% (Campbell, 1974). Oxygen is eliminated by preparing all materials under nitrogen before sealing in glass. Finally, all standards are stored at −20 °C in the dark. Stability testing is normally done using the accelerated degradation method. This involves the storing of ampoules at a range of temperatures, including some at higher temperatures to accelerate the degradation process and obtain measurable losses of activity. The usual range of temperatures is −20 °C (reference), +4 °C, +20 °C, +37 °C and, occasionally, +45 °C. From the losses in potency measured at the higher temperatures, it is possible to predict the degradation rates at −20 °C, using a method based on the Arrhenius equation (Kirkwood, 1984).

Collaborative study. Once suitable candidate preparations have been identified from the preliminary investigations, they are then subjected to an international collaborative study. This is the major part of establishment of a standard and the general principles of such studies have been outlined by the World Health Organization (WHO, 1978). The following represents a brief summary of the guidelines adopted at the National Institute for Biological Standards and Control (NIBSC), though it should be emphasized that many of these have been decided on pragmatic grounds.

Materials. The two main types of material usually included are samples of plasma and one or more purified preparations; these should represent the degree of purity of the test samples against which the standard will be compared. For establishment of a new standard, it is preferable to include more than one purified preparation, prepared by different methods. For studies carried out to replace existing standards, information gained from the previous studies may be used to limit the choice of materials.

Methods. In virtually all studies, each laboratory is asked to use their own assay methods. However, some degree of control is applied in the form of instructions for reconstitution of ampoules, number of dilutions and order of testing.

Comparison with existing unit. When any new standard is established, comparison is always made with the previously accepted unit which, in the case of most clotting factors, is "average normal plasma". Thus participants are asked to collect normal plasma locally for comparison against the proposed standard, and samples of local standards, consisting of frozen or freeze-dried plasma pools, are included. Such comparisons, as well as being the basis of the unitage for the new standard, also serve to illustrate the divergences usually found between different laboratories' concepts of "normal plasma".

Assignment of potency. From the raw data submitted, a mean potency estimate is calculated for each laboratory and the individual laboratory estimates are then combined into an overall mean (Kirkwood and Snape, 1980). It is customary to include all assays except those for which the model assumed in the statistical analysis does not provide a satisfactory fit to the data. For a new standard, the unitage is assigned by comparison with the existing unit, as already mentioned. A replacement standard is usually calibrated against the previous standard, but it may be desirable to compare also against normal plasma, as a check for possible "drift" in the unit over many years. The final assignment of potency and establishment of an international standard is carried out by the WHO in Geneva, on the advice of their Expert Committee on Biological Standardization.

Calibration of national, local and commercial standards

Once an international standard has been established, it acts as the primary reference material and national and local standards should be calibrated against it. Where commercial standards exist, this is particularly important, so that the basis for the unitage is the same for different manufacturers. As in the case of international collaborative studies, few formal rules exist for the calibration process, but some general guidelines can be given. The most important principle is that of repetition, to minimize the errors of the calibration process at each stage. For local standards, it is essential to carry out at least four independent assays, and preferably six. By "independent assay" is meant a completely fresh set of standard and test solutions; for concentrate preparations a new initial dilution should be made and, for freeze-dried standards, a fresh ampoule reconstituted. Since the supply of international standards is often limited to a few ampoules for each laboratory, a useful compromise to obtain the required number of assays is to perform two or more assays from the same ampoule, provided that this can be done within the period of stability of the reconstituted standard (usually 1–2 hours). Repetition of testing of both materials should also be carried out within each assay, using two separate sets of dilutions of each. Ideally, a fresh set of reagents, even if from the same batches, should be used for each assay. In practice, this is not always possible, but some attempt should be made to spread the work over more than one day, to allow for possible day-to-day variation in reagents and environmental conditions. The calibration process is often a good opportunity to involve more than one operator and, indeed, to compare accuracy and precision between operators. For the latter purpose, it is important that the potency and precision of each assay, and of the combined assays, be assessed by appropriate statistical methods.

Concentrate and Plasma International Standards for Factors VIII and IX

Because of the principle of "like versus like" mentioned earlier, a separate series of International Standards has been established for concentrate and plasma for both factors VIII and IX. Brief details of these Standards and their establishment are summarized in Table 4.1.

Factor VIII standards

The development of factor VIII concentrates as articles of commerce in the late 1960s accelerated the need for a stable reference preparation against which these products could be compared, and the 1st International Standard for factor VIII concentrate was established in 1971 (Bangham et al, 1971). This standard was an intermediate purity concentrate (~0.1 iu/mg) and was typical of the products in use at that time. Its replacements, the second and third standards, established in 1978 and 1983, respectively, were similar concentrates, the specific activity of the third standard being around 0.3 iu/mg. When the time came to replace the third standard, however, methods of production had changed dramatically, with the introduction of very high-purity concentrates prepared by monoclonal antibody technology, and even the intermediate-purity concentrates being somewhat purer than before because of the need to introduce viral inactivation techniques. Careful consideration was therefore given to the suitability of different types of product as standards before an intermediate-purity concentrate (3.9 iu/mg) was chosen as the fourth IS. Most recently, a monoclonal antibody preparation was chosen as the 5th IS, because high-purity concentrates, including recombinant factor VIII, have largely replaced intermediate-purity concentrates in clinical use.

Table 4.1 International concentrate and plasma standards for factor VIII and factor IX

Factor VIII		Factor IX	
Concentrate	Plasma	Concentrate	Plasma
1st IS 1971	1st IRP 1983*	1st IS FIX 1974	1st IS 1987†
2nd IS 1978	2nd IS 1989*	1st IS FII, IX, X 1987	2nd IS 1996†
3rd IS 1983	3rd IS 1993*	2nd IS FII, IX, X 1994	
4th IS 1989			
5th IS 1994			

*Calibrated also for von Willebrand factor (vWF). †Calibrated also for FII, VII, X. IS, International Standard; IRP, International Reference Preparation.

For assays of plasma samples, laboratories use either national plasma standards where available, commercial plasma standards, or local plasma pools. Calibration of these plasma standards against the IS for factor VIII concentrate was found to give large discrepancies between laboratories and between assay methods (Kirkwood and Barrowcliffe, 1978; Barrowcliffe and Kirkwood, 1980). Therefore it was decided to establish a plasma standard for factor VIII to co-exist with the concentrate standard. This reference plasma was established in 1982 and calibrated for the other factor VIII-related activities as well as factor VIII:C (Barrowcliffe et al, 1983), i.e. factor VIII:Ag, and von Willebrand factor (vWF) activity and antigen. It has since been replaced by the 2nd IS for factor VIII and von Willebrand factor (vWF) in plasma (Heath and Barrowcliffe, 1992) and more recently by the 3rd IS.

Problems in standardization of factor VIII assays

The principle of "like versus like" has been vindicated in the use of the International Plasma Standard to calibrate successive British Standards; there have been no discrepancies between one-stage and two-stage methods and good agreement between laboratories. The same was true of concentrates in the 1970s and early 1980s (Barrowcliffe and Kirkwood, 1978; Barrowcliffe et al, 1983). However, since 1985 the introduction of viral inactivation procedures, coupled with increased purification by both conventional and monoclonal antibody affinity chromatography and the introduction of recombinant factor VIII, has led to a wide divergence in the composition of concentrates. A survey at NIBSC in 1990 (Barrowcliffe et al, 1990) found that nine of 13 concentrates when assayed against the concentrate IS gave higher potencies in one-stage than in two-stage assays, by 12–40%. Furthermore, collaborative studies of monoclonal and recombinant concentrates gave wide variation between laboratories as well as between assay methods (Barrowcliffe, 1993). Further studies showed that certain technical features were important for assay of these types of concentrates, the main ones being the use of haemophilic plasma rather than artificially depeleted plasma as a substrate in one-stage assays and as a prediluent for all methods and the incorporation of 1% albumin in the assay buffers. When these technical aspects were standardized, agreement between laboratories was greatly improved and the discrepancies between methods reduced, though not eliminated.

The chromogenic method, which is increasingly used by manufacturers and by clinical laboratories in some European countries, was incorporated into the most recent collaborative studies and when the technical features mentioned above were standardized, gave the lowest inter-laboratory variability of the three methods. However, as expected, because it is based on the same principle, it gives largely the same results as the two-stage method; hence discrepancies between the one-stage method and the chromogenic assay still occur and it would be preferable for concentrate manufacturers to standardize on one or other method. A set of recommendations for assay of high-purity factor VIII concentrates was approved by the Scientific and Standardization Committee (SSC) of the International Society on Thrombosis and Haemostasis and recently published (Barrowcliffe, 1994). These recommendations incorporated the chromogenic assay as the reference method. The chromogenic assay has also become the official reference method in the European Pharmacopoeia, replacing the two-stage method in January 1995.

Factor IX standards

The standardization of factor IX followed a similar pattern to that of factor VIII. The first standard to be established was a concentrate of factors II, IX and X (Brozovic et al, 1976).

As with factor VIII, this was found to be unsuitable for calibration of local and national plasma standards, and when the first standard was replaced by a similar concentrate a separate plasma standard was also established (Barrowcliffe, 1988).

The method of predilution was also found to affect the comparison of concentrate and plasma standards, and this created a complication when assigning the potency of the new concentrate standard (Barrowcliffe et al, 1979). Assays of the new concentrate standard against normal plasma using deficient plasma predilution gave potencies 20% higher than against the old concentrate standard. Although the use of buffer predilution gave similar potencies against both the old concentrate standard and normal plasma, the deficient plasma predilution method was preferred because of comparability with ex vivo plasma samples after injection of concentrates, and with the factor VIII situation. Accordingly the potency of the new concentrate standard was assigned against normal plasma using factor IX-deficient plasma as prediluent. This effectively meant a re-evaluation of the factor IX International Unit by about 20%: for instance, bottles labelled 500 iu against the old standard would become approximately 600 iu against the new standard. Although this caused a certain amount of initial confusion, the long-term benefits are a more consistent relationship between the plasma and concentrate standards, and between the dosage and ex vivo response.

Recently "monocomponent" factor IX concentrates, containing minimal quantities of factors II, VII and X, have been produced by several manufacturers using both conventional chromatography and monoclonal antibody technology. By analogy with factor VIII it might be anticipated that assays of such concentrates against the II–IX–X concentrate IS might be subject to more variability than assays of prothrombin complex preparations. In a collaborative study organized by the Food and Drug Administration (FDA), Lamb et al (1991) found that the method of predilution was the main source of variability; when three single factor IX concentrates were assayed against the IS, potencies were significantly higher, and inter-laboratory variability considerably reduced, when either factor IX-deficient plasma or 1% albumin buffer were used as prediluents, compared with buffer alone. For one of the three single factor concentrates, the differences between prediluents were not significant; this concentrate, unlike the other two, was formulated in 1% albumin. It appears therefore that albumin is a sufficiently effective stabilizer for the assay of high-purity factor IX concentrates, and that the use of factor IX-deficient plasma for predilution is not obligatory.

British Standards for Factors VIII and IX

As already mentioned, WHO standards are intended for use throughout the world and hence are only available in limited quantities. The hierarchy of standardization envisages that WHO standards would be used to calibrate National Standards for the most commonly performed assays and this has been the case in the UK for factor VIII and IX, with NIBSC preparing and issuing successive batches of British Standards for many years. As with the International Standards, two separate series of standards have been prepared: plasma standards for assay of patients' plasma samples and concentrate standards for assay of concentrates. The Factor VIII plasma standards were originally calibrated against the WHO concentrate as this was the only International Standard available, but, as already indicated, this gave rise to substantial discrepancies between laboratories and between assay methods. Following establishment of the International Plasma Standard in 1983 (WHO, 1983) this has been used to calibrate all subsequent batches of British factor VIII plasma standards. British factor IX plasma standards were first issued somewhat later than the factor VIII standards and all have been calibrated against WHO Plasma Standards for factor IX.

An advantage of these standards is that they are calibrated in collaborative studies, usually involving six to eight laboratories and therefore the potency is a consensus value, unlike that of commercial standards, which are calibrated in a single laboratory. Another advantage is that they are available in large quantities and therefore can be used as working standards or quality control materials. Because of the high demand, batches of British plasma standards are replaced frequently and the batch size has been increased to 10 000 ampoules.

British concentrate standards for factor VIII have been issued since 1976, and for factor IX since 1980. Like the plasma standards, they are calibrated by collaborative study against the appropriate (i.e. concentrate) International Standards. The British concentrate standards are used as true working standards by the UK manufacturers and by NIBSC, so that all concentrates produced in the UK are assayed using the same working standard.

Table 4.2 summarizes the current British Standards available for factor VIII and IX. As can be seen, the current plasma factor VIII standard is the twentieth, an indication of its high frequency of use.

Table 4.2 Current British working standards for factor VIII and factor IX (1996)

Factor VIII		Factor IX	
Concentrate	Plasma	Concentrate	Plasma
11th BWS	20th BS	3rd BWS*	7th BS†

BWS, British Working Standard; BS, British Standard.
*Calibrated also for FII and FX. †Calibrated also for other coagulation factors (see Table 4.3).

Table 4.3 Standards for other clotting factors and inhibitors

Material	Code no	Description
Antithrombin, Concentrate	88/548	1st IS
Antithrombin, Plasma	93/768	2nd IS
Blood Coagulation Factors Plasma	96/628	7th BS
von Willebrand factor (vWF):RCoF		
von Willebrand factor (vWF):Ag		
Factor IX		
Antithrombin		
Protein C		
Factor VII		
Protein S antigen		
Fibrinogen		
Factor VII Concentrate	89/590	1st BS
Factor VIIa Concentrate	89/688	1st IS
Factor Xa, Bovine	75/595	NIBSC reagent
Flbrinogen, Plasma	89/644	1st IRR
Protein C, Plasma	86/622	1st IS
Protein S, Plasma	93/590	1st IS
Thrombin, α-type, Human	89/588	2nd IS
Thrombin, Human	70/157	1st IS

Other Coagulation Standards

International standards are now available for most of the major clotting factors and inhibitors and in many cases British Standards are also available. Table 4.3 summarizes the various standards available as plasma, concentrates or purified material. Further information on these and other standards in the thrombosis and haemostasis field can be obtained by writing to NIBSC.

Quality Control in Coagulation

Effective quality control in a laboratory involves use of both internal and external quality control measures. Internal quality control measures all aspects of laboratory testing on a day-to-day basis. It allows us to monitor precision so that any errors in procedures may be detected quickly and thus kept to a minimum. External quality control, more correctly termed quality assessment, involves inter-laboratory testing of samples and assessment of performance. In the UK this is organized by an external body: the National External Quality Assessment Scheme (NEQAS); the object of the scheme is to assess between-laboratory comparability of testing procedures. As samples are provided at intervals of approximately 3 months it is a retrospective rather than day-to-day check on performance. Local quality control schemes are also of value and are operated in some areas. They should be used in addition to participation in NEQAS. If well organized, samples may be distributed to laboratories in the region at more frequent intervals than is possible with NEQAS. With the cooperation of participating laboratories it would be hoped that variations occurring in methodology could at least be standardized within the area and hopefully this would show improved overall performance. Both internal quality control and participation in external quality assessment schemes are a vital part of good laboratory practice and are an essential requirement with implementation of laboratory accreditation in the UK. Ultimately it is hoped that a properly managed quality control programme should result in improved diagnosis and monitoring of haemostatic defects and patient care.

Control of Pre-testing Variables

Control of procedures in a laboratory is not isolated to performance of the individual tests – there are several issues to be considered pre-testing.

Anticoagulant

Normally blood is anticoagulated with trisodium citrate for routine coagulation tests. The concentration and proportion of citrate to whole blood is an important point to consider. A concentration of 0.106–0.109 M (or equivalent to 3.13–3.2%) trisodium citrate is generally recommended (Ingram and Hills, 1976b). Higher concentrations have been shown to result in slight prolongation of clotting times. The use of citrate buffered with HEPES (N-2-hydroxyethylpiperazine N-2-ethanesulphonic acid) at a concentration of 0.05 M in plasma has, in recent years, become more popular. The effect of this is to stabilize the pH of plasma resulting in better reproducibility of the prothrombin time (PT) for several hours (Zucker et al, 1970) and to minimize loss of labile clotting factors (V and VIII). It is an acceptable practice to buffer citrate with HEPES pre-venepuncture or to add HEPES to plasma post-separation as is the case with some commercial manufacturers of freeze-dried plasma preparations (Godfrey et al, 1975).

Generally blood is collected into liquid rather than solid citrate for coagulation as minimal delay in anticoagulation of blood is necessary to prevent in vitro activation of the sample. More recently "closed" blood collection systems have become more popular, e.g. Vacutainer, Monovette. These have an advantage over the "syringe" technique as blood flows directly from the vein into anticoagulant thus minimizing problems encountered by delayed anticoagulation of blood.

A 9:1 blood to anticoagulant ratio is normal practice; this should ideally be adjusted for patients with very high or low haematocrits so that the correct concentration of citrate is present in plasma (Ingram and Hills, 1976b).

Whatever blood collection system is used, it should be kept consistent as variation in the anticoagulant used may well affect results obtained. However minor this variation may be, it should be kept to insignificant levels.

Sample collection and preparation

Samples should be collected by clean venepuncture with minimal venous occlusion: tissue from vessel walls can lead to activation of the sample and unnecessary occlusion can lead to a false rise in certain factors, e.g. factor VIII, vWF.

Immediate careful mixing of the blood sample is also required, as delayed mixing may result in activation. Vigorous shaking may lead to haemolysis: substances released from ruptured cells have a secondary effect on coagulation thus testing of samples haemolysed due to poor blood collection should be avoided. Blood samples for coagulation studies should be collected from a vein not an arterial line as may be the case with intensive therapy unit (ITU) patients or with Hickman catheters inserted. Heparin is quite often used to keep the line open, thus resulting in heparin contamination of the sample; it is difficult, if not impossible, to make any judgements about a patient's coagulation status if heparin is present as a contaminant. Receipt by the laboratory of samples for coagulation studies may be difficult to control but should be as short as possible, at most within 2 hours.

The blood should then be centrifuged with minimal delay in order to collect platelet-poor plasma: a speed of 1500–2000 *g* for 10 minutes is generally recommended.

It is well to remember that some factors (V, VIII) are labile and if there is significant delay in preparation of samples for testing then prolongation of clotting times may occur as a result of decay of these labile factors.

Plasma should then be removed from the sample using a plastic transfer pipette and stored in a plastic tube until testing. Glass pipettes and tubes are not suitable as contact activation may occur. Having ensured correct procedures for collection and preparation of blood, plasma samples should be stored at 4 °C on the day of collection and tested with minimal delay. Where batch testing may be performed on frozen samples, store at −40 °C or below.

Control of Technical Variables

No matter what test is to be performed, the equipment to be used and the method of end-point detection must be well controlled.

Equipment

Pipettes used for the transfer of plasma and reagents should be regularly cleaned and calibrated as obviously a variation in volumes dispensed will have an effect on results obtained.

The operational temperature of the water bath or coagulometer should be at 37 °C: variations in temperature have an effect on coagulation time.

Method of end-point detection

Manual methods

In general many haemostasis tests, and specifically those used for diagnosis of haemophilia, result in the formation of a fibrin clot as an end-point. Previously most laboratories used manual methods, but with much development in instrumentation in recent years, currently only 25% of laboratories in the UK still use manual methods. There is much technical variation of methods and this will be discussed in more detail for specific tests but basics such as mixing on addition of reagents, frequency of mixing during an incubation period, whether the end-point is noted to be first formation of fibrin strands or a solid clot may all vary. These factors must be strictly controlled especially when using manual techniques or a variation in results will occur. Though manual methods are open to error, careful control of procedures within one laboratory may significantly reduce error; in experienced hands manual methods may give extremely reproducible results.

Thus, correct training of staff to perform manual techniques in exactly the same way within one laboratory is of vital importance.

Automation

A variety of instruments is available for performance of coagulation tests; in fact, 75% of laboratories in the UK now use some form of automation. Equipment varies from being semi-automated to completely automated and though the method of end-point detection varies from one instrument to another, within one laboratory error levels should be reduced as long as the instrument is consistent and well maintained. In recent years there has been much development in more automated coagulation instruments and these are becoming increasingly popular, e.g. ACL series, MLA Electra, Sysmex CA5000.

Generally, though there will be design differences in the way these instruments operate, they control not only end-point detection but also sampling, thus removing sample and reagent pipetting errors from the operator. Even though use of a coagulometer should improve performance, NEQAS surveys comparing laboratories using similar instrumentation show that samples still vary.

Control of Activated Partial Thromboplastin Time (APTT, PTTK, KCCT)

As the context of this chapter is primarily control of methods for screening and detection of haemophilia and related disorders, only the APTT will be considered as a screening test.

The APTT is a measure of the intrinsic coagulation pathway and thus monitors factors VIII, IX, XI, XII, prekallikrein and high molecular weight kininogen (HMWK) (intrinsic factors). It also monitors factors I, II, V and X though these are also measured by the prothrombin time and are thus termed common pathway factors.

Internal measures of quality control of APTT

Choice of activator and activation time

Previously a non-activated partial thromboplastin time (PTT) was routine procedure though results could be variable owing to varying surface contact activation, thus an activator was introduced to the system in an attempt to control this. Celite was first introduced to provide contact activation though kaolin became more commonly used by laboratories.

Though introduction of an activator such as kaolin to the system standardizes contact activation, the effect is to shorten clotting times compared with a non-activated PTT. The activation time itself is critical as this also has an effect on the clotting time: the longer the activation time the shorter the resultant clotting time.

A 10-minute activation time was originally the recommended method and was thought to have greatest sensitivity to factor VIII deficiency though this is not necessarily the case. Shorter activation times have been shown to have greater sensitivity to detection of prekallikrein and HMWK deficiency, 2 or 3 minutes being ideal; a 10-minute activation time is totally insensitive to even a severe deficiency of these factors.

Activation times vary between laboratories from 2 to 10 minutes though shorter activation times are probably most commonly used. This is just one factor resulting in much variation of results between laboratories.

More recently there has been increased use of non-kaolin activators such as ellagic acid and micronized silica. These combine both activator and phospholipid and are more suitable for use with the automated instruments now available: ACL, MLA Electra; a granular activator such as kaolin is totally unsuitable for these coagulometers.

Whatever the choice, the activator and time of activation should be standardized within a laboratory.

Choice of phospholipid

Phospholipid is required for the conversion of factor VIII to VIIIa and factor II to IIa.

In vivo this is provided by platelets; in vitro it is normal practice to perform tests on platelet-poor plasma as this allows us to add an external phospholipid reagent in an attempt to control the amount of lipid available in the test system. However, such a range of phospholipid reagents are available commercially and it has been shown by many workers that there is variation in sensitivity of both phospholipids and activators, some lacking sensitivity in detecting mild deficiencies of some factors (Poller and Thompson, 1972, 1976; Barrowcliffe and Gray, 1981; Stevenson et al, 1986; Barna and Triplett, 1989).

Guidelines for performance, sensitivity and reproducibility of the PTT have been proposed (Koepke, 1986).

Care should therefore be taken with the choice of phospholipid reagent used for the APTT: it is important that the sensitivity of the reagent to mild factor deficiencies has been established and is acceptable to the laboratory. It should be remembered, however, that the APTT is a screening test only and monitors all factors but VII; it is possible that a mild factor deficiency may be masked by other factors being raised, possibly resulting in a shortening of clotting time to within normal limits. However, this should not generally be the case. Patients with a history of bleeding would normally have factor assays performed in major referral centres even in the presence of a normal APTT.

Normal range

It is of utmost importance that all laboratories performing these tests assess their own normal range rather than using the manufacturer's stated range. This in itself can be a problem as the question then arises how do we define normal and whom do we select as normal donors? The tendency is to bleed staff or collect samples from blood donor sessions from individuals presumed to have no bleeding problems themselves. However, there is the question of whether females on the contraceptive pill should be excluded as it is well known that this causes a rise in factor VIII; this may have the effect of shortening the APTT. Some factors increase with age so should there be an age limit with choice of donors? It is impossible with known variables to collect the "perfect" normal donors but it is important that a realistic assessment of normality is established within each laboratory and that this is checked periodically to make sure that there is no significant change in normal range.

Use of ratio

As discussed previously, variation in activator, phospholipid and incubation time used all have an effect on coagulation times. It would be an impossible task to persuade all laboratories in the UK to use identical reagents and methods, thus variation in results between laboratories has to be accepted to a degree. However, reporting of results in the form of a ratio rather than seconds would provide a part solution to the problem of variation in coagulation times obtained with different reagents and methods: this is normal practice in some laboratories.

The question then arises as to the normal value used for this purpose. Some laboratories test a fresh normal donor each day and base APTT ratios on this. There is generally a reasonable variation in normal range whatever reagent is used, therefore using a single donor each day will not give consistency of results on a day-to-day basis. It is preferable to either use a frozen or lyophilized plasma pool that has been well calibrated and gives consistent results, use the mid-point of the normal range, or assess the geometric mean of normal as is recommended for the PT.

It is obviously important that if we are to try to bring some sort of comparison between laboratories for APTT testing with the range of reagents, incubation times and equipment used, that use of a ratio for reporting results should be standard practice and that the normal value to be used for this purpose is well defined.

Batch testing of reagents

Though generally reagents are obtained commercially and there should be insignificant batch-to-batch variation in these reagents, it is a relatively simple procedure for the user to perform their own internal check on receipt of a new batch to establish for themselves that the sensitivity is as the previous batch. This can be done by performing APTTs on a selection of normal and abnormal samples ranging from mild to severe with both the current and new batch of reagent. There is then assurance that there is no drift in results caused by batch variation. Implementation of laboratory accreditation applies as much to manufacturers as to the users of these reagents, thus strict control over production of consistent batches should also assist in reducing variability of results that may be due to inconsistent batches of phospholipid. If the users of these reagents perform no in-house check for themselves when new batches are received and have no other form of internal quality control procedure, they may be totally unaware of any drift in results.

Monitoring of staff performance

Some laboratories perform exercises to monitor the performance of individual technical staff at regular intervals. This can be a useful exercise, especially in manual laboratories, to ensure consistency of results between operators.

Use of control samples

Many commercial companies marketing coagulation reagents produce lyophilized normal and abnormal plasmas for use as controls. Though generally coagulation times are quoted, it should be remembered that these are only valid if the other reagents used are from the same manufacturer and that their package insert method is strictly followed. Otherwise an in-house assessment of these plasmas using the internal method should be performed before using them as quality control samples.

The purpose of using these controls ideally is to establish the precision or reproducibility of the APTT and then to use the information obtained to set up an internal quality control programme. This should give confidence in the quality of results on a day-to-day basis.

Initially the variation in APTT should be established for each control plasma by repeat testing. Having done this the mean value, variance, standard deviation (SD) and coefficient of variation (CV) may then be calculated.

Ideally the CV should be less than 5% though less than 10% is acceptable. Having established these values within the laboratory, normal and abnormal controls should ideally be processed with each batch of test samples. If the values obtained are within 2 SD of the mean then the batch of patient samples may be reported.

Many laboratories possibly test control plasmas only once in a working day; some use none at all. With gradual implementation of laboratory accreditation it is a requirement that normal and abnormal control plasmas are used throughout the working day. Together with other control mechanisms, this will hopefully lead to greater improvement in performance and more confidence in the quality of results.

Many of the more automated coagulometers, e.g. MLA Electra, ACL series, have in-built quality control programmes thus making monitoring and assessment of data from quality control samples more manageable than with a manual or semi-automated set-up.

External quality assessment of APTT

UK NEQAS surveys assist in highlighting problems of performing APTTs. Recent surveys show that 27 different sources of phospholipid reagents are currently in use in the UK. A total of 465 laboratories currently participate in APTT assessment: of these 25% determine the end-point manually and 75% use a variety of instruments varying from semi-to completely automated; in all 21 different instruments are in use.

For statistical purposes results are assessed for each phospholipid reagent used and are in the form of a median APTT for each user group. For some instruments, as indeed for some phospholipid reagents, there are only a small number of users (one in some instances), thus it is not possible to obtain meaningful statistics of variation in these smaller user groups.

A recent survey included a sample from a donor with mild haemophilia A – the variation in median APTT for each reagent group varied from 30 to 57 seconds. It should be remembered that these results will also reflect different activation times though a breakdown for these data is not given.

Since March 1992 NEQAS has been converting results to the form of a ratio based on the mid-point of each laboratory's stated normal range, thus a local estimation of normal range rather than quoting the manufacturer's normal range is extremely important. Expression of the data in this form appears more meaningful: median APTT ratios for the above sample ranged from 1.0 to 1.47.

However, it should be noted that these are median values only for each reagent group: the actual distribution of results shows that the ratio generally varied from 1.0 to 1.8 with a small number of laboratories reporting ratios of 0.7 and 2.1.

It should be noted that although 85.5% of laboratories in this survey interpreted the result as being abnormal, 10.2% reported results as borderline and 4.3% as normal. Should those laboratories who reported a normal result not automatically also perform a factor VIII assay on a patient with a possible history of haemophilia, then the diagnosis would be missed in the patient.

These figures clearly highlight possible problems in performing APTTs whether it be due to variation in reagent sensitivity or performance problems. Performances were designated unsatisfactory in 4.5% of cases and persistently unsatisfactory in 4.5%. Though this is an example from only one NEQAS survey, data from other surveys show a similar pattern.

It may be of value if more local quality control schemes were in operation; with such variables in reagents and methodology that currently exist, this should result in more local control with the cooperation of participating laboratories in the area, and perhaps then we may begin to see an improvement in NEQAS survey results and improved detection of coagulation disorders.

Control of Factor VIII Assays

Factor VIII may be assayed by one-stage, two-stage or, more recently, chromogenic methods. Currently 97% of laboratories in the UK use a one-stage method, the other 3% being divided between two-stage and chromogenic methods. It would perhaps be useful at this stage to consider each method individually.

One-Stage assay for factor VIII

This is based on the APTT and involves the correction of the APTT of a plasma severely deficient in factor VIII by adding dilutions of a standard or test plasma.

Dilutions are generally made of the standard and test plasma ranging from a 1:5 to a 1:1000 dilution; these represent arbitrary concentrations of 200% to 1%. Glyoxaline buffer is commonly used to prepare these dilutions though a variety of others are in use.

Equal volumes of both plasma dilution and factor VIII-deficient plasma are mixed together and an APTT performed for each mixture. The resultant coagulation times obtained will be inversely proportional to the concentration of factor VIII in each mixture as the only factor VIII in the system is provided by the individual dilutions of standard and test plasma. The factor VIII concentration of the test sample may then be estimated by comparison to a standard graph plotted of factor VIII concentration versus clotting time.

Technical factors affecting one-stage assays

Choice of phospholipid. Generally problems associated with variation in sensitivity of the many phospholipids available for use do not have the same effect on factor assays as they do with detection of factor VIII deficiency by the APTT, as the test sample is being directly compared with a standard.

Activation time. Activation times used for one-stage factor assays vary from 2 to 10 minutes though it was previously thought that a 10-minute activation time was more suitable for assay of factor VIII. The choice of activation time should not have an effect on the factor VIII level obtained on the patient as again there is comparison with a known standard. However, whatever activation time and phospholipid are used, the test samples must be treated in exactly the same manner as the standard for every part of the procedure otherwise inaccuracies will occur.

Deficient plasma. Factor VIII-deficient plasma is available from two sources: individuals with severe haemophilia A or immunodepleted normal plasma.

(a) *Haemophilia A.* This may be obtained commercially from several manufacturers and is normally obtained from HIV-negative individuals. Alternatively some of the larger haemophilia centres may collect blood from suitable registered patients who are HIV negative.

(b) *Immunodepleted plasma.* In recent years factor VIII-depleted plasma has been produced from normal plasma with the use of a monoclonal antibody to factor VIII (Rothschild et al, 1990; Takase et al, 1987). Most of the antibodies used are to vWF, resulting in removal of both factor VIII:C and vWF from the plasma; other factors remaining intact. As plasma is obtained from normal donors who have been HIV tested, it was thought to be a safer alternative for use in factor VIII assays with the onset of HIV-related problems in the haemophilia population. Immunodepleted plasma is available from several commercial companies. However, recent reports have questioned the suitability of these plasmas for assaying factor VIII concentrates (Barrowcliffe et al, 1993). Some immunodepleted plasmas are deficient only in factor VIII and contain normal vWF levels; they may be preferable as they more closely resemble haemophilic plasma.

Whatever the source of factor VIII-deficient plasma used, it is important that the plasma is completely devoid of factor VIII, i.e. less than 1%.

Dilutions of a standard ranging from 100% to 1% when plotted should give a straight line; if flattening of the line occurs at low concentration levels this probably indicates that the substrate plasma is not completely devoid of factor VIII. A "blank" should also be tested with each batch of assays: sample dilution here is replaced by diluent buffer thus the only factor VIII in the system is being provided by the deficient plasma – a blank clotting time should be clearly longer than the 1% standard.

Though use in assays of a factor VIII-deficient plasma that is not completely deficient will probably not have a significant effect on the factor VIII level of patients with normal or mildly reduced factor VIII levels, there will be loss of sensitivity when assaying samples with low levels of factor VIII and it may be impossible to assay accurately levels below 5%. Obviously this is not acceptable to those haemophilia centres where this may be an everyday requirement.

Unfortunately not all sources of commercial factor VIII-deficient plasmas currently available are completely suitable, thus careful choice should be made when selecting the source of deficient plasma to suit the needs of the laboratory.

Whether the factor VIII-deficient plasma is obtained from patients or by immunodepletion of normal plasma, all other coagulation factors should be present at normal levels; if not, the assay system will not be specific for factor VIII. A prothrombin time should be performed as a screen to ensure that extrinsic and common pathway factors are normal.

The substrate plasma should also be free from inhibitors to factor VIII for obvious reasons: when collecting patient-deficient plasma a factor VIII inhibitor screen should be performed to ensure this.

Two-Stage assay for factor VIII

The two-stage factor VIII assay is based on the thromboplastin generation test. In the first stage an incubation mixture is set up that contains all factors required for generation of intrinsic thromboplastin (serum, factor V, phospholipid) except factor VIII. Factor VIII is added to this mixture in the form of dilutions of standard or test plasma. Intrinsic thromboplastin generated is measured in the second stage by subsampling into normal plasma and calcium chloride and noting the clotting time. The amount of intrinsic thromboplastin generated and thus the clotting time in the second stage is inversely proportional to the concentration of factor VIII in the first stage. Results are extrapolated from a graph plotted of factor VIII concentration versus clotting time.

Technical factors affecting two-stage assays

Serum. Serum used for this assay must be carefully prepared. Blood samples should be collected from several normal donors into a plain glass tube. The blood is incubated at 37°C for 4 hours to allow complete coagulation then left overnight at 4°C to ensure that there is no residual thrombin left in the serum. The sera may then be pooled and either frozen at –40°C or lyophilized in aliquots. A batch of serum should store for at least 3 months. For use, one vial of serum is diluted in glyoxaline buffer and stored at 4°C overnight before use. The dilution of serum is critical so that a sufficient supply of factors IX, X, XI and XII are present and this should be carefully optimized for each new batch of serum produced. The serum being at the wrong dilution, incorrectly prepared or simply being too old is probably the most common source of problems with the two-stage assay.

Factor V. Factor V available commercially is of bovine origin. This is normally diluted for use in the assay: this dilution is critical and should be carefully assessed for each new batch of factor V used.

Phospholipid. Many sources of phospholipid are available for use in a two-stage assay: again the concentration used is critical and should be assessed pre-assay. A combined reagent for use in a two-stage assay was reported by Barrowcliffe and Kirkwood (1980); Denson et al (1976) reported use of a combined reagent to simplify a two-stage method as no subsampling is required.

First stage incubation. Both the reagents used for the first stage and the incubation time must be carefully optimized to allow maximal generation of intrinsic thromboplastin. Though methods for two-stage assays vary just as much as those for one-stage assays, on average the first stage incubation is usually in the region of 6–12 minutes. The incubation time is critical in that subsampling should be performed at a time of maximal thromboplastin generation; this may be tested by setting up an incubation mixture including factor VIII and calcium and subsampling at minute intervals. A gradual rise in generation of intrinsic thromboplastin will be observed that eventually forms a plateau. It is at the point of plateau that the system is most reliable and therefore this should be assessed for each new batch of reagents used to ensure reproducibility (Barrowcliffe, 1984).

Chromogenic assay for factor VIII

Chromogenic assays for factor VIII were developed on a commercial basis in the mid-1980s (Seghatchian and Miller-Anderson, 1978; Rosen, 1984). The principle is generally similar to that of a two-stage assay but the end-point involves colour development rather than coagulation time.

Dilutions of plasma supplying factor VIII are incubated with a combination of factor X, activated factor IX, phospholipid, calcium and thrombin. The thrombin causes activation of the factor VIII, which in turn causes activation of factor X in the presence of IXa, phospholipid and calcium. The Xa activity is assessed by hydrolysis of a p-nitroanilide (pNA) substrate specific for Xa. This hydrolysis results in release of pNA and thus colour development. The reaction is stopped by addition of 20% acetic acid.

The colour development (pNA release) is directly proportional to factor VIII concentration, thus the factor VIII level in the test plasma may be established in the normal manner by extrapolation from a graph plotted of factor VIII concentration versus absorbance at 405 nm.

Technical factors affecting chromogenic assays

Reagents for use in this assay are normally in the form of a kit and are available commercially from a range of manufacturers. Optimal conditions for the assay are critical and are normally established by the manufacturer, who will also supply a package insert method. It is therefore important that the users of these kits follow the manufacturer's method exactly in order that reliable results may be obtained.

General Factors Affecting Factor VIII Assays

Source of standard

The standard used for this and any other assays is of great importance as a variety of choices is available. Use of standards is discussed separately in this chapter in detail; however, it should be noted that an incorrectly calibrated standard may have a drastic effect on the factor VIII level obtained in the patient and may lead to misdiagnosis and inaccurate monitoring of therapeutic levels.

Dilutions

Whatever method is used for quantitating factor VIII, it is recommended practice to perform dilutions of a standard ranging from normal to very low levels and at least three dilutions for test samples, though many laboratories perform only two or three dilutions for the standard and one for the test plasma. Some of the more recently developed automated coagulometers are in fact designed to perform a one-point test assay though other coagulometers do allow more flexibility to the user. It should be stressed that though a one-point test assay may be acceptable when screening populations, e.g. donor screening for factor VIII production, for diagnostic purposes it is preferable to perform a minimum of three dilutions on the test sample. This gives more confidence in results plus a view of parallelism which is important to establish. Normally only parallel line assays are acceptable for a valid result. Non-parallelism may occur in some samples owing to the presence of inhibitors, e.g. lupus-type, to activated samples in a one-stage technique or to poor technique. The reason for this non-parallelism, when it occurs, should normally be established; however, if only a one-point assay is performed one is not aware of any problems.

An added variable for assays is the preparation of dilutions pre-assay. It is essential that dilutions are accurately prepared, as "sloppy" technique will only result in increased variability of results. It should also be remembered that factor VIII is labile. Assays should ideally be performed on fresh not frozen samples or some loss in activity will occur. Samples should be stored at 4°C and tested within a few hours of collection. Dilutions should be prepared either as the assay is proceeding so that there is no delay in processing or they may be prepared pre-assay in plastic tubes to avoid contact activation: in this case they should be kept on ice and processed quickly or loss in activity may occur.

Choice of assay

There has been much debate over the years as to the prefered method for factor VIII assay. In diagnostic laboratories in the UK the one-stage assay is most commonly used whereas several manufacturers of factor VIII concentrates use two-stage and chromogenic assays. Discrepancies in factor VIII levels associated with the method used have been noted and there has been much discussion on this subject (Kirkwood et al, 1977; Kirkwood and Barrowcliffe, 1978).

In some instances a two-stage assay may give a higher result than a one-stage when assaying concentrates though this may relate to other aspects of methodology such as whether the standard used was concentrate or plasma (Barrowcliffe, 1993).

In plasma samples the reverse may occur – this may be due to activated factor VIII in the samples which in a two-stage assay would be removed by adsorption of the sample pre-assay with aluminium hydroxide; in a one-stage assay any activated factor VIII would be included as there is no preadsorption of the sample. However, factor VIII may also be removed from a sample by over-adsorption with aluminium hydroxide thus this step must be carefully controlled and could sometimes contribute to discrepancies between the two assay methods.

With the development of the chromogenic method, comparisons have been performed with both techniques. In some instance it has been found to compare well to the one-stage assay when assaying clinical samples (Hutton et al, 1991), the coefficient of variation (CV) being generally lower for the chromogenic assay (<6%) than for the one-stage assay (16%) (Rosen et al, 1985). Other workers have found that the chromogenic assay gives better comparison with the two-stage technique for assay of concentrates, both methods showing similar CVs (Hubbard et al, 1986).

Though few clinical laboratories in the UK use the chromogenic method routinely, it has been established by the European Pharmacopoeia instead of the two-stage method as the reference method. Though this is generally for the assay of concentrate materials, it may well be that in time a gradual increase in usage of the chromogenic assay will be seen in clinical laboratories.

Generally it is accepted that the CV of assays within a laboratory may be 10–20% when performed manually. However, it should be possible to reduce this significantly by carefully controlling methodology and reagents; in fact, in experienced hands the CV is usually lower than quoted. Variables in methodology detail apply to factor VIII assays as much as they do to performance of the kaolin cephalin clotting time (KCCT). Increased usage of automated coagulometers may also serve to reduce the variability apparently inherent in performing factor assays. Some of the recently developed coagulometers, e.g. MLA Electra, ACL, also have programmes to perform chromogenic factor VIII assays, results being generally very reproducible.

Internal quality control plasmas for factor VIII assays

Normal and abnormal control plasmas are available commercially for use in factor VIII assays. As with the KCCT, internal variation in results should be assessed as described previously and control samples ideally included in every batch of assays performed. This will become a standard requirement with the gradual implementation of laboratory accreditation in the UK.

External quality assessment of factor VIII assays

A recent UK NEQAS survey included a plasma sample from a donor with mild haemophilia A. Two hundred and forty-five laboratories participated in this exercise: of these, 238 used a one-stage assay showing a median result of 10.9 iu/dl; five used a two-stage assay with a median result of 7 iu/dl and two used a chromogenic assay showing a median result of 10.5 iu/dl. Assessment of results is mainly for one-stage assay results because of insufficient numbers of laboratories performing two-stage or chromogenic methods.

There were 16 different sources of deficient plasma, 13 sources of reference plasma and 22 sources of phospholipid used. Of 238 laboratories, only 22 used manual methods; the remainder use a variety of coagulometers, approximately 50% of these being of the ACL series. Results were assessed according to platelet substitute: the median of all groups ranged from 3.9 iu/dl to 19.5 iu/dl though the actual spread of overall results was from 3 iu/dl to 30 iu/dl.

There are many factors that influence these results, as previously discussed: primarily they may be due to the reference plasma or standard used for assay, factor VIII-deficient plasma, phospholipid, number of dilutions used or general application of methodology. It is impossible to elucidate the cause of such variation in results, but this survey clearly highlights problems in variability of factor VIII assays.

In this survey 99.2% of participants interpreted the result as abnormal and 0.8% as normal. It is of interest to note that in this particular survey a breakdown was given of normal ranges quoted by participants. Though the mean lower limit is 51 iu/dl, this actually ranges from 34 iu/dl to 82 iu/dl. Clearly this variation in what is considered to be normal contributes to the interpretation of results obtained for diagnostic purposes.

Previous surveys of factor VIII activity show similar disturbing variation in both assessment and interpretation of results.

There have been many attempts to investigate the apparent variability in assay of factor VIII and some of these factors have been identified (Kirkwood et al, 1977; Barrowcliffe and Kirkwood, 1980; Barrowcliffe et al, 1983). However, although problems have been identified and improvement in performance has been demonstrated by standardizing methodology and reagents used, clearly unless all laboratories performing factor VIII assays take note of these variables a large variation will remain, as clearly demonstrated in UK NEQAS surveys. It is of utmost importance for the correct diagnosis and monitoring of haemophilia and von Willebrand's disease (vWD) that these problems are solved and methodology strictly followed.

Control of Factor IX Assays

Factor IX may be assayed by one-stage or, more recently, by chromogenic methods. Most laboratories in the UK currently use the one-stage assay. All methodology variables and internal quality control procedures considered for the assay of factor VIII also apply to the assay of factor IX.

External quality control of factor IX assays

UK NEQAS surveys include factor IX assays at periodic intervals. Two hundred and nineteen laboratories in the UK participated in a recent survey: of these only one laboratory performed a chromogenic assay.

As the assay of factor IX is basically the same as for factor VIII, the same variables in standards and reagents used by participants are seen. The sample for assessment was from a carrier of haemophilia B. According to the phospholipid reagent used, the median factor IX level was 38.8 iu/dl, ranging from 32 iu/dl to 51 iu/dl. However, the actual spread of results ranged from 15 iu/dl to 70 iu/dl with a small number of laboratories assessing the level as 100 iu/dl. When results are assessed according to the reference plasma used rather than the phospholipid, median values ranged from 29 iu/dl to 40 iu/dl.

Results were interpreted as abnormal by 85.7% of participants, as borderline by 9.7% and as normal by 4.6%. It is of interest to note that in this survey a breakdown was given of normal ranges quoted by participants. The lower limit of normal quoted for factor IX ranged from 25 iu/dl to 70 iu/dl showing that there is clear disagreement on what is considered to be the lower limit of normal.

There is a clear indication from this and previous surveys that as many problems apply to the assay of factor IX as they do to the assay of factor VIII, which may include the standard being used, reagents or application to methodology. Clearly these problems should be addressed, not only by the experts but by all laboratories routinely performing these assays to enable more clear diagnosis of factor IX deficiency.

Control of von Willebrand factor (vWF) Assays

For clear differentiation between haemophilia A and von Willebrand's disease, accurate measurement of vWF is an essential requirement for diagnostic laboratories. von Willebrand factor (vWF) may be measured antigenically (vWFAg) or functionally (vWFRiCof) and in general terms levels are normal in haemophilia A and reduced in von Willebrand's disease. In variant forms of von Willebrand's disease, antigenic measurement may be normal and functional vWF reduced.

vWFAg

vWFAg has traditionally been measured by Laurell immunoelectrophoresis (Laurell, 1966) though in recent years ELISA techniques have become increasingly popular. Good comparison is obtained by both methods generally (Bartlett et al, 1976). Both methods involve the use of a rabbit anti-human vWF precipitating antibody. Using the Laurell technique, vWFAg is visualized as a precipitin peak (Laurell rocket), the height of this peak being proportional to vWFAg concentration.

The concentration of antibody used, volume of sample applied and general electrophoretic conditions are critical for maximal sensitivity and should be established in individual laboratories. Antibody suitable for this assay is available from several manufacturers; the concentration required should be carefully established for each batch as incorrect antibody levels will result in peaks that are either ill defined or too short to allow accurate measurement, thus sensitivity will be lost. If carefully established, this method should give results sensitive to a level of approx 5 u/dl with good reproducibility.

Using the ELISA technique, vWF antibody is coated overnight onto a 96-well polypropylene flat-bottomed microplate. Dilutions of test samples and reference standard are applied and incubated. During this incubation vWFAg will bind to the anti-vWFAg bound to the plate. Peroxidase conjugated anti-vWFAg is then applied, which binds to the vWFAg forming an Ab:Ag:Ab layer on the plate. Finally an enzyme substrate is added and hydrolysis occurs resulting in colour development. The reaction is stopped by addition of 1.5M H_2SO_4 and colour measured at 490 nm. The amount of colour is directly proportional to the vWFAg concentration.

At each stage, excess unbound antibody or antigen is washed off the plate: it is important that sufficient thorough washes (three or four) are used and that the plate is properly drained before addition of the next reagent or the result will be poor reproducibility. Use of an automated microplate washer, several of which are now available, may significantly improve reproducibility of results compared with manual washing and reduces the risk to the operator with high-risk samples.

The concentration of both the "coat" and "tag" antibody is critical to obtain maximal binding at each stage and should be carefully established: incorrect antibody concentrations will result in poor sensitivity. Sample dilutions and incubation times used should also be optimized for maximal binding and once established kept consistent.

Though ELISA techniques are probably open to more error than Laurell techniques, when carefully established they generally produce results sensitive to levels below 5 u/dl with high reproducibility. Whichever method is used, careful attention to detail is required for reproducible results.

vWFRiCof

Functional vWF activity may be measured by several techniques based on the ristocetin aggregation of platelets. Platelets washed free of vWF are mixed with a range of dilutions of reference standard and test plasma and the response to ristocetin then monitored. The end-point may be monitored by platelet count (Evans and Austen, 1977), by monitoring optical density change in an aggregometer (Weiss et al, 1973) or by visual agglutination on a tile (Reisner et al, 1978). The response to ristocetin is directly proportional to functional vWF and reflects primarily the presence of large molecular weight vWF multimers.

For platelet count or aggregation techniques, platelets may be prepared locally in which case they may be freshly washed on the day of the assay or fixed with formalin. Freshly washed platelets will only have a few hours shelf-life and must be used on the day of preparation, whereas formalin-fixed platelets allow a large batch to be prepared that have a longer shelf-life for assay use (Allain et al, 1975; Kirby and Mills, 1975). The preparation of platelets for use in these assays is critical and great care must be taken that the platelets have been thoroughly washed free of vWF but that they have not been activated in the process or they will not function efficiently in the assay, resulting in poor reproducibility of results. Problems in preparing suitable platelet suspensions may be overcome by using lyophilized platelets available commercially: these are ready for use after reconstitution and, though expensive, are suitable if only small numbers of vWF assays are being performed.

Commercial kits are also available for vWF measurement; generally these are based on degree of aggregation on a tile and though one worker may produce consistent results, this method is probably open to more variation because of variability in grading the reaction obtained.

Generally vWF measurement by these methods is open to more variability than other coagulation techniques, primarily due to source and preparation of platelets, ristocetin concentration used (generally 1 mg/ml final concentration) and variability in monitoring of the end-point. However, careful control of methodology as with any technique reduces this variation so that in experienced hands the assay should give reproducible results.

More recently, ELISA techniques have been developed for functional vWF measurement based on either the ability of vWF to bind to collagen (Brown and Bosak, 1986; Gilchrist et al, 1990) or by using a monoclonal antibody to the functional vWF binding site (Goodall et al, 1985, modification of). Both methods are similar in principle to the measurement of vWFAg by ELISA and are thus open to the same variables at each stage of the method, i.e. efficient washing, antibody concentration, incubation times, etc. However, these can be carefully controlled and generally ELISA methods produce a lower coefficient of variation than aggregation-based methods.

Generally a good comparison of both types of ELISA techniques to aggregometry methods has been reported in all types of von Willebrand's disease patients (Brown and Bosak, 1986; unpublished report), though discrepancies in some type IIb von Willebrand's disease have been reported (Gilchrist et al, 1990).

The use of normal and abnormal control plasmas as an assessment of variability and quality of results is an essential part of internal quality control of these assays and the same procedures for their assessment should be used as for other assays performed in the laboratory. The source of reference plasma, as with other assays, is of great importance as this will affect the results obtained on patients, thus a properly calibrated plasma standard should be used: these are available commercially or from NIBSC and were discussed earlier in this chapter.

External quality assessment of vWF assays

UK NEQAS surveys regularly include assessment of both vWFAg and RiCof and participation by laboratories regularly performing these assays is important.

A recent UK NEQAS survey for vWFAg showed that approximately 47% of laboratories now use an ELISA technique. The sample for assessment was from a donor with mild vWD. Median results according to reference plasma used varied from 35 u/dl to 63 u/dl though the actual spread of results was from 5 u/dl to 70 u/dl.

Assessment of vWF activity showed that a variety of methods were used. Approximately 50% of participants used aggregometry methods, 20% visual agglutination and 16% ELISA methods.

According to the method used, median results ranged from 12 u/dl to 35 u/dl with an overall CV by ELISA of 16% compared with 53% for aggregometry and agglutination methods, resulting in an actual range of results from 0 u/dl to 45 u/dl though a small number of laboratories reported results of up to 75 u/dl. Normal ranges quoted by each laboratory in a previous survey show a lower limit of normal to be between 38 u/dl and 70 u/dl, showing clearly that there is disagreement over what levels some laboratories consider indicative of von Willebrand's disease. Thus there is also disagreement over interpretation of results in this case.

Although the particular survey quoted shows a patient with mild von Willebrand's disease, a similar spread of results has been obtained in previous surveys where vWF levels were more clearly reduced.

Unsatisfactory performance for both vWFAg and RiCof within UK NEQAS generally tends to be higher than for factor VIII clotting activity, clearly highlighting that though some laboratories have adequate control over performance of technique, there is an unacceptable variation in assessment of vWF, which must be improved if correct diagnosis is to be made.

Factor VIII Inhibitor Detection and Quantitation

Inhibitor Screening

Factor VIII inhibitors are characteristically time dependent and screening for their presence may be tested by a modification of the APTT. Methods used by laboratories vary but generally involve testing the degree of correction of the APTT on mixtures of test and normal plasma that are incubated and non-incubated, the incubated mixture showing an increase in clotting time in comparison to the non-incubated mixture in the presence of an inhibitor to factor VIII. Many laboratories use a 1:1 mix of test to normal plasma though it has been shown that a 4:1 mix of test to normal plasma increases sensitivity to low levels of inhibitor (Kasper, 1982).

The incubation time used for this screening test is of importance as anti-VIII is time dependent; generally 1 or 2 hours is used and should be sufficient for inhibitor detection. Shorter incubation times may result in a lack of sensitivity to low-level inhibitors. It is important that the method used within each laboratory is a standardized technique.

Inhibitor quantitation

A variety of methods for quantitating factor VIII inhibitors have been used in the past though the main methods now used are the Bethesda method (Kasper et al, 1975) and the New Oxford method (Rizza and Biggs, 1973). The principle is the same whichever method is used: dilutions of patient plasma and a negative control are incubated with a standardized source of factor VIII for a specified time at 37°C. At the end of the incubation the residual factor VIII is assayed as a percentage of the control and the inhibitor level calculated from this.

Both the Bethesda and New Oxford methods have the same definition of an inhibitor unit, i.e. one inhibitor unit per ml of plasma destroys 50% of added factor VIII in 2 hours or 4 hours, respectively. Thus it is important that the dilutions of patient plasma resulting in residual factor VIII levels in the region of 50% are used for inhibitor calculation. In fact the Bethesda method states that if a range of dilutions has been incubated with factor VIII then the lowest dilution to give a 50% residual factor VIII be used for this calculation. In patients whose inhibitor shows straightforward kinetics this will not be a problem, however patients with complex kinetics may show two or three dilutions that result in residual VIII activity of around 50%. Obviously this can make a vast difference to the final inhibitor level, thus it is thought more correct to use the first dilution giving a 50% residual factor VIII.

Using the New Oxford method, residual factor VIII activity is plotted against dilution used on log/log paper, a curve is drawn and the dilution that would give a 50% residual factor VIII extrapolated from the graph. Generally the problems experienced with the Bethesda assay in patients with complex kinetics do not arise with the New Oxford method as the incubation time is 4 hours compared with 2 hours for the Bethesda method. It is thought that this overcomes the problems seen in quantitating complex kinetics inhibitors.

Whichever method is used, it is critical that the incubation time and subsequent assay of residual factor VIII is standardized as variation in this will lead to variation in inhibitor levels because factor VIII inhibitors are progressive and thus destruction of factor VIII in vitro will continue.

The New Oxford method uses factor VIII concentrate as a source of factor VIII: concentrate is diluted to approximately 5 u/ml and added to the patient's plasma dilutions to give a final concentration of 1 u/ml. The control should thus contain approximately 1 u/ml of factor VIII but to exclude minor variation the control is also assayed against a calibrated standard and inhibitor levels corrected according to the assayed rather than assumed value of the control. Variables may occur depending on the source of factor VIII concentrate being used for this assay and this may be of particular relevance in recent years with the introduction of a range of higher purity and recombinant factor VIII concentrates. It may be relevant to perform inhibitor assays using the particular concentrate that the patient is receiving. Littlewood et al (1991) have performed studies showing that the source of human factor VIII had a marked effect on the inhibitory activity of a panel of four inhibitors.

The Bethesda method, established in 1976, uses a plasma pool as a source of factor VIII. Some laboratories do not have factor concentrates easily available so this was thought to be a way of overcoming variability between laboratories caused by the source of factor VIII used for the assay. However, it is important that a large donor pool is used so that the factor VIII level is approximately 1 u/ml – small donor pools will have variable factor VIII activity resulting in variation in assessment of inhibitor levels.

An equal volume of plasma pool is added to patients' plasma dilutions so that in fact the actual starting factor VIII level is 50%. Normally no correction is performed to allow for this, as in the New Oxford method, though in some laboratories a correction is made according to the assayed value of the control.

External quality control of factor VIII inhibitors

Samples for quantitation of factor VIII inhibitors have not been included in NEQAS in recent years. However, a collaborative study showed that error between laboratories was much greater than within laboratories (Austen et al, 1982). It is clear that factor VIII inhibitor assays are open to several variables, including the assay of factor VIII. However, by careful control of method conditions used within a laboratory, variation resulting from technical factors may be kept to a minimum. Unfortunately it is not so easy to control variables that occur in methodology between laboratories.

References

Allain JP, Cooper HA, Wagner RH, et al. Platelets fixed with paraformaldehyde: a new reagent for assay of von Willebrand factor and platelet aggregating factor. *Journal of Laboratory and Clinical Medicine* 1975; **85:** 318.

Austen DEG, Lechner K, Rizza CR, et al. A comparison of the Bethesda and New Oxford methods of factor VIII antibody assay. *Thrombosis and Haemostasis* 1982; **47:** 72.

Bangham DR, Biggs R, Brozovic M, Denson KWE, Skegg JL. A biological standard for measurement of blood coagulation factor VIII activity. *Bulletin of the WHO* 1971; **45:** 337.

Barna L, Triplett DA. Use of the activated partial thromboplastin time for the diagnosis of congenital coagulation disorders: problems and possible solutions. *Research in Clinic and Laboratory* 1989; **19:** 345.

Barrowcliffe TW. Methodology of the two-stage assay of factor VIII (VIII:C). *Scandinavian Journal of Haematology* 1984; **41:** (suppl): 25.

Barrowcliffe TW. Standardization of factors II, VII, IX and X in plasma and concentrates. Report of the ICTH sub-committee on factors VIII and IX, Brussels. *Thrombosis and Haemostasis* 1988; **59:** 334.

Barrowcliffe TW. Standardisation and assay. *Seminars in Thrombosis and Haemostasis* 1993; **19:** 73.

Barrowcliffe TW. Recommendations for the Assay of High-Purity Factor VIII Concentrates. Scientific and Standardization Committee Communication. Factor VIII and Factor IX Sub-Committee. *Stuttgart: FK Schattauer* 1994; **70:** 876.

Barrowcliffe TW, Gray E. Studies of phospholipid reagents used in coagulation. 1: Some general properties and their sensitivity to factor VIII. *Thrombosis and Haemostasis* 1981; **46:** 629.

Barrowcliffe TW, Kirkwood TBL. Standardisation of factor VIII. I. Calibration of British standards for factor VIII clotting activity. *British Journal of Haematology* 1980; **46:** 471.

Barrowcliffe TW, Tydeman MS, Kirkwood TBL. Major effect of prediluent in factor IX clotting assay. *Lancet* 1979; **2:** 192.

Barrowcliffe TW, Tydeman MS, Kirkwood TBL, Thomas DP. Standardisation of factor VIII. III. Establishment of a stable reference plasma for factor VIII-related activities. *Thrombosis and Haemostasis* 1983; **50:** 690.

Barrowcliffe TW, Watton J, Tubbs JE, Harman A, Kemball-Cook G. Potency of high purity factor VIII concentrates. *Lancet* 1990; **2:** 124.

Barrowcliffe TW, Tubbs JE, Wong MY. Evaluation of factor VIII deficient plasmas. *Thrombosis and Haemostasis* 1993; **70:** 433.

Bartlett A, Dormandy KM, Hawkey CM, Stableforth P, Voller A. Factor VIII-related antigen: measurement by enzyme immunoassay. *British Medical Journal* 1976; **1:** 994.

Brown JE, Bosak JO. An ELISA test for the binding of von Willebrand antigen to collagen. *Thrombosis Research* 1986; **43:** 303.

Brozovic M, Robertson I, Kirwood TBL. Study of a proposed international standard for blood coagulation factor IX. *Thrombosis and Haemostasis* 1976; **35:** 222.

Campbell PJ. International biological standards and reference preparations. II: Procedures used for the production of biological standards and reference preparations. *Journal of Biological Standardisation* 1974; **2:** 259.

Denson KWE. The simplified two-stage assay for factor VIII using a combined reagent. In: *Transactions of the Conference of the International Committee on Haemostasis and Thrombosis, USA. Stuttgart: FK Schattauer,* 1967: 419.

Denson, KWE. In *Human Blood Coagulation, Haemostasis and Thrombosis.* R Biggs (ed). 1976 Oxford: Blackwell Scientific Publications. pp. 688–692.

Denson KWE, Wilkins T. Semi-automation of the two-stage factor VIII assay. *Clinical and Laboratory Haematology* 1980; **2:** 311.

Evans RJ, Austen DEG. Assay of ristocetin co-factor using fixed platelets and a platelet counting technique. *British Journal of Haematology* 1977; **37:** 289.

Gilchrist M, Stewart M, Etches W, Gordon PA. Rapid diagnosis of von Willebrand's disease using ELISA technology. *Thrombosis Research* 1990; **57:** 659.

Godfrey R, Rhymes IL, Bidwell E, et al. The buffering of anticoagulants for blood collection. *Thrombosis et Diathesis Haemorrhagica* 1975; **34:** 879.

Goodall AH, Jarvis J, Chand S, et al. An immunoradiometric assay for human factor VIII/von Willebrand factor using a monoclonal antibody that defines a functional epitope. *British Journal of Haematology* 1985; **59:** 565.

Heath AB, Barrowcliffe TW. Standardisation of Factor VIII. V. Calibration of the 2nd International Standard for factor VIII and von Willebrand factor Activities in Plasma. *Thrombosis and Haemostasis* 1992; **68:** 155–159.

Hubbard AR, Curtis AD, Barrowcliffe TW, et al. Assay of factor VIII concentrates: comparison of chromogenic and 2-stage clotting assays. *Thrombosis Research* 1986; **44:** 891.

Hutton RA, Kamiguti AS, Matthews KB, Woodhams BJ. The use of a chromogenic assay for factor VIII in patients with factor VIII inhibitors or von Willebrand's disease. *Thrombosis Research* 1991; **63:** 651.

Ingram GIC, Hills M. ICTH reference method for the one stage prothrombin time test on human blood. *Thrombosis and Haemostasis* 1976a; **36:** 237.

Ingram GIC, Hills M. The prothrombin time test: effect of varying citrate concentration. *Thrombosis and Haemostasis* 1976b; **36:** 230.

Kasper C. Experience with the Bethesda assay and other methods of inhibitor detection. In: *Activated prothrombin complex concentrates, Chapter 3 Praeger*, 1982; 17.

Kasper C, Aledort LM, Counts RB, et al. A more uniform measurement of factor VIII inhibitors. *Thrombosis et Diathesis Haemorrhagica* 1975; **34:** 869.

Kirby EP, Mills DCB. The interaction of bovine factor VIII with human platelets. *Journal of Clinical Investigation* 1975; **56:** 491.

Kirkwood TBL. Design and analysis of accelerated degradation tests for the stability of biological standards. III: Principles of design. *Journal of Biological Standardisation* 1984; **12:** 215.

Kirkwood TBL, Barrowcliffe TW. Discrepancy between one-stage and two-stage assay of factor VIII:C. *British Journal of Haematology* 1978; **40:** 333.

Kirkwood TBL, Snape TJ. Biometric principles in clotting and clot lysis assays. *Clinical and Laboratory Haematology* 1980; **2:** 155.

Kirkwood TBL, Rizza CR, Snape TJ, et al. Identification of sources of inter-laboratory variation in factor VIII assay. *British Journal of Haematology* 1977; **37:** 559.

Koepke JA. Partial thromboplastin time test – proposed performance guidelines. *Thrombosis and Haemostasis* 1986; **55:** 143.

Lamb MA, Fricke WA, Rastogi SC. Standardization of factor IX: standards for "purified" factor IX concentrates. *Thrombosis and Haemostasis* 1991; **66:** 548.

Laurell CB. Quantitative estimation of proteins by electrophoresis in agarose gel containing antibodies. *Analytical Biochemistry* 1966; **15:** 45.

Littlewood JD, Bevan SA, Kemball-Cook G, Evans RJ, Barrowcliffe TW. Variable inactivation of human factor VII from different sources by human factor VIII inhibitors. *British Journal of Hematology* 1991; **77:** 535–538.

Poller L, Thompson J. The partial thromboplastin (cephalin) time test. *Journal of Clinical Pathology* 1972; **25:** 1038.

Poller L, Thompson J. Measuring partial thromboplastin time. *The Lancet* 1976; **2:** 842.

Reisner HM, Katz HJ, Goldin LR, et al. Use of a simple visual assay of von Willebrand factor for diagnosis and carrier identification. *British Journal of Haematology* 1978; **40:** 339.

Rizza CR, Biggs R. The treatment of patients who have factor VIII antibodies. *British Journal of Haematology* 1973; **24:** 65.

Rosen S. Assay of factor VIII:C with a chromogenic substrate. *Scandinavian Journal of Haematology* 1984; **33:** (suppl 40): 139.

Rosen S, Andersson M, Blomback M, et al. Clinical application of a chromogenic substrate method for determination of factor VIII activity. *Thrombosis and Haemostasis* 1985; **54:** 818.

Rothschild C, Amiral J, Adam M, et al. Preparation of factor VIII-depleted plasma with antibodies and its use in the assay of factor VIII. *Haemostasis* 1990; **20:** 321.

Seghatchian MJ, Miller-Anderson M. A colorimetric evaluation of factor VIII:C potency. *Journal of Medical Laboratory Sciences* 1978; **35:** 347.

Stevenson KJ, Easton AC, Thompson JM, Poller L. The reliability of activated partial thromboplastin time methods and the relationship to lipid composition and ultrastructure. *Thrombosis and Haemostasis* 1986; **55:** 250.
Takase T, Rotblat F, Goodall AH, et al. Production of factor VIII deficient plasma by immunodepletion using three monoclonal antibodies. *British Journal of Haematology* 1987; **66:** 497.
Weiss HJ, Hoyer LW, Rickles FR, Varma A, Rogers J. Quantitative assay of a plasma factor deficient in von Willebrand's disease that is necessary for platelet aggregation. *Journal of Clinical Investigation* 1973; **52:** 2708.
World Health Organization. *Technical Reports Series* 1978; **626:** 101.
World Health Organization. *Technical Reports Series* 1983; **687:** 23.
Zucker S, Cathey MH, West B. Preparation of quality control specimens for coagulation. *American Journal of Clinical Pathology* 1970; **53:** 924.

5

Replacement Therapy and Other Therapeutic Products

Henry G. Watson and
Christopher A. Ludlam

Introduction

The history of haemophilia and the development of suitable treatment for these deficiency states is a fascinating and topical subject which has attracted attention beyond the realms of science and medicine (Aldhous and Tastemain, 1992); indeed, the development of effective therapy for haemophilia has been a story of great success combined with great tragedy. The range of products currently available for the treatment of haemophilia reflects the advances made in biotechnology and includes several products produced in animal cell culture by recombinant DNA technology as well as highly purified plasma-derived products that have resulted from the development of innovative methods of chromatography. Perhaps the most important issue to have been addressed by concentrate producers is that of the viral safety of products. The thrombogenicity of factor IX concentrates and, more recently, the potential benefits and problems associated with high-purity plasma-derived and recombinant products particularly related to progression of HIV infection and risk of inhibitor development have attracted attention.

In this chapter we will discuss:

- The benefits of replacement therapy.
- Plasma source, donor screening, plasma testing for markers of viral infection.
- Methods of production of concentrates including precipitation, chromatography and recombinant DNA technology.
- Products presently available.
- Side-effects of concentrate use and methods that have been employed to prevent them, such as virus inactivation and purification of factor IX concentrates.
- Discussion of purity and of its effect on HIV disease progression and inhibitor development.

Benefits of Replacement Therapy

The benefits of a therapeutic material that successfully stops painful and life-threatening bleeding crises seem self-evident. Following the introduction of efficacious factor VIII and factor IX concentrates, haemophiliacs have been more able to participate in varied occupational, educational and social pursuits (Levine, 1974; Ingram et al, 1979; Goldsmith, 1986; Pierce et al, 1989). Over the past 20 years, patterns of mortality and morbidity have also changed. In a study of UK haemophiliacs in 1980 it was demonstrated that 44% of haemophilia A patients and 36% of haemophilia B patients were severely affected, with a preponderence of males aged 10–40 years, but a relative paucity of men aged over 40 years when compared with the non-affected population (Rizza and Spooner, 1983). However, even at this point in time a greater proportion of severely affected haemophilic men were reaching middle and old age when compared with earlier studies (Biggs and Spooner, 1977); the calculated median life expectancy at this point approximated that of the non-haemophilic population (69.1 vs 72.8 years) and, indeed, in the USA the median age of death in haemophiliacs rose almost linearly from 35 years in 1968 to 55 years in 1979 (Aronson, 1988). These figures almost certainly reflect the introduction of therapeutic blood products, which succeeded in preventing premature death as a result of bleeding. However, recent reports indicate that the majority of haemophiliac deaths, in the western world are now due to the infectious complications of this same therapy (Eyster et al, 1992; Lee et al, 1995).

History of Treatment of Haemophilia

In 1840 Lane described the first successful treatment of haemophilia, when without any knowledge of the underlying deficiency, he transfused a young haemophiliac with persistent postoperative bleeding with fresh whole blood (Lane, 1840). However, it was following the demonstration that haemophilia was due to a deficiency of a plasma factor by Addis (1911) that citrated plasma was used in bleeding episodes (Feisly, 1923; Payne and Steen, 1929). Around 40 years ago, more specific products for the treatment of haemophilia A were first prepared by cold-ethanol precipitation of factor VIII-rich Cohn fraction I (Cohn et al, 1946; Blomback and Blomback, 1956; Van Creveld et al, 1959). However, at this time, because there were problems obtaining sufficient amounts of human anti-haemophilic globulin (AHG) for clinical use and bovine AHG was easy to prepare in larger amounts and had a much higher AHG content than human plasma, concentrates of bovine factor VIII were used to treat haemophiliacs (Macfarlane et al, 1954). In the late 1950s, concentrates of anti-haemophilic factor derived from human plasma were successfully used to control bleeding from the gastrointestinal tract, into joints and also to cover dental extraction and rectal surgery (Kekwick and Wolf, 1957). The development and refinement of cryoprecipitation and its application to extraction from large plasma pools heralded an increase in the factor VIII content of concentrates (Pool and Shannon, 1965). The concentrates produced by these methods were sterile-filtered to 0.2 μm and freeze dried and were a convenient product free from bacterial contamination. Only a very small proportion of the protein content of these early concentrates was of specific coagulation factor, the majority consisting of other proteins, especially fibrinogen and fibronectin. Progress in the manufacturing of efficacious concentrates of increasing purity continued throughout the 1980s and 1990s. Advances in protein separation technology, including stabilization of clotting factors (Foster et al, 1983) and the development of chromatographic media and processes, have facilitated the production of high-purity plasma-derived concentrates. In addition, advances in molecular biology and the development of suitable vectors has resulted in the relatively recent development of factor VIII:C produced in mammalian cell lines by recombinant DNA technology (Boedeker, 1992; Gomperts et al, 1992).

The development of factor IX concentrates for clinical use followed the early factor VIII concentrates. The earliest factor IX concentrates were produced by calcium phosphate adsorption of EDTA anticoagulated plasma (Didisheim et al, 1959) and soon afterwards such a concentrate was used successfully in the treatment of patients with Christmas disease (Biggs et al, 1961). The prothrombin complex concentrates (PCC) were developed by ion exchange adsorption of the plasma supernatant remaining after either cryoprecipitation or Cohn fraction I using, for example, DEAE sephadex (Hoag et al, 1969). These concentrates contain a mixture of the vitamin K-dependent factors, the exact composition of which is dependent on the ion exchange matrix (Casillas et al, 1969; Hoag et al, 1969; Middleton et al, 1973; Pejaudier et al, 1987). The earlier PCCs contained, in addition, activated coagulation factors and their use was implicated in the development of venous thromboembolism (Blatt et al, 1974; Kasper, 1975) and disseminated intravascular coagulation (Cederbaum et al, 1976). Less thrombogenic concentrates produced by similar methodology are still used in the treatment of factor IX deficiency but recently further purification has been achieved by affinity chromatography (Menache et al, 1984; Burnouf et al, 1989; Feldman et al, 1989) and immunoaffinity chromatography (Hrinda et al, 1991). The factor IX gene has been fully sequenced and cloned and a recombinant factor IX concentrate is presently under clinical trial.

Source of Plasma Used in the Preparation of Therapeutic Coagulation Factor Concentrates

The vast majority of factor VIII and factor IX concentrates are still produced by the fractionation of plasma by both commercial fractionators and not-for-profit organizations. Early observations from the USA demonstrated that the use

Table 5.1 Viruses transmitted by coagulation factor concentrates

HIV
HAV
HBV
HCV
HDV
Parvovirus B19

of pooled concentrates of factors VIII and IX were associated with the transmission of hepatotropic viruses and the development of clinical jaundice (Kingdon, 1970; Boklan, 1971; Hellerstein and Deykin, 1971; Kasper and Kipnis, 1972). It is now clear that plasma-derived concentrates have transmitted hepatitis B virus (HBV) and hepatitis D virus (HDV) (Kingdon, 1970; Kasper and Kipnis, 1972), hepatitis C virus (HCV) (Tedder et al, 1991; Watson et al, 1992b), human immunodeficiency virus-1 (HIV-1) (CDC, 1987a,b), hepatitis A virus (HAV) (Mannucci, 1992; Mannucci et al, 1994b) and parvovirus B19 (Williams et al, 1990a; Azzi et al, 1992) (Table 5.1). This list may be incomplete and concern about others such as the causative agent of Creutzfeldt-Jakob disease, which may be transmissible by blood products (Nau, 1995), has been expressed. Clearly then, measures to prevent viral transmission by concentrates are of primary concern. Efforts to prevent virus transmission by concentrates are presently based on two main principles:

1. Decreasing the virus load in the plasma pool by:
   (i) exclusion of donors at high risk of viral infection;
   (ii) the use of screening tests to detect virus antigens, antibodies or nucleic acid which indicate that a donation is likely to transmit infection.
2. The use of physical or chemical methods to inactivate contaminating viruses and the removal or partitioning of virus during product manufacture.

Volunteer versus remunerated donors

The source of starting plasma, differs in that not-for-profit organizations in general depend on unpaid volunteer donors, whereas commercial companies normally pay for their plasma. One of the main arguments against the use of plasma from remunerated donors is that products from this source have historically been more likely to transmit viral infection such as HBV, HCV and HIV (Leikola, 1993). Studies of single donor units have shown a higher incidence of post-transfusion hepatitis in recipients of products from remunerated donors (Prince et al, 1974; Koretz and Gitnick, 1975). In addition, fractionated products from volunteer donors, prior to the introduction of donor screening, had a lower incidence of HBsAg than commercial products (Hoofnagle et al, 1976). For these reasons it has been recommended within the EEC that all plasma products should be prepared from non-remunerated donors (EEC, 1989). However, with current donor selection procedures, screening of donations and virucidal steps in the manufacturing process, there is little difference between the viral safety of concentrates produced from volunteer and remunerated donors.

New versus established donors

The incidence of infection with transmissible viruses is higher in first-time donors than in those who have previously donated. Studies on donors in the USA show a higher incidence of infection with HBV and HCV as well as HIV and HTLV-1 in newly recruited donors (Myhre and Figueroa, 1995). At present in volunteer British donors the incidence of infection is four times higher in new, compared with established, donors (Gillon, 1995 personal communication).

Donor self-exclusion

Potential blood donors at increased risk of viral infection are first given the opportunity to self-withdraw from donation before being questioned about risk of infection. Individuals with a history of particular activities such as intravenous drug abuse, certain types of sexual activity, and treatment with pooled plasma products and other biological preparations such as growth hormone are not accepted as blood donors. Although the process of donor selection is of great importance, especially given the limitations of the other methods for ensuring viral safety discussed below, it may still fail to detect all donors with potentially transmissible viral infection.

Donor screening

In order to produce virally safe coagulation factor concentrates, testing for potential infection can be performed using antibody, antigen or DNA/RNA-based assays at different stages in concentrate production. The use of surrogate markers of infection such as alanine amino transferase (ALT) has been largely superseded by the development of sensitive assays for the detection of HCV, and the observation that the correlation between surrogate markers and any true infection marker is poor (Myhre et al, 1994). Screening of individual donations for markers of infection is likely to be the most sensitive method of detecting risk of virus infectivity, although screening of plasma pools for antibody (Minor et al, 1990; Simmonds et al, 1990) and viral nucleic acid (Simmonds et al, 1990; McOmish

Table 5.2 Viruses detected by PCR in concentrates

HIV
HCV
HAV
Parvovirus B19

et al, 1993) has been performed. Antibody-based testing of concentrates is almost certainly of no value given their low immunoglobulin content. The polymerase chain reaction (PCR) has been used successfully to detect viral nucleic acid in concentrates (Table 5.2). Ideally assays with a high predictive value should be available for detecting all infectious agents of concern and this would seem to be a reasonable future goal. Presently, plasma donations are screened for markers of infection with anti-HIV 1 and 2, HBsAg and anti-HCV but not for markers of infection with parvovirus B19, HAV and HDV.

Hepatitis B virus

Screening blood donations for HBsAg began in 1969 and has continued since with improved methods. Present screening techniques are probably greater than 99% sensitive and detect antigen levels of 0.1–0.3 iu/ml. However, certain individuals have low levels of HBsAg or may indeed be HBsAg negative but have circulating HBV DNA (Thiers et al, 1988; Lai et al, 1989). As a result, hepatitis B infection may occur in individuals transfused with HBsAg-negative blood products (Hoofinagle et al, 1978; Lander et al, 1978; Katchaki et al, 1981). The current incidence of hepatitis B infection in recipients of single donor screened products in the USA is around 0.002% per transfusion recipient (Dodd, 1989). There has been some debate about the improved sensitivity offered by also performing anti-HB core screening on plasma donations but at present this is not widespread practice.

Human immunodeficiency virus

Testing blood donations for anti-HIV began in most countries in 1985. This is presently done using a combined anti-HIV-1/HIV-2 assay. In established volunteer donors the prevalence of infection is extremely low (Myhre and Figueroa, 1995). Donations repeatedly anti-HIV positive by ELISA are confirmed by western blot technique and in some centres by PCR. Screening of donations for antibodies to HIV does not, however, ensure a completely safe blood supply as a very small minority of HIV-infected donors will be in the so-called window period, being viraemic but without a detectable antibody response at the time of testing (Urbaniek, 1990; Lackritz et al, 1995).

Hepatitis C virus

In the early 1970s it became apparent that the majority of post-transfusion hepatitis was not caused by infection with HAV, HBV or any other virus for which serological tests were available. However, despite continued effort it was not until 1989 that hepatitis C virus (HCV) was discovered and a serological assay to detect antibodies against the virus developed (Choo et al, 1989; Kuo et al, 1989). A great deal of information has been rapidly accrued about HCV despite the fact that no-one has as yet seen or been able to culture the virus (Houghton et al, 1994). A first-generation ELISA which incorporated only non-structural peptides was the first to be commercially available. This assay was capable of detecting most cases of HCV infection but was also complicated by a high incidence of false positive (Skidmore, 1990; Theilmann et al, 1990; McFarlane et al, 1990) and false negative results (Simmonds et al, 1990). In certain high-risk populations the assay performed reasonably well (Ludlam et al, 1989; Makris et al, 1990); however, in blood donors the results were particularly disappointing and difficult to interpret (Skidmore, 1990). Detection of infected blood donations has, however, been improved by the introduction of further screening ELISAs and blot-type confirmatory assays containing both structural and non-structural peptides and by the use of PCR to detect viraemic samples. Recently, type-specific serological and genotyping assays have been developed (Simmonds et al, 1993, 1994). Most western countries now use second-or third-generation tests for screening of blood donations. Using second-generation recombinant immunoblot assays (RIBA) the incidence of HCV infection amongst blood donors varies from 0.02% in Finland to 1.23% in Saudi Arabia (Saeed et al, 1991; Kolho, 1992).

"Window periods" using currently available assays to detect viral infection

As alluded to above, even with the sensitive screening methods available there does exist a "window period" during which infectious donations may be missed. Using the presently available assays, in volunteer donors a window period of 6–38 days is estimated for the anti-HIV-1/HIV-2 assay giving an average annual risk of 1 in 300 000–400 000 infectious donations being missed as a result of being tested in the window period (Urbaniek, 1990; Lackritz et al, 1995). For HBV, using HBsAg tests, the window is 24–128 days with a failed pick-up rate of 1 in 153 194, while for second-generation anti-HCV tests the window period is 56–189 days with a failure rate of 1 in 61 639 (Busch, 1995).

Other agents and screening methods

There is no validated method available at present allowing the exclusion of other viruses such as HAV and parvovirus B19. Clearly, given the high prevalence of seropositivity amongst donors and the arguments in favour of retaining neutralizing antibody in plasma pools, exclusion on the basis of an antibody test is not feasible. The role of PCR has been investigated in these situations and may allow the identification from plasma pools of positive donations (McOmish et al, 1993). However, as in other situations where PCR has been applied, there are problems at present concerning (i) potential cross-contamination in the laboratory; (ii) lack of sensitivity for RNA viruses because of low efficiency of the reverse transcription; (iii) lack of automation and problems with large-scale operations; and (iv) controversy in the interpretation of positive and negative results. At the time of writing, there is no evidence that plasma-derived concentrates of coagulation factors transmit the agent responsible for Creutzfeldt-Jakob disease.

Plasma age and factor VIII content

It has been demonstrated that the age of plasma at the time of initial freezing does affect the factor VIII yield of the cryoprecipitate formed. Plasma frozen within 8 hours of donation produces a higher yield than plasma that is older (Foster and Dickson, 1985). There is, however, difficulty in translating this benefit into a significantly greater factor VIII content at the end of the overall fractionation process due to loss of VIII:C by a variety of different mechanisms.

Methods of Production of Therapeutic Products for Use in Bleeding Disorders

The most common congenital bleeding disorders are haemophilia A and B and von Willebrand's disease (vWD) and therefore most effort has been expended to produce satisfactory concentrates for the treatment of these three conditions. Table 5.3 summarizes the methods used in the production of factor VIII and IX concentrates.

Precipitation

Up until the early 1990s, intermediate-purity lyophilized concentrates produced by precipitation techniques were the cornerstone of haemophilia treatment. Precipitation is dependent on the different solubility of proteins as outlined by

Table 5.3 Methods used in the production of factor VII and IX concentrates

Precipitation
Adsorption
Chromatography
Ion exchange
Chemicoaffinity
Immunoaffinity
Recombinant DNA technology

Cohn (Cohn et al, 1946). These concentrates, in general, contain at most two to five units of factor VIII per milligram of protein along with many other contaminating proteins such as fibrinogen and fibronectin. As a result of the development of satisfactory virucidal methods, there are now safe and efficacious intermediate-purity factor VIII concentrates available (Schimpf et al, 1987; Skidmore et al, 1990; Evans et al, 1991). However, these are going out of favour as the high-purity concentrates produced by improved methods of chromatography and recombinant DNA technology have become available.

Adsorption techniques

The intermediate-purity factor IX concentrates are prepared by adsorption elution with DEAE or tricalcium phosphate. They are in fact prothrombin complex concentrates containing, in addition to factor IX, the other vitamin K-dependent procoagulant proteins, factors II and X, which are concentrated to the same extent as factor IX. Factor VII is not well adsorbed by DEAE and is therefore only present in trace amounts in most currently available PCCs. In addition small amounts of other proteins such as high molecular weight kininogen, C1 esterase inhibitor, factor XII, antithrombin III, α-2-macroglobulin and caeruloplasmin have been demonstrated in PCCs and activated PCCs (Pejaudier et al, 1987).

Chromatographic techniques

The high-purity products now available are the direct results of improvements in protein chemistry. Chromatography has become the central process in nearly all plasma fractionation because it allows the specific isolation of biologically active proteins. Different forms of chromatography are presently used in the production of most plasma-derived factor VIII and IX concentrates.

Ion-exchange chromatography

Ion-exchange chromatography (IEC) is based on the principle that plasma proteins will be differentially absorbed to suitably charged ion-exchange resins. These processes are not specific but proteins can be further purified by differential elution achieved by changing the pH or the ionic strength of the buffers employed.

Chemico-affinity chromatography

Intermediate-purity factor IX concentrates are produced by DEAE or tricalcium phosphate adsorption and elution; however, such concentrates can be further purified by affinity chromatography using heparin agarose, dextran sulphate or metal chelates.

Immunoaffinity chromatography

Factor VIII prepared by immunoaffinity chromatography became available in 1986, and immunoaffinity-purified factor IX concentrates in 1991. Purification of the target protein is achieved using monoclonal antibodies directed against specific epitopes on the molecule. The monoclonal factor VIII concentrates presently available are produced using antibodies against either von Willebrand factor (vWF) to capture the vWF/VIII complex (Monoclate, Armour) or directly against the factor VIII molecule (Hemofil, Baxter). When anti-vWF antibodies are used, elution with calcium is required to improve the recovery of almost pure factor VIII, the majority of the vWF being retained on the chromatography column. Concentrates produced by this method have a factor VIII content of up to 3000 iu/mg of protein but are unstable in this highly purified state until they are diluted and stabilized by human albumin to give a final purity of 10–30 iu factor VIII/mg protein.

Presently only one manufacturer is producing a factor IX for therapeutic use by immunoaffinity chromatography (Mononine, Armour). The process developed uses a murine IgG-1 anti-IX monoclonal antibody, the immunoaffinity chromatography being performed on a prothrombin complex concentrate. After the chromatographic step the factor IX is eluted with sodium thiocyanate, and ultrafiltration as a means of virus removal is followed by aminohexyl sepharose chromatography to remove any residual mouse protein (Hrinda et al, 1991; Kim et al, 1992). Preclinical characterization studies demonstrate the product purity with a factor IX content of around 200 iu/mg of protein and the absence of factors II, VII and X as well as IXa from the concentrate (Hrinda et al, 1991). Further details relating to thrombogenicity are discussed later.

Recombinant DNA techniques

In 1984 the successful cloning and expression of factor VIII was described (Gitschier et al, 1984; Toole et al, 1984). Around this time also the nature and size of the infectious problems associated with the use of plasma-derived products in the treatment of haemophilia became apparent and a rationale for the development of a totally recombinant product free of these problems emerged. The recombinant factor VIII products are prepared by transfecting the cDNA encoding human factor VIII into baby hamster kidney or chinese hamster ovary cell lines. Problems of low-level expression due to low mRNA synthesis and protein instability, because of degradation of the heavy chain following secretion, presently limit the levels of production of recombinant factor VIII. Efforts to improve the efficiency of production have focused primarily on the development of cDNA constructs lacking most of the B domain, which is not required for normal procoagulant function of the protein (Toole et al, 1986). Experiments with different B domainless constructs have demonstrated proteins with the same cleavage patterns with thrombin as plasma-derived factor VIII (Eaton et al, 1986) but with increased yield. Other methods to increase production of recombinant products such as the insertion of translation initiation sequences are being tested and in view of the current rate of progress in biotechnology it is likely that increased amounts of recombinant factor VIII will be forthcoming.

Although the factor IX gene was cloned and sequenced in 1982 (Choo et al, 1982; Kurachi and Davie, 1982), a recombinant factor IX concentrate for clinical use has yet to be licensed. There are specific problems that have hampered the production of a recombinant factor IX protein, which are mainly due to the multiple post-translational modifications that are required to produce functional factor IX, e.g. propeptide cleavage, glycosylation, and carboxylation of the N-terminal glutamic acid residues. Because of the limitations of most expression systems to perform these post-translational modifications, large amounts of non-functional factor IX are produced admixed with biologically active protein. In order to increase the yield of functional factor IX, methods such as immunoaffinity purification using conformation-specific antibodies against the factor IX metal complex have been developed. This process ensures binding to the antibody column of carboxylated factor IX only (Liebman et al, 1985). Alternative strategies to increase expression might include the modification of cell lines to incorporate, for example, vitamin K-dependent carboxylase genes. Animal experiments using a recombinant factor IX have reported plasma half-lives of 12–14 hours, comparable to Mononine (Keith et al, 1994).

Polyelectrolyte fractionation of animal plasma

As products from human plasma became more abundant, the use of non-human factor VIII has diminished and now the only widely used non-human concentrate is a porcine factor VIII, which is indicated for use in individuals with high-level anti-human VIII antibodies. Porcine VIII (Hyate C, Speywood) is produced by polyelectrolyte fractionation of cryoprecipitate of pooled porcine plasma. This separation procedure has the advantage that it removes the majority of the platelet-aggregating activity produced by vWF, which previously hampered the use of this product.

Products Available for the Treatment of Congenital Bleeding Disorders

Guidelines on haemophilia treatment

A number of sets of guidelines to haemophilia treatment have been drawn up to assist with the optimisation of haemophilia care (UK Regional Haemophilia Centre Directors Committee, 1992; Schramm W, 1994). Such guidelines require regular review to keep abreast with the type of developments outlined elsewhere in this chapter. The UK Haemophilia Centre Directors Organisation for example has recently published updated recommendations on many aspects of treatment including guidelines on the management of patients with inhibitors (UK Haemophilia Centre Directors Organisation Executive Committee, 1997; Hay et al, 1996).

Purity of concentrates

Before describing the concentrates available for treatment it is first important to outline some of the controversy surrounding the terminology used to describe their purity. The basic problem relates to the lack of a standard definition of purity, particularly of factor VIII concentrates. To prevent the degradation of factor VIII produced by immunoaffinity and recombinant DNA technology, albumin is added to the final product; however, the specific activity of the concentrate is still quoted by certain manufacturers as that of the coagulation factor prior to albumin addition. Clearly, this is of relevance in the discussion of the effect of product purity on HIV disease progression and anti-factor VIII inhibitor development. The second controversy concerns the vWF content of factor VIII concentrates given its role as the natural carrier of factor VIII and therefore whether or not it is appropriate to consider it as a contaminant when expressing product purity.

These issues do therefore require some attention so that a standard nomenclature can be applied in manufacturers' statements on concentrates giving information on factor VIII, and vWF content as well as the method of preparation of the concentrate.

Fresh-frozen plasma

Fresh-frozen plasma (FFP) is used in the treatment of deficiency states for which there is no suitable concentrate, as well as in the treatment of haemophilia A and B in some developing countries. The advantage of being derived from a single donor source may be more than offset by the high incidence of blood-borne infection in the areas where these products are used. Because of its high protein content it has been hard to incorporate a virucidal method into the production of FFP. However, pasteurization, a solvent detergent and a photo-inactivation method have recently been applied to the manufacture of FFP (Horowitz et al, 1992; Mohr et al, 1992; Burnouf-Radosevich et al, 1992), although there are as yet no studies to demonstrate their efficacy in clinical use.

Cryoprecipitate

The cryoprecipitate of citrated plasma has a high content of fibrinogen, factor VIII and vWF and its use in preventing and stopping bleeding is well documented. However, as a result of problems with storage, circulatory overload, anaphylaxis and viral infections, the guidelines of the United Kingdom Haemophilia Centre Directors (1992) presently do not recommend it for treatment of haemophilia or von Willebrand's disease (vWD), although it does continue to have uses in the treatment of individuals with hypo- or afibrinogenaemia and dysfibrinogenaemia, both congenital and acquired. As is the case with FFP, attempts to improve the viral safety of cryoprecipitate have been made (Smit Sibinga et al, 1988).

Intermediate-purity factor VIII concentrates

These concentrates are produced predominantly by precipitation techniques and have a factor VIII content of between 2 and 5 iu/mg of protein. The half-life and recovery of these products in vivo are similar to the new high-purity concentrates developed using chromatographic techniques (Mannucci and Morfini, 1990). The main problem associated with their use has been transmission of viruses, especially HIV, HBV, HCV and parvovirus B19. Although this problem has been largely overcome by the development of suitable donor screening and effective virucidal techniques, higher-purity concentrates are presently being favoured by many haemophilia treaters for reasons discussed below.

High-purity factor VIII concentrates produced by ion-exchange and gel filtration

Concentrates produced by such methods contain 50–200 iu factor VIII/mg protein and a variable amount of vWF. The factor VIII concentrates produced by these methods do not in general require the addition of stabilizers such as albumin, unlike proteins manufactured using immunoaffinity chromatography. Gel filtration products have a slightly lower content of factor VIII (9–22 iu/mg).

High-purity factor VIII concentrates produced by immunoaffinity chromatography

During the manufacture of concentrates by immunoaffinity methods, a factor VIII purity of 3000 iu/mg protein is achieved. However, the almost pure protein is not suitable for storage or clinical use and albumin and sugars must be added as stabilizers. This results in a final specific activity of factor VIII of 5–30 iu/mg of protein. These products may contain up to 50 ng mouse immunoglobulin per 100 units of factor VIII; however, there is no evidence of immune sensitization to mouse protein in recipients of these concentrates (Haimovich et al, 1990). Studies demonstrate that the half-life of these products is equivalent to plasma-derived intermediate-purity concentrates (Mannucci and Morfini, 1990). Issues relating to the effect of these concentrates on HIV disease progression and inhibitor development are discussed later.

High-purity plasma-derived factor IX concentrates

The high-purity factor IX concentrates, or coagulation factor IX concentrates as they have been called, are produced from PCC by affinity chromatography using heparin, dextran sulphate and metal chelate, or by immunoaffinity chromatography. A study of the comparative compositions of prothrombin complex concentrates, high-purity affinity concentrates and immunoaffinity products demonstrates clear differences in the purity of the products as well as the factor IX content (Berntorp et al, 1993). The PCCs have a factor IX content of around 2 iu/mg protein compared with 89–278 iu/mg protein in the purified products. Other vitamin K-dependent factors such as prothrombin (79–86 iu/ml) and factor X (44–64 iu/ml) that are plentiful in the PCCs are undetectable in most but not all of the high-purity concentrates. Factor VIII:C and vWF:Ag are undetectable in all the high-purity products and are present in only low levels in some PCCs. Of the other proteins found in PCCs, there is still evidence of contamination with fibrinogen and fibronectin in all the high-purity products except the immunoaffinity product, but at greatly reduced levels.

High-purity concentrates produced using a metal chelate developed by BPL also contain minute amounts of factor X but no factor II (Feldman et al, 1989). All of the high-purity products also contain low but detectable levels of IgG and IgA (Berntorp et al, 1993). The factor IX recovery for these products in vivo is equal to (Hampton et al, 1993) or greater than (Mannucci et al, 1990a; Thomas et al, 1994) that seen with conventional PCCs. There is not a great deal of difference between the pharmacokinetics of the PCCs and the high-purity concentrates; the main advantage of the high-purity factor IX concentrates, as discussed below, is their decreased thrombogenic potential.

Recombinant factor VIII concentrates

Characterization studies of the available recombinant factor VIII products show that they are almost identical to plasma-derived factor VIII on SDS polyacrylamide gel electrophoresis and western blot analysis (White et al, 1989; Klein, 1991). Functional comparisons show very similar profiles to plasma-derived factor VIII in terms of correction of clotting times in factor VIII-deficient plasma, rates of factor Xa generation, binding to vWF, thrombin cleavage patterns and inactivation by activated protein C (Klein, 1991). Very low levels of impurity (6 ng/1000 iu mouse IgG, and 51 ng/1000 iu cellular protein) have been reported in these concentrates (Klein, 1991). The specific factor VIII activity of the recombinant products is 3000 iu/mg of protein or greater but, as with the immunoaffinity products, human albumin has to be added as a stabilizer, resulting in final products with specific VIII activity of 1.65–19 iu/mg protein for Recombinate (Baxter) and 8–30 iu/mg for Kogenate (Cutter). Clearly the electrophoretic pattern of the B domainless concentrates is altered but the functional activity, recovery and half-life is equivalent to plasma-derived factor VIII (Berntorp et al, 1995a,b; Peters et al, 1995). In clinical studies the half-life and recovery of the recombinant products is equivalent to plasma-derived factor VIII (White et al, 1989; Schwartz et al, 1990; Morfini et al, 1992) and although recovery has not been as high as predicted in some cases, these have not been associated with a poor clinical outcome (Bray et al, 1994). Clinically recombinant products clearly provide adequate haemostasis in haemophilic bleeding and in surgical prophylaxis. In one study reporting on 810 bleeding events, 92% responded to one or two injections of concentrate and "excellent" haemostasis was documented in nine of 10 invasive or surgical procedures (Bray et al, 1994). In a separate multicentre trial of 540 bleeding episodes in 56 subjects, 74% required only a single dose of concentrate to achieve haemostasis whilst "excellent" haemostasis was provided in all of 22 patients undergoing major surgery (Schwartz et al, 1990). The recombinant factor VIII concentrates developed so far have not been associated with an excess of adverse clinical events. Transient mild allergic symptoms have been reported with both products but these have in general been non-recurring and have not precluded further treatment with the concentrate (Kasper et al, 1991; Lusher et al, 1993; Bray et al, 1994). Two theoretical concerns about recombinant factor VIII that do require close observation and attention are those of infection with viruses from cell line cultures and the theoretical problem of transfection of recipient cells with remaining foreign DNA which might result in oncogenesis. As yet, there is no clinical evidence of these problems but close long-term observation of patients treated with recombinant factor VIII is essential. Issues relating to inhibitor development and HIV infection are discussed below.

Porcine factor VIII

Porcine factor VIII is produced by the polyelectrolyte fractionation of pooled porcine plasma and has a final factor VIII purity of 120–140 iu/mg protein. The use of early porcine concentrates was severely limited by the development of thrombocytopenia caused by an excess of vWF, which resulted in platelet aggregation in vivo. This problem has been overcome to a large degree by the polyelectrolyte fractionation, which removes most of the vWF (Middleton, 1982), and although thrombocytopenia may still be observed it is rarely dangerous or limiting. These concentrates have been used extensively in the treatment of haemophiliacs and non-haemophiliacs with anti-factor VIII antibodies. There is no virucidal step in the manufacture of this concentrate but transmission of porcine viruses has not been reported in recipients.

FEIBA (factor VIII inhibitor bypassing fraction human)

One of the products currently employed in the treatment of high-level inhibitors is FEIBA. This product is produced by Immuno and is stated as containing 0.7–2.5 units FEIBA/mg of protein. In addition it contains factors II, IX and X mainly in non-activated form, as well as activated factor VII. The indications and appropriate doses for its use are discussed elsewhere. The viral safety of this concentrate has not been demonstrated in formal studies conforming to SSC guidelines because all recipients of FEIBA have been exposed previously to other concentrates. However, it is considered that sufficient numbers of individuals with previous concentrate exposure but no markers of hepatitis or HIV infection are now being treated with this concentrate that it should be possible to conduct a study of viral safety (Laurian et al, 1994).

Fibrin sealant

This preparation, which consists of fibrinogen that is activated on wound sites by the addition of thrombin, is gaining in popularity in the management of haemophilia. The most common uses are for bleeding from mucosal surfaces, especially after surgery and dental surgery. There is at present little published information on the viral safety of this material. The constituents of the presently available Scottish National Blood Transfusion fibrin sealant are virus inactivated by solvent detergent (thrombin) and super dry heat (fibrinogen) and this product is presently undergoing studies of viral safety.

Other Therapeutic Concentrates for the Treatment of Congenital Coagulation Factor Deficiency

Individuals with less common congenital coagulation deficiency states were previously treated by infusion of fresh blood or FFP; however, a variety of less commonly used but nevertheless important therapeutic concentrates for their treatment have been developed and are discussed below.

Factor VII deficiency

Hereditary factor VII deficiency is a rare autosomal recessive condition usually associated with normal or reduced levels of a functionally defective molecule. There is little correlation between plasma factor VII levels and bleeding. Because the half-life of factor VII is only 2–3 hours, replacement therapy with plasma is clearly likely to be complicated by volume overload. Concentrates of factor VII are also used in combination with a PCC in the immediate reversal of warfarin therapy associated with haemorrhage and in the treatment of haemostatic failure due to liver disease. However, an increasing number of patients with haemophilia A and acquired anti-VIII antibodies are now treated with factor VII concentrates in order to bypass inhibitor activity. At present there are three plasma-derived factor VII concentrates and one recombinant factor VIIa available.

Plasma-derived factor VII concentrates

These concentrates are produced by absorption of cryoprecipitate supernatant with DEAE sephadex A-50. The VII concentrate is eluted by salt gradient, virus inactivated and further purified (DEAE sepharose CL6B) concentrated, dialysed, sterile filtered and freeze-dried to produce an end-product with 25–30 u factor VII/ml, with only minor contamination with factors II, IX (less than 0.1 u/ml) and X (less than 1 u/ml) The two concentrates currently produced by BPL and LFB differ in their virus inactivation step, the BPL product being dry heated at 80 °C for 72 hours whilst the French product is treated by the solvent detergent method (TNBP 0.3%, Polysorbate 80, 1%).

Plasma-derived factor VIIa

Cryoprecipitate supernatant is adsorbed to an inorganic adsorbent, diluted and concentrated by diafiltration. The resulting concentrate is virus-inactivated by the solvent detergent method (TNBP and Polysorbate 80) before undergoing chromatography on Q-sepharose, being sterile filtered and freeze-dried. Again a pure concentrate is achieved with only minor contamination by the other vitamin K-dependent factors.

Recombinant factor VIIa

The factor VII gene is located in 12.8 kb of chromosome 13. The mRNA predicts a single chain protein of 406 amino acids. Activation, which is by proteolytic cleavage between ^{152}Arg and ^{153}Ile results in a light chain of 152 and a heavy chain of 254 amino acids linked by a disulphide bridge. Recombinant factor VIIa (rVIIa) was first produced from factor VII secreted by baby hamster kidney cells transfected with the cDNA encoding factor VII (Thim et al, 1988). The factor VII is purified by immunoaffinity chromatography using monoclonal antibodies that recognize its Ca^{2+}-stabilized form. Activation occurs spontaneously to factor VIIa during anion exchange chromatography. The rVIIa produced has an identical amino acid sequence with only minor post-translational differences in gamma carboxylation, N- and O-linked glycosylation and beta hydroxylation, when compared with plasma-derived factor VII. These differences are unlikely to be of any significance (Bjoern and Thim, 1986; Bjoern et al, 1991) and at a functional level both plasma-derived VIIa and rVIIa normalize the prolonged APTT in haemophilic plasma and in the plasma of haemophiliacs with inhibitors (Hedner et al, 1990).

Factor VII concentrates, both plasma derived and recombinant, have been successfully used in many clinical situations. The plasma-derived factor VII and VIIa concentrates stop bleeding in patients with anti-VIII antibodies (Hedner and Kisiel, 1983; Hedner et al, 1989) and in patients with factor VII deficiency (Mariani et al, 1978; Caron et al, 1991). Doses up to 100 iu/kg have been used to control haemarthrosis, epistaxis and provide haemostatic cover for dental extraction without thrombotic complications, although one of the early concentrates did transmit HBV infection (Mariani et al, 1978).

By far, the most common indication for the use of rVIIa has been in the treatment of patients with anti-VIII antibodies. The first described use of rVIIa was in a haemophiliac with a high-level inhibitor during synovectomy and débridement (Hedner et al, 1988). It has since been successfully used in many situations and for prolonged periods of up to 48 days without serious adverse effects (Schmidt et al, 1991). Cases where haemostasis has not been achieved with rVIIa have been reported but are few (Gringeri et al, 1991). A plasma half-life of 60–140 minutes has been reported although this may depend to an extent on the haemostatic state of the patient at the time (Schmidt et al, 1991). Initial concerns about the thrombogenic potential of rVIIa have not been realized and large doses have been infused without significant alterations in platelet count, fibrinogen levels or anti-plasmin (Bloom, 1991). Reports of clinical problems with rVIIa have been very few; however, disseminated intravascular coagulation (DIC) has been reported in one case in which rVIIa was used in combination with tranexamic acid in a patient with a massive infected thigh haematoma (Stein et al, 1990).

Factor XI deficiency

Factor XI deficiency is a rare and heterogeneous disorder found predominantly in Ashkenazi Jews in whom the frequency of homozygosity is 1 in 190 as opposed to a global figure of 1 in 1 000 000. Inheritance is autosomal, and there is not always a clear correlation between the bleeding manifestations and the measured factor XI level, although severely affected individuals usually have factor XI:c levels below 15–20 u/dl (Bolton-Maggs et al, 1995). Factor XI does have a long half-life (60 hours) and therefore replacement by fresh frozen plasma is possible but is still potentially complicated by allergic reactions and the risk of viral infection.

Factor XI concentrates

The LFB concentrate is produced by solid-phase adsorption of cryoprecipitate followed by further affinity chromatographic purification. It shows a 10 000-fold enrichment of factor XI over plasma, with a specific factor XI activity of 120–160 iu/mg protein. Virus inactivation is by the solvent detergent method.

The BPL concentrate, which is available for use on a named patient basis, is produced by solid-phase adsorption to DEAE cellulose and affinity chromatography using heparin sepharose. Virus inactivation is by dry heat at 80 °C for 72 hours.

Both products have high levels of factor XI but the BPL product, in addition, contains significant levels of antithrombin III which may serve to neutralize any factor XIa present, and in addition since 1993 has had a small amount of heparin added to it.

Because of the variability of disease severity and its lack of correlation with plasma factor XI levels, it is difficult to know precisely what levels of factor XI are required to ensure haemostasis. However, of 30 factor XI-deficient individuals treated on 31 occasions with the BPL product, normal haemostasis was achieved on all but one occasion with doses ranging from 12 to 62 iu/kg (giving factor XI levels of 59–171% of normal). Only minor allergic reactions were seen in one patient and follow-up for viral safety showed no evidence of seroconversion to HCV, HIV or parvo B19 in 23, 14 and eight patients, respectively (Bolton Maggs et al, 1992). However, arterial thrombosis has been documented in four elderly individuals in the period after receiving the BPL concentrate (Bolton-Maggs et al, 1994).

Published clinical evaluation of the LFB concentrate has shown that haemostatic cover for major surgery could be provided by doses of 50 iu/kg (Mannucci et al, 1994a); however, although this concentrate had not produced thrombosis in the rabbit stasis model, there was evidence of activation of coagulation which was accentuated in one patient by the effects of surgical removal of an adenocarcinoma (Mannucci et al, 1994a). A recent report on an essentially unidentified factor XI concentrate described a dangerous thrombogenic material which produced DIC, severe anaphylaxis and death (Gitel et al, 1991).

The problem of thrombogenicity is one shared by the factor XI concentrates, to the extent that guidelines prepared by the United Kingdom Haemophilia Centre Directors organization suggest that factor XI concentrates should be used only in specialized haemophilia centres with regular monitoring to ensure that therapeutic factor XI levels should be greater than 70 u/dl but less than 100 u/dl.

As with other clotting factors, attempts have been made to produce a recombinant protein by insertion of an expression vector into mammalian cell lines. Secretion of reasonably high levels of factor XI have been achieved using this system. N-terminal sequencing of the protein produced and of the separated chains after proteolytic cleavage has demonstrated normal processing of the recombinant proteins. Furthermore, the ratios of antigen to functional molecule are close to unity and the behaviour of the protein on SDS electrophoresis is identical to plasma-derived factor XI (Kemball-Cook et al, 1994).

Factor XIII deficiency

Factor XIII (fibrin-stabilizing factor) is a tetrameric transglutaminase of about 320 kD, which consists of two a and two b units covalently bonded. It is activated by thrombin cleavage to factor XIIIa, which catalyses the formation of cross-links between fibrin monomers, and further cross-links fibrin to other plasma proteins such as fibronectin and α_2-2 anti-plasmin, inhibiting plasmin-mediated clot dissolution. Factor XIII deficiency is rare. Most commonly, patients lack subunit a and have reduced levels of b. Presentation is often in the neonatal period with bleeding from the umbilical cord being present in about 80% of affected individuals. Spontaneous intracranial haemorrhage and poor wound healing are seen in about 25% of affected individuals and pregnancy is usually complicated by spontaneous abortion (Duckert, 1972; Bohn, 1978). Because of the high risk of intracranial haemorrhage, prophylactic therapy is given, usually on a monthly basis on account of the long half-life of factor XIII. Only low levels of factor XIII are required for normal haemostasis and this can be achieved with fresh blood, plasma or cryoprecipitate; however, the concentrates of factor XIII that are available have been shown to be extremely successful and safe.

Factor XIII concentrates

Behringwerke have, until recently, produced a concentrate (Fibrogammin P) from placentas that are frozen, minced and extracted with sodium chloride. The extract is then purified by adding cetylpyridinium chloride and the factor XIII precipitated with diaminoethxyacridin lactate and ammonium sulphate. The extract is treated at pH 6 and gel filtered on sephadex G-150 (Bohn, 1972).

The resulting product lacks b subunits but has a half-life of 11–12 days. Since 1982 this product has been pasteurized at 60°C for 10 hours. This manufacturer has recently replaced placenta with plasma as the starting source material (Brackmann et al, 1995)

A plasma-derived concentrate (BPL) is produced by precipitation from cryo-poor plasma by cold ethanol. The precipitate is then extracted with sodium citrate and sodium chloride and repeatedly precipitated with trisodium citrate. The concentrate is stabilized with 1% albumin and pasteurized in solution at 60° for 10 hours, concentrated further by diafiltration, filter-sterilized and freeze-dried (Winkelman et al, 1986).

Clinical use of factor XIII concentrates has been extremely successful in preventing and controlling bleeding in patients with congenital factor XIII deficiency (Losowsky and Miloszewski, 1976; Daly and Haddon, 1988; Emrich et al, 1991). The use of factor concentrates in individuals with acquired factor XIII deficiency has also been described (Shirahata et al, 1990; Dempfle et al, 1991) although the role in stopping bleeding in these situations is less clear. Although not followed-up by SSC protocol, there is no evidence of transmission of HIV or HCV infection by either of the concentrates described above (Daly and Haddon, 1988; Emrich et al, 1991).

Complications of Factor VIII and IX Treatment

A variety of complications, differing in severity, have resulted from the use of coagulation factor concentrates (Table 5.4).

Viral infections and methods to ensure viral safety of coagulation factor concentrates

Viral infections are the most widely publicized complications of concentrate use. These are discussed below in the context of development of virus inactivation methods to produce safe concentrates and are considered in greater detail in a later chapter. Suffice to say that at present the management of these problems is among the most difficult, time-consuming and expensive seen in the management of haemophiliacs.

Virus inactivation methods

Clearly the reduction in numbers of high-risk donors and the widespread adoption of screening donations for HIV, HBV and HCV decreases the virus load in plasma pools. However, despite the high level of sensitivity of the screening

Table 5.4 Side-effects of treatment with clotting factor concentrates

Allergic reactions
Haemolytic anaemia
Viral infection
Anti-factor VIII and IX antibody development
Immunomodulation (HIV independent)
Pulmonary hypertension

Table 5.5 Virus inactivation and exclusion techniques

Dry heating
Wet heat in heptane
Pasteurization
Heating with vapour
Solvent detergent
Chaotropic agents
Virus nanofiltration
Dual inactivation method

tests available, it is still inevitable that tests for antibodies will fail to detect donations in the "window period" when circulating virus is present but when testing takes place before a measurable antibody response can be mounted. Direct testing for viral antigens may increase sensitivity of testing for infectious donations. Therefore, because of the limitations of methods used to decrease the virus load in plasma pools, great effort has been channelled into the development of safe methods for the removal and inactivation of contaminating viruses with preservation of the biological activity of the coagulation factors (Table 5.5).

Dry heating

Dry heating was first developed in the early 1980s with a view to decreasing the transmission of hepatitis viruses. It has, in actual fact, been more successful at decreasing HIV transmissions. Terminal dry heat treatment is favoured by many because of its simplicity, its "terminal" position in the production process and because of the comparative sparing of VIII:c when compared with wet heating methods. Although early attempts at heat treatment did decrease hepatitis and HIV transmissions there is good evidence that infection with these viruses continued to be a problem (Colombo et al, 1985; Preston et al, 1985; Allain et al, 1986; van den Berg et al, 1986; White et al, 1986; Mariani et al, 1987;

Lush et al, 1988; Weisser, 1988; Dietrich et al, 1990; Remis et al, 1990; Williams et al, 1990b; Blanchette et al, 1991; Pistello et al, 1991).

With the introduction of virucidal methods in which higher temperatures were used for longer periods it has become clear that earlier regimens were merely suboptimal, and that dry heating can be a very effective method of virus inactivation. Amongst currently available products, dry heating at 80 °C for 72 hours is most preferred and this method has been used by BPL for its products 8Y and 9A, by the Scottish National Blood Transfusion Service for production of its factor VIII and factor IX concentrates and by Cutter for the production of a factor IX concentrate (Konyne 80). Although dry heating at 68 °C has been generally abandoned on account of the failure to inactivate viruses at this temperature, it is still used by Baxter in the production of two prothrombin complex concentrates, Proplex T and Autoplex T. However, whereas concentrates that are known to have transmitted hepatitis and HIV were heated at 60 °C for up to 72 hours, products presently inactivated by this method are exposed for 144 hours. Thus far, products exposed to 68 °C for 144 hours have not been implicated in virus transmission although prospective studies in a treated group are not available.

Studies of concentrate safety using the SSC guidelines (Mannucci et al, 1989) have been performed on the BPL products and also on the Scottish National Blood Transfusion concentrates Z8 and Defix (Study Group of the UK Haemophilia Centre Directors, 1988; Skidmore et al, 1990; Evans et al, 1991; Bennett et al, 1993). These demonstrate an excellent safety record for super dry heat treatment with regard to transmission of the hepatitis viruses and HIV; however, it should be noted that transmission of the non-lipid enveloped virus parvo B19 by concentrates prepared in this way has been reported (Williams et al, 1990a).

Wet heating in heptane

By this method, concentrate is heated in suspension with n-heptane at 60 °C for 20 hours. The potential advantage of increasing the lability of contaminating viruses by this method is offset by the concomitant loss of coagulant protein. There have been no documented cases of HIV transmission by products treated by this method, but five cases of non-A non-B hepatitis have been reported (Carnelli et al, 1987; Kernoff et al, 1987; Kasper et al, 1993). Two concentrates, Profilnine HT and Alphanine high-purity factor IX concentrate, are still manufactured by this process (Alpha). However the new high-purity factor VIII and IX products from Alpha are to be virus-inactivated by solvent/detergent methods (see later).

Pasteurization

Pasteurization was adopted as a method of virus inactivation as early as 1979 in Germany. This method also exploits the increased susceptibility of viruses to heat in a solution, but suffers from the drawback of loss of yield of functional protein. Concentrates treated by pasteurization are therefore artificially stabilized by the addition of sucrose and glycine to minimize loss of yield. Virus spiking experiments performed during the development of Monoclate P demonstrate that pasteurization at 60 °C for 10 hours removes 10.5 $\log^{10}$ viral infective units of HIV and is effective against other lipid and non-lipid enveloped viruses (vaccinia, sindbis, vesicular stomatitis and encephalomyocarditis) (Hrinda et al, 1990).

Fractionators in both Europe and the USA have adopted this method, which is currently used in the production of both intermediate- and high-purity products. Behringwerke adopted this method of inactivation at an early stage and presently use it in the production of an intermediate- and high-purity factor VIII concentrate (Haemate P and Beriate P) and a factor IX complex (factor IX HS). Pasteurization has an excellent record for prevention of HIV infection. A large retrospective study showed that no seroconversions to HIV had occurred in 155 patients treated with almost 16 million units of pasteurized products (Schimpf et al, 1989). Two prospective previously untransfused patient (PUP) studies on Haemate P and Beriate P, with the virus inactivation step applied at different points in the manufacturing process, showed no evidence of hepatitis or HIV infection in 26 patients treated with 32 batches of Haemate P, and in 29 patients receiving 13 batches of Beriate P (Schimpf et al, 1987; Mannucci et al, 1990b). A study of 98 German children treated with 32 batches of Behringwerke pasteurized products over a 10-year period, including 21 followed according to the SSC protocol, showed that none had evidence of hepatitis (Kreuz et al, 1992). However, although in prospective studies there have been no reported hepatitis transmissions, seven sporadic cases of possible transmission of hepatitis B and C have been reported outside studies (Brackmann and Egli, 1988; Gerritzen et al, 1992b; Schulman et al, 1992; Shopnick et al, 1995).

Heating with vapour

By this method moistened lyophilized concentrate is heated at pressure to improve conditions for virus inactivation. Previously, 80 °C for 1 hour at 1370 mbar was used in the production of factor IX and activated prothrombin complex concentrates. Presently, 60 °C for 10 hours at 1190 mbar is used in addition by Immuno in the production of a factor IX concentrate (Bebulin) and an activated factor IX complex (FEIBA). Initial trials of this method prior to modification showed unfavourable results with 4 out of 28 PUPS developing hepatitis B (Mannucci et al, 1988) and 1 out of 28 (co-infected with HBV) HCV infection (Mannucci et al, 1990c). However, a later multicentre study of a further 50 cases showed no evidence for transmission of HIV, HBV or HCV, and it may be that significant improvements have been made in this method (Mannucci et al, 1992c; Shapiro and International Factor Safety Study Group, 1992).

Chemical methods

Solvent detergent method. Solvent detergent treatment is certainly, at present, the method of viral inactivation being most frequently adopted by plasma fractionators. Many of the largest companies, including Alpha, Cutter, Baxter, NYBC, Octapharma, Biotest, Biotransfusion, Aima, and Novo Nordisk as well as not-for-profit organizations, have adopted this method, which was first developed by the New York City Blood Bank (Horowitz et al, 1985).

The method exploits the susceptibility of virus lipid envelope to lysis by organic solvent tri(*n*-butyl) phosphate (TNBP) and a detergent (sodium cholate, Tween 80 or Triton X-100). The solvent detergent method has in its favour a very small loss of yield and an excellent safety record for HIV and hepatitis virus transmission (Ganzengel et al, 1988; Horowitz et al, 1988; Noel et al, 1989; Gonzaga and Boneker, 1990; Mariani et al, 1991; Addiego et al, 1992; Di Paolantonio et al, 1992). Overall in these prospective studies none of the patients receiving solvent detergent treated concentrates prepared by five different manufacturers developed hepatitis. Unlike dry heating it is not, however, a terminal procedure and therefore products may be susceptible to contamination at a later stage in production. A further potential drawback is that, along with many of the other methods described, it does not inactivate non-lipid envelope viruses such as parvo B19 (Azzi et al, 1992). Parvovirus B19 DNA has been detected in solvent detergent-treated concentrates (Lefrere et al, 1994) although detection of viral DNA does not necessarily imply infectiousness (Hart et al, 1993; McOmish et al, 1993). HAV has also been transmitted by high-purity solvent detergent-treated concentrates prepared by or under licence from a single manufacturer in Europe (Gerritzen et al, 1992a; Mannucci, 1992; Temperley et al, 1992; Peerlinck and Vermylen, 1993). In addition to the epidemiological evidence there is corroborating molecular evidence suggesting transmission in the Italian outbreak (Mannucci et al, 1994b). Since the initial series of reports, a further possible cluster of infections has been reported in South African haemophiliacs using solvent detergent-treated concentrates (Cohn et al, 1994). In other groups using similar solvent detergent-treated material there has been no evidence of infection with HAV over a 3-year period (Watson et al, 1994).

Chaotropic agents. The chaotropic agent sodium thiocyanate is presently used as part of the inactivation process in combination with fractionation by immunoaffinity chromatography and virus filtration in the production of the high-purity factor IX concentrate Mononine (Armour). Studies of viral safety are not yet available for this method but preclinical evaluation of the combined virus inactivation steps has shown satisfactory removal of both lipid and protein enveloped viruses and extreme sensitivity of HIV to sodium thiocyanate (Hrinda et al, 1991).

Beta propiolactone and others. Other chemical methods such as treatment with the alkylating agent beta propiolactone and ultraviolet light and chloroform or hydrophobic interaction chromatography are no longer used as the result of serious inactivation failures which have resulted in the transmission of HIV-1 (Kleim et al, 1990). The combination of beta propiolactone and ultraviolet light was one of the earliest attempts made to decrease hepatitis transmissions and in this respect it was successful (Heinrich et al, 1982). However, because of fears about the possible carcinogenic affects of the alkylating agent, its adoption was never widespread.

Immunoaffinity chromatography

The process of immunoaffinity chromatography not only results in a highly purified protein but also in a product with markedly reduced viral load prior to the definitive virus inactivation step. The reduction in viral load in Monoclate P, for example, during the purification alone is of the order of 5 logs of virus (Hrinda et al, 1990). Nevertheless, this process does not provide adequate safety to be used unaccompanied and the products presently produced by affinity chromatography undergo a virus inactivation step in addition: for example, Monoclate P is further treated by pasteurization, Hemofil M by solvent detergent method, and Mononine by virus filtration and sodium thiocyanate. Wheras there are no reports of HIV transmission by presently available immunoaffinity products, possible transmission of HCV by Monoclate, virus inactivated by dry heat at 60°C for 30 hours (Berntorp et al, 1990) and by pasteurization has been reported (Shopnick et al, 1995).

Combined virus inactivation methods and new techniques

As a result of concern about transmission of enveloped viruses, particularly to immunosuppressed (Frickhofen et al, 1990) but also to immunocompetent individuals (Yee et al, 1995) it has been suggested that a combination of virucidal methods be used in concentrate manufacture. It has, for example, been demonstrated that following solvent detergent treatment the addition of a terminal dry heat at 100°C for 30 minutes results in minimal loss of VIII:C activity (Rubinstein et al, 1991). However, early studies of a factor VIII product manufactured by these combined processes suggest that transmission of parvovirus may still occur although the interpretation of these results has been questioned (Prowse, 1994; Santagostino et al, 1994). Double inactivation methods combining the solvent detergent method with 80°C dry heat for 72 hours (Novo

Nordisk), 63°C for 10 hours in solution (Octapharma) and 100°C dry heat for 30 minutes (Aima) have recently been adopted. Experimental methods presently being explored include nanofiltration, which may prove to be of use in the production of factor VIII and IX concentrates (Burnouf-Radosevich et al, 1994).

Evaluation of concentrate safety

As virus inactivation procedures began to be adopted in the early 1980s it became clear that some form of evaluation of concentrate safety was required, especially with regard to non-A non-B transmission for which at that time only surrogate markers of infection were available. In 1984 the International Committee on Thrombosis and Haemostasis assigned a task force to draw up a set of guidelines, which were further revised in 1989 (Mannucci et al, 1989). These guidelines suggested that studies should be prospective, of previously untreated patients, without control groups and should include only individuals with no markers of previous hepatitis or liver damage. However the strict (but essential) protocol for follow-up sampling often resulted in difficulty completing the study period as many of the suitable patients were small babies in whom sampling was difficult to justify by both parents and physicians. Further, because of the development of sensitive assays for HCV infection, including PCR techniques, a re-evaluation of the value of serial ALT measurements is now needed (Myhre et al, 1994). It is now likely that new protocols for the determination of viral safety will soon be drawn up. Additional protocols for the detection of infection with other viruses such as parvovirus B19 have recently been proposed.

Other complications of concentrate use

Allergic reactions

Allergic reactions similar to those experienced with cryoprecipitate were previously commonly seen in association with the use of low-purity concentrates. These varied in degree from slight pruritis and allergic skin rashes to anaphylactic shock. Serious allergic reactions to concentrate are now rarely reported.

Haemolytic anaemia

Haemolytic anaemia caused by isoagglutinins is now rare because of the improved purity of concentrates but has been documented following concentrate infusion, resulting from the infusion of red cell antibodies in plasma-derived concentrates (Ashenhurst et al, 1976; Orringer et al, 1976).

Primary pulmonary hypertension

Primary pulmonary hypertension possibly resulting from concentrate infusion has been reported by American investigators although the exact role of coagulation factor concentrates in these observations is not clear (Goldsmith et al, 1988; Bray et al, 1989).

Venous thromboembolism and DIC

The use of intermediate-purity factor IX concentrates (PCCs) has been linked with an increased incidence of deep vein thrombosis, pulmonary embolism and the development of DIC (Blatt et al, 1974; Kasper, 1975; Cederbaum et al, 1976) and in addition less frequently with serious arterial thrombosis (Aledort, 1977) on occasions in young patients (Agrawal et al, 1981; Fuerth and Mahrer, 1981; Sullivan et al, 1984). Several possible explanations for these observations have been provided and it may be that multiple factors contribute to the increased thrombotic risk. Straightforward overload of other zymogens with a long half-life has been suggested by Magner and Aronson (1979). Other investigators have demonstrated the presence of activated clotting factors Xa (White et al, 1977; Elodi and Varadi, 1978; Hultin, 1979), IXa (White et al, 1977; Elodi and Varadi, 1978) and VIIa (Seligsohn et al, 1979) in PCCs, and a possible role for the contact factors has also been proposed (Chandra and Wickerhauser, 1979). It has also been suggested that the potential thrombogenic affects of activated factors in concentrates are mediated through coagulant-active phospholipids and, indeed, that the major determinant of thrombogenicity of a concentrate containing activated coagulation factors in a rabbit stasis model is its content of these proteins (Giles et al, 1982).

Animal models have been used to demonstrate the thrombogenic effects and to compare concentrates of different purity. Using the Wessler stasis model the doses required to induce thrombosis have been found to vary from 5 to 100 iu/kg factor IX for different thrombogenic products (Kingdon et al, 1975; Giles et al, 1980; Prowse and Williams 1980), whilst higher-purity factor IX products have been shown to be non-thrombogenic in this model (Menache et al, 1984). Using non-stasis models, DIC has been demonstrated following infusion of PCCs (Triantaphyllopoulis, 1972; Prowse and Williams 1980), but was not precipitated by infusion of an early high-purity concentrate produced by dextran sulphate affinity chromatography of DEAE-sephadex eluate (Menache et al, 1984). Recent studies have focused on comparisons of the in vivo thrombogenicity of presently used PCCs and that of the available high-purity concentrates in haemophiliacs. Because of the low sensitivity of commonly used laboratory tests for the detection of DIC, these studies have used more sensitive assays of activation of coagulation such as the prothrombin fragment F1+2 assay, which measures prothrombin cleavage by Xa, fibrinopeptide A assay measuring thrombin cleavage of fibrinogen, factor X activation peptide, and thrombin–antithrombin complexes. In five studies of high-purity factor IX concentrates (four affinity chromatography and one immunoaffinity product) there was consistent evidence of coagulation activation following PCC infusion that was absent or significantly less after high-purity concentrate infusion (Mannucci et al, 1990a, 1991; Kim et al, 1992; Hampton et al, 1993; Thomas et al, 1994).

After initial reports indicated that there was a problem relating to the thrombogenicity of the early PCCs, the factor IX task force of the International Society on Thrombosis and Haemostasis in 1974 suggested that 5–10 units of heparin be added to each millilitre of reconstituted factor IX concentrate prior to use on the assumption that the increased thrombogenicity of these concentrates was due to the presence of activated coagulation factors. Additional measures to prevent thrombotic complications such as giving fresh frozen plasma or small doses of antithrombin (III) along with PCCs have been considered. Cases of venous thromboembolism have continued to be reported in association with intermediate-purity concentrates of factor IX despite these measure, although often these have arisen in situations that per se might be associated with an increased thrombotic risk (Lusher, 1991). However, given the promising nature of the data available on the high-purity concentrates, it might realistically be hoped that serious thrombosis in patients with haemophilia B related to treatment with factor IX concentrates is a thing of the past.

Immunomodulation independent of HIV infection

After the introduction of effective testing for HIV it became apparent that abnormalities suggestive of immunomodulation were not confined to those haemophiliacs infected with this virus (Carr et al, 1984; Brettler et al, 1986; Madhok et al, 1986; Matheson et al, 1986b; Sullivan et al, 1986; Mahir et al, 1988; Chelucci et al, 1992; Cuthbert et al, 1992), and it was proposed that the effect of the massive protein load or alloantigens contained in intermediate-purity concentrates might account for these observations. Furthermore, in vitro studies demonstrate that intermediate-purity concentrates do inhibit normal lymphocyte proliferation in response to broad-spectrum mitogens such as concanavalin-A and phytohaemagglutinin (Lederman et al, 1986; Matheson et al, 1986a) and also inhibit normal monocyte functions such as oxygen radical release, bacterial killing (Eibl et al, 1987) and phagocytosis (Mannhalter et al, 1988; Pasi and Hill, 1990). In contrast, however, to these in vitro demonstrations of an immun suppressive effect of concentrates, investigation of the immune systems of haemophiliacs has produced evidence of both B-cell and T-cell activation (hypergammaglobulinaemia, raised levels of circulating activated T cells, raised IL2-receptor levels and increased B_2-microglobulin levels) in the absence of infection with HIV (Teitel et al, 1989; Cuthbert et al, 1992; Makris et al, 1994). Whether these abnormalities are related only to concentrate use is, however, not clear and it has been suggested, for example, that these abnormalities are related to liver disease (Madhok et al, 1991; Makris et al, 1994).

In vitro studies have demonstrated that infection of CD4+ cells by HIV is facilitated if the cells are in an activated state (Gowda et al, 1989) and that activation of HIV-infected cells may enhance viral replication (Zagury et al, 1986). Therefore if these in vitro observations were to occur in vivo it would follow that haemophiliacs may have been predisposed to HIV infection by the effects of concentrates and that further activation of the immune system might have a deleterious effect on the progression of HIV-related disease. In addition, concern has been voiced about the other possible effects of long-term immunomodulation in haemophiliacs. Several studies have been designed to determine whether, at a clinical level, haemophiliacs are more likely to suffer from significant mortality and morbidity as a result of immunosuppression. Whereas in one study of postoperative wound infection there was no difference in incidence between HIV-negative haemophiliac and non-haemophiliac individuals (Buehrer et al, 1990), another study demonstrated an increased incidence of post-arthroplasty septic arthritis in both HIV-positive and HIV-negative haemophiliacs.

The causes of death in haemophiliacs are changing as a result of transfusion-related illness. However, studies in the pre-AIDS era suggested that haemophiliacs were surviving for longer as deaths from haemorrhage were prevented but had an increased likelihood of dying from infection (Aronson, 1983; Rizza and Spooner, 1983) even after the exclusion of hepatitis as a cause of death (Rizza and Spooner, 1983; Aronson, 1988). There is, in addition, little evidence for an increased incidence of malignancy, and importantly no increase in virus-associated malignancy such as Burkitt's lymphoma (Aronson, 1988). The tuberculosis (TB) outbreak reported in 1985 in which the incidence of TB in exposed haemophiliac children was similar to that in children profoundly immunosuppressed by chemoradiotherapy is without doubt the best documented report of significant morbidity attributable to concentrate related immunocompromise (Beddall et al, 1985) although other events have been reported (Watson et al, 1992a).

Development of inhibitors

One of the most serious and certainly most clinically significant unwanted effects of treatment with factor VIII and factor IX is the development of anti-factor VIII and IX inhibitory antibodies. These IgG antibodies are directed against the coagulant portion of the molecules and therefore prevent normal coagulation despite factor replacement, resulting in a bleeding diathesis that is very difficult to control. The incidence and prevalence of inhibitors is hard to determine as is demonstrated by the huge differences in reported studies (Schwarzinger et al, 1987; McMillan et al, 1988; Lusher and Salzman, 1990). Variables such as disease severity and age of population clearly affect results. The situation is further complicated by the evidence from prospectively followed cohorts that transient low-level inhibitors are common (Ehrenforth et al, 1992). Inhibitors are more commonly found in haemophilia A than in Christmas disease (Ehrenforth et al, 1992) and in general are more common in the severe disease state (Kesteven et al, 1984; Shapiro, 1984b; Ehrenforth et al, 1992). Because inhibitors often develop during the first 5–20 days of concentrate exposure, many of these cases present in very young children and babies (Kasper, 1973; Lusher et al, 1993; Bray et al, 1994). A variety of treatment options exist for the management of haemorrhage in patients with inhibitors; however, their success depends on the level of and the nature of inhibitors (Macik, 1993). These are discussed in detail elsewhere in the text; however, at this point it is appropriate to mention concerns over reports of increased incidence of inhibitor development in individuals treated with recombinant factor VIII and high-purity plasma-derived concentrates, as discussed below.

How Important is Blood Product Purity?

Four main aspects relating to the effect of concentrate require discussion:

- Thrombogenicity of factor IX concentrates
- Concentrate-related immunomodulation
- HIV disease progression
- Inhibitor development.

Thrombogenicity of factor IX concentrates

In view of the reported associations between intermediate-purity factor IX concentrates and thrombosis and DIC, the case for purer factor IX concentrates was clear cut and the developments that have arisen are discussed earlier in this chapter.

Concentrate-induced immunomodulation

The case for introduction of purer (and more expensive) factor VIII concentrates was not so clear cut and was based particularly on the possible detrimental effects of protein impurities on the immune system, particularly in HIV-positive individuals.

The first argument in favour of high-purity concentrates is that based on the degree of purity alone – "purer must be better". There is of course no doubt that products produced by affinity chromatography, ion exchange chomatography and immunoaffinity chromatography are much purer. However, the factor(s) responsible for the in vitro effect of intermediate-purity concentrates on lymphocyte activation and monocyte function have not yet been fully identified, although several studies have isolated protein fractions felt likely to be implicated (Lederman et al, 1986; Mannhalter et al, 1988; Vermot Desroches et al, 1992). Recently, transforming growth factor beta, which is known to have immunosuppressive effects, has been detected in concentrates (Wadhwa et al, 1994); however, it is not entirely clear how important this protein is to these observations (Speirs et al, 1995). In vitro studies suggest a dose-dependent inhibition of lymphocyte activation by concentrates. One of the proposed mechanisms for this is that IL2 secretion is inhibited (Lederman et al, 1986; Thorpe et al, 1989), or that IL2-R expression is down-regulated (Hay et al, 1990). The inhibition of IL2 secretion is less marked with immunoaffinity-produced products than with intermediate-purity and other high-purity products. Further studies suggest that the degree of inhibition of lymphocyte activation is not dependent on product purity but depends on the method of production, with immunoaffinity products appearing to be much less inhibitory than ion exchange high-purity products (Hay and McEvoy, 1992). Monocyte Fc receptor expression and functions such as oxygen radical generation, bacterial killing and phagocytosis all appear to be down-regulated and inhibited by a short incubation with concentrate (Eibl et al, 1987; Mannhalter et al, 1988). Down-regulation of Fc receptor expression may result from exposure to both intermediate-purity and high-purity ion exchange products and immunoaffinity high-purity products, although later studies suggest that monoclonally purified products have less inhibitory affect on monocyte function. What is not yet clear is how these in vitro observations are related to the effects of different products on patients (Pasi and Hill, 1990). However, there are still few reports to confirm that intermediate-purity products alone produce clinically significant immunosuppression.

HIV disease progression

Recently, discussion of the benefits and disadvantages of using high-purity products has focused on the effects of these products on the progression of HIV infection and the risks of inhibitor formation, respectively. With regard to effects on the progression of HIV infection, there is little evidence to suggest that factor VIII or IX usage is an important co-factor for HIV disease progression. Large epidemiological studies suggest that the rate of progression of HIV infection in haemophiliacs is equal to that seen in other risk groups (Eyster et al, 1987) with most studies suggesting similar rates of decline of CD4 counts (Cuthbert et al, 1990; Goldsmith et al, 1991; Phillips et al, 1991; Aledort et al, 1992). Furthermore, comparisons amongst haemophiliacs suggest that the rate of progression is independent of disease severity (and therefore concentrate use) and is the same in individuals with haemophilia A or haemophilia B (Goedert et al, 1989). However, in vitro studies have shown that activation of HIV-infected cells may enhance viral replication (Zagury et al, 1986) and that cell proliferation resulting in virus shedding can be induced by exposure to protein antigens (Margolick et al, 1987). As a result, studies comparing decline of CD4 counts, changes in delayed cutaneous hypersensitivity reactions and rates of clinical disease progression in groups using either high- or intermediate-purity concentrates have been conducted. Of 10 available studies, three prospective and two retrospective show a significant benefit for high-purity concentrates in terms of stabilization of CD4 lymphocyte counts (de Biasi et al, 1991; Goldsmith et al, 1991; Seremetis et al, 1993; Goedert et al, 1994; Sabin et al, 1994). The prospective studies included follow-up on a total of 76 patients over periods varying from 96 to 156 weeks, whilst the retrospective studies analysed 448 patients. One study showed a late stabilization of CD4 counts following addition of AZT (Goldsmith et al, 1991) and two others demonstrated that despite having a beneficial affect on CD4 counts, high-purity concentrates did not affect the development of AIDS or death (Seremetis et al, 1993; Goedert et al, 1994). In all five of these reports the high-purity concentrates were produced by monoclonal antibody technology. Four other studies show no definite evidence for a beneficial effect of high- over intermediate-purity products on CD4 count (Brettler et al, 1989; Fukutake et al, 1991; Mannucci et al, 1992b; Hilgartner et al, 1993). In these studies the high-purity concentrates were immunoaffinity produced in all but one case (Mannucci et al, 1992b), and in an additional study a comparison of two high-purity concentrates showed a non-significant benefit for a monoclonal product over an ion exchange product (Varon et al, 1994). The stabilization of CD4 counts over prolonged periods such as reported in several of these studies is not seen with any presently available specific antiviral agent for the treatment of HIV infection. In the case of the monoclonally produced concentrates it could be hypothesized that their trace amounts of murine protein may be responsible for the stabilization of CD4 counts in these patients. In this respect findings of these studies may have more far-reaching implications for the treatment of other individuals with HIV infection.

Inhibitor development

Whilst a possible beneficial effect has been ascribed to the use of high-purity concentrates on progression of HIV infection, attention has also been drawn to the possible increased incidence of inhibitor development in patients receiving these products. Comparing studies of inhibitor development is complicated by inconsistencies in the reported incidence of inhibitors in patients treated with intermediate-purity products. Many earlier studies almost certainly underestimated the incidence of inhibitor development in intermediate-purity concentrate recipients, so that the higher incidence reported in closely followed high-purity and recombinant users was compared with inaccurate historical data. Following the publication of three prospective studies in which inhibitors were regularly screened for over years of intermediate-purity concentrate use, it has become apparent that previous studies did underestimate the incidence of inhibitor development in this group of patients (Rasi and Ikkala, 1990; Ehrenforth et al, 1992; de Biasi et al, 1994). Further, it is clear that the likelihood of developing inhibitors is related to disease severity and to genetic factors (Shapiro, 1984a; Lippert et al, 1990). It has been suggested that the study of Ehrenforth et al. overestimates the incidence of inhibitor development (Ljung et al, 1992; Lorenzo et al, 1992), however, these studies and others (Rasi and Ikkala, 1990) do agree that the incidence of inhibitors in severely affected individuals is 18–21%.

Against this background the reported incidence of inhibitors in patients treated with high-purity plasma-derived or recombinant concentrates does not appear to be increased. The incidence of inhibitor development in severely affected individuals treated with immunoaffinity plasma-derived products has been reported as 18.5% and 12.5% with Monoclate (Armour) and Hemofil (Baxter), respectively (Lusher and Salzman, 1990; Addiego et al, 1992), whilst in recipients of recombinant products inhibitors developed in 28.5% and 19.8% of patients using Kogenate (Cutter) (Schwartz et al, 1990; Lusher et al, 1993), and 23.9% of those treated with Recombinate (Baxter) (Bray et al, 1994). The concern underlying these prospective studies of recipients of high-purity products and particularly recombinant products is that in the development of these concentrates the factor VIII molecule will have been altered antigenically and will be more likely to produce an immune response. Given the "foreign" nature of functional factor VIII to most severe hemophiliacs it is perhaps surprising that the incidence of inhibitor development is as low as it is, regardless of the type of concentrate used. Therefore with regard to the effect of purity, it is possibly more interesting to note that inhibitors have developed after starting treatment with high-purity plasma-derived and recombinant products in individuals successfully treated for many years with intermediate-purity concentrate (Kessler and Sachse, 1990; Schwartz et al, 1990; Montoro et al, 1991). To date, it is probably reasonable to say that there is not strong evidence that inhibitor formation is more likely in recipients of high-purity concentrates.

Therapeutic Products Other Than Coagulation Factor Concentrates

Desmopressin

The use of the vasopressin analogue desmopressin (deamino-8-D-arginine vasopressin) has revolutionized the treatment of mild and moderate haemophilia and von Willebrand's disease because it can be used therapeutically to raise factor VIII and vWF levels. Used in this way it is effective therapy to treat minor bleeds or to cover surgery. This was particularly important before the era of virally attenuated concentrates because its use avoided exposure to potential viral infection in individuals who otherwise only rarely required to have their factor levels raised. The mechanism by which desmopressin increases factor VIII and vWF remains unclear but the latter is probably released from endothelial cells. In addition desmopressin increases plasma tissue plasminogen activator (tPA), and urokinase (uPA), probably also released from endothelial cells. The response to desmopressin is unimpaired in hypopituitary and anephric subjects. Evidence has been presented to suggest that it may cause monocytes to secrete a mediator, possibly platelet-activating factor, that stimulates endothelial cells to release vWF and tPA (Hashemi et al, 1993); additional studies, however, are needed to further elucidate its mechanism of action. In most patients with severe von Willebrand's disease, not only is the factor VIII and vWF response to desmopressin poor but there is a reduced tPA response (Ludlam et al, 1980). In a proportion of such patients, however, a modest increase in factor VIII may be observed.

Infusion of desmopressin into healthy subjects, as well as individuals with mild haemophilia A and von Willebrand's disease, results in a rise in factor VIII and vWF by about three- to five-fold fold within 30–60 minutes when given in a dose of 0.3 μg/kg; larger doses do not augment the pharmacological effect but do increase the incidence of side-effects. There is a preferential increase in the plasma concentration of high molecular weight multimers of vWF (Ruggeri et al, 1982). Repeat infusions often result in an attenuated response; this tachyphylaxis is more marked in haemophilia A than von Willebrand's disease and may limit its usefulness therapeutically (Mannucci et al, 1992a). Furthermore, the response between individuals is variable and it is therefore advisable to give each patient a test infusion to assess its efficacy. Repeat infusions to the same subject result in a reproducible response. Tachyphylaxis is not observed in the tPA response (Vicente et al, 1993).

In haemophilia A with a basal factor VIII level of over 0.05 iu/ml, a useful rise in its level can often be obtained that is sufficient to allow minor surgery, e.g. dental extraction, to be safely accomplished (Rodeghiero et al, 1991). In circumstances where desmopressin is used a fibrinolytic inhibitor, e.g. tranexamic acid, may be of value given concurrently as it has the potential additional advantage of inhibiting the activity of the released tPA.

For individuals with von Willebrand's disease, desmopressin has a useful place in treating bleeding, e.g. epistaxis, as well as raising vWF levels such that minor, or sometimes major, surgery can be safely accomplished. Desmopressin is particularly effective in the treatment of type I von Willebrand's disease because it results in the release of structurally normal vWF from endothelial cells and there is often a transient shortening of the bleeding time. The factor VIII and vWF rise tends to be more prolonged than in haemophilia A. In type 2A von Willebrand's disease desmopressin is less effective therapeutically because of the structurally abnormal vWF. There is some evidence that it may reduce the platelet count in type 2B disease and for this reason it should be used with caution although there is increasing evidence for its safe use in this situation (Casonato et al, 1994). In those with type 2N von Willebrand's disease (Normandy variant) in which there is reduced binding of factor VIII to a structurally abnormal vWF, desmopressin results in a clinically useful rise in both factors although the duration of the factor VIII increase is reduced.

In individuals with either congenital haemophilia A with an antifactor VIII antibody, or in acquired haemophilia A, desmopressin may be useful if the basal factor VIII level is over about 0.05 iu/ml. In individuals with combined factor V and VIII deficiency, desmopressin only results in a rise in factor VIII.

The response to desmopressin is most predictable when it is administered intravenously; when given subcutaneously the factor VIII response is rather variable. A highly concentrated preparation of desmopressin is available for use intranasally. Although only about 10% of the administered dose is absorbed, the intranasal route has found favour for the treatment of bleeding, e.g. menorrhagia (Chistolini et al, 1991).

Side-effects are uncommon if desmopressin is given slowly intravenously. Facial flushing is the most common symptom; and there may also be a small fall in the blood pressure and rise in the pulse rate; slowing or temporarily halting the infusion allows the symptoms to settle. As a result of its antidiuretic action, water retention is observed for about 24 hours. If the intake of fluids is not monitored and mildly restricted, symptomatic hyponatraemia may occur. This initially manifests as headache but cerebral oedema may be sufficient to result in convulsions, especially in young children. There has been much concern that desmopressin may predispose to arterial thrombosis as several reports have described myocardial infarction (including sudden death) (Hartmann and Reinhart, 1995) and thrombotic strokes shortly after its infusion; it has been suggested that the increase in high molecular weight vWF multimers may increase the tendency of platelets to adhere to atherosclerotic lesions. A systematic review of cardiopulmonary bypass patients who received desmopressin did not reveal any significant excess of arterial thrombotic events. Despite the reassurance offered by this study it is probably prudent to use desmopressin with some caution in individuals at significantly increased risk of arterial thrombosis.

Fibrinolytic inhibitors

Fibrinolytic inhibitors have a well tried and proven place in the treatment of haemophilia A and von Willebrand's disease. EACA has been superseded by tranexamic acid (Cyclokapron) because it is 7–10 times more potent and causes fewer side-effects. Its principal action is to bind to the lysine-binding sites of plasminogen, preventing it binding to fibrin and thus reducing lysis. It also prevents the activation of plasminogen by its specific activators.

Although the use of long-term tranexamic acid alone does not diminish bleeding frequency in severe haemophilia A, it has an important place in the prevention of postoperative bleeding, particularly after dental extraction. To cover dental or other minor surgery the factor VIII level should be raised to about 0.50 iu/ml, either by factor VIII infusion or desmopressin, as appropriate, and tranexamic acid given orally or intravenously at a dose of 15–25 mg/kg. The therapy should be continued thereafter at the same dose four times daily for about 10 days. Mouth washes of tranexamic acid may also be of limited value.

When given intravenously, tranexamic acid should be administered slowly as it may cause nausea and light-headedness. Other side-effects include diarrhoea, rashes, myalgia and muscle weakness. Although tranexamic acid appears safe in pregnancy, EACA should be avoided in this situation because it is teratogenic in rats. Despite its potent ability to inhibit fibrinolysis, there is no evidence that it predisposes to venous thrombosis in individuals with a normal haemostatic system. It should be used with great caution in those with systemic activation of the coagulation system, as in DIC, because it may result in catastrophic thrombosis. It should not be used in patients with haematuria if there is any possibility that the bleeding is originating in the kidney as it may result in obstruction of the ureter by clot and subsequent renal failure from obstructive uropathy. It should not be administered concurrently with prothrombin complex concentrates because it may potentiate their thrombogenic potential and result in DIC and clinical thrombosis.

References

Addiego JE, Jr, Gomperts E, Liu SL, et al. Treatment of hemophilia A with a highly purified factor VIII concentrate prepared by anti-FVIIIc immunoaffinity chromatography. *Thrombosis and Haemostasis* 1992; **67:** 19.

Addis T. The pathogenesis of hereditary haemophilia. *Journal of Pathology and Bacteriology* 1911; **15:** 427.

Agrawal BL, Zelkowitz L, Hletko P. Acute myocardial infarction in a young hemophiliac patient during therapy with factor IX concentrate and epsilon aminocaproic acid. *Journal of Pediatrics* 1981; **98:** 931.

Aldhous P, Tastemain C. Three physicians convicted in French "blood-supply trial" [news]. *Science* 1992; **258:** 735.

Aledort LM. Factor IX and thrombosis. *Scandinavian Journal of Haematology* 1977; **30:** 40.

Aledort LM, Hilgartner MW, Pike MC, et al. Variability in serial CD4 counts and relation to progression of HIV-1 infection to AIDS in haemophilic patients. Transfusion Safety Study Group. *British Medical Journal* 1992; **304:** 212.

Allain JP, Gazangel C, Sultan Y, Verroust F. Clinical evaluation of a heat-treated high purity factor VIII concentrate. *Ricerca in Clinical e in Laboratoris* 1986; **16:** 245.

Aronson DL. Pneumonia deaths in haemophiliacs. *Lancet* 1983; **2:** 1023.

Aronson DL. Cause of death in hemophilia A patients in the United States from 1968 to 1979. *American Journal of Hematology* 1988; **27:** 7.

Ashenhurst JB, Langehennig PL, Seeler RA, Telfer MC. Hemolytic anemia due to anti-B in antihemophiliac factor concentrates. *Journal of Pediatrics* 1976; **88:** 257.

Azzi A, Ciappi S, Zakvrzewska K, Morfini M, Mariani G, Mannucci PM. Human parvovirus B19 infection in hemophiliacs first infused with two high-purity, virally attenuated factor VIII concentrates. *American Journal of Hematology* 1992; **39:** 228.

Beddall AC, Hill FG, George RH, Williams MD, al-Rubei K. Unusually high incidence of tuberculosis among boys with haemophilia during an outbreak of the disease in hospital. *Journal of Clinical Pathology* 1985; **38:** 1163.

Bennett B, Dawson AA, Gibson BS, et al. Study of viral safety of Scottish National

Blood Transfusion Service factor VIII/IX concentrate. *Transfusion Medicine* 1993; **3:** 295.

Berntorp E, Nilsson IM, Ljung R, Widell A. Hepatitis C virus transmission by monoclonal antibody purified factor VIII concentrate. *Lancet* 1990; **335:** 1531.

Berntorp E, Bjorkman S, Carlsson M, Lethagen S, Nilsson IM. Biochemical and in vivo properties of high purity factor ix concentrates. *Thrombosis and Haemostasis* 1993; **70:** 768.

Berntorp E, Brackmann HH, Dechavanne M, et al. Prophylactic treatment with a B-domain-deleted recombinant factor VIII (r-VIII SQ) in previously treated patients with severe haemophilia. *Thrombosis and Haemostasis* 1995a; **73:** 1011.

Berntorp E, Johnsson H, Tengborn L, et al. Deletion of the B-domain in a recombinant factor VIII (r-VIII SQ) does not affect the main kinetic properties. *Thrombosis and Haemostasis* 1995b; **73:** 1014.

Biggs R, Bidwell E, Handley DA, et al. The preparation and assay of a Christmas-Factor (factor IX) concentrate and its use in the treatment of two patients. *British Journal of Haematology* 1961; **7:** 349.

Biggs R, Spooner RJD. Haemophilia treatment in the United Kingdom from 1969 to 1974. *British Journal of Haematology* 1977; **35:** 487.

Bjoem S, Thim L. Activation of factor VII to VIIa. *Research Disclosures* 1986; **269:** 584.

Bjoem S, Foster DC, Thim L, et al. Human plasma and recombinant factor. VII. Characterization of O-glycosylations at serine residues 52 and 60 and effects of site-directed mutagenesis of serine 52 to alanine. *Journal of Biological Chemistry* 1991; **266:** 11051.

Blanchette VS, Vorstman E, Shore A, et al. Hepatitis C infection in children with hemophilia A and B. *Blood* 1991; **78:** 285.

Blatt PM, Lundblad RL, Kingdom HS, McLean G, Roberts HR. Thrombogenic materials in prothrombin complex concentrates. *Annals of Internal Medicine* 1974; **81:** 766.

Blomback B, Blomback M. Purification of human and bovine fibrinogen. *Arkiv For Kemi* 1956; **10:** 415.

Bloom AL. Progress in the clinical management of haemophilia. *Thrombosis and Haemostasis* 1991; **66:** 166.

Boedeker BG. The manufacturing of the recombinant factor VIII, Kogenate. *Transfusion Medicine Reviews* 1992; **6:** 256.

Bohn H. Comparative studies on the fibrin-stabilizing factors from human plasma, platelets and placentas. *Annals of the New York Academy of Sciences* 1972; **202:** 256.

Bohn H. The human fibrin-stabilizing factors. *Molecular and Cellular Biochemistry* 1978; **20:** 67.

Boklan BF. Factor IX concentrate and viral hepatitis. *Annals of Internal Medicine* 1971; **74:** 298.

Bolton-Maggs PHB, Wensley RT, Kernoff PBA, et al. Production and therapeutic use of a factor XI concentrate from plasma. *Thrombosis and Haemostasis* 1992; **67:** 314.

Bolton-Maggs PHB, Colvin BT, Satchi G, Lee CA, Lucas GS. Thrombogenic potential of factor XI concentrates. *Lancet* 1994; **344:** 748.

Bolton-Maggs PHB, Paterson DA, Wensley RT, Tuddenham EGD. Definition of the bleeding tendency in factor XI deficient kindreds: a clinical and laboratory study. *Thrombosis and Haemostasis* 1995; **73:** 194.

Brackmann HH, Egli H. Acute hepatitis B infection after treatment with heat-inactivated factor VIII concentrate. *Lancet* 1988; **2:** 967.

Brackmann HH, Egbring R, Ferster A, et al. Pharmacokinetics and tolerability of factor XIII concentrates prepared from human placenta or plasma: a crossover randomised study. *Thrombosis and Haemostasis* 1995; **74:** 622.

Bray GL, Martin GR, Chandra R. Idiopathic pulmonary hypertension, hemophilia A, and infection with human immunodeficiency virus (HIV). *Annals of Internal Medicine* 1989; **111:** 689.

Bray GL, Gomperts ED, Courter S, et al. A multicenter study of recombinant factor VIII (Recombinate): safety, efficacy, and inhibitor risk in previously untreated patients with hemophilia A. *Blood* 1994; **83:** 2428.

Brettler DB, Forsberg AD, Brewster F, Sullivan JL, Levine PH. Delayed cutaneous hypersensitivity reactions in hemophiliac subjects treated with factor concentrate. *American Journal of Medicine* 1986; **81:** 607.

Brettler DB, Forsberg AD, Levine PH, Petillo J, Lamon K, Sullivan JL. Factor VIII:C concentrate purified from plasma using monoclonal antibodies: human studies. *Blood* 1989; **73:** 1859.
Buehrer JL, Weber DJ, Meyer AA, et al. Wound infection rates after invasive procedures in HIV-1 seropositive versus HIV-1 seronegative hemophiliacs. *Annals of Surgery* 1990; **211:** 492.
Burnouf T, Michalski C, Goudemand M, Huart JJ. Properties of a highly purified human plasma factor IX:c therapeutic concentrate prepared by conventional chromatography. *Vox Sang* 1989; **57:** 225.
Burnouf-Radosevich M, Burnouf T, Huart JJ. A pasteurized therapeutic plasma. *Infusionstherapie und Transfusionsmedizin* 1992; **19:** 91.
Burnouf-Radosevich M, Appourchaux P, Huart JJ, Burnouf T. Nanofiltration, a new specific virus elimination method applied to high-purity factor IX and factor XI concentrates. *Vox Sang* 1994; **67:** 132.
Busch MP. Incidence of infectious disease markers in blood donors: implications for residual risk of viral transmission by transfusion. In: McCurdy PR, Elliot JM (Eds); *Proceedings of NIH Consensus Development Conference on Infectious Disease Testing for Blood Transfusion.* Bethesda, Maryland: National Institute of Health, 1995: 29–30.
Carnelli V, Gomperts ED, Friedman A, et al. Assessment for evidence of non A-non B hepatitis in patients given n-heptane-suspended heat-treated clotting factor concentrates. *Thrombosis Research* 1987; **46:** 827.
Caron C, Goudemand J, Bekri S, Drovin F, Michalski C. Therapeutic trial with a pure factor VII (FVII) in two cases of variant factor VII deficiency. *Thrombosis and Haemostasis* 1991; **65:** 1263.
Carr R, Veitch SE, Edmond E, et al. Abnormalities of circulating lymphocyte subsets in haemophiliacs in an AIDS-free population. *Lancet* 1984; **1:** 1431.
Casillas G, Simonetti C, Pavlovsky A. Chromatographic behaviour of clotting factors. *British Journal of Haematology* 1969; **16:** 363.
Casonato A, Pontara E, Dannhaeuser D, et al. Re-evaluation of the therapeutic efficacy of DDAVP in type IIb von Willebrand's disease. *Blood Coagulation and Fibrinolysis* 1994; **5:** 959.
CDC. Survey of non-U.S. hemophilia treatment centers for HIV seroconversions following therapy with heat-treated factor concentrates. *MMWR Morbidity and Mortality Weekly Report* 1987a; **36:** 121.
CDC. Human immunodeficiency virus infection in the United States. *MMWR Morbidity and Mortality Weekly Report* 1987b; **36:** 801.
Cederbaum Al, Blatt PM, Roberts HR. Intravascular coagulation and the use of human prothrombin complex concentrates. *Annals of Internal Medicine* 1976; **84:** 683.
Chandra S, Wickerhauser M. Contact factors are responsible for the thrombogenicity of prothrombin complex. *Thrombosis Research* 1979; **14:** 189.
Chelucci C, Hassan HJ, Gringeri A, et al. PCR analysis of HIV-1 sequences and differential immunological features in seronegative and seropositive haemophiliacs. *British Journal of Haematology* 1992; **81:** 558.
Chistolini A, Dragoni F, Ferrari A, et al. Intranasal DDAVP: biological and clinical evaluation in mild factor VIII deficiency. *Haemostasis* 1991; **21:** 273.
Choo KH, Gould KG, Rees DJ, Brownlee GG. Molecular cloning of the gene for human anti-haemophilic factor IX. *Nature* 1982; **299:** 178.
Choo QL, Kuo G, Weiner AJ, Overby LR, Bradley DW, Houghton M. Isolation of a cDNA clone derived from a blood-borne non-A, non-B viral hepatitis genome. *Science* 1989; **244:** 359.
Cohn EJ, Strong LE, Hughes WL, et al. Preparation and properties of serum and plasma proteins. A system for the separation into fractions of the protein and lipoprotein components of biological tissues and fluids. *Journal of the American Chemical Society* 1946; **68:** 459.
Cohn RJ, Schwyzer R, Field SP, Fernandes-Costa F, Armstrong D. Hepatitis A in haemophiliacs. *Thrombosis and Haemostasis* 1994; **72:** 785.
Colombo M, Mannucci PM, Carnelli V, Savidge GF, Gazengel C, Schimpf K. Transmission of non-A, non-B hepatitis by heat-treated factor VIII concentrate. *Lancet* 1985; **2:** 1.
Cuthbert RJ, Ludlam CA, Tucker J, et al. Five year prospective study of HIV infection in the Edinburgh haemophiliac cohort. *British Medical Journal* 1990; **301:** 956.

Cuthbert RJ, Ludlam CA, Steel CM, Beatson D, Peutherer JF. Immunological studies in HIV seronegative haemophiliacs: relationships to blood product therapy. *British Journal of Haematology* 1992; **80:** 364.

Daly HM, Haddon ME. Clinical experience with a pasteurised human plasma concentrate in factor XIII deficiency. *Thrombosis and Haemostasis* 1988; **59:** 171.

de Biasi R, Rocino A, Miraglia E, Mastullo L, Quirino AA. The impact of a very high purity factor VIII concentrate on the immune system of human immunodeficiency virus infected haemophiliacs: a randomised, prospective, two year comparison with an intermediate purity concentrate. *Blood* 1991; **78:** 1919.

de Biasi R, Rocino A, Papa ML, Salemo E, Mastullo L, de Biasi D. Incidence of factor VIII inhibitor development in haemophilia A patients treated with less pure plasma derived concentrates. *Thrombosis and Haemostasis* 1994; **71:** 544.

Dempfle C, Magez J, Rokel A, et al. Acquired factor XIII deficiency in exacerbated chronic inflammatory bowel disease (CIBD). *Thrombosis and Haemostasis* 1991; **65:** 1249.

Didisheim PM, Loeb J, Blatrix C, Soulier JP. Preparation of a human plasma fraction rich in prothrombin, proconvertin, Stuart factor and P.T.C. and a study of its activity and toxicity in rabbits and man. *Journal of Laboratory and Clinical Medicine* 1959; **53:** 322.

Dietrich SL, Mosley JW, Lusher JM, et al. Transmission of human immunodeficiency virus type 1 by dry-heated clotting factor concentrates. *Vox Sang* 1990; **59:** 129.

DiPaolantonio T, Mariani G, Chirardini A, et al. Low risk of transmission of the human immunodeficiency virus by a solvent-detergent-treated commercial factor VIII concentrate. *Journal of Medical Virology* 1992; **36:** 71.

Dodd RY. Screening for hepatitis infectivity among blood donors. A model for blood safety? *Archives of Pathology and Laboratory Medicine* 1989; **113:** 227.

Duckert F. Documentation of the plasma factor XIII deficiency in man. *Annals of the New York Academy of Sciences* 1972; **202:** 190.

Eaton DL, Wood WI, Eaton D, et al. Construction and characterization of an active factor VIII variant lacking the central one-third of the molecule. *Biochemistry* 1986; **25:** 8343.

EEC. Council 89/381/EEC. *The Official Journal of the European Communities* 1989; **L181:** 44.

Ehrenforth S, Kreuz W, Scharrer I, et al. Incidence of development of factor VIII and factor IX inhibitors in haemophiliacs. *Lancet* 1992; **339:** 594.

Eibl MM, Ahmad R, Wolf HM, Linnau Y, Gotz E, Mannhalter JW. A component of factor VIII preparations which can be separated from factor VIII activity down modulates human monocyte functions. *Blood* 1987; **69:** 1153.

Elodi S, Varadi K. Activation of clotting factors in prothrombin complex concentrates as demonstrated by clotting assays for factors IXa and Xa. *Thrombosis Research* 1978; **12:** 797.

Emrich HG, Bartels RSM, Kreuz W, et al. Bleeding tendency, long-term substitution therapy and factor XIII determination in patients with congenital factor XIII deficiency. *Thrombosis and Haemostasis* 1991; **65:** 1262.

Evans JA, Pasi KJ, Williams MD, Hill FG. Consistently normal CD4+, CD8+ levels in haemophilic boys only treated with a virally safe factor VIII concentrate (BPL 8Y). *British Journal of Haematology* 1991; **79:** 457.

Eyster ME, Gail MH, Ballard JO, Al-Mondhiry H, Goedert JJ. Natural history of human immunodeficiency virus infections in hemophiliacs: effects of T-cell subsets, platelet counts, and age. *Annals of Internal Medicine* 1987; **107:** 1.

Eyster ME, Schaefer JH, Ragni MV, et al. Changing causes of death in Pennsylvania's hemophiliacs 1976 to 1991: impact of liver disease and acquired immunodeficiency syndrome. *Blood* 1992; **79:** 2494.

Feisly MR. Eludes Sur L'hemophile. *Bulletin et Memoires de la Societe de Hopital de Paris* 1923; **1738**

Feldman PA, Harris L, Evans DR, Evans HE. Preparation of a high purity factor IX concentrate using metal chelate affinity chromatography. In: Rivat C, Stolz JF (Eds), *Biotechnology of Blood Products*. Paris: INSERM/Libbey Eurotext Ltd, 1989: 63–68.

Foster PR, Dickson IH, McQuillan TA, Dawes J. Factor VIII stability during the manufacture of a clinical concentrate. *Thrombosis and Haemostasis* 1983; **50:** 117.

Foster PR, Dickson AJ. Control of large scale plasma thawing. In: Smit Sibinga CT, Das PC, Seidl S (Eds), *Plasma Fractionation and Blood Transfusion*. Boston Martinus Nijhoff, 1985: **57**.

Frickhofen N, Abkowitz JL, Safford M, et al. Persistent B19 parvovirus infection in patients infected with human immunodeficiency virus type 1 (HIV-1): a treatable cause of anemia in AIDS. *Annals of Internal Medicine* 1990; **113:** 926.
Fuerth JH, Mahrer P. Myocardial infarction after factor IX therapy. *Journal of the American Medical Association* 1981; **245:** 1455.
Fukutake K, Fujimaki M, Hanabusa S, Inagaki M, Mimaya J, Shirahata A. Multicentre study on the influence of long-term continuous use of ultrapurified factor VIII preparation on the immunological status of HIV-infected and non-infected hemophilia A patients. *Thrombosis and Haemostasis* 1991; **65:** 996
Ganzengel C, Torcher MF, French Haemophilia Study Group. Virus safety of solvent/detergent treated FVIII concentrate. Results of a French multicenter study. *International Congress of World Federation of Haemophilia* 1988; 59.
Gerritzen A, Schneweis KE, Brackmann HH, et al. Acute hepatitis A in haemophiliacs. *Lancet* 1992a; **340:** 1231.
Gerritzen A, Scholt B, Kaiser R, Schneweis KE, Brackmann HH, Oldenburg J. Acute hepatitis C in haemophiliacs due to "virus-inactivated" clotting factor concentrates. *Thrombosis and Haemostasis* 1992b; **68:** 781.
Giles AR, Johnston M, Hoogendoom H, et al. The thrombogenicity of prothrombin complex concentrates: the relationship between in vitro characteristics and in vivo thrombogenicity in rabbits. *Thrombosis Research* 1980; **17:** 353.
Giles AR, Nesheim ME, Hoogendoom H, et al. The coagulant-active phospholipid content is a major determinant of in vivo thrombogenicity of prothrombin complex (factor IX) concentrates in rabbits. *Blood* 1982; **59:** 401.
Gitel SN, Varon D, Schulman S, Martinowitz U. Clinical experience with a FXI concentrate. Possible side-effects. *Thrombosis and Haemostasis* 1991; **65:** 1157.
Gitschier J, Wood WI, Goralka TM, et al. Characterization of the human factor VIII gene. *Nature* 1984; **312:** 326.
Goedert JJ, Kessler CM, Aledort LM, et al. A prospective study of human immunodeficiency virus type 1 infection and the development of AIDS in subjects with hemophilia. *New England Journal of Medicine* 1989; **321:** 1141.
Goedert JJ, Cohen AR, Kessler CM, et al. Risks of immunodeficiency, AIDS, and death related to purity of factor VIII concentrate. *Lancet* 1994; **344:** 791.
Goldsmith GH, Jr, Baily RG, Brettler DB, et al. Primary pulmonary hypertension in patients with classic hemophilia. *Annals of Internal Medicine* 1988; **108:** 797.
Goldsmith JM, Deutsche J, Tang M, Green D. $CD4^+$ cells in HIV-1 infected hemophiliacs: effect of factor VIII concentrates. *Thrombosis and Haemostasis* 1991; **66:** 415.
Goldsmith MF. Hemophilia, beaten on one front, is beset on others. *Journal of the American Medical Association* 1986; **256:** 3200.
Gomperts E, Lundblad R, Adamson R. The manufacturing process of recombinant factor VIII, recombinate. *Transfusion Medicine Reviews* 1992; **6:** 247.
Gonzaga AL, Boneker C. Follow-up of haemophiliacs using solvent/detergent treated FVIII and FIX concentrates. *Congress of World Federation of Haemophilia* 1990; **25**.
Gowda SD, Stein BS, Mohagheghpour N, Benike CJ, Engleman EG. Evidence that T cell activation is required for HIV-1 entry in $CD4^+$ lymphocytes. *Journal of Immunology* 1989; **142:** 773.
Gringeri A, Santagostino E, Mannucci PM. Failure of recombinant activated factor VII during surgery in a hemophiliac with high-titer factor VIII antibody. *Haemostasis* 1991; **21:** 1.
Haimovich J, Davis HM, Schreiber AB. Human anti-mouse immunoglobulins in sera of patients treated. *Seminars in Hematology* 1990; **27:** 11.
Hampton KK, Preston FE, Lowe GD, Walker ID, Sampson B. Reduced coagulation activation following infusion of a highly purified factor IX concentrate compared to a prothrombin complex concentrate. *British Journal of Haematology* 1993; **84:** 279.
Hart H, McOmish F, Hart WG, Simmonds P, Yap PL. A comparison of polymerase chain reaction and an infectivity assay for human immunodeficiency virus type 1 titration during virus inactivation of blood components. *Transfusion* 1993; **33:** 838.
Hartmann S, Reinhart W. Fatal complication of desmopressin. *Lancet* 1995; **345:** 1302.
Hashemi S, Palmer DS, Aye MT, Ganz PR. Platelet-activating factor secreted by DDAVP-treated monocytes mediates von Willebrand factor release from endothelial cells. *Journal of Cellular Physiology* 1993; **154:** 496.

Hay CR, McEvoy P. Purity of factor VIII concentrates. *Lancet* 1992; **339:** 1613.
Hay CR, McEvoy P, Duggan-Keen M. Inhibition of lymphocyte IL2-receptor expression by factor VIII concentrate: a possible cause of immunosuppression in haemophiliacs. *British Journal of Haematology* 1990; **75:** 278.
Hay CRM, Colvin BT, Ludlam CA, Hill FGH, Preston FE. Recommendations for the treatmant of factor VIII inhibitors: from the UK Haemophilia Centre Disorders' Coagulation Inhibitor Working Party. *Blood Coagulation and Fibrinology* 1996; **7:** 134–138.
Hedner U, Kisiel W. Use of human factor VIIa in the treatment of two hemophilia A patients with high-titer inhibitors. *Journal of Clinical Investigation* 1983; **71:** 1836.
Hedner U, Glazer S, Pingel K, et al. Successful use of recombinant factor VIIa in patient with severe haemophilia A during synovectomy. *Lancet* 1988; **2:** 1193.
Hedner U, Bjoem S, Bernvil SS, Tengborn L, Stigendahl L. Clinical experience with human plasma-derived factor VIIa in patients with hemophilia A and high titer inhibitors. *Haemostasis* 1989; **19:** 335.
Hedner U, Ljundberg J, Lund Hansen T. Comparison of the effect of plasma-derived and recombinant human FVIIa in vitro and in a rabbit model. *Blood Coagulation and Fibrinology* 1990; **1:** 145.
Heinrich D, Kotitschke R, Berthold H. Clinical evaluation of the hepatitis safety of a beta-propiolactone/ultraviolet treated factor IX concentrate (PPSB). *Thrombosis Research* 1982; **28:** 75.
Hellerstein LJ, Deykin D. Hepatitis after Konyne administration. *New England Journal of Medicine* 1971; **284:** 1039.
Hilgartner MW, Buckley JD, Operskalski EA, Pike MC, Mosley JW. Purity of factor VIII concentrates and serial CD4+ counts. *Lancet* 1993; **341:** 1373.
Hoag MS, Johnson FF, Robinson JA, Aggeler PM. Treatment of hemophilia B with a new clotting factor concentrate. *New England Journal of Medicine* 1969; **280:** 291.
Hoofnagle JH, Gerety RJ, Thiel J, Barker LF. The prevalence of hepatitis B surface antigen in commercially prepared plasma products. *Journal of Laboratory and Clinical Medicine* 1976; **88:** 102.
Hoofnagle JH, Seefe LB, Bales ZB, Zimmerman HJ. Type B hepatitis after transfusion with blood containing antibody to hepatitis B core antigen. *New England Journal of Medicine* 1978; **298:** 1379.
Horowitz B, Wiebe ME, Lippin A, Stryker MH. Inactivation of viruses in labile blood derivatives. I. Disruption of lipid-enveloped viruses by tri(n-butyl) phosphate detergent combinations. *Transfusion* 1985; **25:** 516.
Horowitz B, Bonomo R, Prince AM, Chin SN, Brotman B, Shulman RW. Solvent detergent treated plasma: a virus inactivated substitute for fresh frozen plasma. *Blood* 1992; **79:** 826.
Horowitz MS, Rooks C, Horowitz B, Hilgartner MW. Virus safety of solvent/detergent-treated antihaemophilic factor concentrate. *Lancet* 1988; **2:** 186.
Houghton M, Selby M, Weiner A, Choo QL. Hepatitis C virus: structure, protein products and processing of the polyprotein precursor. *Current Studies in Hematology & Blood Transfusion* 1994; **1**.
Hrinda ME, Feldman F, Schreiber AB. Preclinical characterization of a new pasteurized monoclonal antibody purified factor VIII:C. *Seminars in Hematology* 1990; **27:** 19.
Hrinda ME, Huang C, Tarr GC, Weeks R, Feldman F, Schreiber AB. Preclinical studies of a monoclonal antibody-purified factor IX, Mononine. *Seminars in Hematology* 1991; **28:** 6.
Hultin MB. Activated clotting factors in factor IX concentrates. *Blood* 1979; **54:** 1028.
Ingram GI, Dykes SR, Creese AL, et al. Home treatment in haemophilia: clinical, social and economic advantages. *Clinical and Laboratory Haematology* 1979; **1:** 13.
Kasper CK. Incidence and course of inhibitors among patients with classic hemophilia. *Thrombosis et Diathesis Haemorrhagica* 1973; **30:** 263.
Kasper CK. Thromboembolic complications. *Thrombosis et Diathesis Haemorrhagica* 1975; **33:** 640.
Kasper CK, Kipnis SA. Hepatitis and clotting-factor concentrates. *Journal of the American Medical Association* 1972; **221:** 510.
Kasper CK, Inwood M, Scharrer I, Bloom A, Schwartz RS. Safety of recombinant factor VIII in home infusion. *Blood* 1991; **78:** 56.
Kasper CK, Lusher JM, Silberstein LE, et al. Recent evolution of clotting factor concentrates for hemophilia A and B. *Transfusion* 1993; **33:** 422.

Katchaki JN, Siem TH, Brouwer R, et al. Detection and significance of anti-HBc in the blood bank: preliminary results of a controlled prospective study. *Journal of Virological Methods* 1981; **2:** 119.
Keith JC, Ferranti TJ, Misra B, et al. Evaluation of recombinant factor IX. Pharmacokinetic studies in the rat and the dog. *Thrombosis and Haemostasis* 1994; **73:** 101.
Kekwick RA, Wolf PA. A concentrate of human antihaemophilic factor. Its use in six cases of haemophilia. *Lancet* 1957; **647**.
Kemball-Cook G, Garner I, Imanaka Y, et al. High-level production of human blood coagulation factors VII and XI using a new mammalian expression vector. *Gene* 1994; **139:** 275.
Kernoff PBA, Miller EJ, Savidge GF, Machin SJ, Dewar MS, Preston FE. Reduced risk of non-A, non-B hepatitis after a first exposure to "wet heated" factor VIII concentrate. *British Journal of Haematology* 1987; **67:** 207.
Kessler CM, Sachse K. Factor VIII:C inhibitor associated with monoclonal-antibody purified FVIII concentrate. *Lancet* 1990; **335:** 1403.
Kesteven PJ, Holland LJ, Lawrie AS, Savidge GF. Inhibitor to factor VIII in mild haemophilia. *Thrombosis and Haemostasis* 1984; **52:** 50.
Kim HC, McMillan CW, White GC, Bergman GE, Horton MW, Saidi P. Purified factor IX using monoclonal immunoaffinity technique: clinical trials in hemophilia B and comparison to prothrombin complex concentrates. *Blood* 1992; **79:** 568.
Kingdon HS. Hepatitis after Konyne. *Annals of Internal Medicine* 1970; **73:** 656.
Kingdon HS, Lundblad RL, Veltkamp JJ, Aronson DL. Potentially thrombogenic materials in factor IX concentrates. *Thrombosis et Diathesis Haemorrhagica* 1975; **33:** 617.
Kleim JP, Bailly E, Schneweis KE, et al. Acute HIV-1 infection in patients with hemophilia B treated with beta-propiolactone-UV-inactivated clotting factor. *Thrombosis and Haemostasis* 1990; **64:** 336.
Klein U. Production and characterization of recombinant factor VIII. *Seminars in Haematology* 1991; **28:** 17.
Kolho E. Specificity and sensitivity of first and second generation anti-HCV ELISA in a low prevalence population. *Transfusion Medicine* 1992; **2:** 239.
Koretz RL, Gitnick GL. Prevention of post-transfusion hepatitis. Role of sensitive hepatitis B antigen screening tests, source of blood and volume of transfusion. *American Journal of Medicine* 1975; **59:** 754.
Kreuz W, Auerswald G, Bruckmann C, et al. Prevention of hepatitis C virus infection in children with haemophilia A and B and von Willebrand's disease. *Thrombosis and Haemostasis* 1992; **67:** 184.
Kuo G, Choo QL, Alter HJ, et al. An assay for circulating antibodies to a major etiologic virus of human non-A, non-B hepatitis. *Science* 1989; **244:** 362.
Kurachi K, Davie EW. Isolation and characterization of a cDNA coding for human factor IX. *Proceedings National Academy of Sciences USA* 1982; **79:** 6461.
Lackritz EM, Satten GA, Kennedy MB. Residual risk of transfusion-associated HIV transmission. In: McCurdy PR, Eliot JM (Eds), *Proceedings of NIH Consensus Development Conference on Infectious Disease Testing for Blood Transfusion*. Bethesda, Maryland, USA: National Institute of Health, 1995: **21**.
Lai ME, Farci P, Figus A, Balestrieri A, Arnone M, Vyas GN. Hepatitis B virus DNA in the serum of Sardinian blood donors negative for the hepatitis B surface antigen. *Blood* 1989; **73:** 17.
Lander JJ, Gitnick GL, Gelb LH, Aach RD. Anticore antibody screening of transfused blood. *Vox Sang* 1978; **34:** 77.
Lane S. Haemorrhagic diathesis, successful transfusion of blood. *Lancet* 1840; 185.
Laurian Y, Lusher JM, Kessler CM. Viral safety and clotting factor concentrates. *Thrombosis and Haemostasis* 1994; **72:** 649.
Lederman MM, Saunders C, Toossi Z, Lemon N, Everson B, Ratnoff OD. Antihemophilic factor factor VIII preparations inhibit lymphocyte proliferation and production of interleukin-2. *Journal of Laboratory and Clinical Medicine* 1986; **107:** 471.
Lee CA, Sabin CA, Phillips A, Elford J, Pasi J. Morbidity and mortality from transfusion transmitted disease in haemophilia. *Lancet* 1995; **345:** 1309.
Lefrere JJ, Mariotti M, Thauvin M. B19 parvovirus DNA in solvent/detergent-treated antihaemophilia concentrates. *Lancet* 1994; **343:** 211.
Leikola J. Non-remunerated donations. *Developments in Biological Standardization* 1993; **81:** 51.

Levine P. Efficacy of self therapy in hemophilia. A study of 72 patients with hemophilia A and B. *New England Journal of Medicine* 1974; **291:** 1381.
Liebman HA, Limentani SA, Furie BC, Furie B. Immunoaffinity purification of factor IX (Christmas factor) by using conformation-specific antibodies directed against the factor IX-metal complex. *Proceedings of the National Academy of Sciences USA* 1985; **82:** 3879.
Lippert LE, Fisher LMA, Schook LB. Relationship of major histocompatability complex class II genes to inhibitor antibody formation in hemophilia A. *Thrombosis and Haemostasis* 1990; **64:** 564.
Ljung R, Petrini P, Lindgren AC, Tengbom L, Nilsson IM. Factor VIII and factor IX inhibitors in haemophiliacs. *Lancet* 1992; **339:** 1550.
Lorenzo J, Garcia R, Molina R. Factor VIII and IX inhibitors in haemophiliacs. *Lancet* 1992; **339:** 1550.
Losowsky MS, Miloszewski K. Management of patients with congenital deficiency of fibrin stabilising factor (factor XIII). In: Seno S, Takaku F, Irino S (Eds). *Proceedings of 16th International Congress of Haematology*. Kyota, Japan: Excerpta Medica, 1976.
Ludlam CA, Peake IR, Allen N, Davies BL, Furlong RA, Bloom AL. Factor VII and fibrinolytic response to deamino-8-D-argenine vasopressin in normal subjects and dissociate response in some patients with haemophilia and von Willebrand's disease. *British Journal of Haematology* 1980; **45:** 499.
Ludlam CA, Chapman D, Cohen B, Litton PA. Antibodies to hepatitis C virus in haemophilia. *Lancet* 1989; **ii:** 560.
Lush CJ, Chapman CS, Mitchell VE, Martin C. Transmission of hepatitis B by dry heat treated factor VIII and IX concentrates letter. *British Journal of Haematology* 1988; **69:** 421.
Lusher JM. Thrombogenicity associated with factor IX complex concentrates. *Seminars in Hematology* 1991; **28:** 3.
Lusher JM, Salzman PM. Viral safety and inhibitor development associated with factor VIII:C ultra-purified from plasma in hemophiliacs previously unexposed to factor VIII:C concentrates. *Seminars in Haematology* 1990; **27:** 1.
Lusher JM, Arkin S, Abildgaard CF, et al. Recombinant factor VIII for the treatment of previously untreated patients with hemophilia A: safety, efficacy, and development of inhibitors. *New England Journal of Medicine* 1993; **328:** 453.
Macfarlane RJ, Biggs R, Bidwell E. Bovine antihaemophilic globulin in the treatment of haemophilia. *Lancet* 1954; 1316.
Macik BG. Treatment of factor VIII inhibitors: products and strategies. *Seminars in Thrombosis and Hemostasis* 1993; **19:** 13.
Madhok R, Gracie A, Lowe GD, et al. Impaired cell mediated immunity in haemophilia in the absence of infection with human immunodeficiency virus. *British Medical Journal* 1986; **293:** 978.
Madhok R, Gracie JA, Forbes CD, Lowe GD. B cell dysfunction in haemophilia in the absence of presence of HIV-1 infection. *Thrombosis and Haemostasis* 1991; **65** (1): 7.
Magner A, Aronson D. Toxicity of factor IX concentrates in mice. *Developments in Biological Standards* 1979; **44:** 185.
Mahir WS, Millard RE, Booth JC, Flute PT. Functional studies of cell-mediated immunity in haemophilia and other bleeding disorders. *British Journal of Haematology* 1988; **69:** 367.
Makris M, Preston FE, Triger DR, et al. Hepatitis C antibody and chronic liver disease in haemophilia. *Lancet* 1990; **335:** 1117.
Makris M, Preston FE, Ralph S. Increased soluble IL-2 receptor levels in HCV-infected haemophiliacs: a possible indicator of liver disease severity. *British Journal of Haematology* 1994; **87:** 419.
Mannhalter JW, Ahmad R, Leibl H, Gottlicher J, Wolf HM, Eibl MM. Comparable modulation of human monocyte functions by commercial factor VIII concentrates of varying purity. *Blood* 1988; **71:** 1662.
Mannucci PM. Outbreak of hepatitis A among Italian patients with haemophilia. *Lancet* 1992; **339:** 819.
Mannucci PM, Colombo M. Revision of the protocol recommended for studies of safety from hepatitis of clotting factor concentrates. *Thrombosis and Haemostasis* 1989; **61:** 532.
Mannucci PM, Morfini M. Determination of pharmacokinetics of replacement factor VIII. *Seminars in Hematology* 1990; **27:** 8.

Mannucci PM, Zanetti AR, Colombo M. Prospective study of hepatitis after factor VIII concentrate exposed to hot vapour. *British Journal of Haematology* 1988; **68:** 427.

Mannucci PM, Bauer KA, Gringeri A, et al. Thrombin generation is not increased in the blood of hemophilia B patients after the infusion of a purified factor IX concentrate. *Blood* 1990a; **76:** 2540.

Mannucci PM, Schimpf K, Brettler DB, et al. Low risk for hepatitis C in hemophiliacs given a high-purity, pasteurized factor VIII concentrate. International Study Group. *Annals of Internal Medicine* 1990b; **113:** 27.

Mannucci PM, Zanetti AR, Colombo M, et al. Antibody to hepatitis C virus after a vapour-heated factor VIII concentrate. The Study Group of the Fondazione dell'Emofilia. *Thrombosis and Haemostasis* 1990c; **64:** 232.

Mannucci PM, Bauer KA, Gringeri A, et al. No activation of the common pathway of the coagulation cascade after a highly purified factor IX concentrate. *British Journal of Haematology* 1991; **79:** 606.

Mannucci PM, Bettega D, Cattaneo M. Patterns of development of tachyphylaxis in patients with haemophilia and von Willebrand disease after repeated doses of desmopressin (DDAVP). *British Journal of Haematology* 1992a; **82:** 87.

Mannucci PM, Gringeri A, de Biasi R, Baudo F, Morfini M, Ciavarella N. Immune status of asymptomatic HIV-infected hemophiliacs: randomized, prospective, two-year comparison of treatment with a high-purity or an intermediate-purity factor VIII concentrate. *Thrombosis and Haemostasis* 1992b; **67:** 310.

Mannucci PM, Schimpf K, Abe T, et al. Low risk of viral infection after administration of vapor-heated factor VIII concentrate. *Transfusion* 1992c; **32:** 134.

Mannucci PM, Bauer KA, Santagostino E, et al. Activation of the coagulation cascade after infusion of a factor XI concentrate in congenitally deficient patients. *Blood* 1994a; **84:** 1314.

Mannucci PM, Gdovin S, Gringeri A, et al. Transmission of hepatitis A to patients with hemophilia by factor VIII concentrates treated with organic solvent and detergent to inactivate viruses. *Annals of Internal Medicine* 1994b; **120:** 1.

Margolick J, B., Volkman DJ, Folks TM. HTLV III/LAV detection by antigen induced activation of T cells and amplification of direct suppression by virus of lymphocyte blastogenic response. *Journal of Immunology* 1987; **138:** 1719.

Mariani G, Mannucci PM, Mazzucconi MG, Capitanio A. Treatment of congenital factor VII deficiency with a new concentrate. *Thrombosis and Haemostasis* 1978; **39:** 675.

Mariani G, Ghirardini A, Mandelli F, et al. Heated clotting factors and seroconversion for human immunodeficiency virus in three hemophilic patients letter. *Annals of Internal Medicine* 1987; **107:** 113.

Mariani G, DiPaolantonio T, Baklaja R, Mannucci PM. Prospective hepatitis C safety evaluation of a high purity solvent detergent treated FVIII concentrate. *Blood* 1991; **78**(suppl): 55a.

Matheson DS, Green BJ, Poon MC, Bowen TJ, Fritzler MJ, Hoar DI. T lymphocytes from hemophiliacs proliferate after exposure to factor VIII product. *Vox Sang* 1986a; **51:** 92.

Matheson DS, Green BJ, Poon MC, Fritzler MJ, Hoar DI, Bowen TJ. Natural killer cell activity from hemophiliacs exhibits differential responses to various forms of interferon. *Blood* 1986b; **67:** 164.

McFarlane IG, Smith HM, Johnson PJ, Bray GP, Vergani D, Williams R. Hepatitis C virus antibodies in chronic active hepatitis: pathogenetic factor or false-positive result? *Lancet* 1990; **335:** 754.

McMillan CW, Shapiro SS, Whitehurst D, Hoyer LW, Rao AV, Lazerson J. The natural history of factor VIII:C inhibitors in patients with hemophilia A: a national cooperative study. Observations on the initial development of factor VIII:C inhibitors. *Blood* 1988; **71:** 344.

McOmish F, Yap PL, Jordan A, Hart H, Cohen BJ, Simmonds P. Detection of parvovirus B19 in donated blood: a model system for screening by polymerase chain reaction. *Journal of Clinical Microbiology* 1993; **31:** 323–328.

Menache D, Behre HE, Orthner CL, et al. Coagulation factor IX concentrate: method of preparation and assessment of potential in vivo thrombogenicity in animal models. *Blood* 1984; **64:** 1220.

Middleton S. Polyelectrolytes and preparation of factor VIII:C. In: Forbes CD, Lowe GDO (Eds), *Unresolved Problems in Haemophilia.* Lancaster: MTP Press, 1982; 109.

Middleton SM, Bennett IH, Smith JK. A therapeutic concentrate of coagulation factors II, IX and X from citrated, factor VIII-depleted plasma. *Vox Sang* 1973; **24:** 441.

Minor P, Pipkin P, Thorpe R, Thomas D. Antibody to hepatitis C virus in plasma pools. *Lancet* 1990; **336:** 188.

Mohr H, Lambrecht B, KnueverHopf J. Virus inactivated single-donor fresh plasma preparations. *Infusionstherapie und Transfusionsmedizin* 1992; **19:** 79.

Montoro JB, Rodriguez S, Altisent C, Tusell JM. Transient factor VIII inhibitor and treatment with monoclonal-antibody-purified factor VIII. *Lancet* 1991; **337:** 1222

Morfini M, Longo G, Messori A, Lee M, White G, Mannucci P. Pharmacokinetic properties of recombinant factor VIII compared with a monoclonally purified concentrate (Hemofil M). *Thrombosis and Haemostasis* 1992; **68:** 433.

Myhre BA, Jiminez L, Shitabata P, Ukkestad T. The correlations of surrogate markers with anti-hepatitis C virus and other disease markers. *Annals of Clinical and Laboratory Science* 1994; **24:** 76.

Myhre BA, Figueroa PI. Infectious disease markers in various groups of donors. *Annals of Clinical and Laboratory Science* 1995; **25:** 39.

Nau JY. CJD and albumin? *Lancet* 1995; 442.

Noel L, Guerois C, Maisonneuve P, et al. Antibodies to hepatitis C virus in haemophilia. *Lancet* 1989; **2:** 560.

Orringer EP, Koury MJ, Blatt PM, Roberts HR. Hemolysis caused by factor VIII concentrates. *Archives of Internal Medicine* 1976; **136:** 1018.

Pasi KJ, Hill FG. In vitro and in vivo inhibition of monocyte phagocytic function by factor VIII concentrates: correlation with concentrate purity. *British Journal of Haematology* 1990; **76:** 88.

Payne WW, Steen RE. Haemostatic therapy in haemophilia. *British Medical Journal* 1929; 1150.

Peerlinck K, Vermylen J. Acute Hepatitis A in patients with haemophilia A. *Lancet* 1993; **341:** 179.

Pejaudier L, Kichenin-Martin V, Boffa MC, Steinbuch M. Appraisal of the protein composition of prothrombin complex concentrates of different origins. *Vox Sang* 1987; **52:** 1.

Peters M, Fijn van Draat K, Koopman MMW, ten Cate JW. A new B-domain-deleted recombinant factor VIII concentrate (r-VIII SQ): pharmacokinetics and tolerability of three doses. *Thrombosis and Haemostasis* 1995; **73:** 1013.

Philips AN, Lee CA, Elford J, et al. Serial CD4 lymphocyte counts and development of AIDS. *Lancet* 1991; **337:** 389.

Pierce GF, Lusher JM, Brownstein AP, Goldsmith JC, Kessler CM. The use of purified clotting factor concentrates in hemophilia. Influence of viral safety, cost, and supply on therapy. *Journal of the American Medical Association* 1989; **261:** 3434.

Pistello M, Lecherini-Nelli L, Cecconi N, Bendinelli M, Panicucci F. Hepatitis C virus seroprevalence in Italian haemophiliacs injected with virus-inactivated concentrates: five year follow-up and correlation with antibodies to other viruses. *Journal of Medical Virology* 1991; **33:** 43.

Pool JG, Shannon AE. Production of high potency concentrates of antihaemophilic globulin in a closed bag system: assay in vitro and in vivo. *New England Journal of Medicine* 1965; **273:** 1443.

Preston FE, Hay CR, Dewar MS, Greaves M, Triger DR. Non-A, non-B hepatitis and heat-treated factor VIII concentrates. *Lancet* 1985; **2:** 213.

Prince AM, Brotman B, Grady GF, et al. Long-incubation post-transfusion hepatitis without serological evidence of exposure to hepatitis-B virus. *Lancet* 1974; **2:** 241.

Prowse CV. Parvovirus B19 and blood products. *Lancet* 1994; **343:** 1101.

Prowse CV, Williams AE. A comparison of the in vitro and in vivo thrombogenic activity of factor IX concentrates using stasis (Wessler) and non-stasis rabbit models. *Thrombosis and Haemostasis* 1980; **44:** 81.

Rasi V, Ikkala E. Haemophiliacs with factor VIII inhibitors in Finland: prevalence, incidence and outcome. *British Journal of Haematology* 1990; **76:** 369.

Remis RJ, O'Shaughnessy MV, Tsoukas C, et al. HIV transmission to patients with hemophilia by heat-treated, donor-screened factor concentrate. *Canadian Medical Association Journal* 1990; **142:** 1247.

Rizza CR, Spooner RJ. Treatment of haemophilia and related disorders in Britain and Northern Ireland during 1976–80: report on behalf of the Directors of Haemophilia Centres in the United Kingdom. *British Medical Journal* 1983; **286:** 929.
Rodeghiero F, Castaman G, Mannucci PM. Clinical indications for desmopressin (DDAVP) in congenital and acquired von Willebrand disease. *Blood Reviews* 1991; **5:** 155.
Rubinstein AI, Rubinstein DB, Coughlin J. Combined solvent-detergent and 100°C (boiling) sterilizing dry-heat treatment of factor VIII concentrates to assure sterility. *Vox Sang* 1991; **60:** 60.
Ruggeri ZM, Mannucci PM, Lombardi R, Federici AB, Zimmerman TS. Multimeric composition of factor VIII/von Willebrand factor following administration of DDAVP: implications for pathophysiology and therapy of von Willebrand's disease subtypes. *Blood* 1982; **59:** 1272.
Sabin C, Pasi J, Phillips A, Elford J, Janossy G, Lee C. CD4+ counts before and after switching to monoclonal high-purity factor VIII concentrate in HIV-infected haemophilic patients. *Thrombosis and Haemostasis* 1994; **72:** 214.
Saeed AA, AlAdmawi AM, AlRasheed A, et al. Hepatitis C virus infection in Egyptian volunteer blood donors in Riyadh. *Lancet* 1991; **338:** 459.
Santagostino E, Mannucci PM, Grigeri A, Azzi A, Morfini M. Eliminating parvovirus B19 from blood products. *Lancet* 1994; **343:** 798.
Schimpf K, Mannucci PM, Kreutz W, et al. Absence of hepatitis after treatment with a pasteurized factor VIII concentrate in patients with hemophilia and no previous transfusions. *New England Journal of Medicine* 1987; **316:** 918.
Schimpf K, Brackmann HH, Kreuz W, et al. Absence of anti-human immunodeficiency virus types 1 and 2 seroconversion after the treatment of hemophilia A or von Willebrand's disease with pasteurized factor VIII concentrate. *New England Journal of Medicine* 1989; **321:** 1148.
Schmidt ML, Smith HE, Gamerman S, DiMichele D, Glazer S, Scott JP. Prolonged recombinant activated factor VII (rFVIIa) treatment for severe bleeding in a factor-IX-deficient patient with an inhibitor. *British Journal of Haematology* 1991; **78:** 460.
Schramm W. Consensus recommendations for hemophilia treatment in Germany. Hamostaseologie 1994; **14:** 81–83.
Schulman S, Lindgren AC, Petrini P, Allander T. Transmission of hepatitis C with pasteurised factor VIII. *Lancet* 1992; **340:** 305.
Schwartz RS, Abildgaard CF, Aledort LM, et al. Human recombinant DNA-derived antihemophilic factor (factor VIII) in the treatment of hemophilia A. *New England Journal of Medical* 1990; **323:** 1800.
Schwarzinger I, Pabinger I, Kominger C, et al. Incidence of inhibitors in patients with severe and moderate hemophilia A treated with factor VIII concentrates. *American Journal of Hematology* 1987; **24:** 241.
Seligsohn U, Kasper CK, Osterud B, Rapaport SI. Activated factor VII: presence in factor IX concentrates and persistence in the circulation after infusion. *Blood* 1979; **53:** 828.
Seremetis SV, Aledort LM, Bergman GE, et al. Three-year randomised study of high-purity or intermediate-purity factor VIII concentrates in symptom-free HIV-seropositive haemophiliacs: effects on immune status. *Lancet* 1993; **342:** 700.
Shapiro A. International Factor Safety Study Group. A study to determine the safety of virus inactivated factor VIII concentrates in haemophiliacs naive to blood product administration: factor VIII concentrate (human) Immuno, vapor heated. *International Congress of World Federation of Haemophilia* 1992; 25.
Shapiro SS: Genetic predisposition to inhibitor formation. In: Hoyer LW (Ed.), *Factor VIII Inhibitors*. New York: Liss, 1984a: 45.
Shapiro SS. Markers for the factor VIII antibody response in hemophilia A. *Scandinavian Journal of Haematology Suppl* 1984b; **40:** 181.
Shirahata A, Nakamura T, Shimono M, Kaneko M, Tanaka S. Blood coagulation findings and the efficacy of factor XIII concentrate in premature infants with intracranial hemorrhages. *Thrombosis Research* 1990; **57:** 755.
Shopnick RI, Brettler DB, Bolivar E. Hepatitis C virus transmission by monoclonal-purified viral-attenuated factor VIII concentrate. *Lancet* 1995; **346:** 645.
Simmonds P, Zhang LQ, Watson HG, et al. Hepatitis C quantification and sequencing in blood products, haemophiliacs and intravenous drug users. *Lancet* 1990; **336:** 1469.

Simmonds P, Rose KA, Graham S, et al. Mapping of serotype-specific, immunodominant epitopes in the ns-4 region of hepatitis C virus (HCV): use of type-specific peptides to serologically differentiate infections with HCV types 1, 2, and 3. *Journal of Clinical Microbiology* 1993; **31:** 1493.

Simmonds P, Smith DB, McOmish F, et al. Identification of genotypes of hepatitis C virus by sequence comparisons in the E1 and NS-5 regions. *Journal of General Virology* 1994; **75:** 1053.

Skidmore S. Recombinant immunoblot assay for hepatitis C antibody. *Lancet* 1990; **335:** 1346.

Skidmore SJ, Pasi KJ, Mawson SJ, Williams MD, Hill FG. Serological evidence that dry heating of clotting factor concentrates prevents transmission of non-A, non-B hepatitis. *Journal of Medical Virology* 1990; **30:** 50.

Smit Sibinga CT, Schulting PJ, Notebomer J, Das PC, Marrink J, Van De Meer J. Double cryoprecipitated factor VIII concentrate from heparinised plasma and its heat treatment. *Blut* 1988; **56:** 111.

Speirs HJL, Stirling D, Ludlam CA, Steele CM. TGF-B is only a minor immunosuppressive contaminant of factor VIII concentrates. *Thrombosis and Haemostasis* 1995; **73:** 1036.

Stein SF, Duncan A, Cutler D, Glazer S. Disseminated intravascular coagulation (DIC) in a haemophiliac treated with recombinant factor VIIa. *Blood* 1990; **76:** 438a.

Study Group of the UK Haemophilia Centre Directors. Effect of dry-heating of coagulant factor concentrates at 80°C for 72 hours on transmission of non-A, non-B hepatitis. *Lancet* 1988; 814.

Sullivan DW, Purdy LJ, Billingham M, Glader BE. Fatal myocardial infarction following therapy with prothrombin complex concentrates in a young man with hemophilia A. *Pediatrics* 1984; **74:** 279.

Sullivan JL, Brewster FE, Brettler DB, et al. Hemophiliac immunodeficiency: influence of exposure to factor VIII concentrate. LAV/HTLV-III, and herpes viruses. *Journal of Pediatrics* 1986; **108:** 504.

Tedder RS, Briggs M, Ring C, et al. Hepatitis C antibody profile and viraemia prevalence in adults with severe haemophilia. *British Journal of Haematology* 1991; **79:** 512.

Teitel JM, Freedman JJ, Garvey MB, Kardish M. Two-year evaluation of clinical and laboratory variables of immune function in 117 hemophiliacs seropositive or seronegative for HIV-1. *American Journal of Hematology* 1989; **32:** 262.

Temperley IJ, Cotter KP, Walsh TJ, Power J, Hillary IB. Clotting factors and hepatitis A. *Lancet* 1992; **340:** 1466.

Theilmann L, Blazek M, Goeser T, Gmelin K, Kommerell B, Fiehn W. False-positive anti-HCV tests in rheumatoid arthritis. *Lancet* 1990; **335:** 1346.

Thiers V, Nakajima E, Dremsdorf D, et al. Transmission of hepatitis B from hepatitis-B-seronegative subjects. *Lancet* 1988; **2:** 1273.

Thim L, Bjoem S, Christensen M, et al. Amino acid sequence and posttranslational modifications of human factor VIIa from plasma and transfected baby hamster kidney cells. *Biochemistry* 1988; **27:** 7785.

Thomas DP, Hampton KK, Dasani H, et al. A cross-over pharmacokinetic and thrombogenicity study of a prothrombin complex concentrate and a purified factor IX concentrate. *British Journal of Haematology* 1994; **87:** 782.

Thorpe R, Dilger P, Dawson NJ, Barrowcliffe TW. Inhibition of interleukin-2 secretion by factor VIII concentrates: a possible cause of immunosuppression in haemophiliacs. *British Journal of Haematology* 1989; **71:** 387.

Toole JJ, Knopf JL, Wozney JM, et al. Molecular cloning of a cDNA encoding human antihaemophilic factor. *Nature* 1984; **312:** 342.

Toole JJ, Pittman DD, Orr EC, Murtha P, Wasley LC, Kaufman RJ. A large region (approximately equal to 95 kDa) of human factor VIII is dispensable for in vitro procoagulant activity. *Proceedings of the National Academy of Sciences USA* 1986; **83:** 5939.

Triantaphyllopoulis DC. Intravascular coagulation following injection of prothrombin complex. *American Journal of Clinical Pathology* 1972; **57:** 603.

United Kingdom Haemophilia Centre Directors Organisation. Recommendations on choice of therapeutic products for the treatment of patients with haemophilia A, haemophilia B and von Willebrand's disease. *Blood Coagulation and Fibrinolysis* 1992; **3:** 205–214,

United Kingdom Haemophilia Centre Directors Organisation Executive Committee. Guidelines on therapeutic products to treat haemophilia and other hereditary coagulation disorders. *Haemophilia* 1997; **3:** 63–77.
Urbaniek SJ. Adverse effects of transfusion: In: Ludlam CA (Ed), *Clinical Haematology*. Edinburgh: Churchill Livingstone, 1990: 449–459.
Van Creveld S, Veder HA, Pascha CN, Kroeze WF. The separation of AHG from fibrinogen. *Thrombosis et Diathesis Haemorrhagica* 1959; **3:** 572.
van den Berg W, ten Cate JW, Breederveld C, Goudsmit J. Seroconversion to HTLV-III in a haemophiliac given heat-treated factor VIII concentrate. *Lancet* 1986; **1:** 803.
Varon D, Schulman S, Dardik R, Barzilai A, Bashari D, Martinowitz U. High versus ultra high purity factor VIII concentrate therapy. Prospective evaluation of immunological and clinical parameters in HIV-seronegative and -seropositive haemophiliacs. *Thrombosis and Haemostasis* 1994; **72:** 359.
Vermot Desroches C, Rigal D, Blourde C, Bemaud J. Immunosuppressive property of a very high purity antihaemophilic preparation: a low molecular weight component inhibits an early step of PHA induced cell activation. *British Journal of Haematology* 1992; **80:** 370.
Vicente V, Estelles A, Laso J, Moraleda JM, Rivera J, Aznar J. Repeated infusions of DDAVP induce low response of FVIII and vWF but not of plasminogen activators. *Thrombosis Research* 1993; **70:** 117.
Wadhwa M, Dilger P, Tubbs J, MireSluis A, Barrowcliffe T, Thorpe R. Identification of transforming growth factor-beta as a contaminant in factor VIII concentrates: a possible link with immunosuppressive effects in hemophiliacs. *Blood* 1994; **84:** 2021.
Watson HG, Goulden NJ, Ludlam CA. Oesophageal candidiasis in an HIV-negative individual treated with factor VIII concentrate. *Thrombosis and Haemostasis* 1992a; **68:** 782.
Watson HG, Ludlam CA, Rebus S, Zhang LQ, Peutherer JF, Simmonds P. Use of several second generation serological assays to determine the true prevalence of hepatitis C virus infection in haemophiliacs treated with non-virus inactivated factor VIII and IX concentrates. *British Journal of Haematology* 1992b; **80:** 514.
Watson HG, Ludlam CA, McOmish F, Dennis R, Hart H, Simmonds P. Absence of hepatitis A virus transmission by high purity solvent detergent treated coagulation concentrates in Scottish haemophiliacs. *British Journal of Haematology* 1994; **89:** 214.
Weisser J. Transmission of the human immunodeficiency virus by a dry heated Factor VIII concentrate. *Klin Pediatr* 1988; **200:** 375–379.
White GC, Roberts HR, Kingdon HS, Lundblad RL. Prothrombin complex concentrates: potentially thrombogenic materials and clues to the mechanism of thrombosis in vivo. *Blood* 1977; **49:** 159.
White GC, Matthews TJ, Weinhold KJ, et al. HTLV-III seroconversion associated with heat-treated factor VIII concentrate. *Lancet* 1986; **1:** 611.
White GC, McMillan CW, Kingdon HS, Shoemaker CB. Use of recombinant antihemophilic factor in the treatment of two patients with classic hemophilia. *New England Journal of Medicine* 1989; **320:** 166.
Williams MD, Cohen BJ, Beddall AC, Pasi KJ, Mortimer PP, Hill FG. Transmission of human parvovirus B19 by coagulation factor concentrates. *Vox Sang* 1990a; **58:** 177.
Williams MD, Skidmore SJ, Hill FG. HIV seroconversion in haemophilic boys receiving heat-treated factor VIII concentrate. *Vox Sang* 1990b; **58:** 135.
Winkelman L, Sims GE, Haddon ME, et al. A pasteurised concentrate of human plasma factor XIII for therapeutic use. *Thrombosis and Haemostasis* 1986; **55:** 402.
Yee TT, Lee CA, Pasi KJ. Life-threatening human parvovirus B19 infection in immunocompetent haemophilia. *Lancet* 1995; **345:** 794.
Zagury D, Bernard J, Leonard R, et al. Long-term cultures of HTLV-III-infected T cells: a model of cytopathology of T-cell depletion in AIDS. *Science* 1986; **231:** 850.

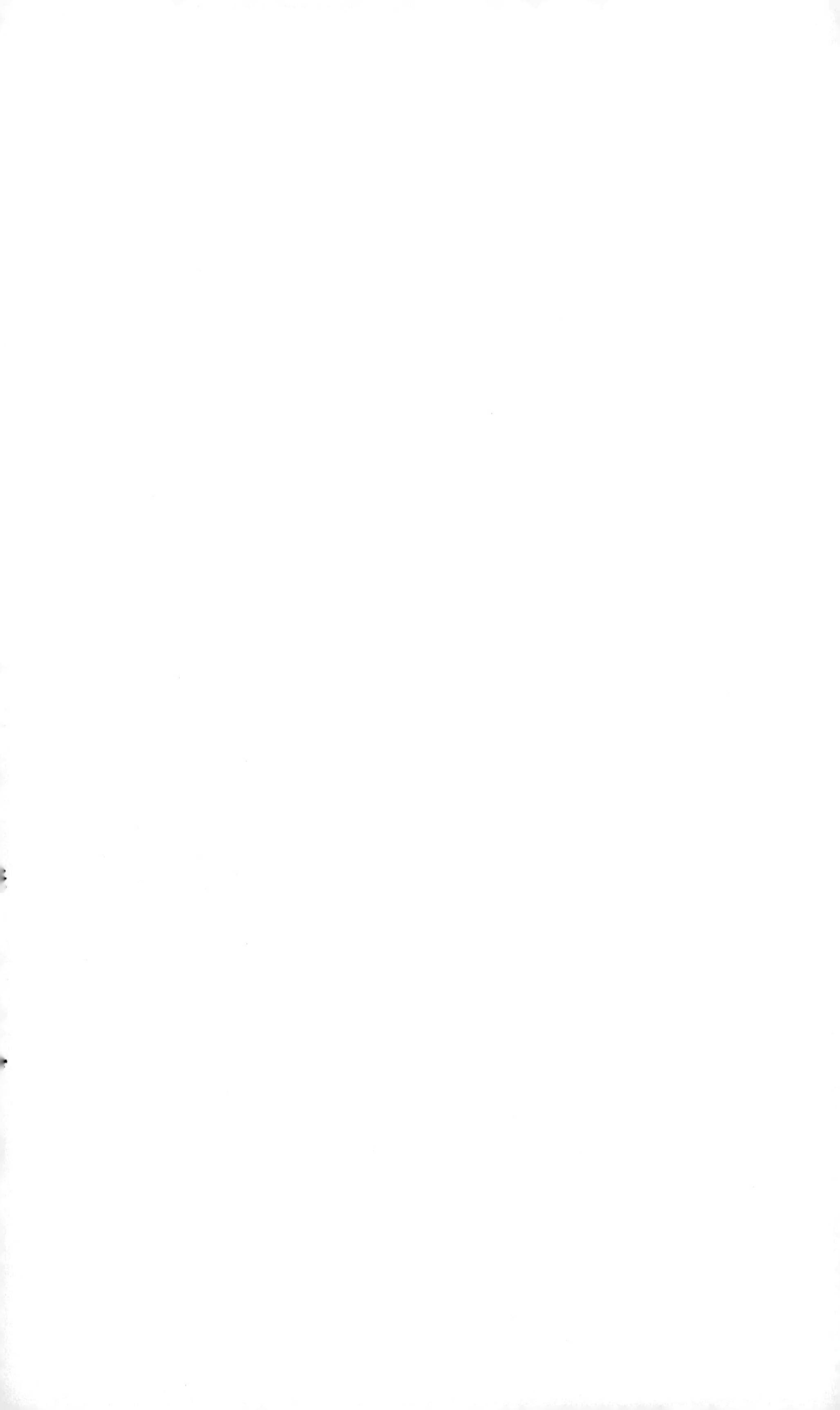

The Management of Haemophilia, Christmas Disease and von Willebrand's Disease

6

PAUL L.F. GIANGRANDE

The goals of treatment of haemophilia, as stated by the World Federation of Haemophilia, are "to minimise disability and prolong life, to facilitate general social and physical well-being and to help each patient achieve full potential, whilst causing no harm" (Kasper et al, 1989). The social and physical consequences of untreated severe haemophilia are well described in a personal account published almost 50 years ago: "I can reply, quite literally, that (haemophilia) is an everlasting bloody nuisance. I cannot emphasize too strongly its everlasting nature, for my friends and relations, and even some doctors who have attended me think that I am not ill except when I am actually bleeding. But in fact the haemorrhages are the final and most dramatic manifestations of a disease whose constant and but less striking physical and mental effects harass the unfortunate sufferer all the days of his life" (Anonymous, 1949). Earlier arcane therapies included an "antihaemophilia" egg-white derivative, topical Russell's viper venom and peanut flour. The subsequent development of blood products such as cryoprecipitate in the 1960s and plasma-derived concentrates in the following decade dramatically altered the outlook for patients with haemophilia. By the early 1980s, life expectancy of patients with haemophilia in developed countries had almost attained that of the normal population.

It is, however, not only the introduction of therapeutic materials that has improved the outlook for patients with severe haemophilia, but also the development of national and international networks of specialized centres devoted to the comprehensive care of people with haemophilia and related disorders of haemostasis. Before turning to the specific therapy of haemophilia, the organization of haemophilia care (with particular reference to the UK) will be outlined.

Table 6.1 Services provided by a Comprehensive Care Centre

- Provision of a 24-hour specialized clinical and laboratory service
- Laboratory service capable of carrying out all tests necessary for the definitive diagnosis of haemophilia and related haemorrhagic disorders
- Provision of an advisory service to patients, their close relatives and general practitioners on matters specific to haemophilia
- Specialist consultant service for dental and orthopaedic surgery; infectious diseases (such as HIV and hepatitis); paediatrics and genetic counselling
- Provision of counselling in privacy
- Provision and organization of home therapy programmes
- Maintenance of satisfactory quality control and assurance for laboratory tests
- Maintenance of medical records and supply of special medical cards
- Participation in appropriate clinical audit
- Provision of a reference laboratory and clinical service to other haemophilia centres
- Educational facilities for medical, technical and nursing staff and other personnel
- Participation in relevant meetings and research programmes

Organization of Haemophilia Care

A network of haemophilia centres has existed in the UK since the early 1950s. Originally, these were few in number and so care was not uniformly available around the country; however, haemophilia centres are now available in every region of the country. There are two tiers of haemophilia centres. 23 centres are currently designated as comprehensive care centres.

A centre should normally provide treatment for 40 or more severely affected patients per year to be designated as a Comprehensive Care Centre, as only centres dealing with patients regularly are likely to maintain the necessary collective expertise. These centres have to satisfy certain strict criteria as regards provision of clinical and laboratory services and are also subject to periodic audit. The specific requirements for comprehensive care centres are set out in a Department of Health circular (HSG (93) 90) and are summarized in Table 6.1.

A larger number of smaller haemophilia centres also exists, which offer more limited clinical and laboratory facilities. These are often located within

Figure 6.1 Example of follow-up clinic notes used at Oxford Haemophilia Centre.

OXFORD HAEMOPHILIA CENTRE
FOLLOW-UP CLINIC

Patient's Surname: .... First Name: ....

Date of Birth: .... Factor VIII or IX ....%

Date of Visit: .... Inhibitors ....

Examining Doctor..................

Home Treatment

Do you have treatment at home: Yes No Record forms returned: Yes No

Type of concentrate used: ....

Where used equipment is disposed ? ....

Who helps with home treatment ? ....

Home Treatment Comments: ....

Vaccination (please circle)

Childhood vaccinations (where applicable): 1st 2nd 3rd

Hepatitis vaccine: Hepatitis A 1st 2nd 3rd
Hepatitis B 1st 2nd 3rd

Urine testing

Blood .... Protein .... Bilirubin .... Glucose ....

Dental

Do you have regular dental check-ups ? Yes No

When was the last visit to the dentist ? ....

Long-standing Problems

Medical problems since last follow-up

Medication/Drugs

Social History

Marital status: .... Employment/school: ....

Accommodation/Housing: ....

Alcohol:

Tobacco:

Has anyone discussed safer sex with you ? ....

Do you receive Disability Living Allowances ? Yes No

Mobility Component: Yes No

Care Component: Yes No

Physical examination

Weight: Height: BP:

CVS:

Respiratory:

Abdomen:

CNS:

ENT:

Musculoskeletal:

1. Most troublesome joints ?
2. Does joint pain disturb sleep ?

Routine Blood Tests

FBC ...... Biochemical profile ..... Inhibitor screen ..... HBV ..... HCV ..... HIV ....

RANGE OF MOTION IN MAIN JOINTS (expressed in degrees of flexion) 0 = Straight

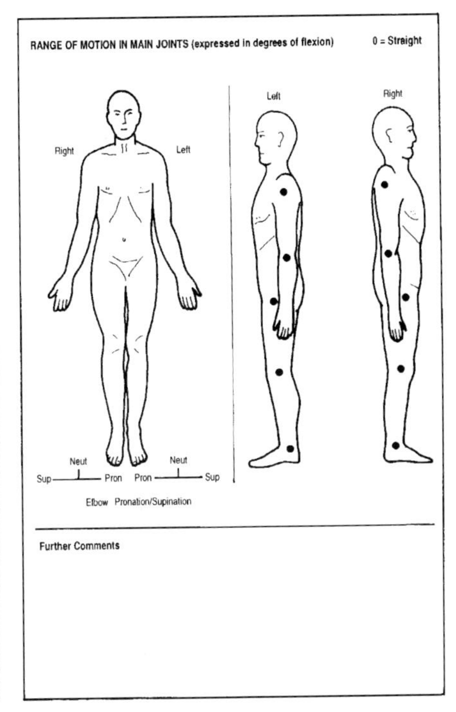

Further Comments

departments of haematology in general hospitals, and are staffed by personnel involved in the treatment of a wide range of haematological disorders.

The United Kingdom Haemophilia Centre Directors' Organization (UKHCDO) is a body composed of nominated directors from all haemophilia centres and comprehensive care centres in the UK. Data are collected and published as a report each year on behalf of the organization (see Chapter 14). Such reports contain information on patient numbers, type and quantity of materials used, patient deaths, adverse events and incidence of inhibitors. The collection of such data also forms the basis for scientific studies. The organization also produces and disseminates guidelines on specific issues. The haemophilia centre should be the natural focus for follow-up treatment of patients with haemophilia. Hospitals with such centres have collective experience of dealing with surgical, obstetric and medical problems. Patients with haemophilia should be followed-up at 6-monthly intervals. Access to orthopaedic surgeons and physiotherapists, dentists, hepatologists and physicians with expertise in infectious diseases such as HIV should be available to all patients when necessary. It is recommended that patients with severe haemophilia should be followed-up at 6-monthly intervals, but yearly follow-up is more appropriate for mildly affected individuals. The purpose of such regular check-ups is to assess the physical condition of the patient, monitor and advise on treatment and to focus on particular related medical problems (such as chronic liver disease and HIV-related problems). The form used at the Oxford Haemophilia Centre is illustrated in Fig. 6.1.

Therapeutic Materials

The various materials available for treatment of patients with bleeding disorders will be described only briefly, as the subject is dealt with in more detail in Chapter 5. National guidelines on the use of these products have been published recently (UKHCDO, 1997)

Cryoprecipitate

The discovery in 1965 of factor VIII activity in cryoprecipitate was a major advance in the therapy of haemophilia. It was subsequently found to contain a substantial amount of von Willebrand factor (vWF), fibrinogen and factor XIII, but not factor IX. However, the content of coagulation factors in bags of cryoprecipitate is very variable and the bags are inconvenient to store and infuse. They also need to be administered with regard to blood group. A further disadvantage with cryoprecipitate is the risk of viral transmission, although chemical means of viral inactivation (for example, through addition of a solvent/detergent mixture) have recently been developed. Cryoprecipitate has been superseded in developed countries by lyophilized coagulation factor concentrate. However, cryoprecipitate remains an important blood product for therapy in many developing countries. Lyophilized cryoprecipitate is used in some countries, which has the advantage that it may be stored at room temperature.

Coagulation factor concentrates

The large-scale development of factor VIII concentrates in the early 1970s was a major advance, and has facilitated the spread of home treatment and prophylactic therapy. It is recognized that the use of products derived from large plasma pools was responsible for the transmision of hepatitis and HIV infection before 1985, when heat treatment (and subsequently other methods) was introduced. Intermediate-purity factor VIII is still widely used. Such products have a good track record as regards viral safety and are cheap compared with high-purity products. They are relatively insoluble, and are not suitable for continuous infusion (e.g. in the setting of surgery). Many patients prefer high-purity concentrates for home therapy because of better solubility. High-purity concentrates have been recommended for treatment of patients seropositive for anti-HIV, as several studies have claimed that the rate of decline in the CD4-lymphocyte count may be slowed by switching to higher-purity products. High-purity concentrates should be used in patients who have had allergic reactions after infusion of less pure products. They may also be useful in patients with severe chronic liver disease associated with ascites, because of the lower sodium content. Recombinant factor VIII is now available, but is considerably more expensive than plasma-derived product. The theoretical advantage is, of course, freedom from the risk of transmission of viral infection. However, it should be appreciated that all such products currently available contain a considerable quantity of human albumin which is added as a stabilizer. Controversy remains about the risk of inhibitor development in patients receiving recombinant factor VIII. Nevertheless, it is very likely that the use of recombinant products will increase markedly over the next few years.

The use of intermediate-purity factor IX concentrates, which also contain factors II and X, has been superseded by high-purity plasma-derived concentrates. Repeated administration of intermediate-purity products at high doses is associated with a risk of thromboembolism, particularly in the setting of surgery, and so such products are no longer regarded as the safest therapeutic material for the regular treatment of patients with haemophilia B. In the UK, the use of such products is restricted to treatment of patients with deficiencies of factors II or X, reversal of the effect of warfarin in selected cases and the treatment of some patients with haemophilia A and inhibitory antibodies. High-purity plasma-derived factor IX concentrates do not contain other vitamin K-dependent coagulation factors and are not suitable for the treatment of these conditions. The infusion of high-purity factor IX concentrate is not followed by an increase in plasma levels of markers of activation of coagulation (such as prothrombin fragment F 1+2) and clinical experience suggests that even administration of high doses to patients undergoing surgery is not associated with an increased risk of thromboembolism. Recombinant factor IX is currently being evaluated in clinical trials, and is likely to become available in the next few years. It does not require the presence of albumin or other stabilizer in the vial.

DDAVP

Desmopressin (1-deamino-8-D-arginine vasopressin, DDAVP) is a synthetic analogue of antidiuretic hormone. The compound boosts the plasma levels of factor VIII and vWF after administration (Mannucci et al, 1977). The mechanism of action by which the levels of factor VIII and vWF in the plasma are boosted is not clear. DDAVP does not release multimers of vWF from cultured endothelial cells, and there appears to be an indirect action which may involve interaction with mononuclear cells (Hashemi et al, 1990).

The most common mode of administration is by intravenous infusion, but it may also be given by subcutaneous injection. A single intravenous infusion at a dose of 0.3 μg/kg can be expected to boost the level of factor VIII three- to six-fold. The peak response is seen approximately 1 hour after infusion. Tachyphylaxis may also be a problem with repeated administration: the rise in factor VIII and vWF levels after further doses may be reduced (Mannucci et al, 1992a). The compound is ineffective in patients with severe haemophilia A, or severe von Willebrand's disease. The factor IX level is unchanged after administration and thus desmopressin is also of no value in haemophilia B. A concentrated spray preparation for nasal insufflation has recently become available: a spray dosage of 300 μg is equivalent to the standard intravenous dose of 0.3 μg/kg (Lethagen et al, 1995). This is likely to prove particularly useful for home treatment of minor bleeding problems.

A decision to use DDAVP must be based on both the baseline concentration of factor VIII and on the nature of the procedure. It would not, for example, be feasible to perform gastrectomy in a patient with a baseline factor VII level of 10% or less as the expected post-infusion level of 30–40% is unlikely to be sufficient to ensure haemostasis and the responses to subsequent doses would be even less. On the other hand, the same patient might be able to have a dental extraction after an infusion. Desmopressin is particularly useful in the treatment of female carriers of haemophilia A. It is the practice of many centres to give a trial infusion of desmopressin in appropriate patients, so that the potential value may be assessed for possible future use.

Desmopressin is also of value in type 1 von Willebrand's disease, which accounts for approximately four-fifths of all cases of this disorder. The compound is, in general, of little benefit in type 2A von Willebrand's disease, and may provoke thrombocytopenia in the type 2B variant. DDAVP is of no value in the treatment of the increasingly recognized type 2N (Normandy variant) (Mazurier, 1992). This form of von Willebrand's disease may masquerade as mild haemophilia: typically, the level of factor VIII is significantly reduced (of the order of 5–20%), whilst the vWF level (assayed both with a functional assay and an antigenic assay) is normal. However, a specific factor VIII-binding assay is abnormal and suspicion may be aroused because of an apparent autosomal dominant pattern of inheritance.

DDAVP is usually diluted in at least 100 ml of physiological saline and given by slow intravenous infusion over 20–30 minutes. Rapid infusion may result in tachycardia, flushing, tremor and abdominal discomfort. Water retention and hyponatraemia is not usually a problem in adults, although concomitant administration of diuretic therapy can exacerbate the risk. However, children appear to be at particular risk of hyponatraemia, which may precipitate seizures (Smith et al, 1989), and it is recommended that DDAVP should not be given to children under the age of 2 years. Similarly, whilst DDAVP is devoid of oxytocic activity it should not be administered to a pregnant woman. DDAVP, unlike the parent hormone, does not increase blood pressure. However, there are case reports of thrombosis and myocardial infarction following infusion of DDAVP, and so it should also be used with caution in elderly patients with signs of arterial disease.

Desmopressin may also be used to control bleeding associated with acquired disorders of haemostasis, including chronic renal failure and liver disease and some platelet disorders (Mannucci, 1988).

Topical thrombin

Topical bovine thrombin is a useful material in controlling superficial bleeds, as it clots the fibrinogen of the blood directly. Once reconstituted, it may be applied directly or soaked into an absorbable gelatine sponge. It may be used, for example, to control epistaxis or bleeding from oozing tooth sockets after extraction. We have also found it useful in controlling persistent bleeding from small superficial cuts in patients with inhibitory antibodies. The material is only intended for topical use. It must not be injected intravenously, as it can provoke fatal intravascular thrombosis. The material is free from any human plasma proteins, and is theoretically free of the risk of infection with human blood-borne viruses. However, there are no published data relating to the viral safety of this material.

The management of patients with inhibitory antibodies is discussed in Chapter 11. However, a brief summary of some of the materials that may be used follows. Guidelines on the choice of product have been published (Hay et al, 1996).

Porcine factor VIII (Hyate:C)

Coagulation factor concentrates of animal origin were originally developed in the 1950s as primary therapeutic materials. The source plasma was readily available, and the factor activity per given volume was often greater than in human plasma. However, severe allergic reactions were not infrequent, particularly after repeated exposure, and such products were abandoned when products derived from human volunteer blood donors became more widely available. Hyate:C (Speywood Pharmaceuticals) is a concentrate derived from porcine plasma, but is manufactured via polyelectrolyte fractionation and is a much purer form than the original material. It is a lyophilized concentrate, but requires storage at −15°C. It is not subjected to a specific viral inactivation procedure, but there are no reports to suggest viral transmission has ever been a problem. Allergic reactions may occur, which are usually only mild (Kernoff et al, 1984; Brettler et al, 1989). However, more serious reactions, including anaphylaxis, have been reported. This should be borne in mind if home therapy with this material is considered. Transient thrombocytopenia has also been reported (Gringeri et al, 1991), and this has been attributed to residual porcine vWF in the concentrate which can directly induce human platelet aggregation (Pareti et al, 1992). Porcine factor VIII is of particular value in acquired haemophilia (Morrison et al, 1993).

Activated prothrombin-complex concentrates

Prothrombin-complex concentrates (such as FEIBA [Immuno] and Autoplex [Baxter]) are useful materials in the treatment of patients with haemophilia A and B and inhibitory antibodies (Lusher et al, 1980). One important potential complication of treatment with these products is precipitation of both venous and arterial thromboembolism. It is particularly important not to exceed the recommended dosage for this reason and concomitant use of tranexamic acid is contraindicated. These plasma-derived products are subjected to heat treatment. Whilst it has not been possible to evaluate them for risk of viral transmission in previously untreated patients, there is no evidence from studies of previously treated patients of transmission of hepatitis or HIV.

Whilst the products do not contain factor VIII, anamnestic responses may occur but these are not usually marked. These products may therefore be particularly useful in the treatment of patients with inhibitory antibodies who are known to be "high responders" with regard to human or porcine factor VIII.

Recombinant factor VIIa

The role assigned to factor VII in the classical coagulation pathway was activation of the so-called extrinsic pathway. Recent work has suggested a single integrated pathway for all coagulation factors, which is initiated by the binding of factor VII to tissue factor (Rapaport & Rao, 1995). Recombinant factor VIIa (Novo) is now licensed for the treatment of patients with haemophilia A and B and inhibitory antibodies, as well as those with acquired haemophilia and congenital factor VII deficiency (Hedner, 1990; Macik et al, 1993). As a genetically engineered product it is theoretically free of the risk of transmission of human blood-borne viruses: it is also subjected to solvent/detergent treatment. Tranetamic acid may be given to patients receiving recombinant factor VIIa.

Recombinant factor VIIa is extremely expensive, which is a barrier to more widespread use. However, it is clearly a valuable therapeutic weapon in patients with an extremely high titre of inhibitory antibody. It has a very short half-life, so that bolus injections need to be given at 2- or 3-hourly intervals to control bleeding. A further problem is that laboratory control or monitoring of therapy is not possible. The manufacturers recommend monitoring of the prothrombin time (which is shortened) and factor VII levels, but these are merely surrogate markers and no therapeutic range has been proposed.

Pharmacokinetics of Factors VIII and IX

The basic rules of drug distribution and elimination can be applied to coagulation factor concentrates, and an understanding of the key issues is of crucial importance in designing new strategies such as continuous intravenous infusion regimes for surgery and protocols for prophylaxis. Computer programmes have been designed that calculate the various pharmacokinetic parameters for individual patients and which suggest treatment schedules for surgery and other procedures.

The volume of distribution is defined as the ratio between the total amount of a drug in the body and its concentration in the plasma. Whilst this may equate to an identifiable physiological volume (such as total body water, or extracellular fluid space), this is certainly not always the case. It should be thought of as the theoretical fluid volume that would be required to contain all of the drug in the body at the same concentration as in the blood or plasma. It is influenced by such factors as tissue binding, partition coefficient of the drug in fat and degree of binding to plasma proteins. The recovery of infused coagulation factor concentrate is an analogous concept, and is based on the peak factor VIII (or IX) level after infusion and an estimate of the patient's plasma volume. It is usually reported as the rise in blood level in iu/dl (or %) per iu/kg of concentrate infused. As a rough and ready rule, the plasma level of factor VIII should rise by 2 iu/dl for each 1 iu/kg of factor VIII concentrate infused. By contrast, the factor IX level will only rise by 1 iu/dl for each iu/kg of concentrate infused. The lower recovery of factor IX has been attributed, at least in part, to binding of factor IX to vascular endothelial cells. The apparent recovery of both factor VIII and factor IX does increase with subsequent doses, probably reflecting saturation of binding sites and equilibration between the various body-fluid compartments. The recovery of both factor VIII and factor IX is also lower than expected in young children.

The clearance is a measure of the body's ability to eliminate a drug. It is the plasma volume that becomes free of drug per unit time (e.g. ml/min), but it can also be corrected for body weight for comparison (e.g. ml/h/kg). A steady state should be achieved when the rate of drug administration equals the rate of drug elimination and this is usually reached after the equivalent of five half-lives of the drug. The elimination of most drugs obeys so-called first-order kinetics, whereby a constant fraction of the drug in the body is eliminated per unit of time. By contrast, a constant amount of drug is eliminated if the mechanism for elimination becomes saturated (zero-order kinetics) and the clearance would vary with time. The fall in plasma factor VIII levels after a single bolus injection of concentrate exhibits the characteristics of first-order kinetics. The half-life is the time it takes for the plasma concentration to fall by 50%. In fact, the picture is complicated by the fact that equilibration takes place as the factor is distributed throughout several compartments, and at least two separate decay curves may be identified. The apparent half-life may thus vary according to the sampling times, although for practical purposes it is a key parameter in clinical practice. Determination of the plasma half-life of infused factor VII or IX remains the most sensitive way of detecting the presence of an inhibitory antibody. International guidelines for the design and analysis of half-life and recovery studies have been published (Morfini et al, 1991). The only significant subsequent modification to these recommendations is that sampling be continued for up to 72 hours in the case of factor IX studies. The pharmacokinetics of intermediate-purity, high-purity plasma-derived and recombinant factor VIII products are, for practical purposes, identical. There is, of course, interindividual variation in the plasma-half-life of infused factor VIII. It has been suggested that such differences might, at least in part, be attributable to variation in levels of circulating vWF which serves as a carrier molecule for factor VIII. It has been observed that the clearance of factor VIII declines with repeated administration, and this is of relevance to continuous infusion protocols.

Dosage of Factors VIII and IX

A simple strategy is to base dosages on the basis of iu/kg of body weight. The total dose, and frequency of treatment, will also be determined by the severity and site of bleeding. Typical doses of factor VIII required for initial treatment of various clinical conditions in patients with haemophilia A but without inhibitory antibodies are given in Table 6.2.

Coagulation factor concentrate is usually supplied in bottles of 250, 500 and 1000 units, and it is usual to "round up" the calculated dose to minimize wastage of this expensive therapeutic material. Most (approximately 85%) joint bleeds will resolve with a single infusion of material, if the bleed is recognized early and treated promptly. It should also be appreciated that bleeding in certain joints may require treatment with more factor to control bleeding. One double-blind study compared doses of 7, 14 and 28 iu/kg for the management of

Table 6.2 Doses of factor VIII required for initial treatment of clinical conditions in haemophilia patients without inhibitory antibodies

	Factor VIII dose (iu/kg)
Early haemarthrosis	15–20
Muscle bleed	20–30
Gastrointestinal bleeding	20–30
Dental extraction	40–50
Surgery	50

haemarthroses in different joints (Aronstam et al, 1980). It was shown that the lowest dose was sufficient to stop bleeding in the ankle, but a dose of 14 iu/kg was required to control bleeds in the elbow and knee. The highest dose (28 iu/kg) did not offer any significant additional benefit. As a general rule, it dose appear that the dose of factor VIII needed to control haemarthroses in the limbs tends to be less in the distal sites than in the proximal. For example, bleeds into the hip joint are relatively rare but do require treatment with a higher dose than a simple knee bleed.

Alternatively, the dose of factor VIII or factor IX needed to achieve a target plasma level can be readily calculated using formulae based on the patient's weight and the recovery of the product. Assuming a typical recovery of factor VIII of 2 iu/ml per iu/kg of concentrate infused, a simple formula for the calculation of a dose to attain a specific target plasma levels is as follows:

$$\text{Dose of factor VIII} = \frac{\text{Wt (kg)} \times \text{Desired rise in factor (iu/dl)}}{2}$$

A greater number of units of factor IX will be required to achieve a target level, reflecting the lower recovery of factor IX after infusion. A formula designed for calculation of dosage of factor IX is as follows:

$$\text{Dose of factor IX} = \text{Wt (kg)} \times \text{Desired rise in factor (iu/dl)}$$

This assumes an average recovery of 1 iu/dl per iu/kg of concentrate infused. However, it is emphasized that these simple formulae are only based on typical, average values. The actual recovery for specific concentrates may be significantly different. For example, high-purity Replenine (BPL) has a recovery of 1.3 iu/ml per iu/kg infused.

It is often helpful to measure the peak plasma factor level after infusion. This is particularly important in the setting of surgery or other invasive procedures. A post-infusion sample should be taken at least 5 minutes after the completion of the bolus infusion to allow for distribution. It should be taken through a fresh needle: a sample taken through the original infusion set, even if flushed with saline, is very likely to contain residual traces of coagulation factor, which will result in spuriously high values. Where possible, the sample should be taken from the contralateral arm. This is particularly important when product is administered by continuous intravenous infusion.

Treatment of Von Willebrand's Disease

The haemorrhagic problems associated with von Willebrand's disease are quite different from those associated with haemophilia. Haemarthrosis is not, of course, a typical feature, although it may occasionally be seen in severely affected patients. Typical features of von Willebrand's disease include easy bruising, prolonged bleeding from cuts and scratches, epistaxis, menorrhagia and bleeding from other mucosal surfaces. Tranexamic acid alone used to treat minor problems, such as recurrent epistaxis or oral bleeding. A syrup preparation is available for children. Aspirin and non-steroidal drugs may exacerbate or provoke bleeding in patients with von Willebrand's disease, and should be avoided. Paracetamol is perfectly acceptable as a simple, alternative analgesic.

The treatment of specific clinical problems is discussed in the following section, but the basic principles are discussed in this section. The choice of product for the treatment of more significant bleeding episodes in patients with von Willebrand's disease depends upon the subtype of the disorder (i.e. type 1 or 2). Approximately 80% of all patients with von Willebrand's disease have the type 1 variant, and are likely to respond well to an infusion of DDAVP (as detailed above). It is often useful to give a test infusion of DDAVP to patients when they are diagnosed as having the disorder in order to assess the potential usefulness of the compound in controlling or preventing bleeding. Patients with type 2 von Willebrand's disease are unlikely to respond to infusion of DDAVP, and are likely to require an infusion of coagulation factor concentrate to control bleeding. An infusion of DDAVP may provoke thrombocytopenia in those with the type 2b variant. Patients with type 1 von Willebrand's disease who undergo surgery are also likely to require such products, because of the limited efficacy of repeated infusion of DDAVP in boosting levels of factor VIII and vWF. Intermediate-purity concentrates differ in their content of high-molecular-weight multimers of vWF. Concentrates with a relatively high content of such multimers are to be preferred for the treatment of von Willebrand's disease, and are more likely to correct the haemostatic defect (Mannucci et al, 1992b). Most bottles of factor VIII concentrates are not labelled to show the content of vWF. The content of factor VIII must be assumed to be roughly equivalent, but even this does not give any indication of the relative proportion of high-molecular-weight multimers. The plasma factor VIII level is used by most centres to monitor therapy in the setting of surgery. If vWF levels are assayed specifically, it is recommended that functional rather than antigenic methods be used. The half-life of infused vWF is around 24 hours, but the disappearance of the largest multimers is more rapid. High-purity factor VIII concentrates do not contain vWF, and are of no value in treating this condition. Concentrates of vWF alone have recently become available. Infusion of such a concentrate will lead to a delayed rise in the plasma level of factor VIII. The peak factor VIII level is seen between 6 and 24 hours after the infusion of vWF concentrate (Mannucci et al, 1992b). As a high level of circulating factor VIII is required for haemostasis in the setting of surgery and other invasive procedures, it is therefore recommended that a dose of factor VIII concentrate be given at the same time if surgery cannot be delayed.

It has been observed that the bleeding time may not be completely corrected after infusion of coagulation factor concentrate. vWF is localized in the alpha granules of platelets, and it has been postulated that the failure to correct the haemostatic defect may reflect poor equilibration between infused vWF and endogenous platelets (Mannucci et al, 1992b). For this reason, there may be a role for additional transfusion of platelets in patients with von Willebrand's disease if bleeding persists and the bleeding time remains prolonged despite adequate doses of coagulation factor concentrate. However, there is a theoretical potential risk of transmission of viral infections associated with transfusion of platelets. The same is true of cryoprecipitate, which is undoubtedly effective in treating bleeding episodes in patients with haemophilia A as well as von Willebrand's disease.

Treatment of Particular Clinical Problems

Orthopaedic complications

Spontaneous and recurrent bleeding into joints are the hallmark of severe haemophilia. The management of bleeds in joints and muscles is described in detail in Chapter 7, but treatment of some of the more common problems will also be described here.

The frequency of bleeding episodes is determined by the baseline factor level. Those with a level of 2 iu/dl or less are labelled as having severe haemophilia. Although some have claimed that the frequency of joint bleeds in haemophilia B is less than that in severe haemophilia A, most accept that the clinical manifestations of both forms of haemophilia are indistinguishable. The principal joints involved are the knees, ankle and elbows. The wrists and shoulders are less frequently involved, whilst bleeds into the hip joint are relatively uncommon. Early symptoms of a bleed include stiffness and pain in the joint. The patient learns to recognize the symptoms of a bleed well before any external signs, such as swelling and warmth, become apparent. Prompt treatment will ensure rapid resolution of an early bleed and, if caught early, a single dose is usually sufficient. A suitable dose would be 15–20 iu/kg for a straightforward haemarthrosis (see below). The patient should be advised to rest the limb, but strict immobilization or encasement in a plaster cast is usually not necessary. A sling will provide considerable relief for elbow and shoulder bleeds. Immobilization in a padded, split plaster cast may, however, be of value in active young children with bleeds where further limb movement is likely to trigger further bleeding. Padded supports, which can be loosely strapped around the joint and perfused with very cold water ("Cryo-cuffs"), also provide very effective pain relief when a joint is swollen and tender. However, bags of ice or even frozen peas packed around the joint may provide just as effective relief! Aspiration is only very occasionally required, and may be of benefit when the joint is very tense and swollen. Obviously, the procedure will need to be covered with higher doses of concentrate (40 iu/kg factor VIII twice daily, or 75 iu/kg factor IX once a day) for 2 or 3 days, and there is a risk of introducing infection (see below). Aspiration should not be carried out if the patient has inhibitory antibodies.

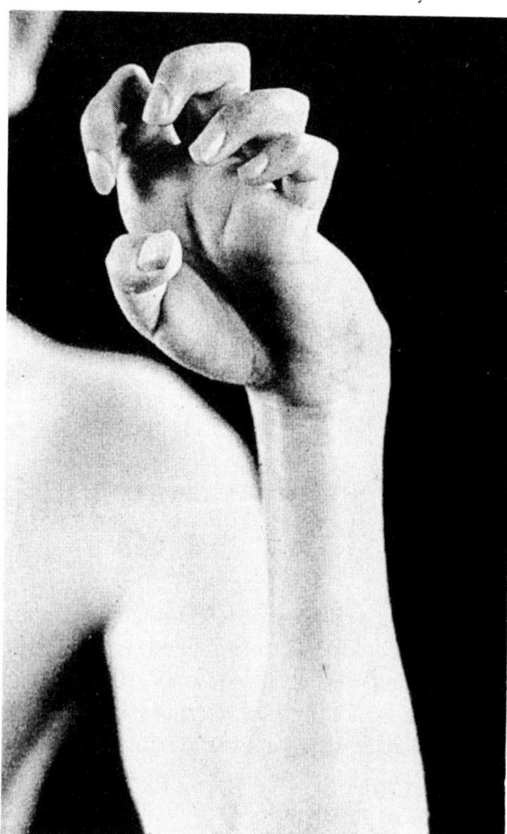

Figure 6.2 Volkmann's ischaemic contracture in the forearm of a patient with haemophilia, as the consequence of a bleed.

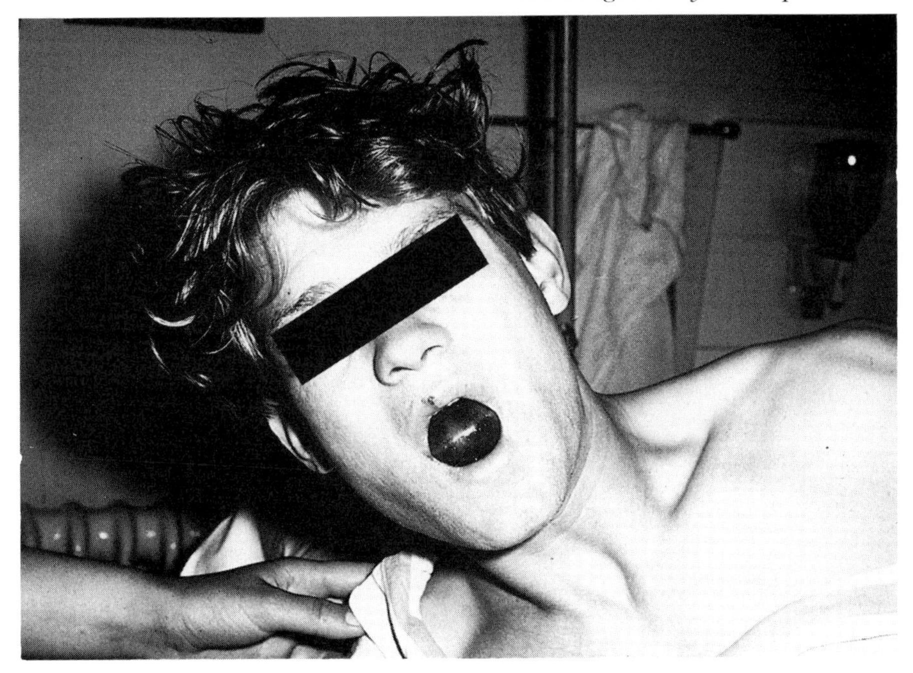

Figure 6.3 Obstruction of the airway due to a bleed into the tongue.

The presence of inhibitory antibodies must be considered if a patient begins to experience unusually frequent bleeds, which do not resolve with the usual dose of concentrate.

A haemarthrosis may very occasionally be complicated by the development of secondary infection. This complication appears to be more frequent in immunocompromised patients seropositive for anti-HIV (Gregg-Smith et al, 1993; Ingram et al, 1994). This should be suspected if the patient has a fever and the pain and swelling in a joint do not improve, or worsen, despite administration of appropriate doses of coagulation factor concentrate. Staphylococcus sp. are the most common organisms isolated. Blood cultures should be taken, and joint aspiration for diagnostic purposes is usually not necessary. The possibility of an associated fracture should also be excluded if what is believed to be a simple haemarthrosis does not resolve rapidly, particularly if there is a history of trauma. Any doubts can be resolved by taking a suitable X-ray.

Muscle bleeds occur less frequently than joint bleeds, and there is often a history of trauma. Intramuscular injections must never be given to patients with haemophilia, or those on anticoagulants such as warfarin and heparin, as an intramuscular haematoma is likely to result. Muscle bleeds are slower to resolve than joint bleeds, and often require a lengthy period of subsequent physiotherapy to ensure restoration of a full range movement in the joint. Bleeds into certain areas are particularly dangerous because of the risk of compression of

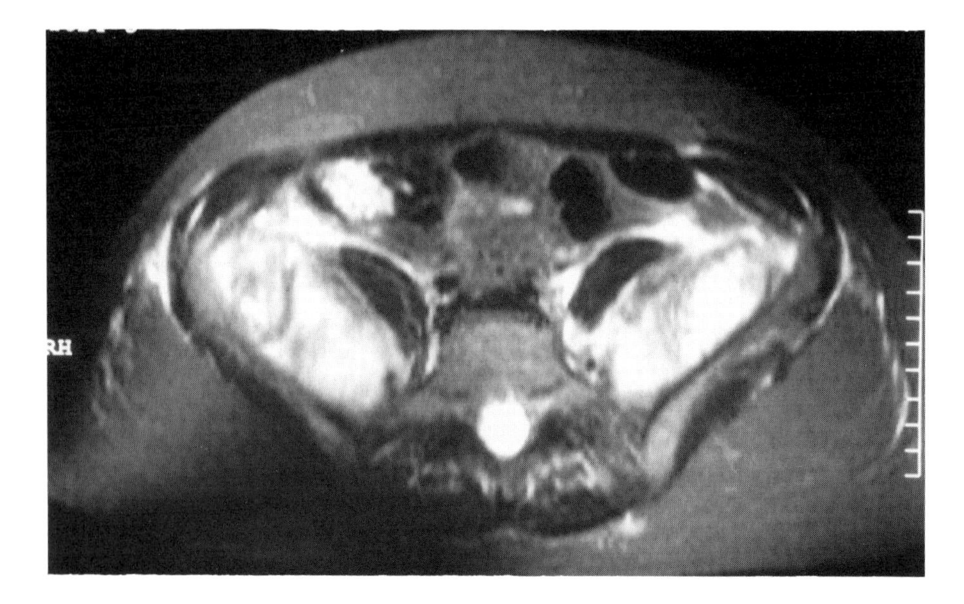

Figure 6.4 MRI scan of a patient with severe haemophilia A and bilateral iliopsoas haemorrhage, which presented with back pain and weakness in both legs.

neighbouring structures. Patients with inhibitory antibodies are particularly at risk in this regard, as bleeds may be more difficult to control. Bleeding into the forearm could result in Volkmann's ischaemic contracture (Fig. 6.2) and bleeds in the tongue can obstruct the airway (Fig. 6.3). Retroperitoneal bleeding within the ilio-psoas muscle (Fig. 6.4) may result in femoral nerve compression, with loss of sensation over the anterior aspect of the leg and rapid onset of quadriceps muscle wasting. Loss of the knee jerk reflex is an early clinical sign.

Haematuria

Painless haematuria is quite a common problem in patients with severe haemophilia, but is relatively rare in von Willebrand's disease (vWD). Haematuria often settles without specific treatment within 2 or 3 days. Infusion of coagulation factor concentrate may provoke ureteric obstruction, which is extremely painful, or hydronephrosis. Antifibrinolytic agents should not be given for the same reason. It is our practice to withhold concentrate initially, and see if the bleeding resolves spontaneously. Patients should be encouraged to keep well hydrated (and drink 2 litres of clear fluids each day) and to keep mobile. If haematuria persists, it is our practice to admit the patient for intravenous hydration overnight followed by morning bolus infusion (25–50 iu/kg) of coagulation factor concentrate. A second dose may be required 8–12 hours later.

It is not usual for there to be a significant drop in the haemoglobin concentration, although this should be monitored and a course of oral iron therapy may be required. Controlled trials have not confirmed the efficacy of prednisolone therapy in controlling bouts of haematuria in patients with haemophilia.

The possibility of underlying pathology should be considered, particularly in elderly patients, subjects with only mild haemophilia and those with recurrent haematuria. Appropriate investigations might include an abdominal ultrasound, microbiological culture and cytological examination of urine, intravenous urogram and/or cystoscopy. Haematuria may occasionally be an accompanying manifestation of retroperitoneal haemorrhage: this presumably results from engorgement and rupture of small intrarenal vessels if the renal vein is compressed.

Gastrointestinal bleeding

A patient who presents with haematemesis or melaena will usually require admission to hospital for investigation and management. Twice daily infusions of concentrate at a dose of around 40 iu/kg should control the bleeding, and a blood transfusion is likely to be necessary.

Haematemesis is often a manifestation of underlying oesophageal varices, secondary to portal hypertension and chronic liver disease. Patients with significant liver disease are likely to require fresh frozen plasma to control bleeding, as well as coagulation factor concentrate: the prothrombin time should be checked. Varices may be injected at endoscopy with sclerosing agents to prevent further episodes. Propranolol and other beta-blockers have been used to reduce portal venous pressure, and reduce the risk of further bleeding episodes. However, the use of beta-blockers may be hazardous as rescuscitation may be more difficult if the patient does have another serious bleeding episode.

Ibuprofen and related non-steroidal anti-inflammatory agents are sometimes very useful in suppressing symptoms of haemophilic arthritis. However, they may (as with aspirin) precipitate the development of gastric erosions and bleeding. If long-term therapy with such agents is felt to be necessary, concomitant prescription of the synthetic prostaglandin analogue misoprostol will minimize the risk of gastrointestinal ulceration.

Bleeding into the gastrointestinal wall, without associated bleeding into the lumen and external blood loss, may occur and cause abdominal pain with symptoms suggestive of abdominal obstruction or appendicitis, with paralytic ileus. It is important to recognize that not all cases of abdominal pain in patients with haemophilia require surgical intervention, and radiological investigations such as computed tomography (CT) may be helpful (McCoy and Kitchens, 1991). Such bleeds rapidly resolve with conservative management ("drip and suck" regime) and infusions of coagulation factor.

An association between von Willebrand's disease (vWD) and angiodysplastic lesions in the gastrointestinal tract is well recognized (Fressinaud and Meyer,

1993). This may cause recurrent melaena. Although the underlying problem can be readily identified at endoscopy the problem is, unfortunately, very difficult to control. The lesions are often very widely disseminated throughout the digestive tract. Surgical excision of parts of the bowel is rarely helpful, as bleeding from other lesions often occurs later. One strategy that may be useful is to attempt to identify particular lesions responsible for active bleeding with angiography or scanning following injection of radiolabelled erythrocytes. There is anecdotal evidence that oestrogen therapy may induce shrinking of lesions.

Liver biopsy

The role of liver biopsy in the management of haemophiliacs infected with hepatitis C (HCV) remains controversial. Whilst it is now recognized that biopsy in haemophiliacs does not entail additional risk compared with other patient groups, many experienced haematologists feel that decisions about treatment may be made on the basis of results of non-invasive tests, such as ultrasound, endoscopy (e.g. to check for the presence of oesophageal varices), viral titre as assessed by polymerase chain reaction (PCR) assay and HCV genotype. However, a liver biopsy may be indicated when a focal lesion has been identified, or when there is doubt about the aetiology of the liver disease.

Liver biopsies should be taken by physicians with considerable experience of the procedure in order to minimize risk. The risks may also be reduced by taking the biopsy under ultrasound guidance, and introducing a sealant plug at the site of the biopsy. Other techniques that have been applied to patients with disorders of haemostasis include laparoscopic biopsy and transjugular biopsy.

Whilst infusion of coagulation factor concentrate may correct the basic haemostatic defect in haemophilia A and B, infusion of concentrate may well not correct the bleeding time in patients with von Willebrand's disease (vWD). Liver biopsy in such patients should be avoided where possible.

A suggested treatment protocol to cover a liver biopsy is as follows (Preston et al, 1995):

Day 0
Pre-biopsy dose of factor VIII/IX concentrate calculated to increase plasma level to 1.0 iu/ml (100%), followed by the same dose 8–12 hours later in the case of haemophilia B.

Day 1
Further morning dose of concentrate calculated to increase plasma factor VIII/IX level to 1.0 iu/ml (100%).

Day 2
Dose of concentrate calculated to increase plasma factor VIII/IX level to 0.5 iu/ml (50%).

A liver biopsy should not be taken from a patient with inhibitory antibodies, and the patient's plasma should be tested before the procedure. It may be necessary to give fresh frozen plasma in addition to coagulation factor concentrate. The need for plasma can be determined on the basis of the prothrombin time. Patients with haemophilia B (Christmas disease) should receive only high-purity factor IX concentrate, in view of the heightened risk of thromboembolism associated with repeated infusions of intermediate-purity factor IX concentrate in subjects with chronic liver disease.

Intracranial haemorrhage and headache

Intracranial haemorrhage was the major cause of death of people with haemophilia before the advent of AIDS. In one study, this complication accounted for 25% of all deaths of patients with haemophilia (Rizza and Spooner, 1983). Bleeding may be subdural, subarachnoid or into the brain substance. Many seem to occur after apparently trivial injuries to the head, but a significant number appear to be spontaneous. The risk is particularly high in patients with inhibitory antibodies, and those patients infected with human immunodeficiency virus (HIV) who have associated thrombocytopenia (Ragni et al, 1990). By contrast, this complication is most unusual in von Willebrand's disease.

Unusual or severe headache, particularly when it follows a blow to the head, must be treated as a potential intracranial haemorrhage. In the case of haemophilia A, a dose of 50 iu/kg of factor VIII should be given and pre- and post-infusion factor VIII assays taken. It is advisable to admit young children as a matter of routine for overnight neurological observations after a blow to the head. Radiological investigations should be considered. A neurosurgical opinion should be sought immediately if an intracranial haemorrhage is diagnosed.

Zidovudine therapy is effective in boosting the platelet count in patients with thrombocytopenia related to HIV infection, and this may minimize the risk of associated intracranial bleeding. Screening for hypertension and control of blood pressure, when necessary, are also important preventative measures. It is also our practice to provide individually-moulded polystyrene helmets to toddlers who seem unduly prone to knocks and bangs during early years.

Subarachnoid haemorrhages and meningitis may also present with headache. Cryptococcal meningitis is not unusual in patients infected with HIV. If lumbar puncture is deemed necessary for diagnostic reasons, this can be carried out if the factor VIII (or IX) level is at least 90 iu/dl or more beforehand, and the level should be maintained at no less than 50 iu/dl for the next 24 hours with further infusions.

Gum bleeding

This symptom is more common in patients with von Willebrand's disease (vWD) than in patients with haemophilia. Persistent bleeding from the gums usually reflects poor dental hygiene and is almost invariably a sign of underlying dental disease. The patient should be referred for a dental opinion. Tranexamic acid is useful in controlling the bleeding. It is usually quite unnecessary to give expensive infusions of coagulation factor concentrate to control this minor problem.

Eruption of new teeth in children only occasionally causes troublesome bleeding. Tranexamic acid in syrup form is particularly useful (and acceptable!) in young children. Topical thrombin may also be useful in this situation.

Menorrhagia

Menorrhagia is a frequent problem in women with von Willebrand's disease and platelet disorders. Oestrogen-containing oral contraceptives boost the levels of both factor VIII and vWF, and often prove very effective. A course of oral tranexamic acid taken during the menstrual period may also reduce blood loss. In more severe cases, the patient can be supplied with the intranasal spray form of DDAVP for domiciliary use.

Patients should avoid all medicines that contain aspirin as a matter of course, although paracetamol is a perfectly acceptable alternative.

Occasionally, severe forms of von Willebrand's disease present with marked bleeding at the menarche. Indeed, one of the very first cases described by von Willebrand in 1926 was a young girl who died from profuse menstrual bleeding. Such cases will require complete suppression of menstrual bleeding with norethisterone, and coagulation factor concentrates may be required.

Menorrhagia is a manifestation of hypothyroidism. It should be borne in mind, particularly when von Willebrand's disease is first diagnosed in older women, that hypothyroidism is associated with an acquired form of von Willebrand's disease and this responds to therapy with thyroxine (Dalton et al, 1987).

Management of pregnancy in female carriers of haemophilia and women with von Willebrand's disease

This subject is reviewed by Walker et al (1994) and Ramsahoye et al (1995) and is dealt with in detail in Chapter 12.

The plasma level of factor VIII rises considerably during pregnancy, and the modestly depressed baseline levels often encountered in female carriers of haemophilia invariably rise to well within the normal range during pregnancy. Plasma levels of vWF also rise significantly during pregnancy. Carrier females or women with mild type 1 von Willebrand's disease are not likely to require any form of replacement therapy during pregnancy, even in the setting of surgery or Caesarean section. However, it is prudent to check the levels at around 34–36 weeks of pregnancy in case emergency admission or Caesarean section are required. Carriers of haemophilia A and women with type 1 von Willebrand's disease are not likely to require haemostatic support if the factor VIII and vWF levels exceed 40 iu/dl. DDAVP should not be given to pregnant women, although it can be given after delivery. If haemostatic support is required, recombinant factor VIII should be used because of the risk of transmission of parvovirus (which can cause hydrops fetalis) associated with plasma-derived products. By contrast, the plasma level of factor IX does not change significantly during pregnancy and carriers of Christmas disease may well require replacement therapy if Caesarean section is required. Recombinant factor IX is not available, only high-purity factor IX concentrates should be used because of the heightened risk of thromboembolism associated with the use of intermediate-purity products.

A frequent dilemma concerns the mode of delivery when the status of the fetus is uncertain, or when the fetus is known to have haemophilia. Is Caesarean section required, or may normal vaginal delivery be permitted? Although it might be imagined that there is a high risk of intracranial haemorrhage associated with the normal vaginal delivery of a child with haemophilia, this is not the case and a normal delivery is not contraindicated (Ljung et al, 1994). It is recommended that oxytocic drugs should not be used to induce delivery, in order to minimize compression of the fetal head. Fetal scalp vein sampling should also be avoided during delivery. Vacuum (ventouse) extraction should be avoided.

There is a documented increased risk of intracranial haemorrhage associated with vacuum (ventouse) extraction. Forceps are not contraindicated, but it is our practice to give a dose of coagulation factor concentrate to neonates proven to have haemophilia who have been delivered by forceps. The child should also, in accordance with standard practice, be vaccinated (via the subcutaneous route) against hepatitis B. There is no contraindication to epidural anaesthesia if the factor VIII (or IX) level is 0.35 iu/dl or more and the bleeding time (in the case of von Willebrand's disease) is normal.

Coagulation factor concentrates are likely to be required to cover delivery in women with types 2A and 2B von Willebrand's disease. Concentrate may be infused at the onset of labour with the aim of achieving factor VIII/vWF levels of at least 40 iu/dl in the case of a normal vaginal delivery. If Caesarean section is required, the levels should be correspondingly higher. Intermediate-purity factor VIII concentrates that contain adequate quantities of higher-molecular-weight vWF multimers should be used, such as 8Y (BPL) or Haemate P (Centeon).

A blood sample should be taken from the umbilical cord after delivery for diagnostic purposes. We recommend a course of oral vitamin K, rather than the usual single intramuscular injection, as prophylaxis against haemorrhagic disease of the newborn if the child is believed to have a significant disorder of haemostasis.

The level of factor VIII and vWF usually return to their former, baseline levels within 48 hours of delivery. Whilst carriers of haemophilia A or women with type 1 von Willebrand's disease are not at undue risk of immediate post-partum haemorrhage, delayed post-partum bleeding may necessitate haemostatic support. In most such cases, an infusion of DDAVP would be suitable.

Analgesia

The use of aspirin in any form is contraindicated in haemophilia and related disorders. Aspirin impairs platelet function irreversibly and this additional haemostatic defect may provoke further bleeding episodes. Aspirin may also precipitate gastrointestinal bleeding as it may cause local irritation of the stomach. Many "over the counter" preparations contain aspirin, and it is important to scrutinize the list of contents before taking any proprietary medicines. By contrast, paracetamol (acetaminophen) does not impair platelet function and may be taken, although regular consumption of large doses is not advisable if liver function is markedly impaired.

Practical Management of a Patient with Haemophilia Scheduled for Surgery

Wherever possible, elective surgery should be carried out in a centre experienced in the management of haemophilia. Patients scheduled for surgery should be admitted 1 or 2 days beforehand for blood tests (Table 6.3). Patients with severe haemophilia are likely to require infusions of concentrate for at least 7–10

Table 6.3 Preoperative check list

1. Check supplies of concentrate are adequate for treatment period
2. Is any other surgical work scheduled?
3. Blood tests for:
    - Baseline factor VIII (or IX)
    - Inhibitory antibody screen
    - Hepatitis HBsAg
    - Anti-hepatitis B antibody (anti-HBs) status
    - Anti-hepatitis C antibody (anti-HCV) status
    - Anti-HIV status
    - Liver function tests
    - Prothrombin time
    - Full blood count
    - Group and save plasma or cross-match as appropriate

days after any type of surgery. They will often need, therefore, to stay in hospital for a longer period than other patients and this must be planned for accordingly. It is all too common to see patients discharged 2 days after "minor" surgery. There is no such thing as "minor" surgery for haemophiliacs.

In some countries where concentrate is not readily available, some centres have achieved considerable savings by good coordination of procedures. If a patient is scheduled to have surgery and will be in hospital and receiving concentrate for some days thereafter, other procedures can be carried out at the same time (e.g. dental work, excision of skin lesions, vasectomy, etc.).

Elective surgery in patients with inhibitory antibodies presents particular problems (see Chapter 11). Surgery is certainly not contraindicated in patients seropositive for anti-HIV. There is no evidence that surgery in such patients accelerates deterioration in the immune system and progression to AIDS. It does appear, however, that the risk of sepsis in certain major operations such as total knee replacement is increased in such patients.

On the day of surgery, concentrate should be infused 1 hour before surgery: a dose of 50 iu/kg of factor VIII or 75 iu/kg of factor IX should suffice to boost the plasma level to within the normal range. Pre- and post-infusion levels should be checked in the laboratory to confirm that a suitable level has been achieved prior to surgery. After surgery, twice-daily bolus infusions of factor VIII will be required for at least 5 days. Further daily doses may be required for a further 5 days or so, until soft-tissue healing is achieved. Factor IX has a longer half-life, and only one infusion a day is necessary. Analgesics must not be given by intramuscular injection, and aspirin is contraindicated.

It is sensible to change dressings after infusion of a dose of concentrate in order to minimize the risk of bleeding from wounds. Similarly, physiotherapy is best scheduled immediately after infusion.

Deep venous thrombosis does not appear to be a problem in patients with haemophilia A and prophylaxis is not necessary, even in the setting of orthopaedic surgery. Thromboembolism is a recognized complication in patients with haemophilia B receiving prothrombin-complex concentrates, and so high-purity factor IX concentrates are recommended to cover surgery in such patients.

Continuous intravenous infusion of concentrates to cover surgery is being employed in many centres. Most high-purity concentrates are sufficiently stable for administration in this way, although they may not actually be licensed by the regulatory authorities for use in this fashion (Schulman et al, 1994). The purported advantage of continuous infusion is the elimination of plasma troughs of factor that may result with bolus administration. As a rough guide, the administration of 2–3 iu/kg/h should be sufficient to achieve satisfactory levels after administration of a conventional loading dose of concentrate. Plasma assays can be used to adjust the infusion rate to maintain a given desired level. Early studies were designed to achieve and maintain a level of 100 iu/dl, but this is certainly not necessary and the aim should be to ensure (as with conventional bolus infusions) that the level does not fall below 50 iu/dl at any time in the critical period after surgery. It has been observed that the clearance of factor VIII declines during continuous infusion, so that a given plasma level may be maintained even though the rate of infusion may be reduced. A steady-state level of factor VIII level will be attained after approximately five half-lives of the infused factor.

Early studies employed concentrate diluted in physiological saline, and undiluted concentrate has been used in association with "mini-pumps." In either case, the product is infused into peripheral veins and it is certainly not necessary to place a long venous catheter. Problems associated with continuous infusion of concentrate include thrombophlebitis and the capital costs of the infusion pumps. Loss of peripheral veins through thrombophlebitis may make subsequent home therapy more difficult, and it is important not to use a patient's "favourite" veins for continuous infusion to cover surgery. One definite advantage of continuous intravenous infusion is that it may result in savings of up to one-third as regards costs of concentrate.

Dental Surgery

It is particularly important for patients with haemophilia to have regular dental check-ups. Many community dental surgeons are reluctant to treat patients with bleeding disorders, not only because of the potential risk of serious bleeding complications but also because of a perceived risk of viral infection and contamination of instruments, and all comprehensive care centres should offer facilities for dental surgery. Regular conservative treatment avoids not only discomfort for the patient, but also considerable expense as regards concentrate use if serious dental disease is allowed to develop unchecked.

Potential hazards from dental work include bleeding into the tongue after cuts from dental instruments and delayed bleeding in the retropharyngeal space after inferior dental nerve block for local anaesthesia. It is essential that the patient is screened for the presence of inhibitory antibodies prior to any significant dental work, just as with any invasive procedure.

Scaling and polishing of teeth usually requires no factor cover. Fillings can often be inserted with papillary nerve block. Extractions are likely to require inferior dental nerve block. In patients with severe haemophilia A, a dose of factor VIII calculated to raise the plasma level to 100 iu/dl should be given by intravenous infusion shortly before the procedure. It is our practice to keep patients in overnight after dental extraction, and a second dose of concentrate is given the following day after an extraction.

Antifibrinolytic therapy is particularly effective in minimizing blood loss in the setting of dental and oral bleeding. Tranexamic acid is given by intravenous infusion prior to the procedure: a dose of 500 mg made up in 100 ml of physiological (0.9% saline) is a standard dose for adults. Tranexamic acid tablets (1 g three or four times daily for adults) are prescribed for up to 5 days after the extraction. A solution of tranexamic acid used as a mouth wash is particularly effective in reducing blood loss as it appears that tranexamic acid given in tablet form is poorly absorbed, and relatively little passes into saliva to inhibit fibrinolysis (Sindet-Pedersen, 1991). A typical regimen would be to use a 10 ml mouth wash of 5% tranexamic acid solution four times daily.

References

Anonymous. Haemophilia. *Lancet* 1949; **ii:** 1050–1051.

Aronstam A, Wassef M, Choudhury DP, McClellan DS. Double-blind controlled trial of three dosage regimens in the treatment of haemarthroses in haemophilia A. *Lancet* 1980; **i:** 169–173.

Brettler DB, Forsberg AD, Levine PH, et al. The use of porcine factor VIII concentrate (Hyate:C) in the treatment of patients with inhibitor antibodies to factor VIII. A multicenter US experience. *Archives of Internal Medicine* 1989; **149:** 1381–1385.

Dalton RG, Dewar MS, Savidge GF, et al. Hypothyroidism as a cause of acquired von Willebrand's disease. *Lancet* 1987; **i:** 1007–1009.

Fressinaud E, Meyer D. International survey of patients with von Willebrand disease and angiodysplasia. *Thrombosis and Haemostasis* 1993; **70:** 546.

Gregg-Smith SJ, Pattison RM, Dodd CAF, Giangrande PLF, Duthie RB. Septic arthritis in haemophilia. *Journal of Bone and Joint Surgery* 1993; **75B:** 368–370.

Gringeri A, Santagostino E, Tradati F, Giangrande PLF, Mannucci PM. Adverse effects of treatment with porcine factor VIII. *Thrombosis and Haemostasis* 1991; **65:** 245–247.

Hashemi S, Tackaberry ES, Palmer DS, Rock G, Ganz PR. DDAVP-induced release of von Willebrand factor from endothelial cells in vitro: the effect of plasma and blood cells. *Biochimica et Biophysica Acta* 1990; **1052:** 63–70.

Hay CRM, Colvin BT, Ludlam CA, Hill FGH, Preston FE. Recommendations for the treatment of factor VIII inhibitors: from the UK Haemophilia Centre Directors Organisation Inhibitor Working Party. *Blood Coagulation and Fibrinolysis* 1996; **7:** 134–138.

Hedner U. Factor VIIa in the treatment of haemophilia (review paper). *Blood Coagulation and Fibrinolysis* 1990; **1:** 307–317.

Ingram A, Inwood MJ, Gregson D, Coppolino M. Multiple pyoarthrosis in human immunodeficiency virus-infected hemophiliacs. *Canadian Journal of Infectious Diseases* 1994; **5:** 33–36.

Kasper CK, Graham JB, Kernoff PBA, Larrieu MJ, Rickard KA, Mannucci PM. Hemophilia: state of the art hematologic care. *Vox Sanguinis* 1989; **56:** 141–144.

Kernoff PBA, Thomas ND, Lilley PA, Mathews KB, Goldman E, Tuddenham EGD. Clinical experience with polyelectrolyte-fractionated porcine factor VIII concentrate in the treatment of hemophiliacs with antibodies to factor VIII. *Blood* 1984; **63:** 31–41.

Lethagen S, Egervall K, Berntorp E, Bengtsson B. The administration of desmopressin by nasal spray: a dose-determination study in patients with mild haemophilia A or von Willebrand's disease. *Haemophilia* 1995; **1:** 97–102.

Ljung R, Lindgren A-C, Petrini P, Tengborn L. Normal vaginal delivery is to be recommended for haemophilia carrier gravidae. *Acta Paediatrica* 1994; **83:** 609–611.

Lusher JM, Shapiro SS, Palascak JE, Rao AU, Levine PH, Blatt PM. Efficacy of prothrombin-complex concentrates in hemophiliacs with antibodies to factor VIII. A multicentre therapeutic trial. *New England Journal of Medicine* 1980; **303:** 421–425.

Macik BG, Lindley CM, Lusher J, et al. Safety and initial clinical efficay of three dose levels of recombinant activated factor VII (rVIIa): results of a phase I study. *Blood Coagulation and Fibrinolysis* 1993; **4:** 521–527.

Mannucci PM. Desmopressin: a nontransfusional form of treatment for congenital and acquired bleeding disorders. *Blood* 1988; **72:** 1449–1455.

Mannucci PM, Lusher JM. Desmopressin and thrombosis (letter). *Lancet* 1989; **2:** 675–676.

Mannucci PM, Ruggeri Z, Pareti FI, Capitanio A. 1-Deamino-8-arginine vasopressin: a

new pharmacological approach to the management of haemophilia and von Willebrand's disease. *Lancet* 1977; **i:** 869–872.
Mannucci PM, Bettega D, Cattaneo M. Patterns of development of tachyphylaxis in patients with haemophilia and von Willebrand disease after repeated doses of desmopressin (DDAVP). *British Journal of Haematology* 1992a; **82:** 87–93.
Mannucci PM, Tenconi PM, Castaman G, Rodeghiero F. Comparison of four virus-inactivated plasma concentrates for treatment of severe von Willebrand's disease: a cross-over randomized trial. *Blood* 1992b; **79:** 3130–3137.
Mazurier C. Von Willebrand disease masquerading as haemophilia A. *Thrombosis and Haemostasis* 1992; **67:** 391–396.
McCoy HE, Kitchens CS. Small bowel hematoma in a hemophiliac as a cause of pseudoappendicitis: diagnosis by CT scanning. *American Journal of Hematology* 1991; **38:** 138–139.
Morfini M, Lee M, Messori A for the Scientific and Standardisation Committee of the International Society for Thrombosis and Haemostasis. The design and analysis of half-life and recovery studies for factor VIII and factor IX. *Thrombosis and Haemostasis* 1991; **66:** 384–386.
Morrison AE, Ludlam CA, Kessler C. Use of porcine factor VIII in the treatment of patients with acquired haemophilia. *Blood* 1993; **81:** 1513–1520.
Pareti FI, Mazzucato M, Bottini E, Mannucci PM. Interaction of porcine von Willebrand factor with the platelet glycoproteins Ib and IIb/IIIa complex. *British Journal of Haematology* 1992; **82:** 81–86.
Preston FE, Dusheiko G, Lee CA, Ludlam CA, Giangrande PLF. Guidelines on the diagnosis and management of chronic liver disease in haemophilia. *Haemophilia* 1995; **1** (suppl 4): 42–44.
Ragni MV, Bontempo FA, Myers DJ, Kiss JE, Oral A. Hemorrhagic sequelae of immune thrombocytopenic purpura in human immunodeficiency virus-infected hemophiliacs. *Blood* 1990; **75:** 1267–1272.
Ramsahoye BH, Davies SV, Dasani H, Pearson JF. Obstetric management in von Willebrand's disease: a report of 24 pregnancies and a review of the literature. *Haemophilia* 1995; **1:** 140–144.
Rapaport SI, Rao VM. The tissue factor pathway: how it has become a "prima ballerina." *Thrombosis and Haemostasis* 1995; **74:** 7–17.
Rizza CR, Spooner RJD. Treatment of haemophilia and related disorders in Britain and Northern Ireland during 1976–1980: report on behalf of directors of haemophilia centres in the United Kingdom. *British Medical Journal* 1983; **286:** 929–933.
Schulman S, Gitel S, Martinowitz U. Stability of factor VIII concentrates after reconstitution. *American Journal of Hematology* 1994; **45:** 217–223.
Sindet-Pedersen S. Haemostasis in oral surgery – the possible pathogenetic implications of oral fibrinolysis on bleeding. *Danish Medical Bulletin* 1991; **38:** 428–443.
Smith TJ, Gill JC, Ambruso DR, Hathaway WE. Hyponatremia and seizures in young children given DDAVP. *American Journal of Hematology* 1989; **31:** 199–202.
United Kingdom Haemophilia Centre Directors' Organisation Executive Committee. Guidelines on therapeutic products to treat haemophilia and other hereditary coagulation disorders. *Haemophilia* 1997; **3**: 63–67.
Walker ID, Walker JJ, Colvin BT, Letsky EA, Rivers R, Stevens R. Investigation and management of haemorrhagic disorders in pregnancy. *Journal of Clinical Pathology* 1994; **47:** 100–108.

7 Musculoskeletal Problems and their Management

Robert B. Duthie

Joint Bleeds

Intra-articular bleeds make up over 85% of all bleeds in the patient with haemophilia and will be considered under acute and chronic haemarthrosis.

Acute Haemarthrosis

The factors affecting the incidence of haemarthrosis are:

1. *The severity of the coagulation defect.* Intra-articular bleeding is the most constant feature of the patient with severe haemophilia (factor VIII level of less than 1% of normal). It is unlikely for such a patient ever to reach adult life without having experienced a haemarthrosis, and in many instances preceding trauma is not often recalled.

Patients with moderate and mild forms of haemophilia (factor VIII more than 1% of normal) rarely present with "spontaneous" intra-articular haemorrhage, but have to be regarded as severely affected for either surgical or accidental trauma. Patients with Christmas disease (haemophilia B) have similar problems.

2. *Nature of the articulation.* Certain joints are more frequently affected by haemarthrosis than others. In a group of 113 patients who were admitted to the Nuffield Orthopaedic Centre in Oxford on one or more occasions for orthopaedic management in the days before home therapy, joint bleeding was present on 366 occasions and was distributed as shown in Table 7.1.

Table 7.1 Distribution of acute haemarthroses in 113 patients over a 3-year period (NOC, Oxford)

	n
Knee	151
Elbow	109
Ankle	73
Wrist	9
Shoulder	8
Foot	5
Hand	5
Hip	5
Sterno-clavicular	1
Total	366

If weight-bearing alone was a major cause, the hip should be involved more often and the elbow less frequently. But in boys the elbow frequently takes leverage of body weight when pushing up from the sitting position, when climbing and in sport. The three most affected target joints – knee, ankle and elbow – are hinge articulations, whereas the "ball and socket" joints, the hip and shoulder, are affected less. Minor angulatory and rotatory strains, which can be accommodated by the hip and shoulder, cause significant stresses on hinge joints and precipitate bleeding.

However, investigation by means of ultrasound has shown that bleeding into the hip joint is more common than previously thought and that bleeding into the hip joint may be misdiagnosed as an ilio-psoas muscle bleed. Gamble et al (1991) have found that during the second decade of life, haemarthrosis occurs more often in the ankle rather than the knee, but that these bleeds may be into an ankle already showing pathological changes.

3. *Previous joint bleeding.* After several acute haemarthroses it is not always possible to restore the joint to normality even by early treatment. The affected joint may remain swollen and warm with synovial thickening on clinical examination and by ultrasound investigation. The presence of a chronically hypertrophied and inflamed vascular synovium predisposes to recurrent haemorrhage and is the most important cause of "bad spells".

4. *Mechanical Factors.* Mechanical factors determine the frequency of bleeding into particular joints. De Andrade et al (1965) demonstrated inhibition of quadriceps function following distension of the knee joint. The presence of muscle wasting, particularly following knee bleeds, adds to the vulnerability of the affected joint. Loss of movement resulting from soft-tissue contractures or

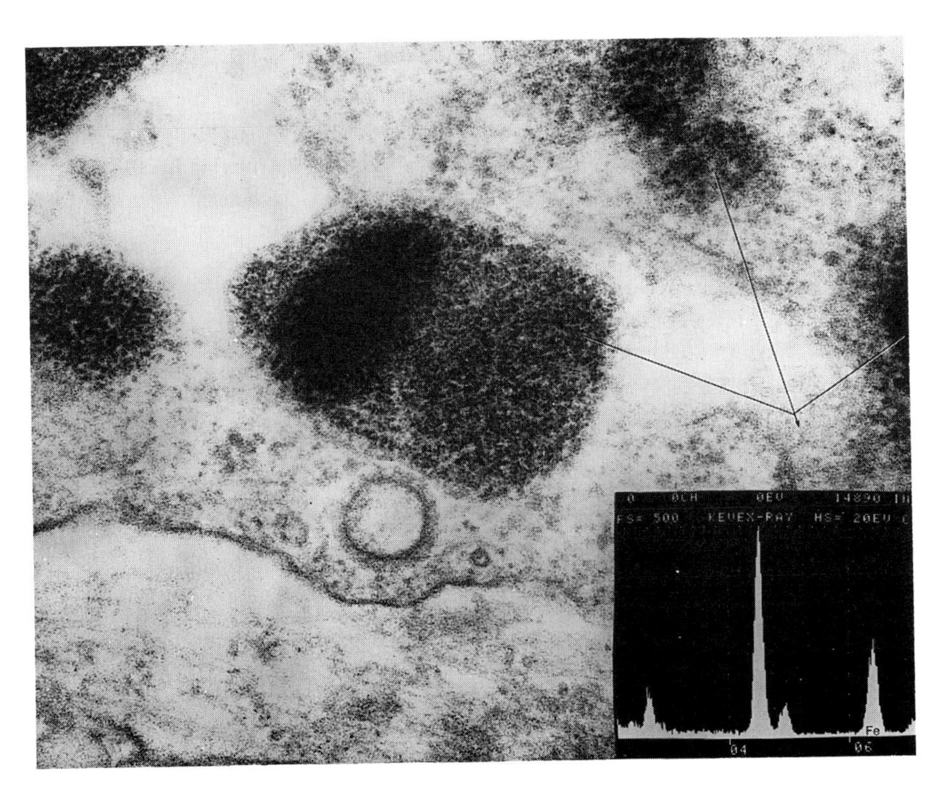

Figure 7.1 Scanning electron micrograph of synovial membrane to show ferritin deposition within cells and in a macrophage (sidersome) (Stein and Duthie, 1981).

intra-articular changes adds further to the susceptibility of the hinge joints to mechanical stresses and strains.

5. *Age.* A greater number of bleeds occur in the younger patients. The greatest incidence is in adolescence, with a decrease in the frequency of bleeding episodes in adults. This is not accompanied by any detectable change in clotting function. As the patient gets older he probably modifies his activities to avoid situations that expose him to risk of injury. Also in later life the joints may be limited by stiffness and reduced mobility.

6. *Antibodies to factor VIII* (see Chapter 3). The development of a circulating antibody to factor VIII is a serious complication, which makes the management of an acute haemarthrosis very difficult since clotting factor replacement has only a limited effect.

Histopathology

Bleeding into a joint is followed within a few hours by a cellular reaction of the synovium with exudation of polymorphonuclear leucocytes and synovitis. Within a few days, hyperplasia of the synovial lining is well established and the inflammatory cells in the stratum synoviale include lymphocytes, histiocytes and polymorphonuclear cells. Haemosiderin pigment accumulates rapidly and is found in the synovial lining, in the subsynovial tissues within a few days of the haemorrhage and in special macrophage-type cells – the siderosome (Fig. 7.1) (Stein and Duthie 1981). The site of haemorrhage may be suggested by the presence of an area of necrosis and ulceration of the synovial membrane with a blood clot firmly adherent to the surface and by extravasation of red blood corpuscles into the surrounding synovial tissue.

Continued breakdown of haemoglobin leads to an increasing content of haemosiderin and ferritin throughout the synovial tissues, with an increase in the number of phagocytic mononuclear cells and lymphocytes. This state may well be permanent when the volume of haemorrhage into a joint has been large, as there is no other mechanism to remove the red cell degradation products. Azorin et al (1985) have described three phases of change in the synovium:

1. Hypertrophic-angiomatous phase with new formation of a dense vascular network in the subintimal layer and hyperplasia of the synovial villi.
2. Hypertrophic-pigmented phase in which there is a large amount of iron pigments within synovial cells, with some decrease in the number and size of the synovial folds with the regular network being submerged in fibrotic material.
3. The fibrotic phase in which the vascular component has disappeared leaving much fibrosis in all layers.

The rich subsynovial plexus of vessels lying in the areolar tissue between the synovium and capsule is the source of the bleeding, but whether there is a general ooze from many small vessels or one major bleeding point is not known. However, once the synovium is hypertrophic and hyperplastic, bleeding can occur over the whole affected area.

The factor or factors that precipitate bleeding from the subsynovial vessels are unclear. External trauma may sometimes cause haemarthrosis in less severely affected haemophiliacs. In the majority of cases, however, there is no such history and in these patients, bleeding is said to be "spontaneous". Unless the subsynovial vessels are unusually susceptible to damage, there seems no reason why minor trauma should not cause a similar high incidence of bleeding from skin, fat and muscle but this is not the case.

As already mentioned, minor rotatory and angulatory strains on hinge joints are an important triggering mechanism. Schumpe (1986) has described the altered biomechanics in the joints of the hip, knee and ankle, in terms of altered gliding and rotating mechanisms. The synovium in the knee, elbow and ankle is arranged in pouches and recesses and is, therefore, more vulnerable to entrapment.

Houghton and Duthie (1978) have pointed out that the larger amounts of synovium and its infolding in the diathrodial hinge joints predispose them to bleeding, unlike the regular sleeve of the synovium in the shoulder and hip. Histological studies have demonstrated small areas of necrosis in the synovium which may be the result of the tissue being nipped by the articular surfaces.

Clinical features

Premonitory symptoms

Before the pain and overt swelling of an acute haemarthrosis develop, the patient may experience a variety of abnormal sensations in the joint, such as a pricking feeling or a sensation of increased warmth, a slight stiffness or of weakness.

Pain

Pain is the main disabling complaint in the acute joint bleed and results from the rapidity of joint distension. Work by de Andrade et al (1965) demonstrated that rapid filling of the knee joint with saline led to severe pain and inhibition of quadriceps function with atrophy of the muscle. On the other hand, synovial effusions, which develop gradually, allow time for the capsule and synovium to distend and pain therefore tends to be less.

Joint swelling

Distension with visible, palpable and tender swelling is the first objective sign of bleeding into a joint. The absence of swelling does not mean that a minor or small haemarthrosis is not present. Absence of tenderness in a swollen joint may signify that the swelling is due to a non-haemorrhagic effusion.

The older haemophiliac with a chronic fibrosed synovium may have a very small joint space. Bleeding into such joints can be extremely painful and distension may be difficult to detect. In the younger haemophiliac, on the other hand, large distended joints are more common and volumes of blood (up to 220 ml) have been aspirated from such knees.

Distension is most easily observed in the knee medial and lateral to the patella. In large haemorrhages the suprapatellar pouch may be distended. The capsule of the ankle joint distends anteriorly and below the malleoli: in the elbow, postero-laterally; and in the shoulder, anteriorly. The diagnosis of bleeding into the hip joint is more difficult and requires ultrasonography.

Loss of movement

Loss of movement in the joint may be marked and is usually accompanied by characteristic deformities. For example, in the case of the knee and elbow the joint is characteristically held at an angle of flexion, of 75–90°. Attempts to correct this protective position will provoke much pain.

Diagnosis

When the patient is a known to be suffering from haemophilia or Christmas disease, the presence of a painful, distended, warm joint in which movement is restricted strongly suggests a haemarthrosis. There may also be an elevation of body temperature to as much as 103°F (38.3°C). A high and sustained fever suggests an alternative diagnosis of an infective arthritis. Gregg-Smith et al (1993) have described septic arthritis in the knees of six haemophilic patients out of a patient population of 800 haemophiliacs, occurring within a 2-year period. Four of these patients were HIV seropositive.

Diagnosis of septic arthritis is by aspiration and culture (fresh aspirate must be plated for both aerobic and anaerobic growth). Acute tenderness is a feature of both haemarthrosis and septic arthritis, but the general well-being of the patient with a haemarthrosis, the rapidity of its onset and the rapid response of haemarthrosis to immobilization and replacement therapy help in the differential diagnosis.

Management

The aim of treatment of acute haemarthrosis is to stop bleeding, to relieve pain, to maintain and restore function and to prevent chronic joint changes.

Replacement therapy

Correction of the basic clotting defect by the infusion of concentrates is the basis of management for acute haemarthrosis and is dealt with in detail in Chapter 6.

Following replacement therapy, relief of pain is often dramatic and function is restored quickly without serious muscle wasting or contractures. In the majority of minor joint bleeds no other measures are necessary.

Early haemarthrosis is best treated as soon as possible after onset of bleeding on an outpatient basis either at home or if necessary at the Haemophilia Centre. Intermediate medical treatment or examination by the family doctor or in accident departments of the local hospital not equipped to provide early replacement therapy delays effective treatment and is not recommended.

Home therapy programmes are now well established, but whether it improves the outcome as regards the development of joint and muscle damage in the long term is not yet clear, but the immediate effect upon the patient in terms of his day-to-day life is obviously beneficial. A single dose of factor of 15–20 iu/kg body weight is usually sufficient to control early joint bleeding. More severe bleeding may require 20–40 iu/kg repeated on several successive days.

If a haemarthrosis is severe, acute and has been present for 12 hours or more without treatment, pain, muscle spasm and loss of movement may be very marked and admission to the combined haemophilia-orthopaedic service is indicated.

Following transfusion of factor, indications that bleeding has stopped are the relief of pain, reduction in capsular tension, the decrease in joint circumference and the relaxation of muscle guarding.

Factor replacement is also required for physiotherapy after severe or protracted bleeding though seldom after haemarthrosis that has resolved promptly. Close cooperation between the physicians, orthopaedic surgeons and physiotherapists is essential in planning the day-to-day requirements.

Immobilization

Splinting of the bleeding joint is indicated in those patients where a tense, painful swelling is accompanied by muscle guarding and flexion contracture. Admission to the orthopaedic unit is usually necessary for such immobilization, replacement therapy and subsequent physiotherapy.

Immobilization of the knee, ankle, elbow, wrist and small peripheral joints is best obtained by padded plaster of Paris splints or by light custom-made orthotic splints. The use of complete casts carries the hazard of vascular obstruction if the bleeding continues.

The joint should be immobilized in the position in which the patient is most comfortable, usually one of flexion, until the muscle guarding has subsided. Too early attempts to move joints into a more functional position will increase intracapsular tension still further, provoke more pain and may precipitate further haemorrhage. Within 24–48 hours it is usually possible to remove the temporary splint and construct a padded plaster of Paris splint or plastic splint in a more functional position. These splints are changed at intervals to achieve gentle and gradual correction of any flexion contraction. Elevation of the limb and application of ice packs to the affected joint can help to relieve pain.

Bleeding into the hip joint might be treated by the use of a Thomas splint but in practice this may not be tolerated in the acute period. The patient usually adopts a position of hip flexion either on his side or on his back with his leg supported on pillows. In severe bleeding, comfort may sometimes be achieved by immobilization in a hip spica.

The shoulder joint may be effectively immobilized by a sling and body bandage without the need for a shoulder spica, or by means of an abduction aeroplane splint.

Pain is usually relieved by factor replacement, splinting and analgesics, but in the patient with antibodies to factors VIII or IX, pain may persist.

Aspiration

In the smaller haemarthrosis without severe pain, blood is rapidly absorbed following standard replacement therapy but the larger and more severe joint bleeds may take several weeks to resolve completely. For these, aspiration may minimize joint damage and shorten the period of disability. Severe unremitting pain in a tense joint is an important indication for aspiration. Having said that, the decision to aspirate should not be taken lightly and requires considerable experience by a senior member of the orthopaedic team in consultation with the physician from the Haemophilia Centre. Adequate replacement therapy must be given before and for several days after the procedure.

Aspiration may be effectively performed without the use of a general anaesthetic, except in children who are obviously frightened or in whom difficulty is anticipated.

The skin is prepared and draped and the surgical procedure is carried out with full aseptic technique. The skin and joint capsule are infiltrated with a small volume of local anaesthetic using a fine needle. Coagulation factor replacement is given simultaneously by intravenous infusion. The joint should be aspirated to dryness if possible and supported by a Robert Jones compression bandage.

Arthroscopy and wash out

With the development of arthroscopy it is now possible to wash joints free of blood and clots. This may help in "deloading" the joint of ferritin and haemosiderin particles. The procedure requires a general anaesthetic and full factor replacement like any other operation, to be followed by compression bandaging and progressive physiotherapy.

Rehabilitation

The purpose of early treatment of acute joint haemorrhage is to arrest bleeding and to return the child to his home and school environment or the adult to his work, as soon as possible. Prolonged immobilization by splintage or bed rest is to be avoided because it results in atrophy of muscles (Young et al, 1987), joint instability and further bleeds. Static exercises are commenced with factor replacement as soon as the joint is pain-free and if there is no flare-up of pain or joint swelling, active exercises begun at the earliest opportunity, usually within 48 hours of the controlling of bleeding. The joint is rested in a posterior plaster slab or polythene splint between physiotherapy sessions for protection and to prevent contracture. Unprotected weight-bearing in the case of knee or ankle bleeds is delayed until the joint swelling has subsided. Synovial thickening, indicating a reactive synovitis, may be present for up to 14 days or even 3 weeks after a major joint bleed. Bearing weight during this time may provoke further haemorrhage and non-weight-bearing exercises are preferred until this hypertrophic synovitis has subsided. Active exercises and walking in the hydrotherapy pool provide a graduated preparation for normal activity. Protection by external plaster or polythene splints such as a quadriceps enhancing splint, or the use of a long leg orthoses, is necessary following a severe haemarthrosis of the knee accompanied by quadriceps wasting.

Chronic Haemophilic Arthropathy

Although Otto (1803) in his description of the disease and Legg (1872) in his classical monograph on haemophilia described joint deformities, neither author suggested any association of arthropathy with recurrent haemorrhage. However, Konig (1892), in a study of eight cases, noted the association of joint bleeding and haemophilic arthropathy.

Aetiology

Although chronic joint changes in haemophilia are related to intra-articular bleeding, the actual pathogenesis is not clearly understood. Descriptions from post-mortem material (de Palma and Cotler, 1956; Rodnan, 1959) gave little information on the causative process. In spite of increasing numbers of surgical procedures that are safely performed on haemophilic joints, macroscopic observations and biopsy material remain scanty.

Experimental evidence has proved to be important. Swanton (1959) observed, in haemophilic dogs, that the earliest pathological change was an inflammatory reaction of plasma cells and lymphocyte infiltration following small haemorrhages in the synovial tissues. Haemosiderin deposition was observed in the synovial cells with phagocytosis of iron pigment by macrophages. Organization of the fibrinous exudate led to synovial adhesions, reduction in size of the joint space and limitation of movement. The articular cartilage was discoloured with softening of its surface.

Young and Hudacek (1954) injected blood into the knee joints of dogs over a period of 1 year producing moderate to severe villous hyperplasia and capsular fibrosis. By electron microscopic studies of synovial membrane in human haemarthrosis, Roy and Ghadially (1967) have shown that synovial cells can phagocytose erythrocytes.

In 1967 Hoaglund successfully produced the synovial and cartilaginous changes characteristic of haemophilic arthropathy by injecting the knees of puppies with 1–4 ml of blood six times a week. Radiographs showed enlargement of the distal femoral epiphyses and patella, and deformity of the joint surfaces. The usual synovial pigmentation, hypertrophy and fibrosis were observed. Hoaglund suggested that previous experiments had failed to demonstrate cartilaginous changes because they were of insufficient intensity and duration. In discussing the joint changes he implicated immobilization as causing the observed osteoporosis.

Plasminogen, activated by cytokinase from leucocytes, was suggested by Lack (1959) as a factor producing cartilage damage, but in Hoaglund's experiments, epsilon-aminocaproic acid (a potent inhibitor of plasminogen activation) afforded no protection against cartilage change. Other proteolytic enzymes, as found in rheumatoid arthritis (Luscombe, 1963), might be present in the hypertrophied synovium which could cause degradation of chondromucoprotein.

Azorin et al (1985) have developed an ingenious animal model of recurring haemarthrosis by producing a popliteal arteriovenous malformation with bleeding into the knee. This lasted up to 48 hours, before becoming thrombosed, producing a haemarthrosis as well as an increased intra-articular pressure of 120–140 mmHg. After 6–8 weeks these joints exhibited the advanced stages of haemophilic arthropathy with articular cartilage destruction, subchondral bone resorption and necrosis.

Histopathological changes

Synovium

The hyperplasia and hypertrophy of the synovial lining cells with large numbers of macrophages and lymphocytes and deposition of haemosiderin leads to thickening of the synovial membrane with further haemorrhages. The phagocytic reaction is replaced by fibroblastic activity with collagen deposition in the synovium (Fig. 7.2).

Post and Telfer (1975) have shown that these synovial changes affect the secretion of glycosaminoglycans and hyaluronic acid, which are involved in the maintenance of articular cartilage, and Stein (1975) demonstrated that the layer of hyaluronic acid that is normally present in articular cartilage is absent in haemophilic arthropathy.

Itokazu et al (1988) have shown lectin binding on haemophilic synovial membrane, both on the surface as well as intracytoplasmic, in response to haemosiderin particles. Multinucleate giant cells appear in the hyperplastic synovium. Larger giant cells, resembling the classical type of foreign-body giant cell, contain haemosiderin and are called siderosomes (Stein and Duthie, 1981).

Other changes may be observed in the synovium such as patchy areas of necrosis, which probably result from the mechanical trapping by disintegrated fragments of the cartilaginous and bony tissues. This material in itself induces a cellular response, with multinucleate giant cells and mononuclear phagocytes.

Articular cartilage

The surface of the cartilage may be covered partially or wholly by fibrous tissue in which there are deposits of haemosiderin and chronic inflammatory cells. The cartilage under this pannus is irregularly fibrillated and some cartilage cells may be totally absent, having undergone necrosis and autolysis. Chondrocytes can be seen irregularly distributed throughout the matrix and often aggregated in cell

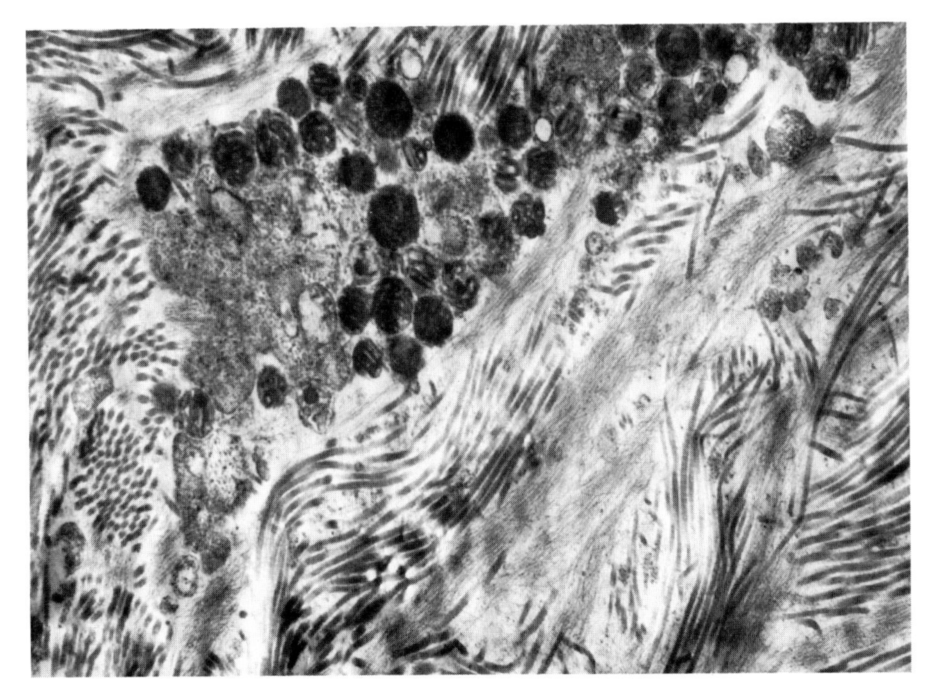

Figure 7.2 Photomicrograph showing intracytoplasmic deposition of ferritin and haemosiderin particles with fibroblastic activity and deposition of collagen fibrils.

clusters indicating a proliferative stage. The chondrocytes are loaded with intracellular iron deposits (Fig. 7.3). Stein (1975) has suggested that the lysosomal membranes are damaged chemically in response to the intracellular accumulation of iron.

High levels of cathepsin D and prostaglandin E are found in haemophilic synovium (McLardy-Smith et al, 1984). Cathepsin D is a proteolytic enzyme of lysosomal origin and has a marked chemotactic effect, perpetuating chronic inflammatory changes and articular cartilage destruction. Prostaglandin E is known to increase vascular permeability and promote bone resorption (Robinson et al, 1976). McLardy-Smith et al (1984) have shown that haemophilic synovium in culture produces prostaglandin E at markedly higher levels than normal but less than that found in rheumatoid arthritis. Haemophilic synovium conditioned medium causes a significant loss of chondroitin sulphate from human cartilage, and such changes are likely to contribute to the loss of matrix stability and increased fibrillation. The cartilage becomes more susceptible to subsequent mechanical disruption. The beneficial effects of non-steroidal anti-inflammatory drugs in haemophilia are probably due to their potent inhibition of the biosynthesis of these humoral substances.

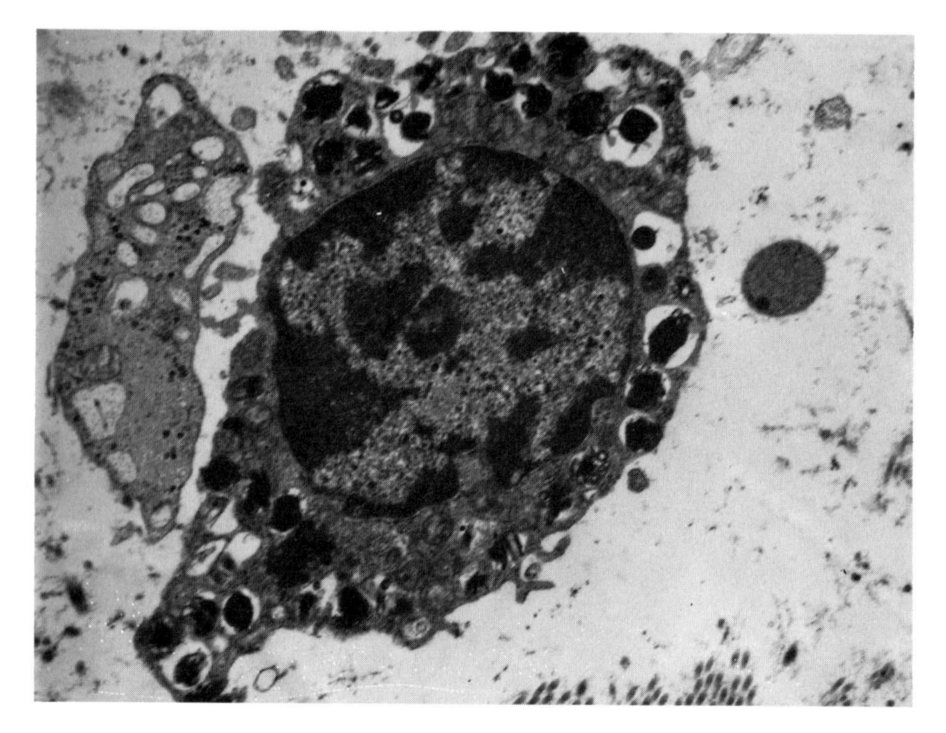

Figure 7.3 Photomicrograph of a cartilage cell undergoing necrosis with loss of cytoplasm and contents and condensation within the nucleus.

The pathogenesis of chronic haemophilic arthritis has been described by Stein and Duthie (1981) (Fig. 7.4).

Radiological changes

Many authors have described the typical changes of chronic haemophilic arthropathy as seen on radiographs. Boldero and Kemp (1966) emphasize that all or certain radiological features may result from a single or, far more commonly, repeated haemorrhages into the joint cavity, or non-specific changes resulting from the immobilization of the limb, or from reactive hyperaemia.

Radiological changes include osteoporosis, condylar enlargement (Blount, 1960), degenerative changes, widening of the intercondylar notch, patellar abnormalities and disturbance of alignment with deformity (Kingma, 1965).

The late changes of loss of cartilage space (Lack and Ali, 1967), subchondral collapse, cystic changes and osteophyte formation signify the development of secondary degenerative arthritis and the features are those often seen in osteoarthrosis. Some prominence was given by earlier observers (Bourdon et al, 1963) to para-articular cysts, which were attributed to intraosseous bleeding.

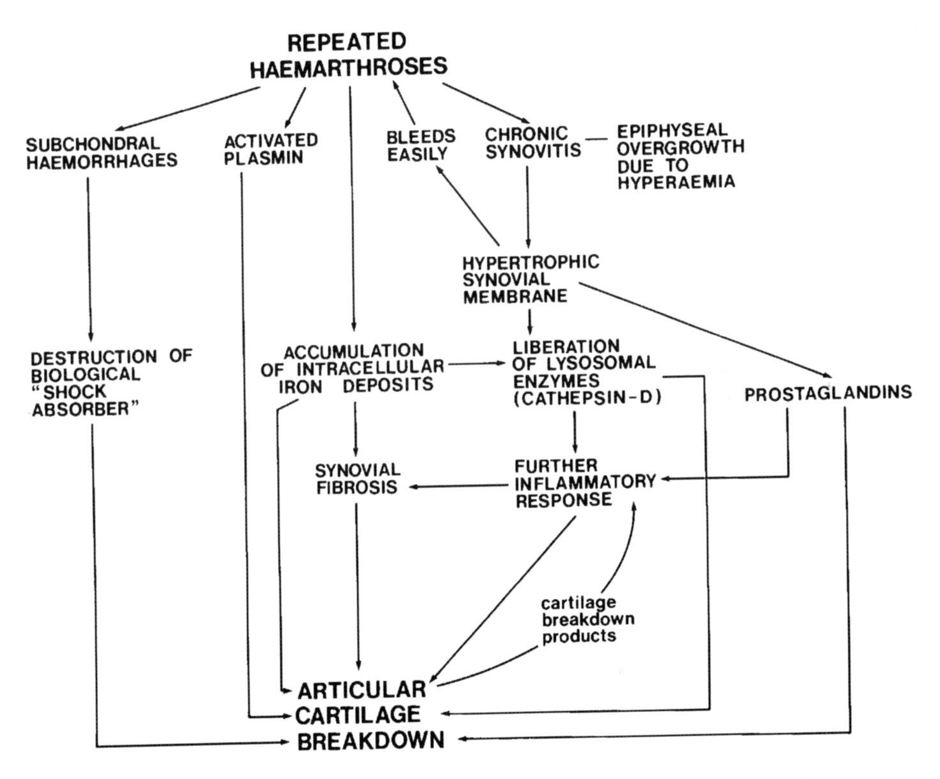

Figure 7.4 A diagram to show the pathogenesis of chronic haemophilic arthritis. (Reproduced from Stein and Duthie, 1981, with permission of the authors and the Editor of the *Journal of Bone and Joint Surgery*, UK.)

Abnormalities in the patello-femoral compartment are frequently found in haemophilic arthropathy with narrowing of the joint space, loss of congruity of the joint surfaces and the more particular feature of squaring of the inferior pole of the patella (Fig. 7.5a). The changes observed in the tibio-femoral joint include condylar squaring, depression of the tibial plateau, narrowing of the cartilage space, incongruity of joint surface and, in the late degenerative cases, cyst formation and osteophytosis (Fig. 7.5b). All changes tend to be more severe in the medial compartment than in the lateral compartment despite the frequent presence of a valgus deformity.

De Palma (1967) stated that the most frequent deformities in the haemophilic knee were flexion, valgus and external rotation. In addition, two other abnormalities of alignment may be observed: posterior subluxation of the tibia and lateral shift of the tibia on the femur. The lateral radiographic views will show posterior subluxation only if taken in maximum extension. These deformities appeared in about 25–50% of the patients in all age groups. External rotation of the tibia may play a considerable part in the progression of deformity

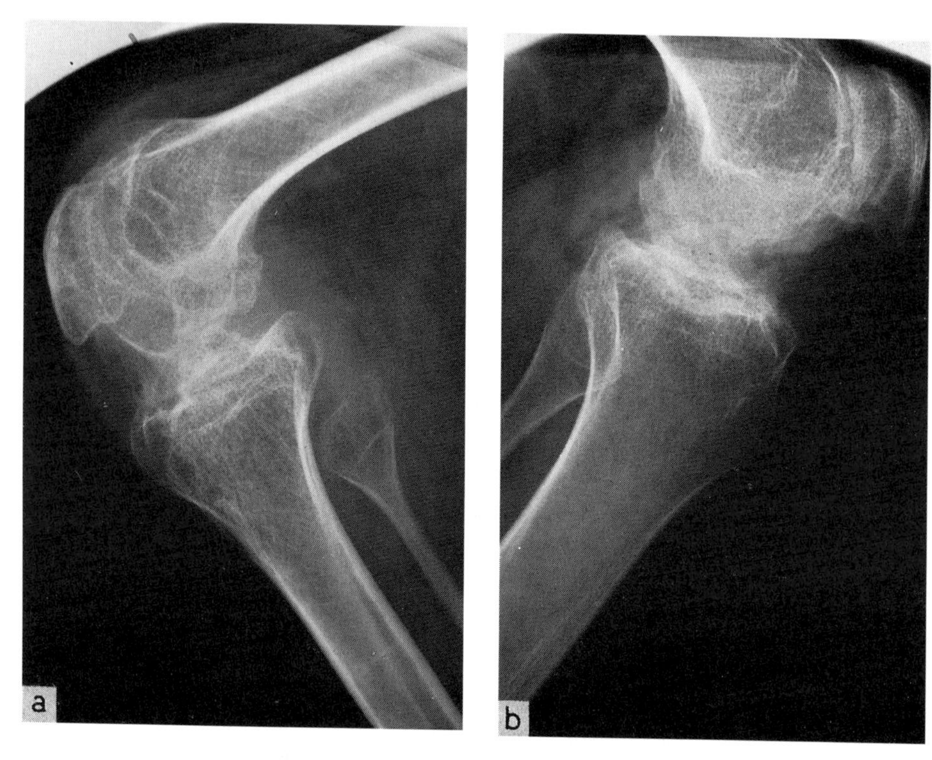

Figure 7.5 (a,b) Radiographs to show the squaring of the patella, loss of congruity of the joint surfaces and loss of intra-articular space with attenuation of bone on the left and development of osteophytes.

(Fig. 7.6). It is frequently underestimated because of not being adequately demonstrated on X-rays and may result from the deforming forces exerted by the tensor fasciae latae and lateral hamstrings compensating for weakness of the quadriceps.

Petersson et al (1980) have described a radiological classification of haemophilic arthropathy based on a points system (Table 7.2).

Distribution

Ahlberg (1965) in a study of the Swedish haemophilic population confirmed that the distribution of chronic arthropathy in the different joints was similar to that of acute haemarthrosis, with the knee, elbow and ankle joints being most often affected.

Clinical features

The most frequent finding is loss of movement, occurring many years before pain and gross deformity are noted. In the knee, flexion is lost initially. Where

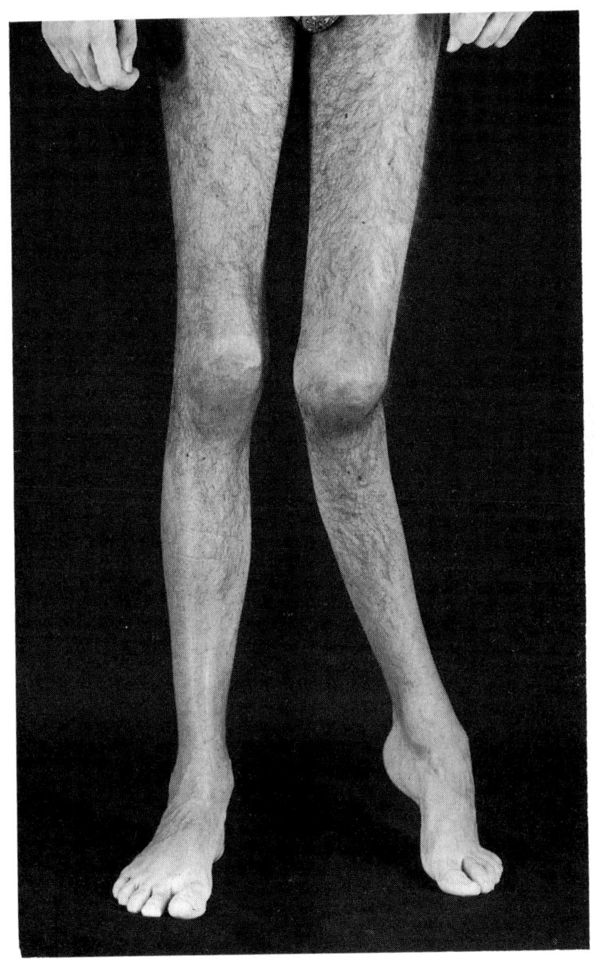

Figure 7.6 Photograph to show the classical long-standing deformities of sub-luxation of the left tibia with external rotation of the tibia and prominence of the left medial malleolus.

moderate or severe radiological changes are present, 80% of the knees have a fixed flexion contracture which can be corrected initially, but as the joint changes progress of this correction becomes more difficult.

The elbow joint shows a loss of extension. Limitation of flexion is less evident. Ankle motion seems to be less restricted than knee or elbow motion for a given degree of joint damage.

When radiological changes such as reduction in cartilage space, cysts and osteo-phyte formation appear, the clinical picture resembles that of osteoarthrosis. There is chronic aching in the joint punctuated by periods of more acute pain. Swelling, which may be chronic, may denote an effusion rather than a haemarthrosis. The range of movement of the joint may progressively decrease and the joint eventually become ankylosed. The patient may be severely crippled,

Table 7.2 Radiological classification of haemophilic arthropathy by Petersson et al (1980)

Type of change	Finding	Score (points)
Osteoporosis	Absent	0
	Present	1
Enlarged epiphysis	Absent	0
	Present	1
Irregular subchondral surface	Absent	0
	The surface partly involved	1
	The surface totally involved	2
Narrowing of joint space	Absent	0
	Present: joint space >1 mm	1
	Present: joint space <1 mm	2
Subchondral cyst formation	Absent	0
	1 cyst	1
	>1 cyst	2
Erosions at joint margins	Absent	0
	Present	1
Gross incongruence of articulating bone ends	Absent	0
	Slight	1
	Pronounced	2
Joint deformity (angulation and/or displacement between articulating bones)	Absent	0
	Slight	1
	Pronounced	2
Possible joint score: 0–13 points		

(Reproduced from Petersson et al, 1980, with permission.)

particularly when both knees are involved, and in such cases crutches or even a wheelchair are necessary for getting about.

Management

Once established joint changes are present, treatment falls into the following four categories.

1. *Physiotherapy*. The most important aspect of physiotherapy in chronic haemophilic arthropathy is the maintenance of good muscle power, especially of the quadriceps femoris in the case of the knee. This is difficult

because of the severe wasting that follows each haemarthrosis. Furthermore the presence of a flexion contracture will put this muscle at a mechanical disadvantage. Active exercises to maintain joint movement may delay the progress of ankylosis, but in the face of repeated haemarthroses are unlikely to alter the final outcome.

2. *Bracing, orthotic and corrective devices* (Stein and Dickson, 1975).
3. *Plaster correction* is rarely required now. Correction by dynamic sling or Flowtron techniques is much more commonly used. The dynamic sling method is gentle and slow, and is unlikely to succeed in the more severe and more rigid deformities. The plaster of Paris casts used are well padded and changed twice weekly with gradual straightening of the plaster. No clotting factor replacement therapy is given. It is dangerous to use closed plasters in haemophiliacs for fear of the pressure effects of recurrent haemorrhage within the cast. The patient should therefore be under close supervision.
4. *Surgery*. Ultimately in severe arthropathies, where pain, fixed deformities or disability are interfering with the patient's life and work, it may be decided to carry out joint stabilization procedures such as ankylosis or an arthroplasty.

Muscle Bleeds

The incidence of intramuscular haemorrhage is much less than intra-articular bleeding; nevertheless it is the second most frequent type of spontaneous bleeding in haemophilia.

Favre-Gilly (1964), from an analysis of 130 haemophilic patients, found a distribution of 147 bleeds in the upper limbs, 101 in the lower limbs and 60 in the neck or trunk. Galindo et al (1986) have reported the use of ultrasonography in defining anatomically 48 intramuscular haematomas. They found the iliopsoas was affected in 27 patients, glutei in four, quadriceps femoris in seven, gastrocnemius in seven, forearm muscles in two and pectoralis major in one.

Aetiology

Like haemarthrosis, intramuscular haemorrhage is frequently spontaneous and may result from unguarded stresses and strains of the muscle during activity or sleep. Another important and avoidable cause of deep haematomas are intramuscular injections. These are forbidden in the management of haemophiliacs and all drugs must be given by the oral, subcutaneous or intravenous route.

Pathology

When blood is forced into muscle tissue the muscle fibres die and within a few hours may be observed as anuclear structures embedded in blood clot. An exudation of polymorphonuclear leucocytes is seen, followed by the appearance of phagocytic mononuclear cells and immature fibroblasts. Resorption of blood clot and necrotic muscle fibres occurs and is followed by fibrosis. There is no effective regeneration of muscle fibres following large haematomas.

Large accumulations of blood in muscle, when too large for phagocytic cells to remove, may become encapsulated and sealed-off from surrounding viable tissue, with the formation of a persistent cystic lesion containing blood clot, haemoglobin degradation products and lipid material. This is an important complication of muscle haemorrhage and is dealt with in more detail below.

Clinical features

Bleeding into muscle may present more insidiously than bleeding into joints, but pain again is the predominant symptom accompanied by swelling and induration. The size, shape and fascial confines of the muscle group will determine the eventual limit of the haematoma and its tension. A small haemorrhage into the iliacus, rigidly confined on one aspect by the pelvis and on the other by the strong iliacus fascia, leads to rapidly increasing pain, whereas in the quadriceps, calf or buttock more extensive haemorrhage is required to produce pain.

Intramuscular haematomas may press on peripheral nerves causing loss of function. This is particularly so in iliacus haematomas where femoral nerve palsies are a common complication (Goodfellow et al, 1967).

Table 7.3 Prevalence of muscle contractures following intramuscular bleeding

	Small haematoma without contracture	Major haematoma without contracture or only transient deformity	Contracture lasting 1 month or more	Permanent contracture	Total
Buttock	0	3	0	0	3
Iliopsoas	0	19	0	0	19
Thigh	7	3	1	1	12
Calf	7	1	1	5	14
Shoulder girdle	0	4	0	0	4
Arm	5	1	0	0	6
Forearm	4	3	3	2	12
Total	23	34	5	8	70

(Reproduced from Duthie et al, 1994, with permission.)

Vascular ischaemia is a rare but important complication of intramuscular haemorrhage. A lesion resembling Volkmann's contracture results from haemorrhage into the flexor muscles of the forearm, with a contractural fibrosis. A Volkmann's contracture can also arise when increasing swelling is rigidly confined by a tight plaster cast. Careful observation on the circulation must always be carried out in cases of haemorrhage into the muscle compartments of the forearm and calf for any increase in the intracompartmental pressure.

Contractures are fairly common following intramuscular bleeds and our experience of this complication is shown in Table 7.3. This table shows the distribution of muscle haematomas in our Oxford series. Eleven per cent caused permanent contractures but in the majority of the bleeds no significant deformity resulted. Where contractures did occur, either permanently or lasting for several months, the site of haemorrhage was most commonly in the calf or forearm. Neurological involvement was found in half of the cases. No contractures were seen following haemorrhages into the buttock. Hip flexion deformity is found initially in all iliacus haematomas but these resolve within a week or two without the need for special orthopaedic treatment. Haematomas of the thigh, upper arm or shoulder girdle caused no permanent deformity.

Physical examination

Early in the course of the haemorrhage the haematoma is likely to be indurated, or tense, but later it may become fluctuant. Tape measurements are taken at two or three levels over the mass at marked sites. Bruising and ecchymosis should be looked for over the swelling and the condition of the skin and its circulation noted.

The peripheral nervous system is carefully examined for sensory, motor and reflex changes. The extent of a sensory defect should be marked on the skin with a pencil and photographed. A muscle power chart of the affected limb is completed and dated. Measurements of the size of the mass and the neurological examination should be repeated weekly or more frequently to determine the progression of the lesion. The peripheral pulses are examined and the evidence noted of any signs of venous occlusion such as distended veins, slow venous emptying, oedema or skin discoloration.

Ultrasonographic examination

Ultrasonography has proved to be most valuable, not only in demonstrating where the lesion is anatomically but also its dimensions and volume, and its resolution during treatment. Kinnas et al (1984) have described the technique for determining the volume of the blood collection. Wilson et al (1989), by using ultrasonographic examination, have demonstrated two types of bleeding with two differing echo patterns, the blood either splitting the soft-tissue muscle planes or interdigitating between the actual muscle fibres where the borders are relatively difficult to define. Computed tomography (CT) and Magnetic resonance imaging (MRI) may also give further valuable information, although in the early stages of bleeding and pain, abnormal positioning of the limbs may make these investigations impossible.

Treatment

Replacement therapy, as in the case of haemarthroses, is essential and should be given as soon as possible. A dosage regimen similar to that used for acute haemarthrosis is usually effective.

It is important that the damaged bleeding muscle be kept at complete rest until resolution and healing have taken place. Splinting may be used to permit healing to take place in the optimum functional position. Failure to splint the limb may lead to undesirable fixed contractures. A much longer period of immobilization is usually required for muscle haematomas than for haemarthroses because of the slower process of resolution and fibrous scarring after a deep haematoma.

The initial position of immobilization will be that in which the patient is most comfortable but this will not necessarily be the position of optimum function. As soon as bleeding has ceased, as judged by the relief of pain, a programme of frequent, gentle, gradual changes of plaster splints should be instituted, aiming at gradual correction of the contracture before it becomes fixed.

Aspiration of muscle haematomas is not effective and is contraindicated because intramuscular bleeding is not confined within a cavity like a haemarthrosis. For the same reasons evacuation of the intramuscular haemorrhage by a surgical approach is unlikely to be any more useful than aspiration. Surgical procedures such as fasciotomy or division of the muscle sheath to bring about decompression are rarely indicated.

The time at which it is safe to begin static exercises is judged by the disappearance of tenderness, the absence of pain on static or isometric contraction, softening of the haematoma and a progressive decrease in size as determined by frequent measurements of the limb girth or by ultrasonography. Later during the period of corrective splintage the limb should be removed daily from the plastic support to begin joint mobilization, which will also correct any contracture. At this stage exercises in the pool are begun. Weight-bearing on the affected limb should be delayed until the haematoma is no longer firm and tender.

Fractures and Soft-Tissue Injuries

Fractures in patients with haemophilia are uncommon (Flatmark, 1964; Ahlberg and Nilsson, 1967; Kemp and Matthews, 1968) but most haemophilic patients without HIV are now leading ordinary lives with normal activities and therefore are at risk. The percentage and the types of injuries sustained by haemophiliacs are no different from those seen in the normal population. Several authors have emphasized the association of fractures with haemophilic cysts and pseudotumours. Jordan (1958), in a review of 110 patients, reported fractures in 12, and indicated that fractures in haemophilia unite with solid bony union, usually in less than the average time. This has not been our experience in Oxford. From the Oxford series of over 25 patients with fractures, the healing time was similar to that in the normal population and is related to the severity of the fracture, its stability, the efficiency of factor control and the orthopaedic treatment.

The majority of authors (Ikkala, 1960; Kemp and Matthews, 1968; Feil et al, 1974) reported that fractures often occurred from trivial injuries. The combination of poor muscle function, limitation of the joint movement and osteoporosis secondary to repeated haemarthrosis predisposes to such fractures.

Plain radiography is usually diagnostic. Ultrasonography is very useful in diagnosing associated soft-tissue injuries, for example muscle tears and avulsion of the lower pole of the patella.

Management of fractures

Emergency treatment is splintage and immediate, adequate factor replacement, with analgesia and sedation. Definitive treatment includes reduction of the fracture, immobilization in plaster of Paris or fixation under general anaesthesia followed by prolonged rehabilitation.

Factor VIII or IX infusion is administered to maintain the circulating levels of factor above 40% for at least 14 days because of the considerable risk of recurrent bleeding during this period. Immobilization of the fracture is usually secured by the safest method to reduce further haemorrhage unless the fracture is unstable or involves joint surfaces. Skeletal traction with percutaneous pin is rarely practised because of the risk of infection, the likelihood of subsequent joint stiffness, lack of tolerance and the risk of further haemorrhage and greater factor requirement. With modern external fixation devices, it is now possible to control the unstable long bone fracture, e.g. in both bones of the forearm or in tibial fractures (Fig. 7.7) where there is potential skin and soft-tissue damage. Internal fixation for example by AO plating is required only when there is no alternative and more conservative means to maintain an acceptable position. Fractured neck of femur is a particular example when internal fixation devices are required and allow mobilization of adjacent joints. This type of fracture will become more frequent with the ageing of the haemophilic population (Duthie et al, 1994).

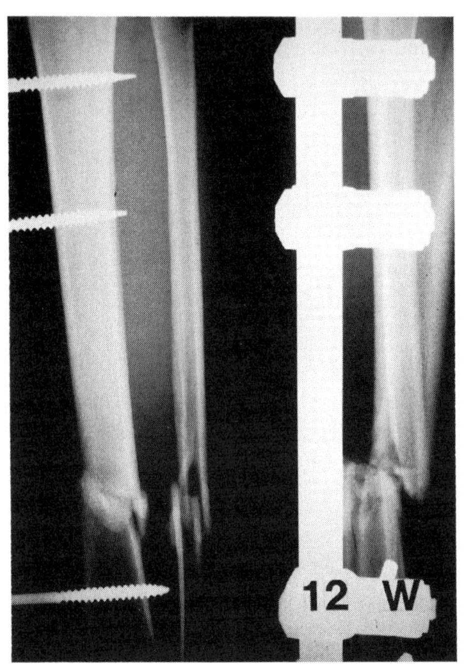

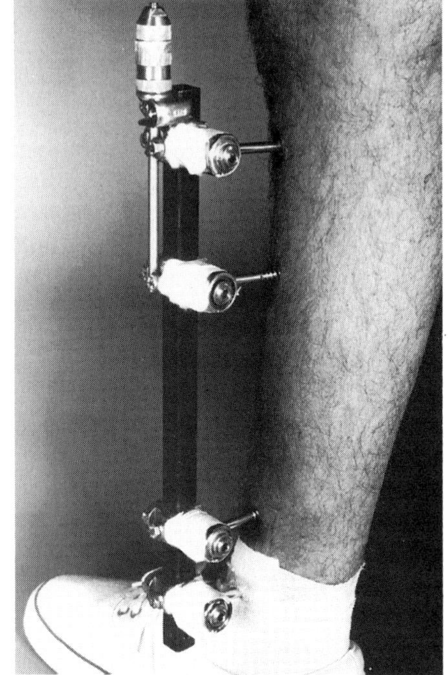

Figure 7.7 (a) Radiographs of an unstable fracture at the junction of the middle and distal thirds of the tibia with the external fixation device. (b) A photograph of the same leg to show the external fixation device in position for walking.

Peripheral Nerve Lesions

Incidence

Involvement of peripheral nerves commonly accompanies intramuscular bleeding in the haemophiliac. Early reports by Bulloch and Fildes (1911), Lord (1926) and Seddon (1930) first drew attention to this problem in isolated cases, and Silverstein (1964) in a survey of 206 haemophiliacs found nerve involvement in 31 cases.

Katz et al (1991) have reported on 61 peripheral nerve lesions in 1351 admissions to the Nuffield Orthopaedic Centre Oxford in 54 haemophilic patients. The femoral nerve was most commonly involved followed by the median, ulnar and sciatic nerves (Table 7.4). In 30 (49%) of the 61 lesions, the nerve had a full motor and sensory recovery; in 21 (34%), there was a residual sensory deficit; and in 10 (16%), both a persistent motor and sensory deficit resulted. Patients who had antibodies to factor VIII were significantly less likely to recover full motor or sensory function and the time for full recovery in these patients was significantly longer than in patients without antibodies.

Table 7.4 Anatomical distribution of peripheral nerve lesions

Nerve	Number of lesions
Femoral	31
Median	10
Ulnar	7
Sciatic	4
Radial	3
Posterior interosseous	2
Lateral popliteal	1
Posterior tibial	1
Sural	1
Thoracic/sacral nerve roots	1
Total	61

Aetiology

Peripheral nerve lesions are most commonly caused by intramuscular haemorrhage, an external compression of the nerve with a neuropraxia. Intraneural bleeding causing nerve palsy can occur but is rare. The clinical course is that of a neuropraxia (a transient physiological interruption of nerve conduction due to compression or slight stretching of the nerve). The recovery of function is usually complete but may take many months.

Clinical features

In the common iliacus haematoma syndrome the patient may complain of acute pain in the groin some hours before femoral nerve palsy becomes evident. Difficulty may be experienced in distinguishing a right-sided iliacus haematoma from acute appendicitis. In both, there may be pain and tenderness in the right iliac fossa, loss of appetite, constipation, fever and leucocytosis, and flexion of the hip. In the iliacus haematoma maximal tenderness is usually over the mid inguinal point and a mass in the iliac fossa just within the pelvic brim may be felt. A progressive fall in haemoglobin and the onset of femoral nerve palsy are in keeping with the diagnosis of a haemorrhage and not of appendicitis in a haemophiliac.

As the haematoma is formed the patient rapidly develops an acute contraction of the hip in 60–90° of flexion due to tension within the iliacus sheath.

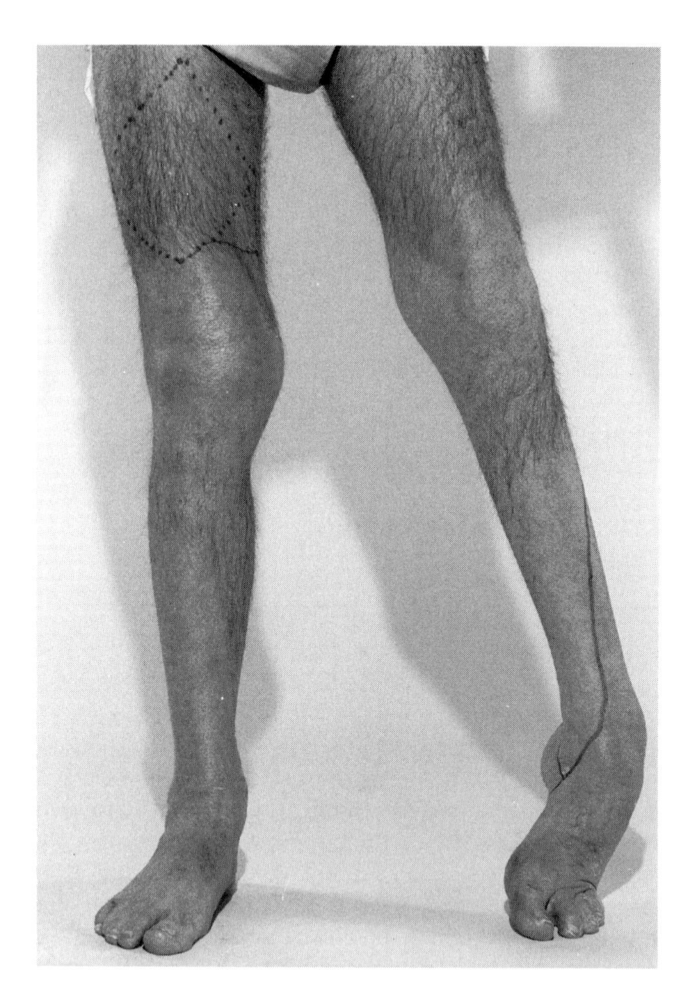

Figure 7.8 Photograph of the lower extremities showing the patch of local anaesthesia caused by a right femoral nerve palsy with an iliacus bleed. On the left side the area of anaesthesia and a dropped foot deformity are due to a sciatic nerve bleed.

Attempts to extend the hip may cause much pain. Ultrasonography is the most helpful investigation in differentiating this condition from bleeding into the hip joint.

The neurological disorder is heralded by a localized impairment of sensation over the front of the thigh. In the complete neuropraxia, total anaesthesia over the front of the thigh rapidly develops with quadriceps paralysis and the loss of the patellar tendon reflex (Fig. 7.8).

In the series of Katz et al (1991), sciatic nerve palsies with sensory, motor and reflex loss developed after bleeding into the buttocks in four patients. Three of these patients still had impaired motor and sensory function at 1 year. In the fourth patient, complete motor recovery occurred, but with impaired sensation in the first sacral root dermatome.

Median nerve lesions have occurred after massive bleeds into the anterior flexor compartment of the forearm. All of the median nerve lesions described by Katz et al (1991) resolved fully, at a mean of 7 months (range 3 weeks to 12 months).

Ulnar nerve lesions have developed after bleeding into the forearm or after a bleed into the elbow joint. One patient required transposition of the ulnar nerve 1 month after an injury because of a small, persistent haematoma around the ulnar groove and severe haemophilic synovitis of the elbow joint (Duthie et al, 1994). This patient eventually had a full recovery although was left with interosseous muscle atrophy. In most patients, full recovery occurred at a mean of 7 months (range 3 days to 23 months).

Radial nerve lesions have occurred after bleeding into and around the elbow joint. They present with a drop wrist deformity and sensory loss. Full recovery usually takes place.

Factors affecting outcome

Neither the mechanism of bleeding (spontaneous or traumatic) nor the type of haemophilia (A or B) significantly affected the time to recovery. However, the presence or absence of antibodies to factors VIII or IX appears to have a significant prognostic effect (Katz et al, 1991).

Treatment

The management of the neurological complications of haemophilia is by factor replacement, initial analgesia and splintage and care of the recovering neurological lesions. Splinting is more prolonged than that required for an acute haemarthrosis and is continued until contraction of the affected muscle groups can be carried out without pain or local tenderness. To prevent contractures, splinting must also include joints that are normally moved by the paralysed muscle. The management of neurological lesions in haemophilia is similar to that of the more familiar peripheral nerve lesions seen after trauma.

Haemophilic Cysts and Pseudotumours

Haemophilic cysts are a rare complication of haemophilia. Fernandez de Valderama and Matthews (1965) have described three main types:

Table 7.5 Anatomical distribution of haemophilic bone cysts

Site	–
Femur	20
Pelvis	12
Calcaneus	4
Tibia	3
Foot	1
Thumb	2
Others	4
Total	47

1. Simple cysts which are confined within the fascial envelope of a muscle without involvement of bone.
2. Cysts arising in muscles with extensive periosteal attachments, which may cause cortical thinning of bone, actual destruction of bone and, in some, the response of new bone formation.
3. True pseudotumours arising from subperiosteal haemorrhages, some of which may also arise from intraosseous haemorrhage.

Incidence

Cyst formation is a rare occurrence in haemophilia. Forty-seven published examples were traced in the world literature by Steel et al (1969) and, more recently, Dohring and Hofmann (1985) discovered 104 haemophilic patients who had 110 pseudotumours. The common distribution of bone cysts in the skeleton is shown in Table 7.5 (Steel et al, 1969).

Dohring and Hofmann (1985) found pseudotumours of long tubular bones in 69 cases (femur, tibia/fibula, humerus, ulna and radius); of the ilium in 37 cases; cysts of spongy bone in 22 cases (calcaneus, talus, scapular, vertebrae); and of small tubular bones in seven cases (metacarpals, metatarsals and phalanges).

Prior to 1961, when only fresh blood or plasma was available, the mortality from this lesion was over 50%. As the name suggests, pseudotumours in haemophilia were often thought to be sarcomatous in nature and this sometimes resulted in unnecessary exploratory biopsies and aspirations, frequently with fatal haemorrhage or infection. Without treatment, however, progressive enlargement leading to skin necrosis, ulceration, infection and haemorrhage resulted in an equally dangerous situation in those days.

Since the 1960s, with the availability of adequate replacement therapy, the mortality rate has fallen considerably. Since 1970 we in Oxford have had no mortality due to the pseudotumour or its complications. Döhring and Hofmann (1985) reported from their own series a 75% mortality rate up to 1959, a 77% mortality rate up to 1969 and since 1970 a 20% mortality rate.

Aetiology

Muscle cysts

As already mentioned, these simple cysts arise uncommonly as a consequence of massive intramuscular haemorrhage. A small collection of blood is readily absorbed and the damage done to tissues by the haemorrhage readily healed by granulation tissue and fibrosis. A large volume of blood and clot by its size alone will tend to persist and eventually become encapsulated. The critical factor is the progressive nature of the lesion as a result of further haemorrhage, which may occur spontaneously in the untreated patient or after ill-advised surgical interference by aspiration, incision or evacuation. The iliacus muscle is well recognized as one of the most common sites of intramuscular bleeding and development of cysts in haemophiliacs. Some of these iliac cysts have been present for very long periods of time, varying from 2 years in the case reported by Nelson and Mitchell (1962) to 19 years in that described by Eibl et al (1965).

Bone cysts

The first reported haemophilic pseudotumour (Starker, 1918) demonstrated elevation of the periosteum of the femur. Most examples of pseudotumours arising in adults have occurred in relation to the pelvis or femur where there are extensive muscle attachments. Many of the cases recorded in children have involved cancellous areas where periosteal stripping is unlikely (Favre-Gilly, 1964). Subperiosteal bleeding is certainly not the only cause of haemophilic bone cysts. We have described a calcaneal bone cyst and a tibial lesion in which there was no evidence of periosteal elevation or reaction (Fig. 7.9). The cyst in the calcaneus and one in the tibia showed massive destruction of the internal trabeculae by intraosseous bleeding.

Pathology

Longitudinal sections of an amputated pseudotumour of the radius in one of our patients showed that the haemorrhage was chiefly extraosseous with only limited involvement of the medullary cavity by haemorrhage (Fig. 7.10). There was extensive subperiosteal bleeding and reactive new bone formation. Extension of the haemorrhage into the subcutaneous tissues, the metaphysis of the radius,

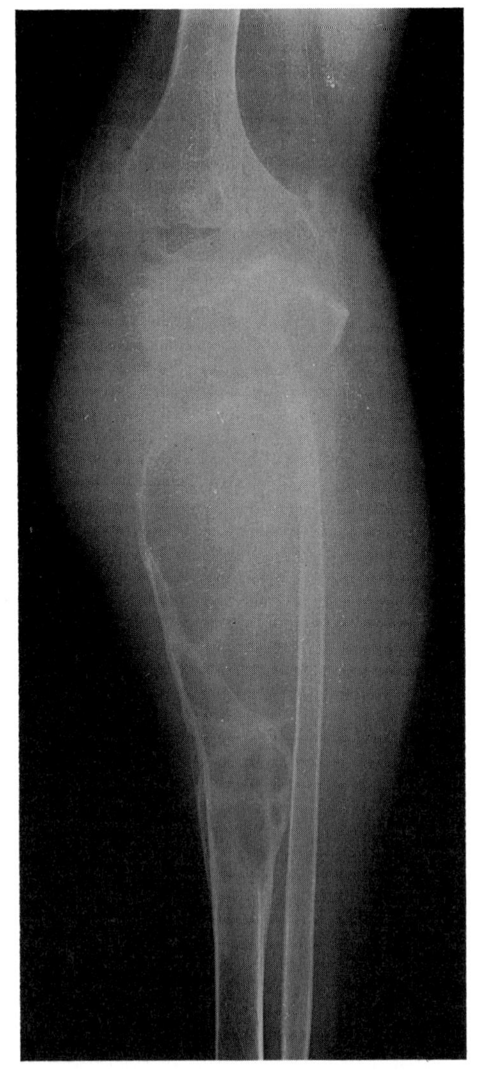

Figure 7.9 An anteroposterior radiograph of the upper tibia showing a multilocular osteolytic haemophilic cyst but no periosteal reaction.

the epiphyseal plate and the proximal carpal joints was observed. The areas of haemorrhage contained granulation tissue, fibrous tissue and accumulations of inflammatory cells, many of which were histiocytes containing haemosiderin. There were areas of resorption of bone in contact with the expanding haemorrhage, and areas of regenerating new bone formation. The epiphyseal plate was invaded by the massive bleeding process leaving only islands of fragmented cartilage.

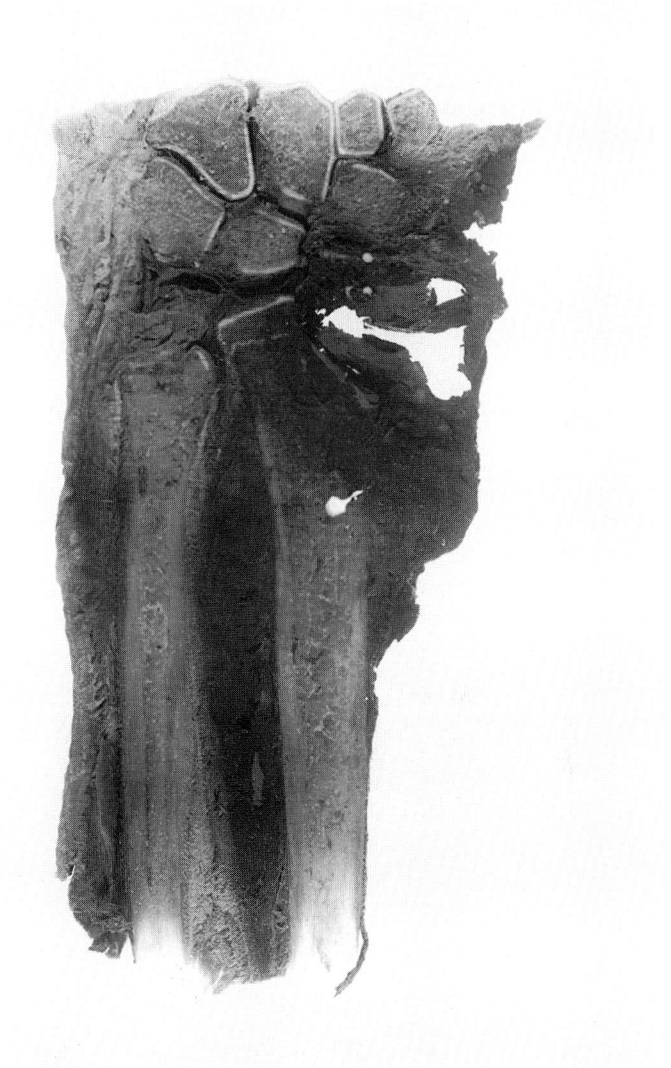

Figure 7.10 Haemophilic bone cyst affecting the lower end of the radius.

An attempt was made to demonstrate the local vasculature by injecting Micropaque into the vessels of the amputated part. Numerous thin-walled vessels were seen in the periosteum proximal to the lesion with a large number of "blow outs" and vascular irregularities. These may well explain how factor replacement and immobilization may fail to halt the progression.

Diagnosis

The presence of a persistent or increasing mass in a limb or in the pelvis in a haemophiliac, with or without radiological evidence of bony involvement, should raise suspicion of a haemophilic cyst. Simple haematomas usually resolve rapidly with specific replacement therapy. The differential diagnosis includes malignant tumours such as sarcomas, benign tumours such as chondroma and haemangioma, and infections such as osteomyelitis. Sarcomas have been reported in haemophiliacs, and in one report a chondrosarcoma of the scapula was thought to be a pseudotumour (Koepke and Brower, 1965).

Radiological features

A haemophilic pseudotumour is clearly not a single pathological entity but the response of bone to a haemorrhagic process. Osteolysis is the predominant feature, especially if the haemorrhage is intraosseous or from muscle attachments, with or without new bone formation. The margin of the lesion is ill-defined, the integrity of the cortex is lost, and there is a surrounding soft-tissue shadow. Where haemorrhage is subperiosteal the features will be those of

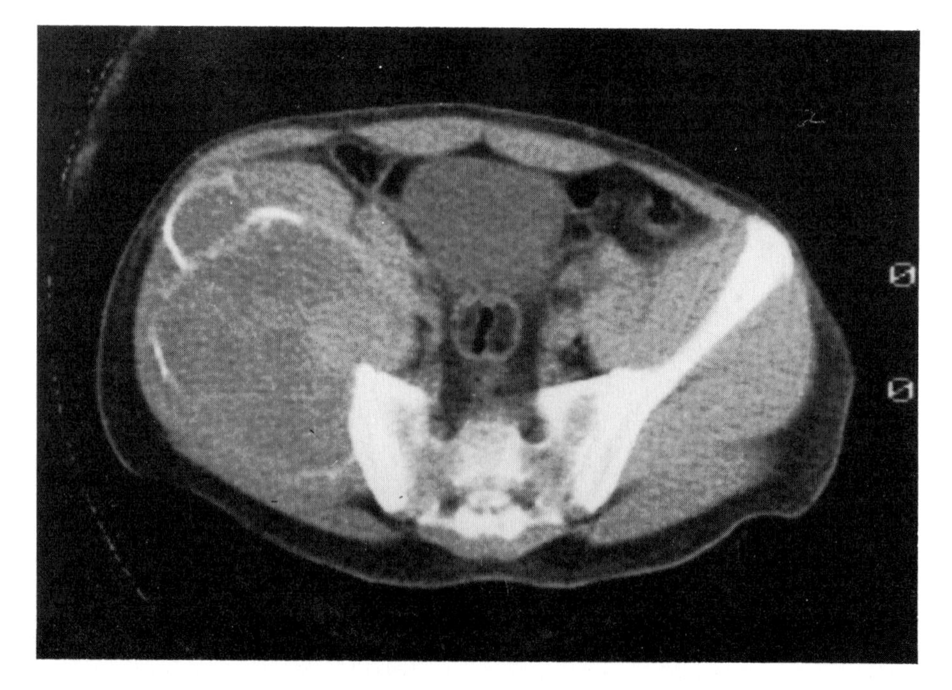

Figure 7.11 CT scan of the pelvis to show the destruction of the leaf of the ilium containing a pseudotumour.

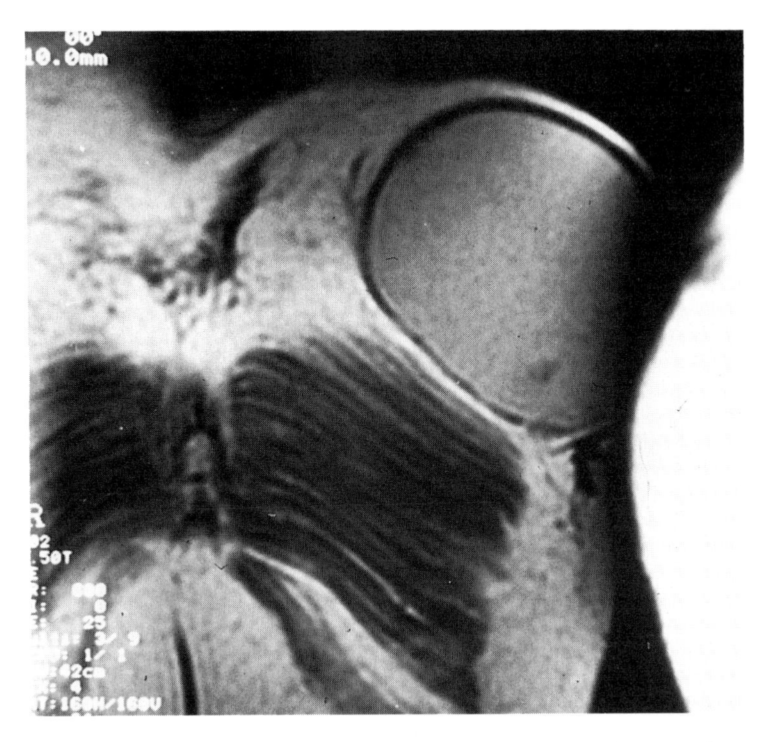

Figure 7.12 An MRI transverse scan through the pelvic floor to show a large intramuscular buttock cyst with a very thickened capsule, thick fluid contents and the sciatic nerve posterolateral in position.

periosteal stripping, new bone formation and remodelling. These changes are non-specific and will follow any condition where periosteum is elevated by blood, pus or tumour.

With CT (Fig. 7.11) and, even better, MRI the soft-tissue component of the cyst, its contents and "wall" and the adjacent tissues are all clearly defined (Fig. 7.12). Multilocular cysts are outlined and are commonly seen in the pelvis and in the femur. Scintigraphy with technetium radio isotope (T99) is of only some help in delineating the mineral derangement of the bone structure. Ultrasonography is very useful for following change over periods of time (Fig. 7.13).

Treatment

Amputations have been successfully carried out in the early days for removal of a cyst of the thumb (Ghormley and Clegg, 1948) and a pseudotumour of the foot (Davidson et al, 1949). The survival of these patients probably depended on the peripheral situation of their lesions (Jones, 1965).

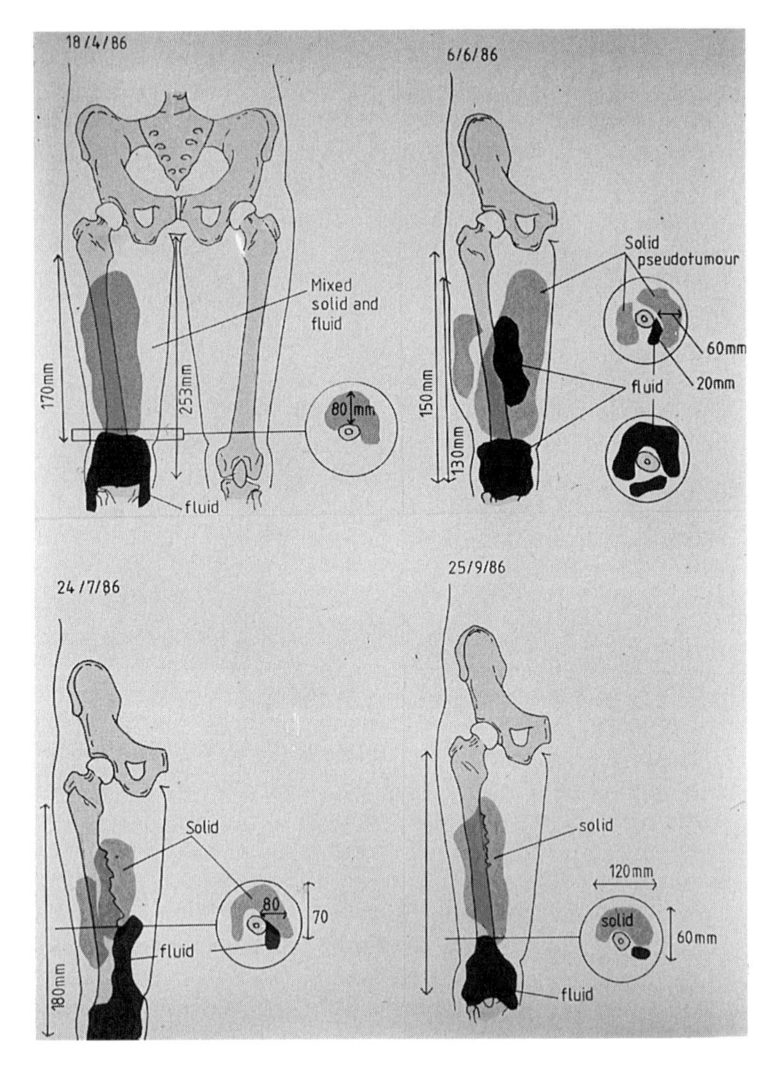

Figure 7.13 A diagram of ultrasound scans taken over a 5-month period showing a decrease in the mass of the pseudotumour and reduction in the fluid from the haemarthrosis of the knee. (Reproduced from The pathogenesis of chronic haemophilic arthroplasty. *J. Bone. Joint Surgery* 1981, **63B**:606–609, with permission of the authors and Oxford University Press.)

Our experience with both muscle cysts and pseudotumours leads us to advocate a conservative approach in all early cases. Initially, the part is rigidly immobilized and factor VIII or factor IX should be given until there is evidence that bleeding has ceased. Thereafter, immobilization is continued and progress is assessed by regular clinical, radiographic and ultrasonographic examinations. Any evidence that bleeding has recurred, for example sudden onset of pain, should lead to a further course of replacement therapy. A successful policy of non-intervention has also been reported by Favre-Gilly et al (1965). Nevertheless, there is clearly a stage in the progress of these cysts when resolution cannot be achieved or the continuity of the bone shaft is at risk of a pathological fracture or the skin at risk of necrosis with infection. In circumstances where the lesion is progressing despite adequate immobilization and replacement therapy, excision of the cyst should be undertaken. Complete excision should be the aim with excision of the wall and obliteration of any dead space.

In the limb bones, pseudocyst formation may progress in spite of factor replacement and rigid immobilization. In order to prevent a pathological fracture it may be necessary to stabilize the shaft by an intramedullary rod fixation and then proceed to an excision of the pseudotumour mass if possible. An unstable mobile pathological fracture resulting from a pseudotumour will rarely, if ever, heal and either requires amputation for a life-threatening situation or, preferably, stabilization.

In the pelvic wall, once there has been bony destruction, excision is required as a massive life-saving procedure. Careful visualization of the exact perimeters and involvement of the surrounding soft tissues, particularly blood vessels, is essential. The support of a general surgeon is recommended for such major dissections. In certain cases it is possible to divide the pelvic bone rim front and back and retract it with its muscle attachments and afterwards resuture it down into its old bed. Dead spaces should be avoided by compressive haemostatic sponges, bandaging and plaster of Paris casting.

Radiotherapy has been used in a child by Hilgartner and Arnold (1975) for a pseudotumour of the femur, but it is no longer appropriate except in the presence of high levels of inhibitors (Castaneda et al, 1991). The outcome is unpredictable and healing of tissues is very slow.

Since Hall et al (1962) reported the successful removal of a loin cyst and recorded the excision of a calf cyst, several personal cases have been successfully and safely excised. In cases with progressive enlargement, delay may be dangerous, and spontaneous rupture is potentially lethal (Eibl et al, 1965). Fernandez-Palazzi and Rivas (1985) have reported on their early successful experience in the use of "fibrin seal" (Tissucol-Tisseel (R) Immuno AG) in pseudotumours of the tibia, the foot and the iliacus and in cysts of the humerus and ischium. This material consists of fibrinogen, factor VIII, albumin and globulin as well as a solution of thrombin and calcium chloride. When injected into the cyst it undergoes coagulation with formation of fibrin to provide a matrix for stimulating the ingrowth of fibroblasts and cicatrization.

Orthopaedic Surgical Management

Although, with factor replacement, any orthopaedic operation is technically feasible in haemophiliacs, in general only tried and tested surgical procedures with predictable outcomes should be carried out. HIV infection in haemophilic patients with or without AIDS, hepatitis B and hepatitis C infection have all added further difficulties to surgical management regimens. The patients are usually young and will make heavy demands on their joints for many subsequent years.

Surgery should only be carried out in a specialized unit accustomed to caring for haemophiliacs. The orthopaedic surgeon should always work closely with the haematologist, nursing staff, physiotherapists and social workers who all have been trained in this field. The amount of factor required for the pre- and post-operative periods must be available and reserved for that particular patient. Full HIV and/or hepatitis precautions are used by all theatre and nursing staff for every operative procedure and for wound dressings in the wards.

Preoperatively, all patients are carefully screened for any evidence of factor VIII inhibitor, HIV or hepatitis B and C as well as for any medical contraindications to elective, reconstructive surgery. The presence of antibodies to factors VIII or IX remains a contraindication to elective surgery.

Immediately before surgery a dose of factor sufficient to raise the patient's level to 100% of normal is administered. Postoperatively, "bolus" therapy is administered every 8–12 hours for 2 weeks aiming to keep the level of factor VIII or IX to at least 60% of normal. Rigid immobilization of the operation site is maintained during the first few postoperative days to ensure primary wound healing without complications and to minimize the risk of reactive bleeding.

The progression of haemophilic arthropathy from haemarthrosis to chronic synovitis with extensive joint surface destruction cannot be predicted even in the face of good medical treatment (Fig. 7.14). Chronic haemophilic arthropathy is initially managed by conservative treatment, namely analgesia, physiotherapy, orthotics and corrective devices, before surgery is ever considered. Patients who are well motivated and without medical contraindications are considered for reconstructive surgery, but only when the symptoms and signs are significant (Luck, 1981).

Surgical principles

Standard surgical approaches and techniques are used and pneumatic tourniquets applied where appropriate to obtain a bloodless field. Meticulous attention to haemostasis is essential, and electro-cautery is used for all tissue dissection except skin. Exposure is kept to a minimum, as is the stripping of tissue planes as this will predispose to haematomas. Wounds are closed by co-aptation of tissue planes by continuous haemostatic polyglycolic acid sutures or by clips. The dissected areas are not usually drained but a firm compression bandage is applied and often

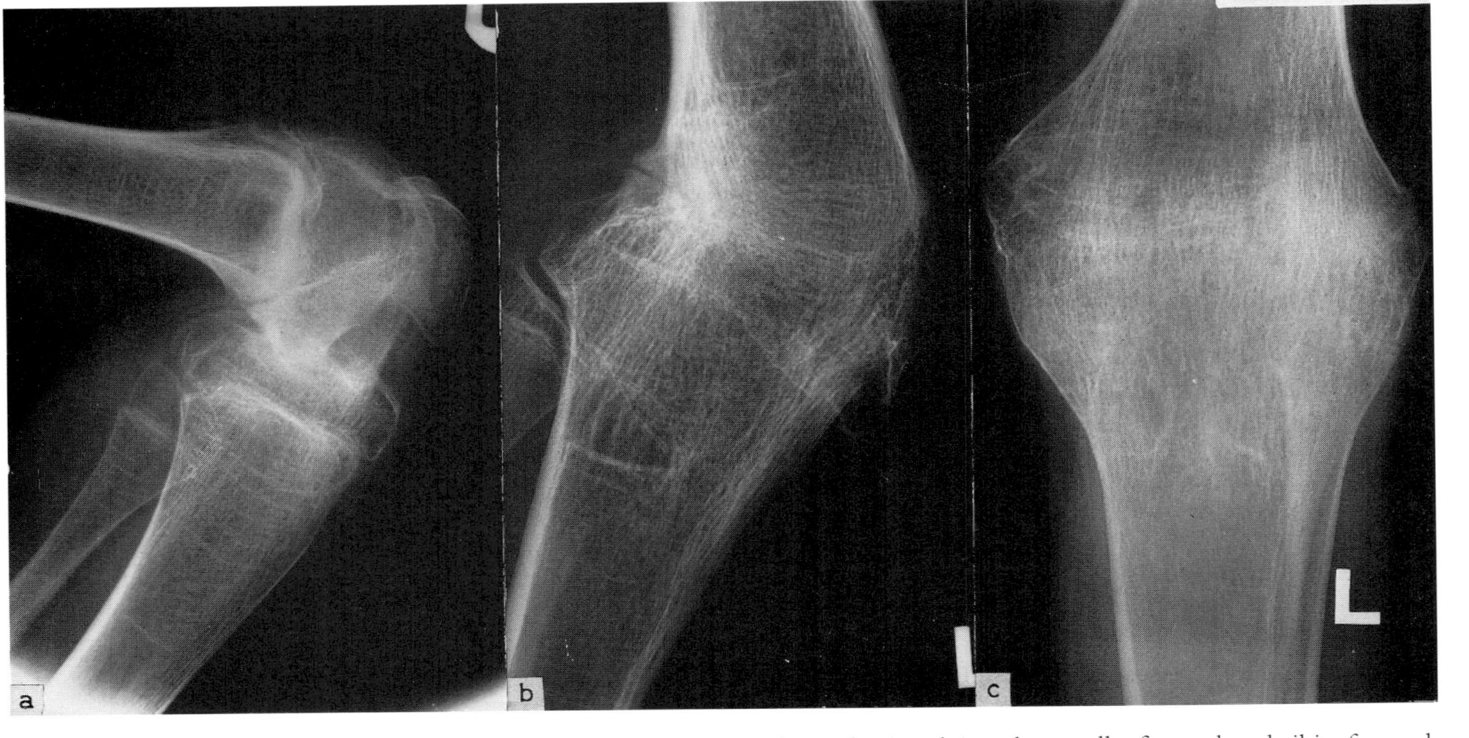

Figure 7.14 (a) Lateral radiograph showing gross haemophilic arthropathy involving the patello-femoral and tibio-femoral joints resulting in severe contracture. (b,c) Radiographs showing successful arthrodesis 2 years later.

rigid immobilization is achieved with a plaster of Paris splint. Splintage discourages haematoma formation, allows soft-tissue healing, reduces factor requirement and is continued until primary wound healing is achieved. Prophylactic antibiotics are administered pre- and postoperatively until the wound appears normal in its healing.

Summary of surgical procedures by anatomical location

Shoulder

Pain is the primary indication for surgical intervention and the traditional approach has been for arthrodesis, which gives predictable and durable results (Luck and Kasper, 1989). A prosthetic shoulder replacement in the severely damaged shoulder has been reported by Luck and Kasper (1989) but long-term follow-up results of shoulder joint replacement are still required.

Elbow

End-stage elbow arthropathy is common in the haemophiliac. Synovectomy with radial head excision has been described by Le Balch et al (1985) for frequent painful bleeds and chronic swelling or pain. Results are impressive with reduction in the frequency of bleeds; the range of motion was not lost. However other authors (Post et al, 1986) have reported loss of a significant degree of mobility in the joint and progression of radiographic changes.

The Oxford experience of patients who underwent synovectomy and radial head excision for a stiff, painful elbow (Houghton, 1983) and followed-up for 10 years confirmed that this procedure was the treatment of choice for management of chronic arthropathy of the elbow. The procedure produces predictable pain relief with an increased range of motion, reduced bleeding episodes and has held up well over time.

Luck and Kasper (1989) have described a few total elbow replacement prostheses for severe haemophilic arthropathy with poor results and this procedure is not recommended for routine use.

Hip

The hip joint is frequently affected by chronic haemophilic arthropathy. Total hip replacement will relieve the pain of the haemophilic hip joint. A large series of total hip replacements in haemophiliacs has been presented by the Oxford Centre. Nelson et al (1992) described a total of 39 patients, 23 total hip replacement operations in 22 patients, with a mean follow-up of 7.5 years (range 2.6–13.1 years). Cemented Charnley prostheses were used in all patients. The mean hospital stay was 5 weeks. There was one intraoperative death from cardiac arrest, one dislocation and three haematomas, one of which went on to a deep infection, all occurring in the early period of the learning curve. The average factor replacement per operation was nearly 60 000 units which has to be contrasted with an arthrodesis of the knee requiring 30 000 units, arthrodesis of the ankle 22 000 units. The operation consistently reduced pain and increased the range of motion and therefore is regarded as a very worthwhile procedure. At follow-up, five patients in our series had required revision surgery: two for sepsis and three for aseptic loosening. Three further cases showed radiological signs of loosening. There was therefore a 27% incidence of loosening at a 10-year follow-up. These figures are comparable to other series describing total hip replacements in a young patient for other conditions.

Knee

Haemophilic arthropathy of the knee is the most frequent cause of severe pain and disability requiring surgery.

Synovectomy is reserved for persistent synovial thickening and recurrent bleeding of the knee joint. Synovectomy can either be performed surgically as an open procedure or as an arthroscopic technique using a radiochemical synovioarthesis.

Storti et al (1969) first described synovectomy as a new approach in the management of early haemophilic arthropathy, in order to reduce the demand for available clotting factor concentrates and reduce the frequency of further bleeding. Duthie et al (1972), from a large series, defined accurately which patient required this procedure. Forty-one patients with persistent chronic synovial swelling and recurrent bleeding were submitted to bed rest, compression bandaging that was frequently reapplied, and adequate factor replacement for a period of 2–3 weeks. Only eight patients did not respond satisfactorily to the above conservative treatment regimen with resolution of swelling and the regaining of adequate movement. These eight patients subsequently underwent an anterior two-thirds synovectomy (Matsuda and Duthie, 1984). However, only four patients, in spite of intensive physiotherapy under factor control, and some manipulation, achieved more than 75° of normal flexion.

Traldi et al (1985) have reported their 20-year experience with synovectomy. All patients encountered a marked reduction in the amount of factor products subsequently required. In 1979 Aritomi (personal communication) described the use of arthroscopy for debridement and synovectomy in order to reduce the extent of the open surgical exposure, with a better recovery, less factor usage and regaining more movement. Weidel et al (1986) described their experience of using arthroscopic synovectomy in 20 knees from several centres. They emphasize that this procedure had a low morbidity and allowed rapid rehabilitation. Storti and Ascari (1975) and Montane et al (1986) felt that there was radiological improvement in the arthropathy following a synovectomy, but other series have not confirmed this observation.

Radioactive nucleo synoviorthesis

Ahlberg and Pettersson (1979) were the first to report on the use of radioactive gold in 27 haemophiliac patients with a 3–9-year follow-up, with under half having no further bleeds. The arthropathy tended to progress. Fernandez-Palazzi and his co-workers (1984) using radioactive gold found that 88% overall were improved with 28% having reduced bleeding, but 6% of patients reported increased bleeding.

Other radionuclear fibrosing agents such as radioactive rhenium and yttrium 90 have been used. The basic principles are the same as for gold, but these substances are less likely to leak and cause any chromosomal breakages. The underlying effect appears to produce fibrosis in the synovial folds and the underlying subsynovial tissue plane with its vulnerable blood vessels. Erken (1985) carried out a controlled trial of 15 patients who had received injections of yttrium 90 compared with another 15 matched patients and the only difference was a marked decrease in bleeding frequency in the yttrium 90 group.

Patellectomy

Patellectomy is a good and simple procedure when carried out for extensor mechanism problems of pain, crepitus, poor quadriceps function and sudden episodes of instability. It can be performed with or without synovectomy but Luck and Kasper (1989) found that some patients required further reconstructive surgery, e.g. fusions or total knee replacement procedures. One would expect this because the arthropathy is not usually limited to the patello-femoral surface.

Osteotomy

High tibial osteotomy is occasionally performed for haemophilic arthropathy (Smith et al, 1981; Luck and Kasper, 1989). Their indications were painful limited movement, high frequency of bleeds, degenerative changes and a varus deformity. Complications of postoperative infection, severe arthrofibrosis and limited motion have all been recorded.

Arthrodesis

Knee fusion in the haemophiliac patient remains a sound procedure with predictable lasting results and few complications. In Oxford arthrodesis is the preferred method of treatment for end-stage haemophilic arthropathy of the knee (Houghton and Dickson, 1978). In this series the mean time to bony union was 5.7 months, including three patients who took 7, 11 and 12 months, respectively.

Luck and Kasper (1989) described their experience of primary knee fusions performed in seven cases of end-stage arthropathy, with five fusing without problems and with good long-term results.

Total knee replacement

Total knee replacement is gradually becoming more acceptable, but most authors emphasize that this is a technically difficult operation in the presence of severe contractures, posterior and lateral subluxations of the tibia, as well as the poor quality of the subchondral bone due to osseous necrosis and cyst formation (Giangrande et al, 1994).

McCullough et al (1979) had a 50% complication rate in 10 total knee replacements including one loosening and one deep sepsis after only 23 month average follow-up.

In 1983 Wilson et al reported on 24 cases with a short mean follow-up of 19 months in which five patients had early complications of haemarthrosis, haematoma, common peroneal nerve palsies and deep infection which required removal of the component. The remainder achieved knee scores comparable to those expected in this procedure for osteoarthrosis. Lachiewicz et al (1985) also reported 24 replacements in 14 patients with an average age of 35 years. There was a 20% complication rate including deep sepsis in two patients.

Weidel et al (1989) have presented their experience from several centres in the USA. Between 1974 and 1989, 93 prosthetic knee replacements were performed in 76 patients between the ages of 21 and 62 years. Maintenance of a range of motion differed depending upon the type of prosthesis used, some losing 10° and some gaining 25°. Early complications included massive haemarthrosis, recurrent haemarthrosis, Coombs' positive haemolysis and wound dehiscence. Later complications included cases of haematogenous infection, loosening of the tibial component, loosening of the femoral component and loosening of the patellar component. These workers commented upon the increasing occurrence of acute infections after total knee arthroplasties due to the high incidence of HIV infection in their patient population.

With its higher complication rate, this procedure in the haemophiliac requires to be carefully evaluated, especially as there are less severe and less complicated surgical procedures available, especially in the younger age groups (Duthie, 1975). A less severe and demanding procedure is a MacIntosh intercondylar insertion, which gives good pain relief and retention of a functional range of motion of 30–60° of flexion, with far fewer complications

Ankle

Fourteen per cent of all haemarthroses are into the ankle joint with resulting arthropathy. In addition, bleeds into the calf musculature may result in contracture and equinus deformity at the ankle. As in the elbow, only a small percentage

of such patients have symptoms severe enough to require surgery (Lovering, 1988).
Arthrodesis is the usual procedure of choice and is commonly performed. Houghton and Dickson (1978) have described the results after an Royal Air Force (RAF) fibular onlay fusion. A 2-month mobilization period in plaster of Paris followed by a Yates splint was required and the mean union time was 3–9 months. Skin necrosis with delayed healing was the only complication. More recently, Duthie et al (1994) have used successfully the intra-articular dowel method of arthrodesing the ankle. This is simple to perform with less factor requirement and fewer postoperative complications.

Infection with HIV, hepatitis B and hepatitis C: implications for surgery

HIV

In view of the fact that more than 50% of haemophiliacs have been infected with HIV, an important consideration arises from the suggestion of Konotey-Ahulu (1987) that surgery may hasten the progression of AIDS in seropositive

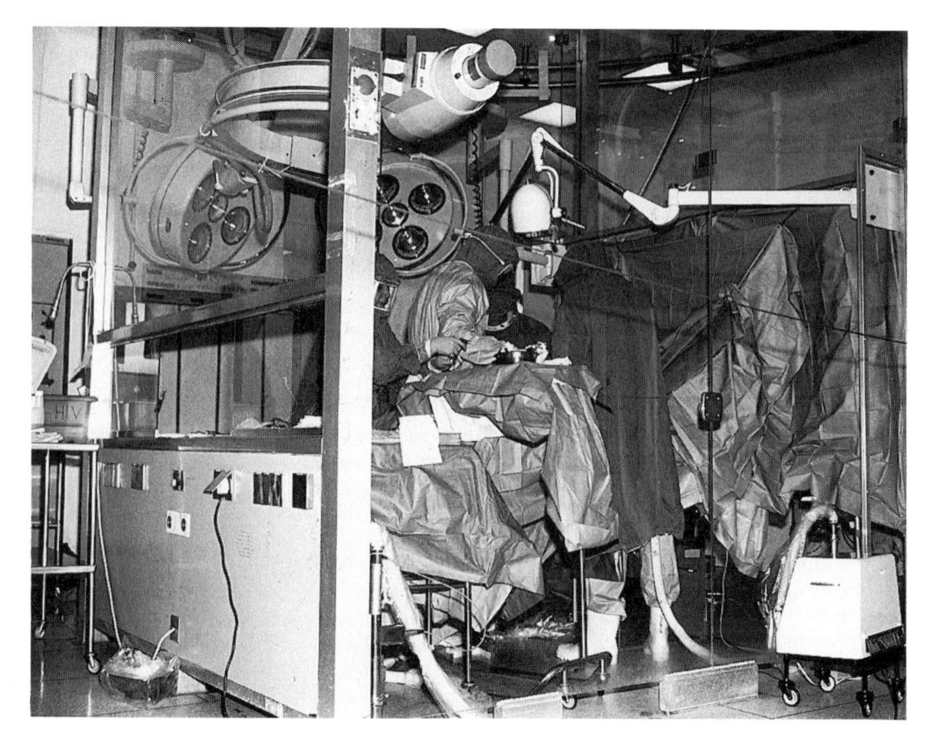

Figure 7.15 The vertical laminar flow, isolation operating room with exhaust system, disposable drapes, etc.

patients. There have been anecdotal reports on HIV patients who had undergone total joint replacements, and who had developed clinical AIDS within 2 to 3 years of surgery. One of the first observations made about HIV-positive patients was that they had a decreased natural killer cell activity with a reduced number of CD4 helper cells (Gottlieb et al, 1983). A similar immunological response of reduction in helper and lymphocytic populations has been recorded in the perioperative period after major surgery in patients not infected with HIV (Hansbrough et al, 1984; Lennard et al, 1985). However, Tonnensen and Wahlgreen (1988) described this depression of the immune system after surgery in "normal" patients as being transient. Obviously these interesting and important observations must be carefully considered before operating upon any haemophilic patient (Scannell, 1989).

With regard to special precautions during surgery on patients who are HIV positive, rigorous precautions are essential and comprise isolation of the operating team and patients within a vertical laminar flow operating room (Fig. 7.15) to allow control of contaminated materials, decontamination at the end of the procedure, restriction of staff and of all movement during procedures. A manual of general principles must be available for immediate reference by all staff, with details of the preparation of operating and anaesthetic rooms, equipment, handling of swabs and their disposal, instrument cleansing, and management of all spillages, donning and removal of disposable protective clothing.

The value of zidovudine prophylaxis after accidental exposure to HIV is yet to be established. However, Aboulafia (1992) has suggested that strong indications for its use are massive parenteral exposure or a deep penetrating injury, whereas weak indications are mucous membrane or subcutaneous exposure.

Hepatitis B and C

According to the Center for Diseases Control, Atlanta (Marcus, 1988), occupationally transmitted hepatitis B virus (HBV) occurred in an estimated 18 000 health care workers annually, and about 250 of those die each year as a result of the acute and chronic sequelae of HBV. Infection with HIV-1 has occurred in a much smaller number (fewer than 75) of health care workers who do not have non-occupational risk factors for the disease. Therefore the risk to health care workers of acquiring HIV from patient care activities is very low. The documented episodes of seroconversion have usually followed percutaneous exposure (80% were accidental needle sticks, 8% cuts with sharp objects, 7% open wound contamination and 5% mucous membrane exposures) to infected blood. The risk of seroconversion after an accidental needle stick exposure to blood from a patient carrying HIV-1 is thought to be about 0.5%. This has to be compared with the 30% infection rate after similar exposure to HBV-infected blood. Universal precautions are easy to implement (Regnier, 1991). The use of hepatitis B vaccine is imperative in the prevention of HBV infection in high-risk groups.

In the orthopaedic surgery of total hip replacements, osteotomies, etc., the incidence of glove perforation can be as high as 20% per operation, therefore double and protective gloving is required. Inspection of hands for blood staining after removing of gloves is sensible and thorough washing of the hands with an antiseptic soap should be carried out. Wound dressing at the end of the surgical procedure should be with a water repellant, impervious dressing to contain any exudate. Redressing of wounds should be carried out in designated areas, which can be decontaminated and where dressings and discharged material can be "bagged" for incineration. The health care team should be properly dressed and protected with impervious aprons, gloves, eye and mouth protection shields.

Physiotherapy

Physiotherapy has an important role in the treatment of bleeding disorders affecting the musculoskeletal system. The physiotherapist with a special interest and experience in haemophilia is a member of a team of people involved in the management of haemophiliacs and she/he must liaise closely with all other members. The physiotherapist should have a thorough understanding of the nature of the disease, its behaviour and the purpose and limitations of physical treatments as well as an understanding of the psychology of these patients.

Aims of physiotherapy

Allen (1994) has described the overall aim of physiotherapy, which is to restore and improve muscle and joint function, relieve pain and assess the need for supportive or corrective devices as well as in the education of the patient and his family. Exercise is important for all haemophiliacs to prevent the long-term disastrous effects of repeated bleeding. Haemophiliacs who maintain levels of general fitness with good musculature have fewer spontaneous haemorrhages (Weissmann, 1977).

Physiotherapy techniques

Exercise

1. Passive movements do not really have a place in the treatment of haemophiliacs except where a bleed has resulted in a peripheral nerve lesion and paralysis. The affected joints need to be put through their full range of movement several times a day with factor replacement, without causing any stress, but all forced passive movements are contraindicated in haemophiliacs (Desmarres and Laurian, 1984).

2. Static exercises contract a muscle without producing any movement at the joint and are very important in helping to avoid muscle atrophy when a joint is immobilized. Wasting is not simply a disuse atrophy but is exaggerated by reflex neuromechanisms which aggravate the process of muscle wasting (Haggmark et al, 1978).

3. Active assisted exercises. These are useful in the early stages of joint mobilization or where joint stiffness is a particular problem. Assistance can be given by the therapist's hands, the patient's contralateral limb (auto-assisted) or by pulley systems, or less indicated is a continous passive motion machine (usually insufficient supervision results).

4. Resisted exercises. Weights, springs and pulley systems, when used for resistance, should be placed so that their effect is felt upon one joint only and progressed by small increments gradually.

Hydrotherapy

The water is kept at between 35.5° and 36.6°C (96–98°F). The warmth of the water helps to relieve pain, decrease muscle spasm and induce relaxation. The effects of buoyancy adds to both passive and active assisted movements following peripheral nerve lesions or more commonly when muscles are weak and joints stiff after prolonged immobilization.

Hydrotherapy is not indicated after an acute bleed whilst the joint is still warm and swollen or in the presence of a large, boggy synovitis.

HIV infection is not a contraindication to treatment in a chlorinated hydrotherapy pool (Zucherman, 1986; Harrison and Davies, 1988), but with all patients it is important to check that the patient does not have open cuts or sores, or any discharge, before they enter the pool as these are contra-indications.

Ice therapy

Ice therapy is often used to help decrease pain and reduce swelling following an acute muscle or joint bleed. Short applications of 5–15 minutes cause a reduction in blood flow due to vasoconstriction and increased blood viscosity. Ice has a place in the treatment of chronic joint arthropathy, especially when associated with synovitis or following surgery.

Deep heating

Deep heating by short-wave diathermy is contraindicated for haemophiliacs. Pulsed short-wave diathermy can be effective in acute bleeds as, unlike conventional short-wave diathermy, no heat is discharged. Pulsed short-wave diathermy, by increasing metabolism, helps to decrease the rate of haematoma formation as

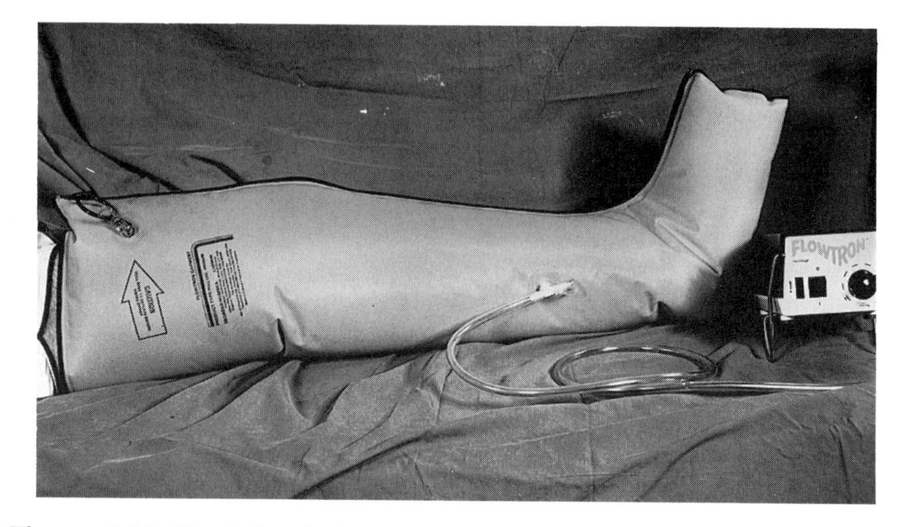

Figure 7.16 The inflated Flowtron orthotic splint with attached pump and control box.

well as relaxing muscle spasm to give pain relief and early resolution of acute bleeds (Buzzard and Jones, 1988).

TENS

Transcutaneous electrical nerve stimulation (TENS) has proved to be a useful modality for the treatment of chronic pain in haemophilic arthropathy (Roche et al, 1985), in the postoperative period to assist rehabilitation and in painful bleeds, especially when the patient has inhibitors and pain is difficult to control. A study by Marhnowicz et al (1986) has shown that TENS hastens the resolution of acute haemarthrosis.

Flowtron

The Flowtron (Huntleigh Technology, Luton) intermittent compression system (Fig. 7.16) may be used to correct fixed flexion deformities of less than 40°. Initially treatment is limited to 20 minutes at a starting pressure of 30 mmHg so that the patient feels a gentle stretch but no pain. With increased tolerance the pressure can be steadily increased to a maximum of 90 mmHg and prolonged for 60 minutes or longer two or three times a day.

In between sessions with the Flowtron, the patient is encouraged to exercise his quadriceps in the new range to help maintain the passively increased range of movement (Boone et al, 1975). Patients have found it beneficial to have a Flowtron unit for home use. It is important that they fully understand the necessity of continuing an active exercise programme and do not just rely on the machine (Allen, 1988; Nelson et al, 1989).

References

Aboulafia DM. Aids and surgery: risks and precautions. *Surgery* 1992; **1:** 89–93.
Ahlberg A. Haemophiliac in Sweden. *Acta Orthopaedic Scand.* (suppl) 1965.
Ahlberg A, Nilsson IM. Fracture in haemophiliacs with special reference to complications and treatment. *Acta Chirurgica Scandinavica* 1967; **133:** 293–301.
Ahlberg A, Pettersson H. Synoviorthesis with radioactive gold in haemophiliacs. *Acta Orthopaedica Scandinavica* 1979; **50:** 513.
Allen AL. Use of "Flowtron" in haemophiliac patients and others with fixed flexion deformity problems. *Journal of Chartered Society of Physiotherapy* 1988; **74:** 581–582.
Allen AL. The role of physiotherapy. Chapter 13. In: *The Management of Musculoskeletal Problems in the Haemophilias*, 2nd edn. Oxford: Oxford University Press, 1994.
Atkins RM, Henderson NJ, Duthie RB. Joint contractures in the haemophiliacs. *Clinical Orthopaedics and Related Research* 1967; **219:** 100–105.
Azorin L, Marques F, Gomar F. Morphology of haemophilic joints. In: Dohring S, Schulitz KP (Eds), *Orthopaedic Problems in Haemophilia.* München, Bern, Wien: W. Zuckschwerdt Verlag; 1985: 12–23.
Backmayer E, Hodredge S. Developmental activities, sports and games. *Haemophilic World* 1991; **7:** 5–6.
Blount WP. Unequal leg length. *Instructional Course Lecture, American Academy of Orthopaedic Surgery*, St Louis, 1960; **17:** 218.
Boldero JL, Kemp HS. The early bone and joint changes in haemophilia and similar blood dyscrasias. *British Journal of Radiology* 1966; **39:** 172.
Boone DC, Greenberg R, Perry J. The energy expenditure of walking in haemophiliac patients with knee motion restriction. Presented at 51st Annual Conference, American Physical Therapy Association, Anaheim, CA, 1975.
Bourdon R, Bernard J, Caen J, Bard M, Patrux C. Donnees evolutives des lesions osteo-articulaires radiologique de L'Hemophile. *Semaine des Hopitaux de Paris* 1963; **58:** 2818.
Bulloch W, Fildes P. Hemophilia. In: *Treasury of Human Inheritance Francis Galton Eugenics Laboratory Memoirs, University of London.* London: Cambridge University Press, 1911: 169.
Buzzard BM, Jones PM. Physiotherapy management of haemophilia, an update. *Journal of Chartered Society of Physiotherapy* 1988; **74:** 224.
Castaneda VL, Parnley R-T, Bozzini M, Feldmeier JF. Radiotherapy of pseudotumours of bone in haemophiliacs with circulating inhibitors to factor VIII. *American Journal of Haematology* 1991; **36:** 55–59.
Davidson CS, Epstein RD, Miller GF, Taylor FHL. Hemophilia. A clinical study of forty patients. *Blood* 1949; **4:** 97.
De Andrade JR, Grant C, Dixon AStJ. Joint distension and reflex muscle inhibition in the knee. *Journal of Bone and Joint Surgery* 1965; **47A:** 313.
De Palma AF, Hemophilic arthropathy. *Clinical Orthopaedics* 1967; **52:** 145.
De Palma AF, Cotler JM. Haemophilic arthropathy. *Clinical Orthopaedis* 1956; **8:** 163.
Desmarres Ch, Laurian Y. From top to toe. An alternative approach to physiotherapy for haemophiliacs. *Scandinavian Journal of Haematology* 1984; **33** (Suppl 40): 469–470.
Dohring S, Hofmann P. Haemophilic pseudotumours. In: Dohring S, Schulitz KP (Eds), *Orthopaedic Problems in Haemophilia.* Munchen, Bern, Wien: W. Zuckschwerdt Verleg, 1985.
Duthie RB. Reconstructive surgery in haemophilia. *Annals of the New York Academy of Sciences* 1975: 240–295.
Duthie RB, Matthews JM, Rizza CR, Steel WM. *The Management of Musculoskeletal Problems in the Haemophilias.* Oxford: Blackwell Scientific, 1972.
Duthie RB, Rizza CR, Giangrande PCF, Dodd CAF. *The Management of Musculoskeletal Problems in the Haemophilias.* Oxford: Oxford University Press, 1994.
Eibl M, Fisher M, Kuhbock J. Pseudotumour des Darmbeins bei Hamophile A. *Deutsche Medizinische Wockenschrift* 1965; **90:** 1864.
Erken EH. Radiocolloids: joint protection. In: Dohring S, Schulitz KP (Eds), *Orthopaedic Problems in Haemophilia.* München, Bern, Wein: W. Zuckschwerdt Verlag, 1985.
Favre-Gilly J. Experience de cinq ans du Centre Emile Remigy de Montain (Jura) pour jeunes garcons hemophilies. *Hemostase* (1964); **4:** 231.
Favre-Gilly J, Chatain R, Trillat A, Saint-Paul E. Pseudotumeur du calcaneum chez un

hemophile. *Hemostase* 1965; **5:** 95.
Feil E, Bentley G, Rizza CR. Fracture management in patients with haemophilia. *Journal of Bone and Joint Surgery* 1974; **56B:** 643–649.
Fernandez de Valderama JA, Matthews JM. The haemophilic pseudotumour or haemophilic subperiosteal haematoma. *Journal of Bone and Joint Surgery* 1965; **47B:** 256.
Fernandez-Palazzi F, Rivas S. The use of "fibrin-seal" in surgery of coagulation diseases with special reference to cysts and pseudotumours. In: Dohring S, Schulitz KP (Eds), *Orthopaedic Problems in Haemophilia.* Munchen, Bern, Wein: W. Zuckschwerdt Verlag, 1985.
Flatmark AL. Fracture union in the presence of delayed blood coagulation. *Acta Chirurgica Scandinavica* 1964; Suppl 343.
Galindo E, Merchon CR, Gage J, Orban A. Ultrasonics in the diagnosis and assessment of the effect of treatment of intramuscular haematomas in haemophiliacs. In: Dohring S, Schulitz KP (Eds), *Orthopaedic Problems in Haemophilia.* München, Bern, Wien: W. Zuckschwerdt Verlag 1986.
Gamble JG, Bellah J, Rinsky LA, Bleder B. *Journal of Bone and Joint Surgery* 1991; **73A:** 1008–1015.
Ghadially FN. *Ultrastructural Pathology of the Cell.* London: Butterworths, 1975.
Ghormley RK, Clegg RS. Bone and joint changes in hemophilia. *Journal of Bone and Joint Surgery* 1948; **30-A:** 589.
Giangrande PLF, Dodd CAF, Gregg-Smith SJ. Knee replacement in haemophilia. *Journal of Bone and Joint Surgery* 1994; **76B:** 166.
Goodfellow JW, Fearn CBD'A, Matthews JM. Iliacus haematoma. A common complication of haemophilia. *Journal of Bone and Joint Surgery* 1967; **49B:** 748–756.
Gottlieb MS, Groopman JE, Weinstein WM, Fahey JL, Detels R. The acquired immunodeficiency syndrome. *Annals of Internal Medicine* 1983; **99:** 208–220.
Gregg-Smith S, Giangrande PLF, Pattison R, Dodd CR, Duthie RB. Septic arthritis in haemophilia. *Journal of Bone and Joint Surgery* 1993; **75B:** 368–370.
Haggmark T, Jansson E, Svane B. Cross-sectional area of the thigh muscle in man measured by computed tomography. *American Journal of Clinical Laboratory Investigations* 1978; **38:** 355–360.
Hall MRP, Handley DA, Webster CU. The surgical treatment of haemophilic blood cysts. *Journal of Bone and Joint Surgery* 1962; **44B:** 781.
Hansbrough JF, Bender EM, Zapata-Sirvent R, Anderson J. Altered helper and suppressor lymphocyte populations in surgical patients. *American Journal of Surgery* 1984; **148:** 303–307.
Harrison RA, Davis BC. *Hydrotherapy in Practice.* Edinburgh: Churchill Livingstone, 1988: 169.
Hilgartner MW, Arnold WD. A haemophilic pseudotumour treated with replacement therapy and radiation. *Journal of Bone and Joint Surgery* 1975; **57A:** 1145.
Hoaglund FT. Experimental hemarthrosis. The response of canine knees to injections of autologous blood. *Journal of Bone and Joint Surgery* 1967; **49A:** 285.
Houghton GR. Joint surgery in haemophilia. In: Forbes CD, Lowe GDO (Eds), *Unresolved Problems in Haemophilia.* Lancaster: MTP Press, 1983.
Houghton GR, Dickson RA. Lower limb arthrodesis in haemophilia. *Journal of Bone and Joint Surgery* 1978; **60B:** 143–144.
Houghton GR, Duthie RB. Orthopaedic problems in haemophilia. *Clinical Orthopaedics and Related Research* 1978; **138:** 197–216.
Ikkala E. Haemophilia. *Scandinavian Journal of Clinical and Laboratory Investigation* 1960; **12:** (Suppl 46).
Itokazu M, Bradley J, Francis MJO, Duthie RB. Localisation of specific carbohydrate configurations in the haemophilic synovial membrane. *Clinical Orthopaedics and Related Research* 1988; **230:** 284–288.
Jones DM. Haemophilic blood cyst. *Journal of Bone and Joint Surgery* 1965; **47B:** 266.
Jordan HH. *Hemophilic Arthropathies.* Springfield, Illinois: Charles C. Thomas, 1958.
Katz SG, Nelson IW, Atkins RM, Duthie RB. Peripheral nerve lesions in haemophilia. *Journal of Bone and Joint Surgery* 1991; **73A:** 1016–1019.
Kemp HS, Matthews JM. The management of fractures in haemophilia and Christmas disease. *Journal of Bone and Joint Surgery* 1968; **50B:** 351–358.
Kingma MJ. Overgrowth in hemophilia. *Clinical Orthopaedics* 1965; **39:** 199.

Kinnas PA, Woodham CH, Maclarnon JC. Ultrasonic measurement of haematomata of joints and soft tissues in the haemophiliac. *Scandinavian Journal of Haemotology* 1984; **33** (Suppl 40): 225–235.
Koepke JA, Brower TW. Chondrosarcoma mimicking pseudotumour of hemophilia. *Archives of Pathology* 1965; **80:** 655.
Konig F. Die gelenkerkrankungen bei Blutern mit besonderer Berucksichtigung der Diagnose. *Klinische Vortrage* 1892; **36:** 233.
Konotey-Ahulu FID. Surgery and risk of AIDS in HIV-positive patients. *Lancet* 1987; **ii:** 1146.
Lachiewicz PF, Inglis AE, Insall JN, Sculco TP, Hilgartner MW, Bussell JB. Total knee arthroplasty in hemophilia. *Journal of Bone and Joint Surgery* 1985; **67A:** 1361.
Lack CH. Chondrolysis in arthritis. *Journal of Bone and Joint Surgery* 1959; **41B:** 384–387.
Lack CH, Ali PY. The degradation of cartilage by enzymes. In: Barrett CAC (Ed.), *Cartilage Degradation and Repair.* Washington DC: National Academy of Engineering, 1967: 67–71.
Legg JW. *A Treatise on Haemophilia.* London: HK Lewis, 1872.
Le Balch T. Synovectomy of the elbow in young haemophilic patients. *Journal of Bone and Joint Surgery* 1985; **69A:** 264–269.
Lennard TWJ, Shenton BK, Borzotta A. The influence of surgical operations on components of the human immune system. *British Journal of Surgery* 1985; **72:** 771–776.
Lord JP. Hemophilia with Volkmann syndrome. *Journal of the American Medical Association* 1926; **87:** 406.
Lovering J. The ankle joint. *The Bulletin of the Haemophilia Society* 1988; No. **1:** p. 14–15.
Luck JV Jr. Surgical management of advanced hemophilic arthropathy. In: Dohring S, Schulitz KP (Eds), *Orthopedic Problems in Hemophilia.* Münich: W. Zuckschwerdt Verlag, 1981: 145–149.
Luck JV Jr, Kasper CK. *Surgical Management of Advanced Haemophilic Arthropathy* 1989.
Luscombe M. Acid phosphatase and catheptic activity in rheumatoid synovial tissue. *Nature* 1963; **197:** 1010.
Marcus R. Surveillance of health care workers exposed to blood from patients infected with the human immunodeficiency virus. *New England Journal of Medicine* 1988; **319:** 1118–1123.
Marhnowicz U, Beeton K, Heim M, Tuddenham EGD, Kernoff PBA. Transcutaneous electrical nerve stimulation in the treatment of haemarthroses in haemophilia: a double-blind controlled study. *XVIIth International Congress of the World Federation of Haemophilia* Milan, 1986.
Matsuda Y, Duthie RB. Surgical synovectomy for haemophilic arthropathy of the knee joint: long-term follow-up. *Scandinavian Journal of Haematology* 1984; **33:** 237.
McCullough NC III, Enis JE, Lovitt J, Lian EC-Y, Niemann KNW, Loughlin EC Jr. Synovectomy or total knee replacement of the knee in haemophilia. *Journal of Bone and Joint Surgery* 1979; **61A:** 69.
McLardy-Smith PD, Ashton IK, Duthie RB. A tissue culture model of cartilage breakdown in haemophilic arthropathy. *Scandinavian Journal of Haematology* 1984; **33** (Suppl 40) 215–220.
Montane I, McCollough NC III, Lian EC-Y. Synovectomy of the knee for hemophilic arthropathy. *Journal of Bone and Joint Surgery* 1986; **68A:** 210.
Nelson IW, Atkins RM, Allen AL. Brief report. The management of knee flexion contractures in haemophilia. *Journal of Bone and Joint Surgery* 1989; **71B:** 327.
Nelson MG, Mitchell ES. Pseudotumour of bone in haemophilia. *Acta Haematologica* 1962; **28:** 137.
Nelson ID, Swamuruga S, Latham PD, Matthews J. Total hip arthroplasty for haemophilic arthroplasty. *Clinical Orthopaedic Related Research* 1992; **276:** 210–213.
Otto JC. An account of an haemorrhagic disposition existing in certain families. *Medial Repository* 1803; **6:** 1.
Palazzi FF. *Sinoviortesi radioactura en hemopilicos.* 1981. pp. 225–232. FK Schattauer: Stuttgart.
Petersson H, Ahlberg A, Nilsson IM. A radiologic classification of hemophilic arthropathy. *Clinical Orthopaedics and Related Research* 1980; **140:** 153–159.
Post M, Telfer MG. Surgery in haemophiliac patients. *Journal of Bone and Joint Surgery* 1975; **57A:** 1136–1145.
Post M. Synovectomy in hemophilic arthropathy. A retrospective review of 17 cases. *Clinical Orthopaedics and Related Research* 1986; **202:** 139–146.

Regnier SJ. Symposium probes risks and future concerns of operating room staff. *Bulletin of the American College of Surgeons* 1991; **76:** 110.
Robinson DR, Smith H, McGuire HB, Levine L. Prostaglandins stimulated bone resorption by rheumatoid tissue. *Prostaglandin* 1976; **10:** 67.
Roche PA, Gijsberg K, Belch JJF, Forbes CD. Modification of haemophilia haemorrhage pain by transcutaneous electrical nerve stimulation. *Pain* 1985; **21:** 42.
Rodnan GP. Some observations on experimental hemarthrosis and the pathogenesis of hemophilic arthritis. *Laboratory Investigation* 1959; **8:** 1278.
Roy S, Ghadially FN. Ultrastructure of synovial membrane in human hemarthrosis. *Journal of Bone and Joint Surgery* 1967; **49A:** 1636.
Scannell KA. Surgery and human immunodeficiency virus disease. *Journal of AIDS* 1989; **2:** 43–53.
Schumpe G. Biomechanic aspect of the haemophiliac arthropathy. In: Dohring S, Schulitz KP (Eds), *Orthopaedic Problems in Haemophilia.* München Bern Wien: W. Zuckschwerdt Verlag, 1986: 24–32.
Seddon HJ. Haemophilia as a cause of lesions in the nervous system. *Brain* 1930; **53:** 1.
Silverstein A. Neuropathy in hemophilia. *Journal of the American Medical Association* 1964; **190:** 554–555.
Smith MA, Urquhart DR, Savidge GF. The surgical management of varus deformity in haemophilic arthropathy of the knee. *Journal of Bone and Joint Surgery* 1981; **63B:** 261.
Steel WM, Duthie RB, O'Connor BT. Haemophilic cysts. *Journal of Bone and Joint Surgery* 1969; **51B:** 614.
Stein H. The inter-relationship of Synovium and Articular Cartilage, PhD Thesis, University of Oxford 1975.
Stein H, Dickson RA. Reversed dynamic slings for knee-flexion contractures in the haemophiliac. *Journal of Bone and Joint Surgery* 1975; **57A:** 282–283.
Stein H, Duthie RB. The pathogenesis of chronic haemophilic arthropathy. *Journal of Bone and Joint Surgery* 1981; **63B:** 601.
Storti E, Ascari E. Surgical and chemical synovectomy. *Annals of the New York Academy of Sciences* 1975; **240:** 316.
Storti E, Traldi A, Tosatti E, Davoli PG. Synovectomy, a new approach to haemophilic arthropathy. *Acta Haematologica* 1969; **41:** 193.
Swanton MC. Hemophilic arthropathy in dogs. *Laboratory Investigation* 1959; **8:** 1269.
Tonnensen E, Wahlgreen C. Influence of extradural and general anaesthesia on natural killer cell activity and lymphocyte subpopulations in patients undergoing hysterectomy. *British Journal of Anaesthiology* 1988; **60:** 500–507.
Traldi A, Melanotte PL, Africano A, et al. Twenty years experience with synovectomy for haemophilic arthropathy. In: Dohring S, Schulitz KP (Eds), *Orthopaedic Problems in Hemophilia.* Munich: W. Zuckschwerdt Verlag, 1985: 180–183.
Weidel JD, Gilbert MS, Berson BL, Hofmann A. Arthroscopy of the knee in hemophilia. In: Dohring S, Schulitz KP (Eds), *Orthopaedic Problems in Hemophilia.* Munich: W. Zuckschwerdt Verlag, 1986: 121–127.
Weidel JD, Luck JV, Gilbert M. Total knee arthroplasty in the patient with hemophilia: evaluation of the long term results. In Gilbert MS, Green WB (Eds), *Musculoskeletal Problems in Hemophilia.* New York: National Hemophilia Foundation, 1989: 152–157.
Weissman. Rehabilitation medicine and the haemophiae patient. *Mt Sinai J. of Medicine* 1977; **44:** 363–370.
Wilson FC, Mahew DE, McMillan CW. Surgical management of musculoskeletal problems in hemophilia. In Evarts CM (Ed.), *AAOS Instructional Course Lectures: The Management of Musculoskeletal Problems in Hemophilia*, vol 32. St Louis: CV Mosby, 1983: 233–241.
Wilson IW, Atkins RM, Allen AL. Brief report. The management of knee flexion contractures in haemophilia. *Journal of Bone and Joint Surgery*, 1989; **71B:** 183–186.
Young A, Stokes M, Iles JF. The effect of joint pathology on muscle. *Clinical Orthopaedics and Related Research* 1987; **219:** 21–27.
Young JM, Hudacek AG. Experimental production of pigmented villo-nodular synovitis in dogs. *American Journal of Pathology*, 1954; **30:** 799.
Zuckerman AJ. Aids and swimming pools. *British Medical Journal* 1986; **293:** 221.

8 The Haemophilias in Childhood

MARGARET W. HILGARTNER

During childhood, the true haemophilic identification of disease must be made, whether factor VIII or factor IX deficiency, and plans initiated for care of the child that incorporate haemophilia care and routine normal practices of age-specific health care. Each age has different problems and priorities that parents and physicians must learn. The principles referred to in this chapter for health care measures are those recommended by the American Academy of Pediatrics. Time schedules may vary for the UK and other countries, but principles are similar.

Implications for Delivery

Improved identification of the haemophilic carrier has increased the ability to detect the affected fetus in utero. Identification of the sex and the presence of haemophilia can now be accomplished with a small sample of cells taken from the edge of the implanting fetus. This chorionic villus sampling (CVS) can be done at 9–12 weeks of gestation. Chromosome analysis of these cells will give the gender. In addition, the DNA extracted from the cells can identify the haemophilic fetus in 80% of gestations where informative markers are present (Miller, 1989a). Although CVS has been considered a relatively safe procedure, limb disfigurement has been seen recently in a very small percentage of cases. Many physicians, therefore, wait until 15–16 weeks of pregnancy when sufficient amniotic fluid can be obtained for both sex determination and disease status. Should these methods not be successful, fetal blood sampling can be done at 16–18 weeks of gestation for factor VIII antigen and activity. The latter is not possible for factor IX, as normal levels of factor IX antigen are not present in the non-haemophilic child until 6 months after birth.

The determination of fetal disease has prompted the discussion of the method of delivery and the mode that may give greatest safety for the haemophilic fetus.

When prenatal testing is taken advantage of, alternate avenues may be followed concerning the pregnancy. However, Miller has pointed out the concern that only 30% of mothers with an affected son prefer to have prenatal testing done (Miller 1989b). It is hoped that the genetic counsellor can inform more carrier women of the hazard of delivery and the potential advantage of fetal identification.

The information concerning fetal in utero bleeding is very sparse with only anecdotal reports of intracranial bleeding that may or may not be related to haemophilia. There is a similar lack of good scientific data concerning intracranial bleeding at birth following normal vaginal delivery. However, Caesarean section for the known fetus with haemophilia has been considered the preferred method of delivery by some haematologists and obstetricians. A survey conducted by Goldsmith in 1990 of 104 distinct treatment centres in the USA and Canada found that 18 of 1070 (1.8%) newborn infants with haemophilia had intracranial haemorrhage at birth and 20 (1.9%) had an intracranial haemorrhage at 1 month of age. As haemorrhage in the non-haemophilic newborn is stated to be 1–2% (Goldsmith and Kletzel, 1990), the rate of 1.8% at birth and a total of 3.7% after 1 month does not seem to be excessively high. His conclusion, therefore, was that insufficient information was available to recommend Caesarean sections routinely for women at risk for the delivery of a haemophilic fetus.

Older data from the German literature reported more abnormalities on an electroencephalogram (EEG) in a group of 1-year-old haemophilic boys compared with non-haemophilic children, which the authors believed were due to bleeding at birth or within the neonatal period. These findings were not found when the EEG was repeated at 3 years of age, suggesting that the earlier changes were not significant. In the USA the Hemophilia Growth and Development Study of haemophilic boys has carried out Magnetic Resonance Imaging (MRI) and obtained a birth history on 347 boys greater than 6 years of age at entry to the study. It was hoped this study would add information concerning the bleeding at birth and, thereby, add support for a recommendation of delivery method, but the data do not seem to be helpful (Wilson et al, 1992).

The recommendations for delivery, therefore, can only be generalized. These gestations should be managed as high-risk pregnancies, and the method of delivery determined by the specialist in this field as indicated. Larger studies remain to be done to support these recommendations. However, as the knowledgeable reader will recognize, measures for protection of the haemophilic fetus may be taken for only a small percentage of newborns because of the high new mutation rate for haemophilia and widespread lack of prenatal diagnosis.

Following delivery, circumcision is not recommended until diagnosis is confirmed and then only if deemed essential for religious reasons. Routine universal circumcision is no longer recommended in the USA. The parents must understand that circumcision for the *known* haemophiliac is an operative procedure and should be performed with factor replacement for a minimum of 5 days, although older data have shown that up to 30% of severe haemophiliacs have not bled when the procedure was performed without factor replacement.

Immunizations

Routine immunizations are recommended for all children irrespective of haemophilic status. Although schedules may vary from one country to another, and vaccine types vary, most countries vaccinate against similar diseases. The schedules are consolidated in Tables 8.1 and 8.2, and are taken from that recommended by the American Academy of Pediatrics and the Center for Disease Control (CDC) in October, 1996. In the USA today, children are immunized against 11 different agents with varicella vaccine close to licensure. Combinations of these vaccines are obviously desired without increased morbidity.

Hepatitis B vaccine should be given to all children who may have a life-long need for blood products (Buchanan et al, 1986; Hoots, 1989). In fact, in the USA it has now been mandated by the CDC to be given at birth to all babies in an effort to control spread of this virus that is projected with the new migration patterns from countries where hepatitis B is endemic. Repeat injections to complete the series should be given at 2- and 3-month intervals.

At 2 months of age, DPT (diphtheria, pertussis and tetanus) are begun in the USA (Table 8.1). Repeat injections are given at 4, 6 and 18 months as intramuscular injections: for the haemophiliac, a small needle (number 27) should be used with steady pressure applied for 5 minutes thereafter. Replacement factor is not usually given and does not seem necessary as long as the volume is small and the needle is fine. In the UK subcutaneous injection is the preferred route. Boosters are given at 15–16 months and at 4–6 years prior to entry to school. Diphtheria and tetanus boosters are given at 14–16 years of age. Polio, either Salk or Sabin, should be given at 2 and 4 months with boosters at 15–18 months and 4–6 years.

Influenza B (HIB) vaccine is much more complicated. The schedule depends upon which of the manufacturers' vaccine is used, i.e. PedraxHIB (Merck), HIBITITER (Lederle) or PROHIBIT (Connaught). Alternatives may be available in the UK. Lederle recommends starting at 6 months, Merck at 12–15 months and both Lederle and Connaught at 15 months. Because problems with pneumonia, sepsis and meningitis, due to *Haemophilus influenzae*, occur in the younger months of life, immunization at the earlier years may have merit.

Measles, mumps and rubella (MMR) may be given subcutaneously (s.c.) to the patient with haemophilia to avoid intramuscular haematoma. The schedule begins at 6 months, in some cases, with a booster at 15 months and 11–12 years, or may start at 15 months only. Because of the resurgence of measles in the USA, the recommendation for MMR has recently been changed to 6 months and repeated at 12 months in areas of high risk.

Additional immunization such as Bacille-Calmette-Guérin (BCG) may be given at birth in those countries where tuberculosis is still considered to be a public health problem. Alternatively, a tuberculin screening test for exposure to tuberculosis, mandated in New York City where the disease appears to be reappearing, should be done at 6 months and repeated annually until 5 years of age. The Tine test, a skin test for exposure to *Mycobacterium tuberculosis*, may be

Table 8.1 Recommended vaccine schedule, October, 1996

Age	Vaccines	Notes
Birth – 2 months	Hepatitis B #1	If mother HbSAg +, initial dose given at birth with HBIG. Second dose given at 1 month.
2 months	Hepatitis B #2 DPT/Hib #1 OPV or IPV #1	Interval between Hepatitis #1 and #2 must be ⩾ 4 weeks, preferably 8 weeks.
4 months	DPT/Hib #2 OPV or IPV #2	Minimal interval between dose #1 and #2 of DPT/Hib and OPV is 6 weeks
6 months	DPT/Hib #3	
6–18 months	Hepatitis B #3	Hepatitis #3 may be given no sooner than 4 months after the 2nd dose. Preferred timing is at an interval of 6–12 months after dose #2.
	OPV #3 or IPV #3	Interval between OPV #2 and OPV #3, must be ⩾ 6 weeks. Interval between IPV #2 and IPV #3 must be ⩾ 6 months.
> 12 months	MMR #1 (NYC Residents)	MMR #1 must be given after first birthday or not accepted by NYC day care, schools, etc. Some jurisdictions may require MMR #1 at ⩾ 15 months, check local requirements
	*Varicella	*Currently optional. Must be given after first birthday. Two doses are given 4–6 weeks apart to patients ⩾ 13 years.
15–18 months	DTaP #4 Hib #4 *OPV #3	If DPT/Hib #4 not given earlier. Give OPV #3 by 18 months if not given earlier.
4–6 years	DTaP #5 OPV #4 or IPV #4 MMR #2	
> 7 years	Adult dT	Adult dT booster is given every 10 years after 7 years of age.

Table 8.2 Recommended vaccine schedule for immune suppressed children, 1996

Birth – 2 months	Give all vaccines (as in Table 8.1); give only IPV for all doses
4 months – 6 months	All vaccines as stated in Table 8.1
> 12 months	MMR, do not give if child has AIDS; can give if CD_4 > 200 per uL no varicella vaccine
> 2 years	Pneumococcal vaccine. Repeat annually
2 years	Hep. A
4–6 years	MMR. Repeat annually in older HIV+ patient with CD_4 > 200 per uL

used in the younger child for testing of immunity to tuberculosis; however, the tuberculin test is considered to be more accurate.

The CMI multitest is a combined multiple skin test for immunity which tests the presence of T cell immunity *in vivo*, specifically delayed type hypersensitivity and reflects general immune competence as well as specific protection against opportunistic infections. The antigens are tuberculin tetanus toxoid, Candida, Streptococcus, Proteus, mumps, control (glycerin), tricophytan and diphtheria toxoid. Varicella vaccine is currently offered to all patients at age 1 but is considered optional (Table 1).

In summary, schedules of vaccines vary worldwide; however, as long as the age of the child and the dose of the immunogen are recorded, the protective immunization can be verified and accepted wherever the child may travel (Pokalo, 1993).

For the HIV-positive child or the child living in a household with an HIV-infected parent, killed polio (Salk) vaccine, further enhanced and inactivated, has been recommended to prevent passage of live virus in the household. The American Academy of Pediatrics Committee on Vaccines has recommended the continued use of live measles vaccine as deleterious side-effects have *not* been reported in such families, nor have they been reported with live polio vaccine. Booster injections of DPT are given at 18 months and 4–6 years as with HIV-negative children.

One of the effects of the HIV virus appears to be on B lymphocyte cell function manifesting as an inability to make or maintain protective titres of childhood vaccinations. Many investigators have noted a loss of hepatitis B titres in HIV-positive haemophiliacs that appears to correlate with the CD4 level (Bray et al, 1993). Protective titres for diptheria and tetanus, MMR and HIB have been assessed by the US Hemophilia Growth and Development Study. Data reported by Jason et al (1993) have shown no difference between HIV-positive and HIV-negative boys for diphtheria, tetanus and influenza B. Loss of measles protection has been significantly greater in the HIV-positive (41.7%) than in the HIV-negative (57.1%) groups, as has mumps (HIV+, 60.8%; HIV–, 81%). Again, the change in the loss of protective titre to rubella has been in the HIV-positive boys (36.1% vs. 83.9% in the HIV-negative), with a marked difference in the 6–9 years and 10–13 years age groups (46.1% vs. 80.0%) but little difference in the older 14+ age boys (44.7% vs. 56.0%). The loss has varied more with the age of the child from the time of immunization, as expected. The level of titres in HIV-positive individuals has also been inversely correlated with CD4 lymphocyte numbers, i.e. the percentage without a protective titre has been lower in those with a low CD4 count. The ability to immunize the HIV-positive boys to the degree seen is probably due to the fact that they were immunized prior to infection and, therefore, have a different response to those infants infected in utero or soon after birth.

The ability to respond to boosters by both the HIV-positive and HIV-negative haemophilic boys is being analysed for a report on haemophilic boys in the growth and development study.

Education

Schooling for children with coagulation abnormalities should be appropriate for all ages through High School, or the equivalent requirements for each country (Dimercurio, 1991). Higher education can be obtained in most countries as desired, with the necessary capabilities. No restrictions need to be made for haemophilia that is well controlled, as these children should not be classed as disabled and need not be educated with others who may be mentally or physically disabled (Markova et al, 1980); haemophiliacs have a median intelligence quotient (IQ) above normal (Loveland et al, 1996).

When the time approaches for pre-school and kindergarten, it may be necessary for the haemophilia treatment team to assist the school in understanding haemophilia and the possible problems the child may have to face while recovering from a bleeding episode. These may include coming to school with crutches or a sling. The manner in which these episodes are dealt with, both by school staff and peers, will have an impact on the development of the child's self-esteem and ultimate ability to cope with the disease. The programme of teacher education and classmates' education is of vital importance in these early years.

Some data from the US Hemophilia Growth and Development Study seem to suggest that both HIV-positive and negative haemophilic boys appeared to perform below their IQ level on neuropsychological adaptive behaviour and academic achievement measures (Wide Range Achievement Tests) (Loveland et al, 1996). It has been recognized for some time that support measures were necessary for a family to help teach the child coping skills for the chronic illness of haemophilia and thereby allow the boy to achieve sufficient self-esteem to achieve his potential. This was one of the goals of the psychosocial component of the Comprehensive Care Team. With coping skills in early childhood, it was hoped the child would be able to perform maximally according to his potential. The current data suggest this has not been achieved in this US cohort, and that greater emphasis needs to be put into this component of care.

Should transient synovitis or other orthopaedic problems occur with swelling and pain necessitating the use of crutches, arrangements can usually be made with the school for temporary accommodation. For those unusual children with dysfunctional families, a boarding school such as La Queue-les-Yvalines in France or the Lord Mayor Treloar school in the UK may be a better way to arrange for schooling in a protective setting where the child can learn about haemophilia and home care with the skills of self-infusion, as well as obtaining his basic education.

Schooling for the HIV-infected child carries with it the double problem of haemophilia and HIV (Weiner, 1991). The disease of haemophilia "came out of the closet" about 25 years ago with the development of concentrate, home therapy and self-infusion, but with the introduction of HIV disease in older children, secrecy, isolation and fear of alienation with rejection have reappeared and are now common themes (Bussing and Johnson, 1992). Parents are afraid to tell the school about haemophilia for fear of the synonymous identification of haemophilia and AIDS. There is realistic concern for abandonment by family and friends for the haemophiliac and sibling alike. Although guidelines and recommendations for the HIV-positive child have been published by the CDC and The American Academy of Pediatrics and statutory and case law protects these children, entrance into public or private school may still be a problem in the USA. Fortunately, litigation has been almost universally successful, to date, but the parents must be made aware of the potential problem. Withholding the information is usually not the best decision, but the decision for revelation may require additional help from the child's health care team to deal with the school board, teachers and other school personnel, even classmates and their parents.

When the information is withheld, the result may be disastrous for the child. Negative psychological sequelae are certain to appear (Loveland et al, 1996). We have had one teenager who did relatively well with his haemophilia as a young child who became a recluse with a severe school phobia when told of his HIV status, and who now remains home day after day with sparse home tutoring and no interaction with friends or peers. The fear of loss of confidentiality is too great for him to handle.

There may be problems with the HIV-positive child when he begins to progress to AIDS and possibly with development of AIDS dementia. There are data to suggest that additional supportive measures may be necessary to help the HIV-positive child cope with the second chronic illness, which may impede his learning abilities.

The child and family both need assistance in designing a programme with the school that will allow the child to move forward and develop to his greatest potential.

Sporting Activities

Sports should be played by all children, even the boy with haemophilia.

A child learns by interacting within his environment, by touching and exploring it. Development of physical ability depends upon the variety of experiences for the haemophilic child, as with any non-haemophilic child (Seeler et al, 1977; Kelley, 1991a). Orthopaedists and physical therapists have noted for many years that the people with a well-developed musculoskeletal system have less joint bleeding and subsequent destruction and are better able to withstand the minor trauma of daily living.

The baby with haemophilia will have developed bruises in his crib as he rolled over on his toys or pacifier. The crawling infant may even have bruises on the outer aspect of his arms and knees or even bleeding within the knee and elbow joint. The toddler, as he learns to gain his balance, may have many falls and increased bruising on head or buttocks. At this time, the parental anxiety increases and should be dealt with to allow for normal increased activity. It is at this time in the infant's life that the parents must learn their role in allowing the child to explore the new activities that lead to good muscular development, even though more bruising may occur. Double or triple nappies, padding sewn or tucked into elbow or knee pockets of the clothing and a helmet can be excellent protective measures during play periods. However, good parental supervision must accompany the learning child in the playground. The haemophilic child must learn to swing, run, climb, kick a ball, throw and catch a ball, ride the small low "tricycle" for the 2 year old, the tricycle for the 3–4 year old and the bicycle for the 6 year old. The attainment of these skills will help him in his choice of sports beginning at 4–5 years of age. As pointed out by Bachmayer and Holdredge (1991), the child need not be restricted in his choice of activities, although potentially harmful, because the challenge of the activity is a learning experience which may teach him motor development or may show him the risk is such that he may be physically unable to engage in the activity. The risk may come from the sport itself or from the size of his peers competing in the sport.

The effects of physical activities have additional benefits for the haemophiliac that are purely psychosocial in nature and allow him to develop along with his peers in a near normal mode (Weiner, 1991). This may even have a positive effect with a decrease in spontaneous bleeding. As he matures, it is enormously helpful for him to compete, win or lose, with his peers and, thereby, learn teamwork, as well as independence and self-reliance. It is for these reasons that the child with haemophilia must be allowed to develop his motor skills in the same manner and to the same extent as the non-haemophilic child.

Several generalities are worth considering. Non-contact sports or those carried out by the individual by himself are preferred over contact sports. For example, swimming, golf and tennis are preferred over American football, soccer and basketball. As peers increase in age, they also increase in size, so that sports such as baseball, basketball or even ice hockey that were enjoyed by the haemophiliac as a young boy may not be safe as a teenager. In countries where continuous prophylaxis is used, all sports except those with most physical contact, such as American football, can be engaged in without fear of injury. In countries where prophylaxis for sports can be used, again, all but American football can be played. For those living in countries where treatment is not so plentiful, sports should be learned correctly from an instructor rather than from peers.

A very important aspect of sports participation has been pointed out by Gilbert et al (1984), which pertains to the present condition of the joints and the past history of bleeding when choosing a sport. A child with elbow arthropathy should reconsider tennis and the boy with severe ankle arthropathy should consider swimming rather than athletics and basketball. In addition, both child and parent should investigate a training or muscle-conditioning programme before entering into the playing of the sport itself, such as professional athletes must do. The extent to which this extra conditioning is necessary depends upon the general body condition of the child. It is far better to be in good physical condition for a sport that will lead to successful competition rather than early injury which may lead to defeat. Finally, the child must accept that bleeding may occur requiring treatment, and only if repeated bleeds occur, which may lead to severe joint disability, must he reconsider his choice and perhaps abandon his choice of sport. This decision should be made by him with the help of his family and not by his family alone.

When the child enters school, the physical education teacher may be a great help for the child once the teacher has been educated about haemophilia and the needs of the child. The orthopaedist and/or the physical therapist from the child's haemophilia team may frequently be of great assistance in the education of the physical education teacher. Once the instructors have been alerted to the needs of the haemophiliac, they are often a great ally for the boy as they see him as a challenge for their own skills and training in physical education.

The choice of sports activities varies with age, location of the family and the sport itself, as already mentioned. Thought should be given to the life-long use of a sport, such as tennis, swimming and golf, and to the sports prominent in the family location, i.e. skiing, horseback riding for the boy raised on a farm. A very thorough and convenient evaluation of all sports, along with the areas of the body that are stressed, and whether a sport is or is not recommended, has been compiled by Gilbert et al (1984) and published under the auspices of the American Red Cross for the National Hemophilia Foundation, from whom it can be obtained. Sports are divided into three categories and are grouped for the boy with severe or moderate disease. It is an excellent guide for parents, boys, teachers and physical education instructors alike and should be used very early in the life of the child as a guide for life-long good musculoskeletal development and maintenance.

Prophylaxis

Prophylaxis is defined as that regimen of therapy which attempts to convert the patient with severe disease to one with moderate disease. This is accomplished by raising the plasma level from less than 1% to approximately 5–10% or that level where spontaneous bleeding will not occur. Prophylaxis may be given as routine to maintain the higher level of plasma factor level to prevent bleeding in the deficient patient or prophylaxis may be given for a short period of time to allow healing of damaged tissue to occur (Nilsson et al, 1992).

Prophylaxis for all children with haemophilia is available as a routine form of treatment early in childhood in many countries where socialized medicine is available and is considered the right for all patients with this chronic illness. The schedule of infusions to maintain plasma levels above that of severe disease, as well as the amounts used, vary with the country of origin. Unfortunately, few countries assay the patient prior to the subsequent infusion; therefore, exact levels that are achieved are not known. Most have attempted, in general, to convert the patient with severe disease to one with moderate disease. The dose may vary from 20 to 40 units/kg every other day or three times per week. A small survey carried out by an international group of paediatricians associated with the World Federation of Hemophilia (WFH) in 1984 found wide variability in the dose, schedule and age when programmes were begun, i.e. within the first year of life or following the first bleeding episode. Only in the centres in Malmo and Stockholm have plasma levels been followed to know that plasma levels of 2–5% of factor VIII have been attained (Petrini et al, 1991; Nilsson et al, 1992). A study is underway for the World Federation of Hemophilia Pediatric Child Care Committee to ascertain the varied dose schedules and the amount of bleeding occurring within each schedule to be able to recommend the most appropriate method for prophylaxis as many patients and clinicians alike are coming to realize the value of some form of permanent treatment. The 20-year data from Sweden, The International Multicenter Orthopedic Outcome Study and many others have shown the value of joint preservation which may be obtained from such prophylactic programmes (Aledort, 1992).

Permanent prophylaxis has been reserved in this clinic for those children who have had repeat central nervous system bleeding or whose joint bleeding has been more than once per week and interfered with any semblance of normal living (Hilgartner, 1989).

Limited or short-term prophylaxis has been used by many clinicians as the medical therapy to heal chronic synovitis. The regimen used at the New York Hospital Hemophilia Treatment Center includes prednisone 2 mg/kg daily for 2 weeks with factor replacement at 50 units/kg three times weekly for 6 weeks. Intensive physical therapy is initiated at the same time to improve atrophied muscles. A repeat course may be indicated if healing does not occur or there is recurrence of boggy swelling within 2 weeks. This short-term prophylaxis is used for 3–6 months prior to referral to the orthopaedist for arthroscopic débridement. Other centres may wait 6–9 months before referral for surgical treatment. The use of both steroids and prednisone have come under discussion for the HIV-positive patient. The immunologist is concerned about the infectious complications when steroids are used for prolonged time periods, but admits their usefulness in the patient with CD4 counts above 300×10^6/l.

As already stated in this chapter, limited prophylaxis for sports is worthy of consideration in those countries where universal prophylaxis is not available. Where routine prophylaxis is available, additional factor may be necessary before a game or practice depending on the level attained by the infusions. For example, maintenance above 1% may not be sufficient for sports in the Gilbert category of two such as baseball and basketball and may require an additional infusion, whereas in those areas where maintenance is closer to 10% or if the game is close to the time of the infusion, an additional infusion may not be necessary.

Where routine prophylaxis is not used, additional infusions before undertaking the sport are worth considering to ensure a minimum number of bleeding episodes, as bleeding episodes might discourage both the boy and his coach and discredit him in the eyes of his peers and negate all of the advantages one hopes to gain by participation.

Cost and availability of product in any one country and the third-party payer is of great importance, particularly with the current emphasis on home care costs. In many countries it will be increasingly difficult to justify broad expensive programmes of support for sports alone. It can only be hoped that the wisdom of preventing bleeding and joint destruction in childhood with the subsequent benefits of a productive adult will be addressed and recognized by health care planners of today. The cost of products has risen at least four-fold since the first survey in 1984, making programmes extremely difficult to initiate at the current time. Theoretically, the development of recombinant factor VIII should provide a product at one-tenth the cost of the plasma-derived virally inactivated products of today. However, until the reduction in price is realized, widespread use of the recombinant products is not likely to occur.

The length of time for prophylaxis to be maintained is also of concern. If a boy has never known the warning signs of a bleeding episode, or the caution of his actions that has developed in the older boy or man who has only been treated as necessary with episodic treatment, or if he has never known the pain, anxiety and discomfort of a bleeding episode, he will never be willing to have his product reduced and his plasma level allowed to sink to its own level. Scheibel (personal communication) has stated emphatically that she has been unable to get her older patients off of prophylaxis at any age. The fear and anxiety that appears on the faces of parents and patient alike give the answer to the question. The answer found in Denmark was "No, we will not stop prophylaxis". This is another aspect of the disease that must be addressed for the future.

Venous Access

At the present time, the haemophiliac can only receive his factor replacement material intravenously. Therefore, venous access is of prime importance lifelong. The skill of the infusor is also important at all times, particularly the first few years of life.

In the past, children were encouraged to learn the skill of catching and throwing a ball early in life to improve arm musculature and ultimately venous size. In the 1960s, venous size was enhanced with the surgical manipulations of arterial-venous anastomosis or arterial grafting. These procedures were not always successful, as the grafts often closed or venous engorgement was disfiguring and gave an undue burden to the heart. Vessel size made surgery difficult in very young children. For most children today, vessel size is not a problem for the skilled phlebotomist and parents may become skilled when the child is quite young.

The development of deep venous catheters in the early 1970s has changed the mode of management for many haematological disorders. The Broviac catheter for children or the Hickman catheter for adults have revolutionized the delivery of antibiotics, intravenous fluids, hyperalimentation fluids, haemodialysis fluids, blood transfusions and blood product infusions (Mullan et al, 1992). For the younger haemophiliac these devices may be used for those needing daily infusions for immune-tolerance programmes or for small babies or children with exceedingly poor venous access. For the adult with HIV infection these devices may be used for hyperalimentation and intravenous antibiotics in addition to blood products. Recently, the single-lumen devices have increased to double- and triple-lumen devices. The introduction of deep implantable devices such as the Infusaport or Port-a-cath have further enhanced this modality of care. However, the complication rate with these devices was as high as 17.6% (Hockenberry et al, 1989).

Port-a-cath or Infusaport devices have been put into peripheral or deep veins such as the cephalic or subclavian or into the right atrium for almost 10 years with improved access and some decrease in complications over the Broviac or Hickman external catheters attributed to the deep tunnelling of lines. However, infections and thrombotic complications have continued to occur but to a somewhat lesser degree in the healthy haemophiliac child. In one series, the overall complication rate has been as low as 5% in 18 812 days of use, and in a more recent series, the complication rate was the same as with the Broviac or Hickman device (Essex-Carter et al, 1989; Sariego et al, 1993). As expected, the immunocompromised children tend to have more infectious complications (David and Andrew, 1993). Access is gained by a needle inserted directly into the subcutaneously implanted bladder. For the child with a clotting disorder, complications include haematoma at the time of implantation, particularly in those patients with inhibitors, thrombosis and sepsis. We have found daily therapy for at least 14 days post-surgery to be necessary with insertion of the Huber access needle at surgery.

Thromboses are best treated with insertion of 4000–5000 units of urokinase for 12–24 hours and repeated as necessary. Infections are treated with antibiotics through the catheter continuing for 14 days after the first negative blood culture and the ports are removed only if two infections cannot be cleared. Local infections also may occur around the port and are treated in a similar manner.

Irrespective of the device used, these assisted routes for venous access have given the patient with haemophilia an additional improvement in his lifestyle and access to medical care not previously available. We have begun to use the subcutaneous implants more often than the Broviac, as they have less complications and better patient acceptability, although skin puncture is still necessary.

Home Therapy

Infusion therapy given at home, work or on holiday away from the patient's hospital base by the patient or family member has become the accepted mode of treatment for this chronic illness. The first official programme was put into place when the mother of a patient of Dr Fred Rabiner at the Hemophilia Center of Michael Reese Hospital in Chicago, Illinois, confessed that she was a nurse and had been infusing her young son at home for some time. With this confession, home therapy became a reality and an established form of treatment (Rabiner and Telfer, 1970). In addition to the above, guidelines have been developed that detail criteria for admission to the home therapy programmes. They include severe haemophilia A and B and severe von Willebrand's disease without the presence of inhibitors, although inhibitor patients are now included. Parents must be trained for patients over 4 years of age; boys over 12 years of age who show sufficient maturity to assume the responsibility and manage self-infusion may be trained themselves. These guidelines for education of the family or patient were drawn up by the physicians for the National Hemophilia Foundation (Agle et al, 1977). They also include the philosophy of care, recognition of bleeding episodes and early infusion, as well as the teaching of sterile technique for administration of blood product factor, calculations for dosage based on size and severity of bleeding episode. Strict psychosocial requirements pertaining to the fitness of the parents/patient to assume the role of decision-maker in the medical care have to be met and certain responsibilities have to be accepted by the family/patient.

Patient inclusion is based on acceptance of responsibility and agreement to send the Center an account of how the blood product was used, type of bleeding treated and the amount of time away from normal daily activities. These records or bleeding logs relay information to the center about the amount of bleeding the patient was having and his success in treatment. In addition, the patient agrees to be seen at his center annually or biannually. If these conditions are not met, the center could remove the patient from the home therapy roles and he would have to return to the clinic for treatment.

The center agrees to supervise the allotment of product with necessary infusion equipment to each patient or family. Various means have been devised: home delivery, postal delivery or collection by the patient at his hospital or clinic or home therapy companies. Collection of waste materials has been recently added to this center's responsibility.

Procedures were originally drawn up for the use of frozen blood products (cryoprecipitate or fresh frozen plasma) at home. When lyophilized concentrates were developed, dedicated freezers were no longer necessary and products were maintained in the standard home refrigerator at 4°C. Multiple teaching guides, including booklets and videos, have been developed as instruction manuals by the fractionation industry to make this modality of care a regular part of comprehensive care given for this disease.

Data from the bleeding logs collated annually for national statistics in many countries have documented a marked improved in lifestyle and disease outcome for patients (Rabiner and Lazerson, 1976; Sergis-Davenport and Varni, 1983; Smith and Levine, 1984). These data show a marked decrease in time lost in school and work, an improved functional outcome that has allowed the patient to pursue higher education and improved vocational achievements. This resulted in decreased unemployment until the advent of the AIDS epidemic. Lifestyle as a whole, however, has continued to improve for the patient who may have this form of treatment at home or work where he is independent of physician and clinical staff and may have a greater sense of control over his life (Lazerson, 1972; Markova et al, 1983).

Effect of Haemophilia on Normal Siblings

Haemophilia affects all members of a family. The adjustment of a family to chronic illness varies with time and the point of life at which each family member may be. The effect of the diagnosis of a new sibling with haemophilia may appear to have no effect on an older sibling, but, inadvertently, the sibling will feel the loss of his or her "place in the sun" far more than if the new sibling did not have an illness to which his mother and father will react more strongly (Salk et al, 1972; Handford and Strickler, 1982).

The siblings, inevitably, have psychological difficulties and very conflicting feelings towards the sibling with the chronic illness and their role in the family structure. There is certainly jealousy over the increased attention given to the ill child at all times and rejection of the well child by the parents. In addition, there is guilt by the well child about their feelings and guilt that they are well and their sibling may have the pain and suffering. One investigator has found that the well siblings feel they must fulfil their parents' expectations for the ill child and again feel frustration and depression when they cannot receive, from the parents, the praise they look for (Sherman, 1993). Others have observed that these well siblings feel they must help the parents take care of the ill siblings at the expense of their own desires and expectations (Mattsson, 1984; Simon, 1989).

Female siblings have an additional burden as a possible carrier. It is because of this additional burden, and the probability that these young girls might be treated differently by their parents, that genetic counsellors have agreed to wait until the carrier status is important to the young girl for reproductive choices before determination of the carrier status and imparting this information to her is carried out (Salk et al, 1972). We have found many of these carrier female siblings to be very ambivalent about marriage and children and insistent on prenatal diagnosis to avoid the birth of a child with haemophilia. The scar of growing up with a haemophilic sibling is a very deep one for most young women.

The identification of these multiple problems leads to the development of psychosocial programmes as an integral and necessary part of the comprehensive care programme (Handford and Strickler, 1982; Jones, 1990; Kelley, 1991b).

References

Agle DP, Hilgartner MW, Lazerson J and Van Eys J. *Home Therapy for Hemophilia: A Manual for Physicians*. New York: National Hemophilia Foundation, 1977.

Aledort LM. Prophylaxis: the next hemophilia treatment. *Journal of Internal Medicine* 1992; **232:** 1–2.

Bachmayer E, Holdredge S. Developmental activities, sports and games. Hemophilia World. *World Federation of Hemophilia* 1991; **7:** 5–6.

Bray GL, Kronner B, Arkin S, et al. Loss of high responder inhibitor in patients with severe hemophilia A and HIV infections. *American Journal of Hematology* 1993; **42:** 375–379.

Buchanan GR, Richards N, Sexauer CL, Stevens B. Serologic response to hepatitis B vaccine in children receiving multiple blood transfusions. *Pediatric Infectious Diseases* 1986; **5:** 68–70.

Bussing R, Johnson SB. Psychosocial issues in hemophilia before and after the HIV crisis: a review of current research. *General Hospital Psychiatry* 1992; **14:** 387–403.

David M, Andrew M. Venous thromboembolic complications in children. *Journal of Pediatrics* 1993; **123:** 337–346.

Dimercurio D. School and the child with hemophilia. Hemophilia World. *World Federation of Hemophilia* 1991; **7:** 9–10.

Essex-Carter A, Gilbert J, Robinson T, Littlewood JM. Totally implantable venous access systems in paediatric practice. *Archives of Disease in Childhood* 1989; **64:** 119–123.

Gilbert MS, Schorr JB, Holbrook T, Tiberio D. *Hemophilia and Sports* New York: 1984 American Red Cross, National Hemophilia Foundation.

Goldsmith JC, Kletzel M. Risk of birth related intracranial hemorrhages in hemophilic newborns: results of a North American survey. *Blood* 1990; **76:** 421.

Handford H, Strickler EM. Psychosocial programs. In: Hilgartner M (Ed.), *Hemophilia in the Child and Adult*. New York: Masson, 1982: 231.

Hilgartner MW. Factor replacement therapy. In: Hilgartner M, Pochedly C (Eds), *Hemophilia in the Child and Adult*, 3rd edn. New York: Raven Press, 1989: 1–26.

Hockenberry M, Schultz WH, Bennett B, Bryant R, Falleta JM. Experience with minimal complications in implanted catheters in children. *American Journal of Pediatric Hematology/Oncology* 1989; **11:** 295–299.

Hoots WK. Hemophilic liver disease. In: Hilgartner M, Pochedly C (Eds), *Haemophilia in the Child and Adult*, 3rd edn. New York: Raven Press, 1989: 69–87.
Jason J, Murphy J, Sleeper L, et al. Hemophilia growth and development study: report on baseline immunology analysis. *Journal of Acquired Immune Deficiency Syndrome* 1994; **96:** 29–32.
Jones P. *Living With Hemophilia* New York: Oxford University Press, 1990.
Kelley LA. Raising a child with hemophilia. *Sports Activities* 1991a; 153.
Kelley LA. Raising a child with hemophilia: *Your children Without Hemophilia. Published by the National Hemophilia Foundation.* 1991b: 169–174.
Lazerson J. Hemophilia home transfusion program: effect on school attendance. *Journal of Pediatrics* 1972; **81:** 330–332.
Loveland K, Stehbans J, Contant C, Bell T, Schiller M, et al. Hemophilia growth and development study: baseline neuropsychological findings. *Journal of Pediatric Psychology* 1994; **19:** 223–228.
Markova I, Macdonald K, Forbes C. Integration of hemophilic boys into normal schools. Child: *Care Health and Development* 1980; **6:** 101–109.
Markova I, Forbes CD, Rowlands A, Pettigrew A, Willoughby M. The hemophiliac patient's self-perception of changes in health and lifestyle arising from self-treatment. *International Journal of Rehabilitation Research* 1983; **6:** 11–18.
Mattsson A. Hemophilia and the family: life-long challenges and adaptation. *Scandinavian Journal of Haemotology* 1984; **33** (Suppl 40): 65–74.
Miller CH. Genetics of hemophilia and von Willebrand's disease. In: Hilgartner M, Pochedly C (Eds), *Hemophilia in the child and adult*, 3rd edn. New York: Raven Press, 1989a: 297–345.
Miller CH. Genetic counseling. In: Hilgartner M, Pochedly C (Eds), *Hemophilia in the Child and Adult* 3rd edn. New York: Raven Press, 1989b: 161–172.
Mullan FJ, Hood JM, Barros D'Sa. Use of the Hickman catheter for central venous access in patients with haematological disorders. *British Journal of Clinical Practice* 1992; **46:** 167–170.
Nilsson IM, Berntorp E, Loquist T, Pettersson H. Twenty-five years' experience of prophylactic treatment in severe hemophilia A and B. *Journal of Internal Medicine* 1992; **232:** 25–32.
Petrini P, Lindvars N, Egberg N, Blomback M. Prophylaxis with factor concentrates in preventing hemophilic arthropathy. *American Journal of Pediatric Hematology/Oncology* 1991; **13**(3): 380–387.
Pokalo CL. Foreign Vaccines OK. If They Meet US Standards. *Infectious Diseases in Children* 1993; **6:** 1–7.
Rabiner SF, Telfer MC. Home transfusions for patients with hemophilia A. *New England Journal of Medicine* 1970; **283:** 1011–1015.
Rabiner SF, Lazerson J. Home management and prophylaxis of hemophilia. In: Brown ED (Ed.), *Progress in Hematology*, 3rd edn. New York: Grune and Stratton, 1976: 226–236.
Salk L, Hilgartner M, Granich B. The psychosocial impact of hemophilia on the patient and his family. *Social Science and Medicine* 1972; **6:** 491–505.
Sariego J, Bootorabi B, Matsumato T, Kerstein M. Major long-term complications in 1422 permanent venous access devices. *American Journal of Surgery* 1993; **165:** 249–231.
Seeler RA, Ashenhurst JB, Langehennig PL. Behavioral benefits in hemophilia as noted at a special summer camp. *Clinical Paediatrics* 1977; **16:** 525–529.
Sergis-Davenport E, Varni J. Behavioral assessment and management of adherence to factor replacement therapy in hemophilia. *Journal of Pediatric Psychology* 1983; **8:** 367–377.
Sherman C. *The Psychosocial Impact of Acquired Immune Deficiency Syndrome on Mothers of Hemophiliacs.* New York University, PhD Thesis, September 1993.
Simon RM. The family and hemophilia. In: Hilgartner M, Pochedly C (Eds), *Hemophilia in the Child and Adult*, 3rd edn. New York: Raven Press, 1989: 213–226.
Smith PA, Levine PH. Benefits of comprehensive care of hemophillia. *American Journal of Public Health* 1984; **74:** 616–617.
Weiner L. School and the HIV-infected child with hemophilia. Hemophilia World. *World Federation of Hemophilia* 1991; **7:** 6–7.
Wilson D, Nelson M, Fenstermacher M, et al. Brain abnormalities in male children and adolescents with hemophilia: detection with MR imaging. *Radiology* 1992; **185:** 553–558.

9 Other Inherited Disorders of Blood Coagulation

PAUL L.F. GIANGRANDE

Haemophilia and von Willebrand's disease are the most common congenital disorders of blood coagulation. Other congenital disorders of coagulation are considered in this chapter. Isolated congenital deficiencies of other coagulation factors are quite rare, and an impression of the incidence in the UK can be gained from Table 9.1.

Fibrinogen Deficiency

Biochemistry

Fibrinogen (factor I) is a 340 kD protein encoded on chromosome 4 and synthesized by hepatocytes. It is composed of two identical subunits, each containing three dissimilar polypeptide chains (Aα, Bβ, γ) which are linked by disulphide bonds (Fig. 9.1). Thrombin cleaves fibrinopeptides A and B from fibrinogen, resulting in the formation of strands of insoluble fibrin monomer, which consists of three paired α, β and γ chains. Afibrinogenaemia (or hypofibrinogenaemia) is due to production of decreased levels of normal fibrinogen. Dysfibrinogenaemia is a condition associated with production of structurally abnormal fibrinogen. More than 250 structural variants have been described that are associated with a bleeding tendency (Ebert, 1991). Most of these variants exhibit impaired thrombin-catalyzed release of fibrinopeptides, or impaired fibrin polymerization. Some variants of fibrinogen are associated with a thrombotic tendency rather than a bleeding tendency, and this has been attributed to impaired binding of plasminogen or tissue plasminogen activator (tPA) to the abnormal fibrinogen molecule.

Fibrinogen is also essential for aggregation of platelets. Activation of platelets results in conformational changes in the glycoprotein IIb/IIIa membrane complex, which is subsequently able to bind plasma fibrinogen and thus cross-link adjacent platelets.

Table 9.1 Numbers of patients with rare congenital disorders of coagulation registered with Haemophilia Centres in the UK (1994)

Coagulation defect	Number of patients
Fibrinogen deficiency	74
Prothrombin deficiency	11
Factor V deficiency	48
Factor VII deficiency	146
Factor X deficiency	78
Factor XI deficiency	530
Factor XII deficiency	476
Factor XIII deficiency	27

(Reproduced with permission of the UK Haemophilia Centre Directors' Organization.)

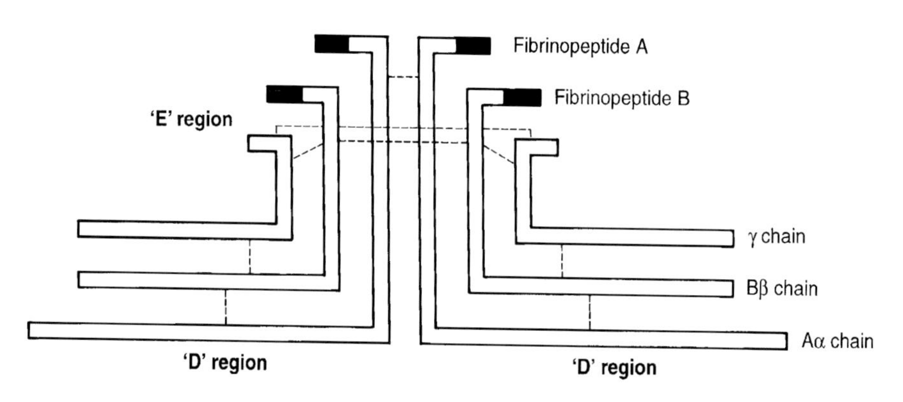

Figure 9.1 The fibrinogen molecule.

Clinical and laboratory features

Congenital afibrinogenaemia is inherited as an autosomal recessive trait. There is often a history of parental consanguinity. Complete deficiency of fibrinogen is likely to result in bleeding episodes from an early age. A typical feature is persistent bleeding from the umbilical stump. Bleeding from mucosal surfaces such as epistaxis, menorrhagia and melaena are also common. Intracranial haemorrhage has also been reported. By contrast, bleeding into muscles and joints is unusual.

Laboratory features include marked prolongation of the prothrombin time, thrombin time and activated partial thromboplastin time (APTT). The platelet count is normal, which helps to exclude the differential diagnosis of disseminated intravascular coagulation (DIC). The bleeding time may be prolonged, reflecting the requirement for fibrinogen in platelet aggregation. In dysfibrinogenaemia the Reptilase time is often markedly prolonged, and there is usually a considerable discrepancy between immunological and functional assays of fibrinogen.

Treatment

A lyophilized, heat-treated concentrate of fibrinogen is available (Immuno). Only small amounts of fibrinogen are required to obtain a sustained correction of the bleeding time (Cattaneo et al, 1992). A single infusion of 3–4 g is usually sufficient to control bleeding episodes. Fresh frozen plasma and cryoprecipitate also contain fibrinogen, and may also be used as alternative therapeutic materials if heat-treated concentrate is not available. Afibrinogenaemia in females is often associated with menorrhagia, recurrent abortions and post-partum haemorrhage. Regular infusions of fibrinogen concentrate have been used successfully to prevent complications during pregnancy in congenital afibrinogenaemia (Grech et al, 1991).

Prothrombin Deficiency

Biochemistry

Prothrombin (factor II) is a single-chain 72 kD glycoprotein encoded on chromosome 11 and synthesized by hepatocytes. Vitamin K is essential for post-translational gamma-carboxylation of the molecule, which renders the molecule functionally active. Prothrombin is activated by factor Xa on the surface of platelets in the presence of factor V and calcium through selective hydrolysis of two peptide bonds, yielding thrombin. Prothrombin fragment F1+2 is cleaved from prothrombin during this step: assays for this fragment have been developed and used as an indicator of activation of the coagulation cascade in prothrombotic states.

Laboratory and clinical features

Prothrombin deficiency is a rare condition, inherited as an autosomal recessive disorder, which was first recognized in 1950 (Landwehr et al, 1950).

Approximately 50% of normal activity is required to ensure haemostasis. Marked prothrombin deficiency may result in a bruising tendency, menorrhagia and haemorrhage following surgery, dental extractions or childbirth. Spontaneous bleeding into joints is not a feature of this disorder.

The prothrombin time and APTT are both prolonged. These may be corrected by mixing with aged plasma, but not with serum or plasma adsorbed with alumina. The thrombin time is normal. Several exogenous, non-physiological activators of prothrombin have been described, including proteinases in several snake venoms. Specific assays for prothrombin activity may be performed in a one-stage assay using the venom of the Taipan snake (*Oxyuranus scutellatus*) (Denson et al, 1971). Type I prothrombin deficiency is characterized by reduced levels of prothrombin activity and antigen, reflecting decreased synthesis of a structurally normal prothrombin molecule (hypoprothrombinaemia). Type II prothrombin deficiency is somewhat rarer, and is characterized by normal levels of immunologically detectable prothrombin which has reduced functional activity (dysprothrombinaemia). Snake venoms have been used not only to study the mechanism of prothrombin activation in detail, but also to permit identification and classification of specific prothrombin variants (Rosing and Tans, 1991). The possibility of vitamin K deficiency should be excluded before making a diagnosis of congenital prothrombin deficiency (as with factors VII, IX and X) and the use of *Echis carinatus* venom may also be useful in this regard (Solano et al, 1990).

Treatment

Bleeding is rarely severe in these patients, and treatment with blood products is required relatively infrequently. By contrast with high-purity factor IX concentrates, prothrombin-complex concentrates contain adequate amounts of prothrombin for therapeutic use. For example, the Bio Products Laboratory concentrate 9A contains approximately 600 iu of factor II (prothrombin) per vial. The half-life of prothrombin is approximately 3 days, so that if repeated infusions are required (e.g. to cover surgery) prothrombin-complex concentrates do not have to be administered as regularly as for patients with haemophilia B. This minimizes the risk of thromboembolism. Such concentrates are, in general, preferable to fresh plasma as the concentrates have been subjected to virucidal treatment such as heat treatment. However, packs of fresh frozen plasma that have been subjected to treatment with a solvent/detergent mixture are now becoming available.

Factor V Deficiency

Biochemistry

Factor V is a single-chain 300 kD glycoprotein encoded on chromosome 1, and synthesized by both hepatocytes and megakaryocytes. Approximately 80% of the whole blood factor V circulates freely in the plasma, and the remaining 20% is stored within α-granules of platelets (Tracy et al, 1982). Circulating factor V is activated by thrombin, and activated factor Va serves as a co-factor for activation of prothrombin by factor X. The activation of prothrombin is achieved by assembly of a prothrombinase complex of factor X, factor Va, phospholipids and calcium on cell membrane surfaces, including platelets. There is evidence to suggest that the platelet-associated fraction of factor V is particularly important for haemostasis. In one study, the severity of the bleeding tendency was poorly correlated with the plasma level of factor V but there was a relationship with the number of Xa binding sites on platelets (Miletich et al, 1978). Furthermore, a family with a significant bleeding tendency has been described in which a modest reduction in the plasma factor V level is associated with a marked reduction in platelet-associated factor V activity (Tracy et al, 1984).

Factor V, like factor VIII, is inactivated by protein C. A specific mutation (^{506}Arg→Gln) results in resistance to activated protein C (Dahlback et al, 1993). This is associated with a thrombotic tendency, rather than a bleeding tendency, as the mutation does not involve the thrombin cleavage site.

Clinical and laboratory features

A bleeding disorder due to deficiency of factor V was first described in 1947, and was called "parahaemophilia". (Owren, 1947). The disorder is inherited as an autosomal recessive condition. The bleeding tendency is usually not severe. Typical manifestations include easy bruising, epistaxis and menorrhagia, as well as bleeding after trauma, dental extractions or surgery. An unusually high incidence of congenital abnormalities, often involving the cardiovascular system or urogenital tract, has been reported in association with factor V deficiency (Seeler, 1972).

The usual laboratory findings are of a prolongation of both the prothrombin time and APTT. These are corrected by the addition of normal plasma adsorbed with alumina but not by addition of serum or aged normal plasma. Factor V deficiency is the only coagulation defect in which a prolonged prothrombin time is associated with deficient function of the plasma reagent in the thromboplastin generation test. The thrombin time is normal. The bleeding time is found to be prolonged in approximately one-third of cases. An association between factor V deficiency and factor VIII deficiency is well recognized, but the basis for this is unknown (Hultin and Eyster, 1981; Soff and Levin, 1981).

Factor V deficiency secondary to development of inhibitory antibodies has also been reported, usually associated with exposure to blood products (Feinstein et al, 1970; Crowell, 1975; Zehnder and Leung, 1990).

Treatment

Plasma-derived concentrate of factor V is not available. Fresh frozen plasma may be used to control or prevent bleeding in these patients. Infused factor V has a half-life of approximately 12–15 hours, and so twice-daily infusions are advisable for patients with severe deficiency undergoing surgery (Melliger and Duckert, 1971). The relative importance of the platelet pool of factor V has been demonstrated by the observation that transfusion of fresh, normal platelets alone may correct the haemostatic defect for several days, even though the plasma level is not raised significantly (Borchgrevink and Owren, 1961). The administration of platelets may be particularly effective in controlling bleeding associated with the presence of inhibitory antibodies (Chediak et al, 1980).

Factor VII Deficiency

Biochemistry

The role assigned to factor VII in the classical coagulation pathway was activation of the so-called extrinsic pathway. Recent work has suggested a single integrated pathway for all coagulation factors, which is initiated by factor VII, which in turn can activate both factor X and factor IX (Broze et al, 1990) (Fig. 9.2). Factor VII is a single-chain 50 kD glycoprotein, encoded on chromosome 13 and synthesized in the liver. Synthesis of active factor VII requires the presence of vitamin K. Factor VII is activated upon contact with tissue factor, exposed by vascular injury, to form factor VIIa through cleavage of a single bond (Rao and Rapaport, 1988). Factor VIIa is in turn responsible for activation of both factor IX and factor X. Tissue factor pathway inhibitor (TFPI) is a physiological inhibitor of factor VII which is associated with the lipoprotein fraction of plasma (Broze and Miletich, 1987).

Laboratory and clinical features

The clinical manifestations of factor VII deficiency are rather variable, and there is a poor correlation between the level of factor and the bleeding tendency. Haemorrhagic symptoms include easy bruising and bleeding from mucosal surfaces, but joint bleeds are also a recognized manifestation (Marder and

Schulman, 1964; Ragni et al, 1981). Typical laboratory findings include a prolonged prothrombin time, but a normal bleeding time, APTT and Russell's viper venom (Stypven) time. The prothrombin time is corrected by addition of serum or aged plasma, but not by addition of plasma adsorbed with alumina. A specific factor VII assay using deficient plasma confirms the diagnosis. The prolongation of the prothrombin time may vary significantly according to the source of the thromboplastin reagent used, and this has been used to define particular variants (Triplett et al, 1985; Poggio et al, 1991). If plasma is left to stand at 4°C for some hours, "cold activation" may occur and this may result in spurious elevations of the factor VII level (Gjonnæss, 1972; Poggio et al, 1991). Immunological assays, employing monoclonal antibodies directed against functional epitopes of the factor VII molecule, circumvent this problem and are now available. Deficiency of vitamin K should be excluded before a diagnosis of congenital deficiency is made.

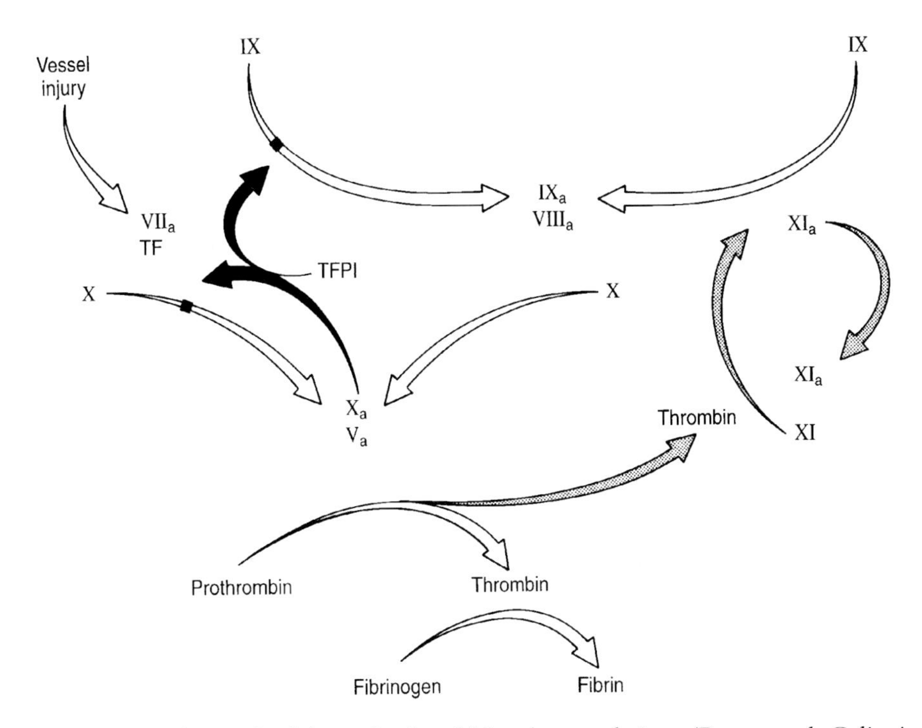

Figure 9.2 The revised hypothesis of blood coagulation (Broze and Galiani, 1993). Coagulation is initiated at a site of vessel damage when factor VIIa is exposed to tissue factor. Factors VII, IX and XI are required for the production of additional factor Xa due to feedback inhibition of the factor VIIa/tissue factor complex by tissue factor pathway inhibitor (TFPI). The hatched arrows show the potential thrombin-mediated pathway for factor XI activation.

Treatment

Most prothrombin-complex concentrates contain only negligible quantities of factor VII, and are not suitable for replacement therapy in deficient individuals. However, a specific heat-treated, plasma-derived factor VII concentrate is now available for clinical use (Bio Products Laboratory). A factor VII level of only 10–15% of normal is sufficient to secure haemostasis, even in the setting of surgery. The recovery of infused factor VII is almost complete, so an infusion of 5–10 iu of factor VII/kg body weight should be adequate. Factor VII has a relatively short half-life of around 4 hours so frequent infusions may be required in the setting of invasive procedures. Recombinant factor VIIa is only licensed for treatment of patients with haemophilia and inhibitory antibodies. Fresh frozen plasma may be used as a source of factor VII if concentrate is not available.

Factor X Deficiency

Biochemistry

Factor X is a 59 kD glycoprotein, composed of a 17 kD light chain and 42 kD heavy chain. It is synthesized in the liver, and the gene is located on chromosome 13. Factor X may be activated by both factor IX (in a reaction which requires the presence of factor VIII) or a complex of tissue factor and factor VII. Activation of factor X involves cleavage within the heavy chain. Activated factor X forms a complex with factor V and calcium on membrane surfaces, and the resultant complex cleaves prothrombin to form thrombin. Several point mutations have been described in patients with factor X deficiency. Some of these give characteristic results with tests of haemostasis (see below). For example, factor X_{Friuli} (^{343}Pro→Ser) is associated with a prolonged prothrombin time when tissue thromboplastin is used, but the variant is activated normally by Russell's viper venom (Girolami et al, 1970).

Clinical and laboratory features

Factor X is also known as Stuart-Prower factor after the two families in whom this rare defect was first reported (Telfer et al, 1956; Hougie et al, 1957). Inheritance of factor X defects is autosomal recessive. Heterozygotes usually have only a mild bleeding tendency, but may bleed in the setting of surgery or dental extractions. Complete deficiency is associated with a marked bleeding tendency, and apparently spontaneous bleeding into joints and muscles may occur. Intracranial haemorrhage has also been reported.

The typical initial findings in factor X deficiency are a prolonged prothrombin time and APTT, but a normal thrombin time. However, different patterns may occasionally be encountered, so that an isolated prothrombin time or APTT may be the only indication (Denson et al, 1970). For example, Factor X_{Padua} (^{304}Arg→Gln) is associated only with a prolonged prothrombin time, and the APTT is normal (Girolami et al, 1985). The abnormalities in the screening tests are corrected by mixing with serum or aged normal plasma, but not alumina-adsorbed plasma. Russell's viper venom (previously also known by its commercial name of "Stypven") activates factor X directly and this reagent has been adopted for one-stage assay of factor X activity. Factor X is dependent upon availability of vitamin K, and deficiency of this vitamin should be excluded before a diagnosis of congenital deficiency is made. Acquired deficiency of factor X has also been reported in association with amyloidosis (Furie et al, 1981).

Treatment

No specific factor X concentrate is manufactured, but prothrombin-complex concentrates contain an adequate quantity of factor X for therapeutic use (e.g. 9A (Bio Products Laboratory), which contains approximately 500 iu of factor X per vial). Such products are preferable to fresh frozen plasma as a source of factor X as concentrates are subjected to physical treatment to minimize the risk of transmission of viral infections. Infused factor X has a half-life of around 36 hours so that frequent infusions are not necessary, which minimizes the risk of thromboembolism which has been associated with repeated administration of prothrombin-complex concentrates. Prophylactic therapy with such concentrates may be useful in severely affected individuals who have frequent bleeding episodes.

Factor XI Deficiency

Biochemistry

Factor XI is a serine protease enzyme, encoded by a gene located on chromosome 4 and synthesized in the liver. It circulates as a dimer of two identical 80 kD subunits, which are linked by disulphide bonds. In the original "cascade" model of coagulation, factor XI was believed to have a role in initiation of the intrinsic pathway through contact activation. However, it appears that thrombin can also activate factor XI and it has been proposed (Fig. 9.2) that the principal role of factor XI is to support factor IX generation after primary activation of factor IX by the factor VII/tissue factor complex (for a review, see Broze and Galiani, 1993). The principal inhibitor of activated factor XIa in the circulation is α_1-antitrypsin.

The human factor XI gene consists of 15 exons spread out over 23 kb. Several mutations have been described in deficient individuals, and there appears to be a relationship between specific defects and the severity of the bleeding tendency (Hancock et al, 1991; Pugh et al, 1995).

Clinical and laboratory features

Deficiency of factor XI is associated with a bleeding tendency, but the correlation between the plasma level and the severity of the haemorrhagic manifestations is poor. Whilst levels of less than 15% are very likely to be associated with bleeding problems, bleeding in the setting of surgery may be problematic even in heterozygotes with factor XI levels of 50–70% (Bolton-Maggs et al, 1988, 1995). The bleeding tendency shows variable penetrance in a family, and does not breed true. Factor XI deficiency is particularly common amongst Ashkenazi Jews, but has been reported in many other ethnic groups. By contrast with the haemophilias, spontaneous bleeding is very rare and the usual problem is persistent bleeding after trauma or surgery (for a review, see Seligsohn, 1993). Bleeding after dental extractions is a particularly common problem. Menorrhagia is a frequent problem in women. Spontaneous haemarthroses are not a feature of this condition.

The prothrombin time and thrombin times are normal. The APTT is prolonged and is corrected after mixing with alumina-adsorbed normal plasma or aged plasma. Coincidental inheritance of low levels of factor VIII and von Willebrand factor may in part explain the variation in bleeding tendency in some cases, and these levels should be checked (Bolton-Maggs et al, 1995). The development of inhibitory antibodies has been described in congenitally deficient patients who have received blood products, as well as in other previously normal patients (Reece et al, 1984; Schnall et al, 1987).

Treatment

It is often possible to control bleeding in association with dental surgery with tranexamic acid alone, even in severely affected patients (Berliner et al, 1992). A heat-treated, plasma-derived concentrate of factor XI is available (Factor XI, Bio Products Laboratory) (Bolton-Maggs et al, 1992). This is an unlicensed product, and is available only on a named-patient basis. The half-life of the infused factor XI is approximately 50 hours. This should be used in patients with a definite bleeding history and severe deficiency undergoing surgery. It is of particular value in major surgery or when fibrinolysis is a particular problem (e.g. tonsillectomy, prostatectomy). Despite the fact that the concentrate contains a small amount of both heparin and antithrombin III, isolated instances of thromboembolism have been reported following repeated infusions of the concentrate, usually in the setting of surgery (Bolton-Maggs et al, 1994; Mannucci et al,

1994). The risk of thromboembolism appears to be higher in elderly subjects, and those with a history of cardiovascular disease. Factor XI concentrate should be reserved for use in patients with severe factor XI deficiency only. Haemostasis is achieved with levels of around 70% and particular care should be taken to ensure that the peak post-infusion level does not rise above 100%. It is recommended that the initial dose of concentrate should not exceed 30 iu/kg body weight. Patients with only mild deficiency or who are felt to be at risk of thromboembolic sequelae should be treated with fresh frozen plasma. Cryoprecipitate does not contain factor XI, and is of no value.

Factor XII Deficiency

Biochemistry

Factor XII is also known as Hageman factor, after the first patient with this defect to be studied (Ratnoff and Colopy, 1955). Factor XII is a plasma single-chain glycoprotein of molecular weight 80 kD. It is encoded on chromosome 5 and synthesized in the liver. Factor XII may be activated in vitro by contact with negatively charged surfaces, although kallikrein is probably the principal enzyme responsible for activation in vivo. Factor XII is activated after being cleaved by kallikrein into heavy (52 kD) and light (28 kD) chains held together by a single disulphide bridge. Activated factor XII converts factor XI into its active form, which in turn activates factor IX in the intrinsic coagulation cascade.

Clinical and laboratory features

The prothrombin and thrombin times are normal. The APTT is prolonged, often markedly so. However, isolated factor XII deficiency is not associated with a bleeding tendency. Indeed, complete deficiency of factor XII appears to be associated with a modest thrombotic tendency and it is of note that the original patient described with factor XII deficiency did not have a bleeding tendency but died of pulmonary embolism (Ratnoff et al, 1968; Lämmle et al, 1991; von Känel et al, 1992). Factor XII deficiency has been reported in (presumably fortuitous) association with significant haemorrhagic disorders such as von Willebrand's disease (Cramer et al, 1976). It is thus important to exclude concomitant deficiencies of other significant coagulation factors, particularly if there is a suggestive history, which could be masked by the greatly prolonged APTT due to factor XII deficiency.

Treatment

Patients with isolated factor XII deficiency are not at risk of bleeding, even in the setting of surgery. There is absolutely no need to cover such procedures by administration of blood products.

Factor XII deficiency does not confer protection against thrombosis. Despite the prolonged APTT, individuals with factor XII deficiency may be treated with anticoagulants if such treatment is deemed necessary, e.g. heparin prophylaxis to cover surgery. Of course, the International Normalized Ratio (INR) may be used to monitor warfarin therapy in factor XII deficient individuals as the baseline prothrombin time is normal.

Factor XIII Deficiency

Biochemistry

Fibrin monomers produced by the action of thrombin upon fibrinogen are bound merely by hydrophobic bonds. The initial fibrin clot is subsequently stabilized by factor XIII, a transglutaminase enzyme which forges covalent bonds between adjacent strands of monomeric fibrin. Factor XIII is found in plasma as a 320 kD tetramer composed of two 75 kD "a" subunits linked non-covalently to two 80 kD "b" subunits (Schwartz et al, 1973). The "a" subunit is encoded on chromosome 6 and is synthesized in the liver. The "b" subunit is encoded on chromosome 1 and is not synthesized in the liver, but principally by macrophages. Factor XIII is activated by thrombin in a calcium-dependent reaction, resulting in dissociation of the "b" subunits and the cleavage of activation peptides from the active "a" subunits. The "a" subunit is responsible for forging covalent bounds between lysine and glutamine residues of adjacent gamma chains of monomeric fibrin strands which results in greatly enhanced clot stability. The precise role of the "b" subunit is unclear, but it appears to function merely as a carrier for the active "a" subunit. The relative importance of the "a" subunit is emphasized by the fact that in the great majority of clinical cases of factor XII deficiency, only the "a" subunit is found to be functionally abnormal, but a bleeding disorder due to deficiency of "b" subunits has been described (Saito et al, 1990).

Clinical and laboratory features

Factor XIII deficiency is an extremely rare disorder, with an estimated prevalence of only 1 in 5 million individuals. The disorder is inherited as an autosomal recessive trait, and so females as well as males are affected. There is often a history of parental consanguinity. Factor XIII deficiency results in a life-long bleeding tendency in homozygotes, and this is associated with poor wound healing (Duckert et al, 1960; Lorand et al, 1980). Typically, a clot appears to form normally after injury or surgery but this soon breaks down and further bleeding occurs. Such cycles may be repeated at the same site of injury for weeks or months, and unsightly scars may form. Easy bruising, prolonged bleeding from superficial wounds and poor wound healing are common features. A common early manifestation is bleeding from the umbilical stump. Spontaneous bleeding from mucosal surfaces and into joints are not typical clinical features. However, there is a high risk of intracranial haemorrhage associated with this disorder. This complication often arises spontaneously and without any history of previous head injury. Recurrent spontaneous abortion has been reported in affected females (Kitchen and Newcomb, 1979). An acquired form of factor XIII deficiency due to the development of inhibitory antibodies has been reported. In several of the published cases there was an association with isoniazid therapy (Lorand et al, 1968; Graham et al, 1973; Otis et al, 1974).

All the basic laboratory investigations are completely normal, including the bleeding time, prothrombin time, thrombin time and APTT. A simple screening test for the disorder involves assessing clot solubility in either 5M urea or 1% monochloroacetic acid. Normal fibrin clot remains insoluble after incubation with either reagent for up to 8 hours, but in factor XIII deficiency the clot is unstable and dissolves within a few hours. Quantitative assay is now possible by radioassay measuring the incorporation of radiolabelled putrescine into dimethylated casein, and a chromogenic assay has recently become available.

Treatment

Plasma-derived concentrates of factor XIII are now available (Factor XIII, Bio Products Laboratory; Fibrogammin, Centeon) (Winkelman et al, 1986; Daly and Haddon, 1988) Low plasma levels of factor XIII confer protection against bleeding episodes, including intracranial haemorrhage, and the half-life of factor XIII is of the order of 10 days. For these reasons, it is recommended that patients with factor XIII deficiency should receive prophylactic infusions of factor XIII (50–75 units/kg) at monthly intervals. The interval between infusions should be shortened if there are episodes of "break-through" bleeding. Surgical procedures may be covered with a single infusion of concentrate (50–70 units/kg immediately before surgery) in view of the long half-life of the product. Cryoprecipitate is also rich in factor XIII, and could be used when concentrate is not available.

α_2-Antiplasmin Deficiency

Biochemistry

α_2-Antiplasmin was identified in 1976 as the principal inhibitor of plasmin (Collen, 1976). It is a single-chain glycoprotein of molecular weight 70 kD. It is a serpin and shows sequence homology to other members of this group such as antithrombin III. The gene is encoded on chromosome 7 and the molecule is synthesized in hepatocytes. α_2-Antiplasmin binds with high affinity to circulating plasmin, which it inactivates. It also promotes clot stability by binding to fibrin during coagulation, in a reaction promoted by factor XIII, where it also inactivates α_2-antiplasmin bound to fibrin.

Clinical and laboratory features

A bleeding disorder attributable to congenital deficiency of α_2-antiplasmin was first reported in 1978 (Koie et al, 1978; Aoki et al, 1979). It is a very rare condition, inherited as an autosomal recessive trait. Parental consanguinity has been noted in several cases. Typical features include prolonged bleeding, epistaxis and bruising after minor trauma, and haemarthroses have also been reported (Stormorken et al, 1983).

The prothrombin time, APTT and thrombin time are all normal as are the bleeding time, platelet count and fibrinogen level. A typical laboratory finding is a marked shortening of the whole blood clot lysis time. The euglobulin clot lysis time is also shortened, but less markedly so as α_2-antiplasmin does not precipitate in the euglobulin fraction. Both functional and immunological assays for α_2-antiplasmin have been developed which permit the identification of this rare disorder. It should be borne in mind that liver disease may also result in a significant reduction in the plasma level of α_2-antiplasmin. The plasma level may also be low in conditions associated with increased consumption, such as disseminated intravascular coagulation. This can be distinguished from primary deficiency by the detection of plasmin–α_2-antiplasmin complexes in the circulation.

Treatment

This is a rare disorder, and there are few published case reports on which to base advice on management of bleeding episodes in these patients. Fresh frozen plasma is a good source of α_2-antiplasmin, which has a half-life of 3 days. Tranexamic acid could theoretically be of value, and was observed to reduce the incidence of spontaneous haemarthroses in the original case report (Koie et al, 1978).

References

Aoki N, Saito H, Kamiya T, Koie K, Sakata Y, Kohahura M. Congenital deficiency of α_2-plasmin inhibitor associated with severe hemorrhagic tendency. *Journal of Clinical Investigation* 1979; **63:** 877–884.

Berliner S, Horowitz I, Martinowitz U, Brenner, Seligsohn U. Dental surgery in patients with severe factor XI deficiency without plasma replacement. *Blood Coagulation and Fibrinolysis* 1992; **3:** 465–468.

Bolton-Maggs PHB, Wan-Yin BY, McCraw AH, Slack J, Kernoff PBA. Inheritance and bleeding in factor XI deficiency. *British Journal of Haematology* 1988; **69:** 521–528.

Bolton-Maggs PHB, Wensley RT, Kernoff PBA, et al. Production and therapeutic use of a factor XI concentrate from plasma. *Thrombosis and Haemostasis* 1992; **67:** 314–317.

Bolton-Maggs PHB, Colvin BT, Satchi G, Lee CA, Lucas GS. Thrombogenic potential of factor XI concentrate. *Lancet* 1994; **344:** 748–749.

Bolton-Maggs PHB, Patterson DA, Wensley RT, Tuddenham EGD. Definition of the bleeding tendency in factor XI-deficient kindreds – a clinical and laboratory study. *Thrombosis and Haemostasis* 1995; **73:** 194–202.

Borchgrevink CF, Owren PA. The hemostatic effect of normal platelets in haemophilia and factor V deficiency. *Acta Medica Scandinavica* 1961; **170:** 375–383.

Broze GJ, Galiani D. The role of factor XI in coagulation. *Thrombosis and Haemostasis* 1993; **70:** 72–74.

Broze GJ, Miletich JP. Characterization of the inhibitor of tissue factor in plasma. *Blood* 1987; **69:** 150–155.

Broze GJ, Girard TJ, Novotny WF. Regulation of coagulation by a multivalent Kunitz-type inhibitor. *Biochemistry* 1990; **29:** 7539–7546.

Cattaneo M, Bettega D, Lombardi R, Lecchi A, Mannucci PM. Sustained correction of the bleeding time in an afibrinogenaemic patient after infusion of fresh frozen plasma. *British Journal of Haematology* 1992; **82:** 388–390.

Chediak J, Ashenhurst JB, Garlick I, Desser RK. Successful management of bleeding in a patient with factor V inhibitor by platelet transfusions. *Blood* 1980; **56:** 835–841.

Collen D. Identification and some properties of a new fast-acting plasmin inhibitor in human plasma. *European Journal of Biochemistry* 1976; **69:** 209–216.

Cramer AD, Melaragno AJ, Phifer SJ, Hougie C. von Willebrand's disease San Diego, a new variant. *Lancet* 1976; **ii:** 12–14.

Crowell EB. Observations on a factor-V inhibitor. *British Journal of Haematology* 1975; **29:** 397–404.

Dahlback B, Carlsson M, Svensson PJ. Familial thrombophilia due to a previously unrecognized mechanism characterized by poor anticoagulant response to activated protein C. *Proceedings of the National Academy of Sciences USA* 1993; **90:** 1004–1008.

Daly HM, Haddon ME. Clinical experience with a pasteurized human plasma concentrate in factor XIII deficiency. *Thrombosis and Haemostasis* 1988; **59:** 171–174.

Denson KWE, Lurie A, De Cataldo F, Mannucci PM. The factor X defect: recognition of abnormal forms of factor X. *British Journal of Haematology* 1970; **18:** 317–327.

Denson KWE, Borrett R, Biggs R. The specific assay of prothrombin using Taipan snake venom. *British Journal of Haematology* 1971; **21:** 219–226.

Duckert F, Jung E, Schmerling DH. Hitherto undescribed congenital haemorrhagic diathesis probably due to fibrin stabilising factor deficiency. *Thrombosis et Diathesis Haemorrhagica* 1960; **5:** 179–186.

Ebert RF (Ed.) *Index of Variant Human Fibrinogens*. Boca Raton: CRC Press, 1991.

Feinstein DI, Rapaport SI, McGehee WG, Patch MJ. Factor V anticoagulants: clinical, biochemical, and immunological observations. *Journal of Clinical Investigation* 1970; **49:** 1578–1588.

Furie B, Voo L, McAdam KPWJ, Furie BC. Mechanism of factor X deficiency in systemic amyloidosis. *New England Journal of Medicine* 1981; **304:** 827–830.

Girolami A, Molaro G, Lazzarin M, Scarpa R, Brunetti A. A new congenital haemorrhagic condition due to the presence of an abnormal factor X (factor X_{Friuli}). Study of a large kindred. *British Journal of Haematology* 1970; **19:** 179–192.

Girolami A, Vicarioto M, Ruzza G, Cappelato G, Vergolani A. Factor X_{Padua}: a 'new' congenital factor X abnormality with a defect only in the extrinsic system. *Acta Haematologica* 1985; **73:** 431–436.
Gjonnæss H. Cold promoted activation of factor VII. *Thrombosis et Diathesis Haemorrhagica* 1972; **28:** 155–205.
Graham JE, Yount WJ, Roberts HR. Immunochemical characterization of a human antibody to factor XIII. *Blood* 1973; **41:** 661–669.
Grech H, Majumdar G, Lawrie AS, Savidge GF. Pregnancy in congenital afibrinogenaemia: report of a successful case and a review of the literature. *British Journal of Haematology* 1991; **78:** 571–582.
Hancock JF, Wieland K, Pugh RE, et al. A molecular genetic study of factor XI deficiency. *Blood* 1991; **77:** 1942–1948.
Hougie C, Barrow HM, Graham JB. Stuart clotting defect. Segregation of a hereditary hemorrhagic state from the heterozygous heretofore called 'stable factor' (SPCA, proconvertin factor VII) deficiency. *Journal of Clinical Investigation* 1957; **36:** 485–493.
Hultin MB, Eyster ME. Combined factor V/VIII deficiency: a case report with studies of factor V and VIII activation by thrombin. *Blood* 1981; **58:** 983–985.
Kitchen CS, Newcomb TF. Factor XIII. *Medicine* 1979; **58:** 413–429.
Koie K, Ogata K, Kamiya T, Takamatsu J, Kohakura M. Alpha-2-plasmin inhibitor deficiency (Miyasoto disease). *Lancet* 1978; **ii:** 1334–1336.
Lämmle B, Wuillemin WA, Huber I et al. Thromboembolism and bleeding tendency in congenital factor XII deficiency–a study on 74 subjects from 14 Swiss families. *Thrombosis and Haemostasis* 1991; **65:** 117–121.
Landwehr G, Lang H, Alexander B. Congenital hypoprothrombinemia: a case study with particular reference to the role of non-prothrombin factors in the conversion of prothrombin. *American Journal of Medicine* 1950; **8:** 255–261.
Lorand L, Jacobsen A, Bruner-Lorand J. A pathological inhibitor of fibrin cross-linking. *Journal of Clinical Investigation* 1968; **47:** 268–273.
Lorand L, Losowsky MS, Miloszewski KJM. Human factor XIII: fibrin-stabilizing factor. *Progress in Hemostasis and Thrombosis* 1980; **5:** 245–290.
Mannucci PM, Bauer KA, Santagostino E, et al. Activation of the coagulation cascade after infusion of a factor XI concentrate in congenitally deficient patients. *Blood* 1994; **84:** 1314–1319.
Marder VJ, Schulman NR. Clinical aspects of congenital factor VII deficiency. *American Journal of Medicine* 1964; **37:** 182–194.
Melliger EJ, Duckert F. Major surgery in a subject with factor V deficiency: cholecystectomy in a parahaemophilic woman and review of the literature. *Thrombosis and Haemostasis* 1971; **25:** 438–446.
Miletich JP, Majerus DW, Majerus PW. Patients with congenital factor V deficiency have decreased factor X_a binding sites on their platelets. *Journal of Clinical Investigation* 1978; **62:** 824–831.
Otis PT, Feinstein DI, Rapaport SI, Patch MJ. An acquired inhibitor of fibrin stabilization associated with isoniazid therapy: clinical and biochemical observations. *Blood* 1974; **44:** 771–781.
Owren PA. Parahaemophilia. Haemorrhagic diathesis due to absence of a previously unknown clotting factor. *Lancet* 1947; **i:** 446–448.
Poggio M, Tripodi A, Mariani G, Mannucci PM. Factor VII clotting assay: influence of different thromboplastins and factor VII-deficient plasmas. *Thrombosis and Haemostasis* 1991; **65:** 160–164.
Pugh RE, McVey JH, Tuddenham EGD, Hancock JF. Six point mutations that cause factor XI deficiency. *Blood* 1995; **85:** 1509–1516.
Ragni MV, Lewis JH, Spero JA, Hasiba U. Factor VII deficiency. *American Journal of Hematology* 1981; **10:** 79–88.
Rao LVM, Rapaport SI. Activation of factor VII bound to tissue factor: a key step in the tissue factor pathway of blood coagulation. *Proceedings of the National Academy of Sciences USA* 1988; **84:** 6687–6691.
Ratnoff OD, Colopy JE. A familial hemorrhagic trait associated with a deficiency of a clot-promoting fraction of plasma. *Journal of Clinical Investigation* 1955; **34:** 602–613.
Ratnoff OD, Busse RJ, Sheon RP. The demise of John Hageman. *New England Journal of Medicine* 1968; **279:** 760–761.

Reece EA, Clyne LP, Romero R, Hobbins JC. Spontaneous factor XI inhibitors. Seven additional cases and a review of the literature. *Archives of Internal Medicine* 1984; **144:** 525–559.

Rosing J, Tans G. Inventory of exogenous prothrombin activators. *Thrombosis and Haemostasis* 1991; **65:** 627–630.

Saito M, Asakura H, Yoshida T, et al. A familial factor XIII subunit B deficiency. *British Journal of Haematology* 1990; **74:** 290–294.

Schnall SF, Duffy TP, Clyne LP. Acquired factor XI inhibitors in congenitally deficient patients. *American Journal of Hematology* 1987; **26:** 323–328.

Schwartz ML, Pizzo SV, Hill RL, McKee PA. Human factor XIII from plasma and platelets. *Journal of Biological Chemistry* 1973; **248:** 1395–1407.

Seeler RA. Parahemophilia: factor V deficiency. *Medical Clinics of North America* 1972; **56:** 119–125.

Seligsohn U. Factor X deficiency. *Thrombosis and Haemostasis* 1993; **70:** 68–71.

Soff GA, Levin J. Familial multiple coagulation factor deficiencies. *Seminars in Thrombosis and Haemostasis* 1981; **7:** 112–148.

Solano C, Cobcroft RG, Scott DC. Prediction of vitamin K response using the Echis time and Echis-prothrombin time ratio. *Thrombosis and Haemostasis* 1990; **64:** 353–357.

Stormorken H, Gogstad GO, Brosstad F. Hereditary α_2 antiplasmin deficiency. *Thrombosis Research* 1983; **31:** 647–651.

Telfer TP, Denson KW, Wright DR. A 'new' coagulation defect. *British Journal of Haematology* 1956; **2:** 308–316.

Tracy PB, Eide LL, Bowie EJ, Mann KG. Radioimmunoassay of factor V in human plasma and platelets. *Blood* 1982; **60:** 59–63.

Tracy PB, Giles AR, Mann KG, et al. Factor V (Quebec): a bleeding diathesis associated with a qualitative platelet factor V deficiency. *Journal of Clinical Investigation* 1984; **74:** 1221–1228.

Triplett DA, Brandt JT, Batard MA, Dixon JLS, Fair DS. Hereditary factor VII deficiency: heterogeneity defined by combined functional and immunochemical analysis. *Blood* 1985; **66:** 1284–1287.

von Känel R, Wuillemin WA, Furlan M, Lämmle B. Factor XII clotting activity and antigen levels in patients with thromboembolic disease. *Blood Coagulation and Fibrinolysis* 1992; **3:** 555–561.

Winkelman L, Sims GE, Haddon ME, Evans DR, Smith JK. A pasteurized concentrate of human plasma factor XIII for therapeutic use. *Thrombosis and Haemostasis* 1986; **55:** 402–405.

Zehnder JL, Leung LLK. Development of antibodies to thrombin and factor V with recurrent bleeding in a patient exposed to topical bovine thrombin. *Blood* 1990; **76:** 2011–2016.

Complications of Replacement Therapy: Transfusion-transmitted Disease

10

CHRISTINE A. LEE

Human Immunodeficiency Virus (HIV)

The history of the epidemic in haemophilia

The first cases of acquired immune deficiency syndrome (AIDS) in haemophilic patients were reported in 1982 (Centers for Disease Control, 1982). In the UK the first reported seroconversion to HIV occurred in October 1979 following infusion with concentrate of American source plasma in August 1979 (Lee et al, 1990). In a well-studied cohort of haemophilic patients in London the dates of seroconversion were between 1979 and 1985 (Fig. 10.1) It is likely that in the USA seroconversions occurred a year earlier (Eyster, et al 1987) and overall in the world there were some late seroconversions occurring in 1986 following treatment with early heated concentrate. The advent of virally inactivated therapeutic materials has successfully prevented further transmission of HIV infection and no new cases following transfusion of sterilized clotting factor concentrate have been reported since 1986 (Mannucci, 1996). AIDS has significantly changed the life expectancy for individuals with haemophilia (Chorba et al, 1994; Darby et al, 1995). Chorba et al examined recent changes in longevity and the cause of death among patients with haemophilia A in the USA between 1968 and 1989 when there were 2792 deaths reported. The death rate increased from 0.5 to 1.3 per 1 000 000 deaths reported. The median age at death decreased from 57 years in 1979–1981 to 40 years in 1987–1989 (Fig. 10.2). A similar study in patients on the UK haemophilia Directors Registry by Darby *et al* showed that among 1227 individuals infected between 1979 and 1986, the death rate rose steeply from 8 per 1000 in 1985–1992 in seronegative individuals, reaching 81 per 1000 in 1991–1992 in seropositive individuals (Fig.10.3). Patients with haemophilia have provided, and will continue to provide, information about the natural history of HIV infection because the time of seroconversion is known,

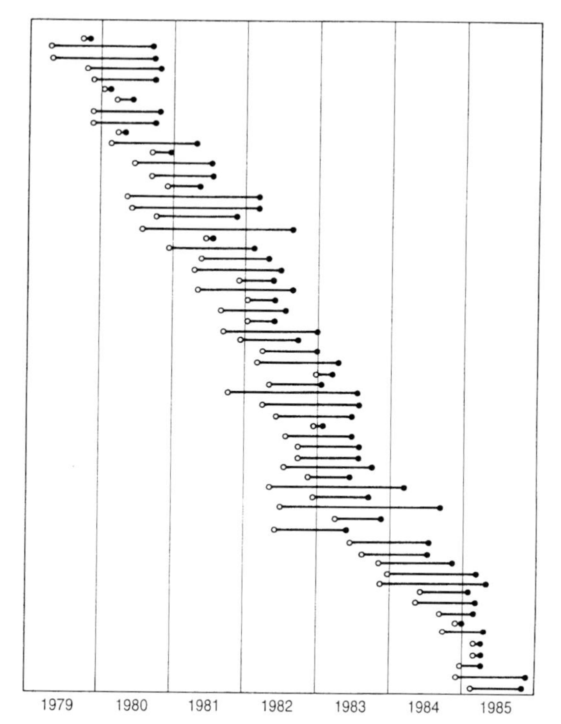

Figure 10.1 Dates of seroconversion of 63 haemophiliacs. ○, anti-HIV negative serum; ●, anti-HIV positive serum. (Reproduced, with permission, from HIV infection in Haemophilia. Far East Symposium Series, No. 44, 1991, p. 2. Excerpta Medica, Elsevier Company.)

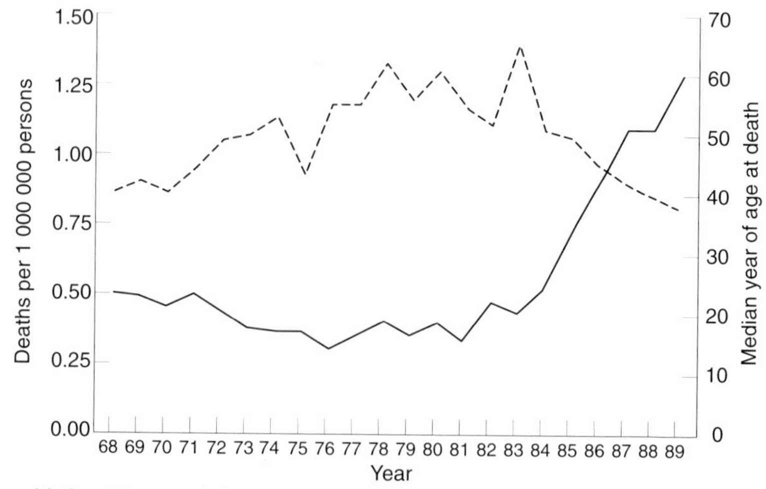

Figure 10.2 Haemophilia A death rates (——) and median age at death (········) by year, United States, 1968–1989. (Reproduced, with permission, from *Clinical Haematology* 1996, **9**, 370.)

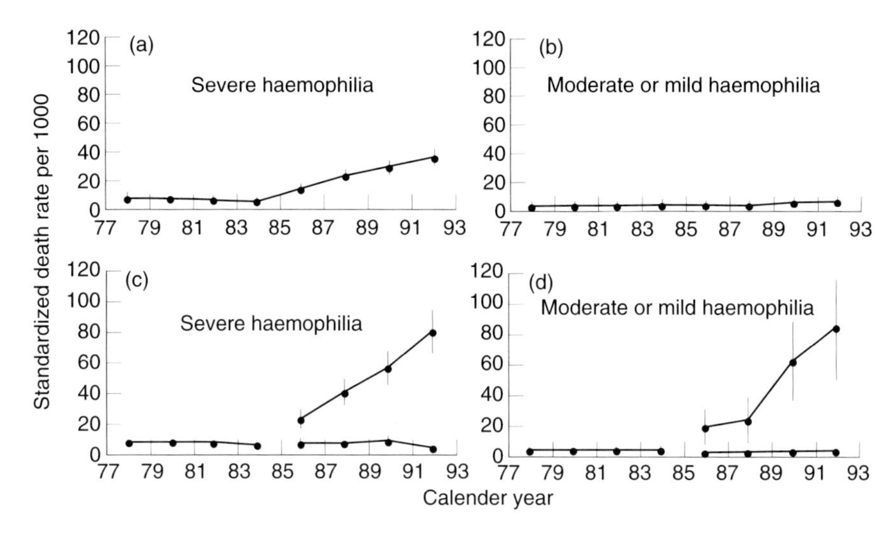

Figure 10.3 Annual death rates per 100 in patients with haemophilia in the UK. –△–, all patients; –□–, HIV positive; –■–, HIV negative. (Reproduced, with permission, from *Clinical Haematology* 1996; **9**: 370).

the age at seroconversion is wide and, because of their haemophilia, patients are under regular follow-up.

CD4 counts are related to disease progression

The relationship between the CD4 count and time since seroconversion is shown in Fig. 10.4. A linear regression model showed a slope of –85 cells/μl/year. In a study of 111 patients followed 11 years from seroconversion, progress to AIDS could largely be explained by differences in rates of decline of CD4 lymphocyte counts (Fig. 10.5) (Phillips et al, 1991a).

The percentages of patients with slopes within a given range are shown in Fig. 10.6. Only 6% of patients had slopes around zero and none of them developed AIDS. Most patients (94%) had negative slopes. AIDS was more common among patients with steeper negative slopes (Fig. 10.5). To assess the strength of the relation between the CD4 count and the progression to AIDS, a simple model has been proposed for the natural history of HIV infection. Since it has been observed that AIDS developed in 50% of untreated patients before the CD4 count falls to 50, in this model it was assumed that the decline in CD4 count is near linear and that when a count of 50 is reached the patient manifests AIDS (Phillips et al, 1989). By fitting a straight line to the CD4 counts of each patient and calculating when the line would cross the count of 50 it could be estimated when the patient would get AIDS. In this way it was possible to classify correctly 84% of patients. It has thus been possible to

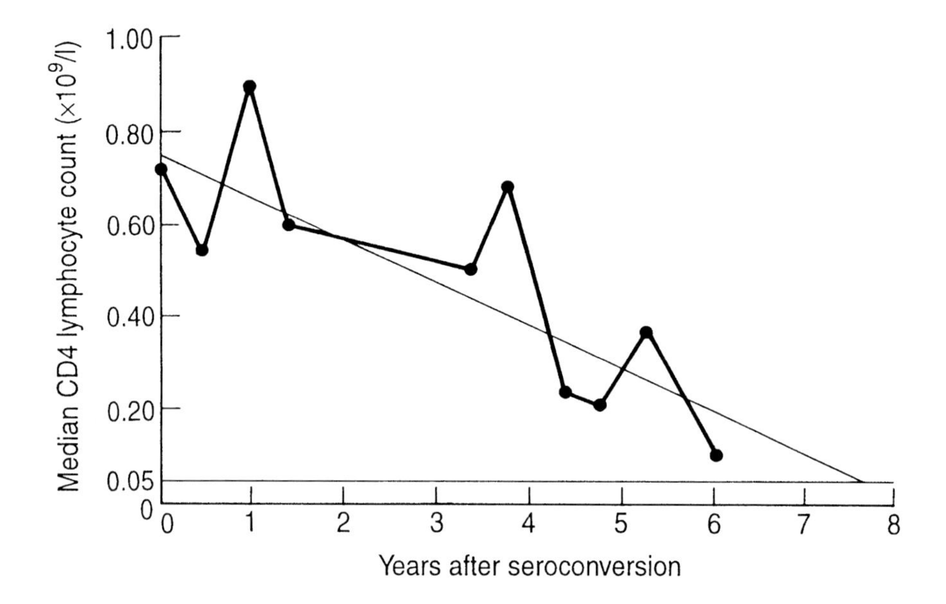

Figure 10.4 Serial CD4 lymphocyte counts over time since seroconversion for one HIV-infected patient. Root mean-square-error fitted about slope = 0.16 $\times 10^9$/l. (Reproduced, with permission, from Phillips AN, Lee CA, Elford J, et al. Serial CD4 lymphocyte counts and development of AIDS. *Lancet* 1991; **337**: 389.)

estimate that at least a quarter of individuals will remain AIDS-free 20 years from seroconversion (Phillips et al, 1994).

The effect of age

It was shown by Eyster et al, in 1987 that older age at the time of seroconversion was associated with an increased risk for AIDS in haemophilic patients (Fig. 10.7). Many other studies in haemophilic patients have confirmed these findings (Darby et al, 1989; Goedert et al, 1989; Lee et al, 1989; Ragni et al, 1990). A large study in the total UK population of patients with haemophilia has shown this effect persists over a long timescale (Darby et al, 1989) (Fig. 10.8). In order to understand the significance of changes in CD4 count during HIV infection amongst patients of different ages, the CD4 count by age should be appreciated in anti-HIV negative haemophilic patients (Fig. 10.9). When the mean CD4 count by years from seroconversion according to four age categories is plotted (Fig. 10.10) after the age of 10 years the decline of the CD4 count is the same in all three age groups. After adjustment for the CD4 count the relative risk of developing AIDS for each 10-year increase in age is 1.31 (confidence interval (CI) 1.03,1.67; $p < 0.05$) Thus older patients

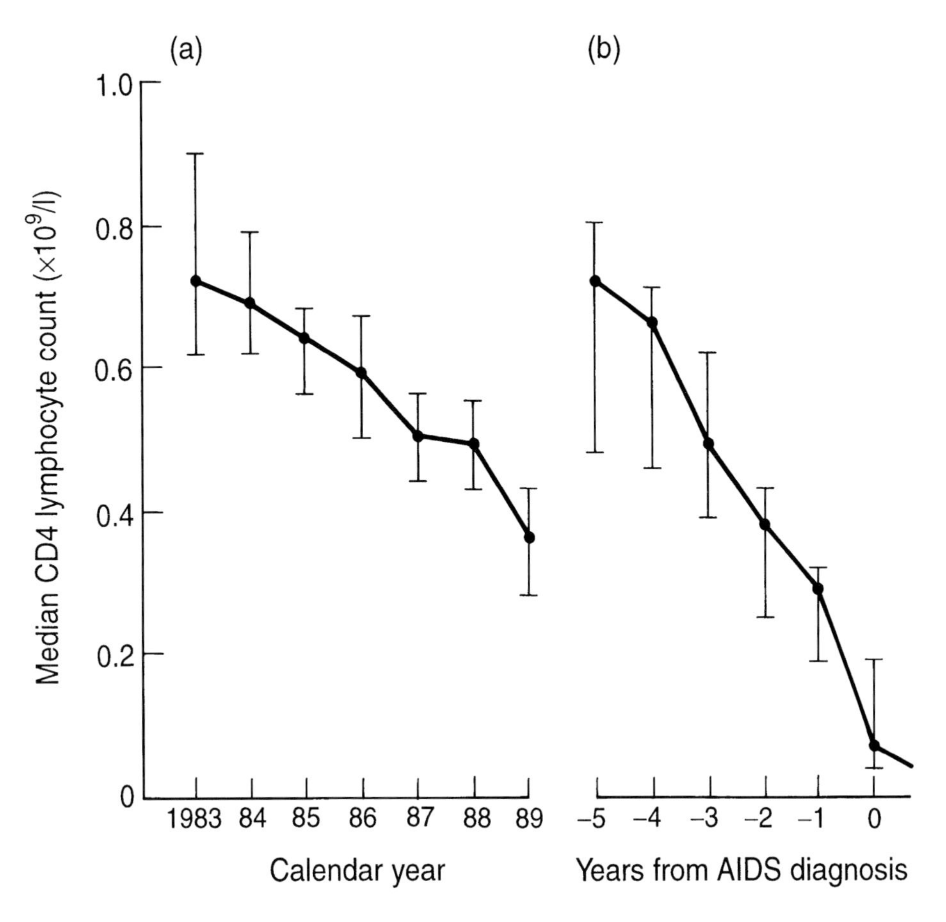

Figure 10.5 Median CD4 lymphocyte count (with 95% confidence intervals). (a) Patients AIDS-free at 1 January 1990; (b) patients with AIDS by 1 January 1990. (Reproduced, with permission, from Phillips AN, Lee CA, Elford J, et al. Serial CD4 lymphocyte counts and development of AIDS. *Lancet* 1991; **337**: 389.)

are at higher risk of progression to AIDS than their younger counterparts even if the CD4 count is the same (Phillips et al, 1991c).

P24 antigenaemia

Allain et al in 1987 reported a study of 96 haemophilic patients and showed that the decline of p24 antibody and the appearance of HIV antigen are predictive of HIV-related clinical complications including AIDS. In another study of 88 haemophilic patients a high titre of p24 antibody response at seroconversion was

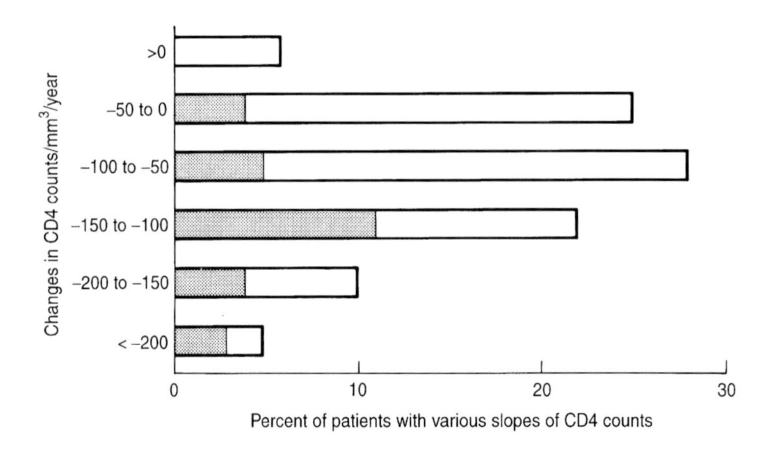

Figure 10.6 The percentages of patients with CD4 slope within a given range. ■, with AIDS; □, without AIDS. (Reproduced, with permission, from Janossy G, et al (Eds) *Immunodeficiency in HIV Infection and AIDS*. Basel: S Karger AG).

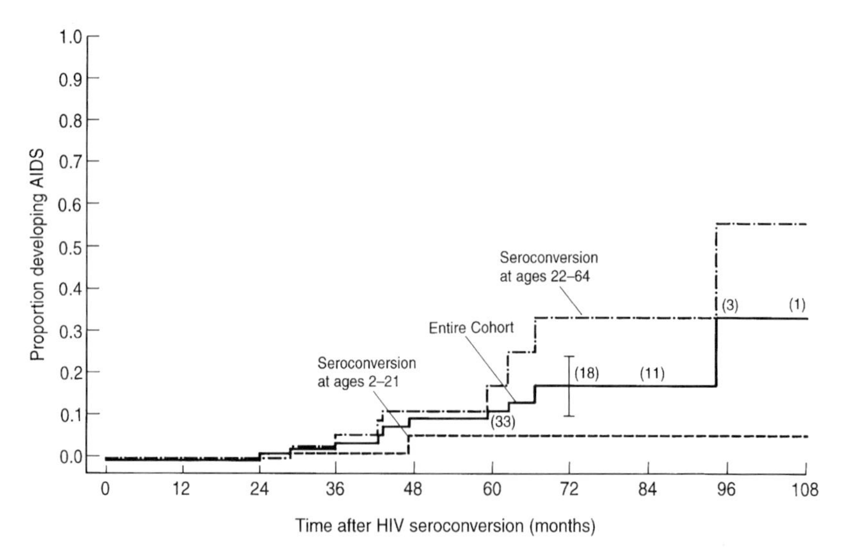

Figure 10.7 Actuarial incidence of AIDS in 84 haemophiliacs who developed antibodies to HIV. Data are computed according to the Kaplan–Meier survival curve technique, with each individual patient's seroconversion date (midpoint between last seronegative and first seropositive specimens) being used as time 0. Numbers in parentheses indicate number of patients still being followed at years 5 to 9 after seroconversion. Vertical bar at 72 months indicates ±1 SE. (Reproduced, with permission, from Eyster ME, Gail MH, Ballard JO, et al. Natural history of HIV infections in haemophiliacs: effects of T-cell subsets platelet counts and age. *Annals of Internal Medicine* 1987; **107**: 1).

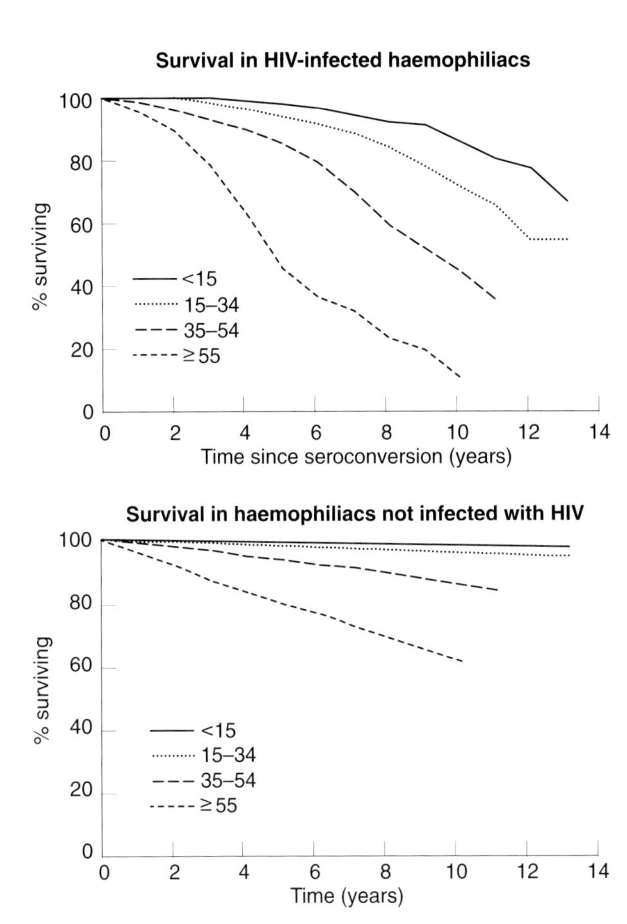

Figure 10.8 Survival in HIV-infected seropositive haemophilic patients by age at seroconversion and expected survival based on mortality rates for uninfected patients subdivided by age. Within each age-at-seroconversion group estimates are censored when fewer than five HIV-seropositives remain at risk. (Reproduced, with permission, from *Lancet* 1996; **347**: 1575).

associated with a longer time to the development of HIV related disease. In contrast higher titres of gp120 at seroconversion correlated with more rapid clinical deterioration (Cheingsong-Popov et al, 1991). The significance of this study is that it would suggest the possibility of post exposure immunotherapy with a p24 construct to boost the p24 antibody response. Several studies have shown in patients with haemophilia that the presence of p24 antigenaemia is associated with a markedly increased risk of progression to AIDS (Allain et al, 1987; Eyster et al, 1989; Goedert et al, 1989). In a cohort of haemophilic patients in London (Phillips et al, 1991b), p24 antigenaemic patients were more likely to develop

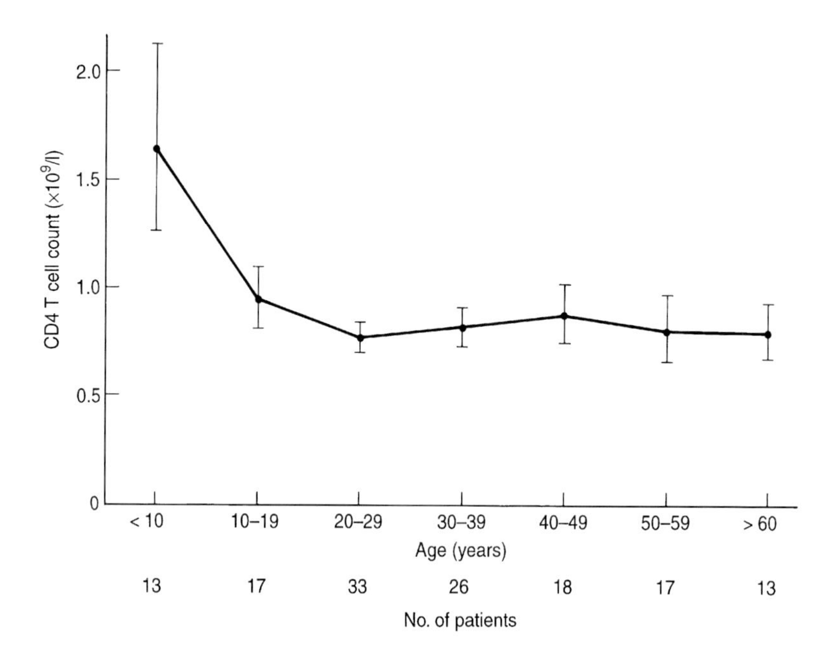

Figure 10.9 Geometric mean (and 95% confidence limits) CD4+ T-cell count by age for 137 anti-HIV-negative haemophiliacs. (Reproduced, with permission, from Phillips AN, Lee CA, Elford J, et al. More rapid progression to AIDS in older HIV-infected people: the role of CD4+ T-cell counts. *Journal of Acquired Immune Deficiency Syndromes* 1991; **4**: 970.)

AIDS (Table 10.1). However p24 positive patients were also more likely to be older and cytomegalovirus (CMV) positive. When the relative risk for development of AIDS was calculated in p24-positive individuals, it was 5.42 even after adjustment for age and CMV (Table 10.2). It was found that CD4 lymphocyte counts declined more rapidly in p24 positive patients than in p24 negative patients (Fig. 10.11). Since detectable p24 antigenaemia is probably a marker for increased viral load, the major part of the pathological effect of increased viral replication is mediated through a progressive decrease in CD4 lymphocyte count. Therefore anti-HIV therapy should be introduced earlier in p24 positive individuals.

The introduction of viral load measurements into clinical practice has enabled an assessment of the long-term incidence of AIDS in relation to HIV-1 RNA levels measured early in HIV-1 infection. HIV-1 RNA levels measured 12–36 months from seroconversion showed higher levels in older haemophilic patients and 10 years from seroconversion and were a strong age-independent predictor of clinical outcome, low levels defining individuals with a high probability of long-term AIDS-free survival (Mellors et al, 1996; O'Brien et al, 1996) (Fig. 10.12).

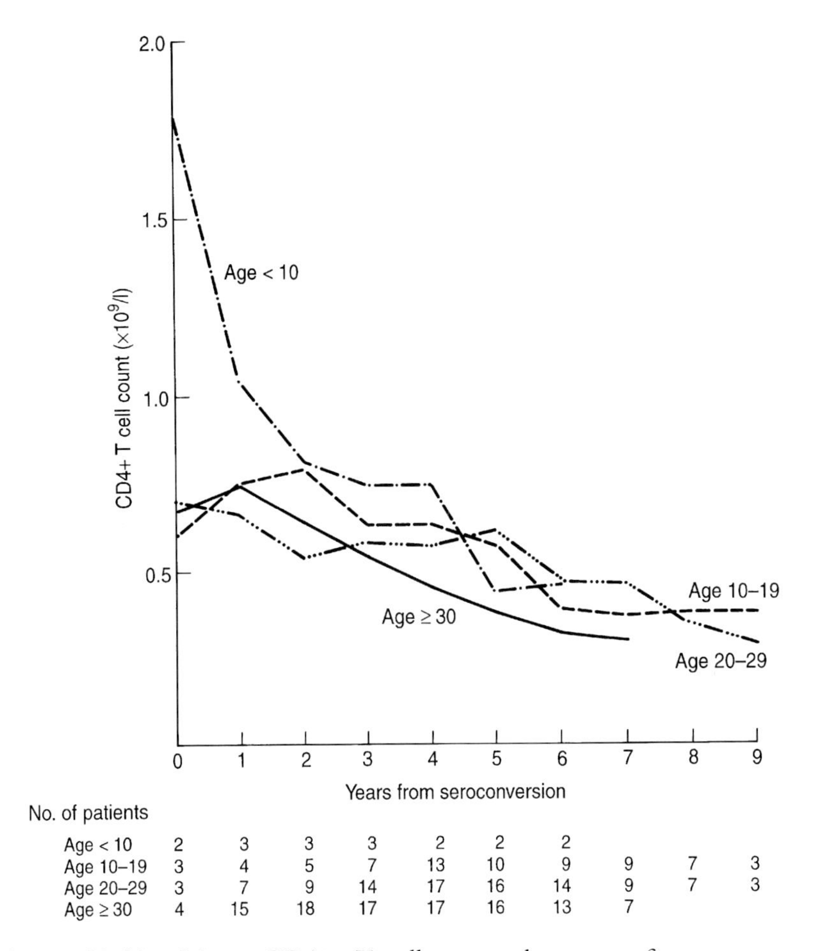

Figure 10.10 Mean CD4+ T-cell count by years from seroconversion, according to four age categories. The patients included at any time point after seroconversion are those for whom CD4+ T-cell counts were available before and after that point. The count at the time point was estimated by linear interpolation. The numbers beneath indicate the number of patients involved for each point estimate. (Reproduced, with permission, from Phillips AN, Lee CA, Elford J, et al. More rapid progression to AIDS in older HIV-infected people: the role of CD4+ T-cell counts. *Journal of Acquired Immune Deficiency Syndrome* 1991; **4**: 970.)

Early predictors of disease progression

Markers of immune function present before infection may determine the subsequent course of disease in HIV-infected individuals. The HLA haplotype A1 B8 DR3 was first shown by Steel et al, in 1988 to distinguish which individuals

Table 10.1 Classification of patients according to whether or not p24 antigen was detected in serum during the follow-up and whether AIDS developed

	p24 antigenemia		
AIDS	Yes	No	Total
Yes	16	17	33
No	11	67	78
Total	27	84	111

(Reproduced, with permission, from Phillips et al, 1991).

Table 10.2 Relative risk associated with the presence of p24 antigenaemia estimated from a Cox proportional hazards model with p24 antigen status fitted as a time-dependent covariate. Adjustment is made for age, cytomegalovirus (CMV) serostatus and CD4 lymphocyte count, also fitted as a time-dependent covariate

	After adjustment for:		
Unadjusted	Age	Age and CMV	Age, CMV and CD4 lymphocyte count
7.24 ($p < 0.0001$)	6.11 ($p < 0.0001$)	5.42 ($p < 0.0001$)	1.97 ($p = 0.2$)

(Reproduced, with permission, from Phillips et al, 1991).

amongst the 18 haemophilic patients in Edinburgh who were infected with HIV would progress to AIDS. In a study of French haemophiliacs progression to AIDS was associated with HLA-B35 (Sahmoud et al, 1993). Thus the pathogenesis of HIV disease is strongly related to the nature and degree of the host immune response. In a study where CD8 counts and IgA levels were measured soon after seroconversion, while the CD4 count remained relatively high individuals with high CD8 counts and high IgA levels experienced a more rapid rate of CD4 loss than those with low baseline levels (Phillips et al, 1993). In a study of 202 haemophilic children in Europe rising IgA concentrations were markers of disease progression (Aronstam et al, 1993) and Simmonds et al (1991) have also shown in 18 Scottish haemophilic patients that the IgA specific HIV response rose gradually in the year after exposure in most individuals. In a patient who was symptomatic at the time of seroconversion, there was a much greater and more prolonged IgA response (Fig. 10.13). Thus immune activation as reflected by raised CD8 counts and raised IgA levels appears to be linked to the process of CD4 depletion. It is possible that the raised CD8 and IgA levels may not only reflect early immune activity but also the higher viral load of such patients. This would be supported by the study from Edinburgh where the group

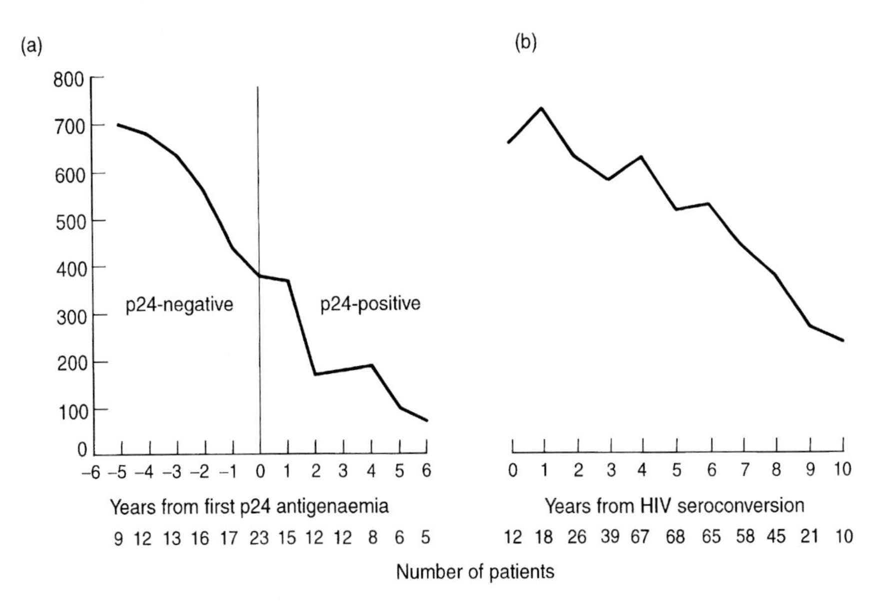

Figure 10.11 Median CD4 lymphocye count ($\times 10^6$/l). (a) Years from the first p24 antigen-positive test in p24-antigenaemic patients; (b) years from first anti-HIV-positive test in patients persistently p24-antigen-negative. (Reproduced, with permission, from Phillips AN, Lee CA, Elford J, et al. *AIDS* 1991; **5**: 1217.)

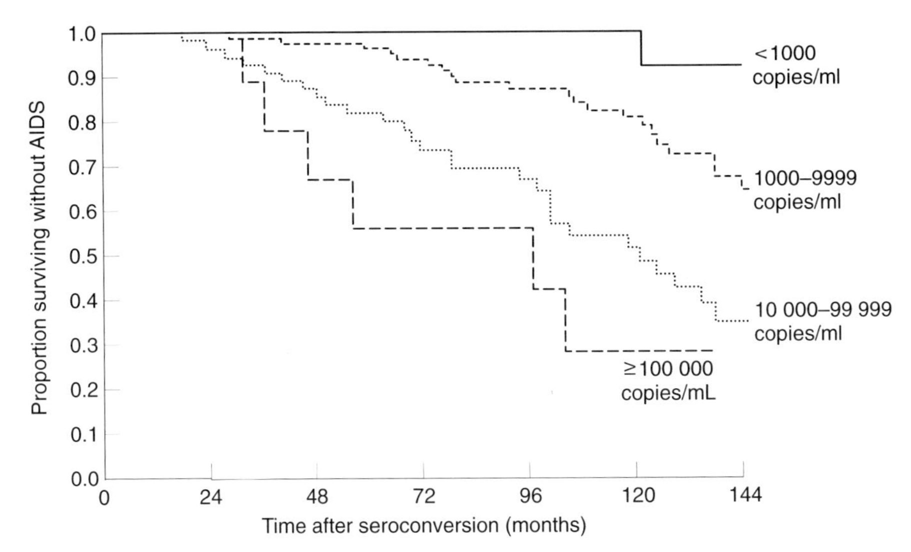

Figure 10.12 Proportion of subjects surviving without AIDS, by HIV-1 RNA level (in copies/ml) 12 to 36 months after the estimated date of HIV-1 seroconversion, Multicenter Hemophilia Cohort Study, 1979 to 1995 ($P < 0.01$). Data were truncated at 144 months of follow-up for 3 RNA categories because there were few remaining subjects in each HIV-1 RNA category. (Reproduced, with permission, from *Journal of American Medical Association*, 1996; **276**: 108.)

of 18 patients who seroconverted after exposure to a single batch of concentrate had received higher amounts than the 14 who had remained negative for HIV antibody (mean 43 (range 9–109) vs. mean 15 (range 3–30) phials, $p < 0.01$) (Cuthbert et al, 1990).

The CKR5 receptor facilitates the entry of HIV-1 into the CD4 cell and those individuals who have a gene deletion for the coding of this protein are relatively protected from infection. This may explain why some individuals who were exposed to large amounts of clotting factor concentrate did not become infected with HIV (Pasi et al, 1996). Furthermore it has been shown in both non-haemophilic and haemophilic individuals that homozygous and heterozygous gene deletions result in slower progression rates to clinical disease.

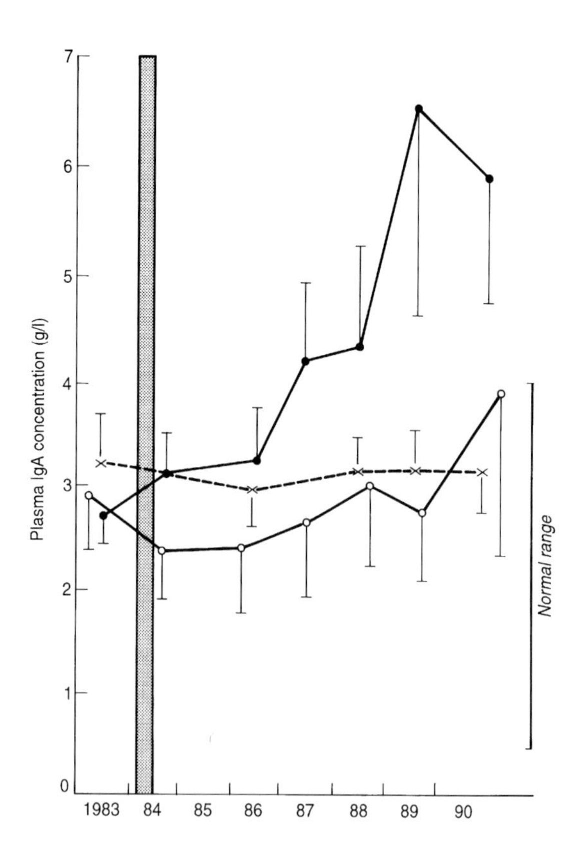

Figure 10.13 IgA concentration in members of Edinburgh haemophilic cohort. ×, Patients negative for HIV antibody (n = 14); ●, patients positive for HIV antibody with CDC IV disease 5 years after exposure (n = 10); ○, patients positive for HIV antibody with CDC category I or II disease (n = 8). (Reproduced, with permission, from *Lancet* 1991,338, p. 1160).

CMV as a co-factor

It has been demonstrated in a group of haemophilic patients that CMV infection is associated with a more rapid progression to AIDS (Webster et al, 1989). Such an observation is possible in haemophilic individuals who, in contrast to homosexuals, are not universely infected with CMV. In a further study in this group of patients (Webster et al, 1992) it was shown that the CD4 count was not affected by the CMV status but that individuals who were CMV positive developed AIDS at a higher CD4 count (Fig. 10.14). This suggests that additional mechanisms mediated by CMV, such as a functional deficit in surviving CD4 lymphocytes or entry of HIV into other cell types, may facilitate the onset of AIDS. For example, CMV may expand the tropic range of HIV disease, perhaps via the induction of Fc receptors, or may have a bystander effect by causing secretion of cytokines that can drive HIV replication in other cells. However although CMV has consistently demonstrated a co-factor effect in this group of patients others have looked in haemophilic individuals, but have failed to demonstrate such an effect.

Thrombocytopenia

The association of immune-mediated thrombocytopenia (ITP) in HIV infected haemophiliacs was first recognised by Ratnoff et al, in 1983 who described ITP in five multiply transfused patients infected with HIV. Thrombocytopenia may be the first manifestation of HIV infection, and occurs in 5–10% of asymptomatic people infected with HIV compared with 25–45% of people affected with AIDS (Pottage et al, 1988). ITP usually occurs as an isolated manifestation of HIV infection unrelated to CD4 count and does not increase the risk for development of AIDS (Ratner, 1989). Thrombocytopenia associated with HIV infection has been described in all risk groups for HIV: homosexual men (Karpatkin, 1988), haemophiliacs (Eyster et al, 1987; Karpatkin 1988) and intravenous drug users (Savona et al, 1985; Karpatkin, 1988). Although ITP rarely results in bleeding complications in HIV-infected homosexuals or intravenous drug users, there may be a significant risk of bleeding when ITP complicates the course of a seropositive haemophiliac (Ragni et al, 1990). This report showed that four of 11 seropositive haemophilic ITP patients suffered intracranial haemorrhage, and in two of these patients the platelet counts were above $30 \times 10^9/l$. The mechanism of HIV associated thrombocytopenia is thought to be due to either non-specific deposition of circulating immune complexes and complement on platelets (Karpatkin, 1988) and/or a specific anti-platelet antibody to a platelet antigen of 25 000 D (Stricker et al, 1985).

Treatment for HIV related thrombocytopenia has included intravenous immunoglobulin, steroids, zidovudine, interferon and splenectomy. Intravenous immunoglobulin is limited because the response is only transient and is therefore mainly used for a pre-splenectomy procedure (Beard & Savidge 1988) and in profound thrombocytopenia.

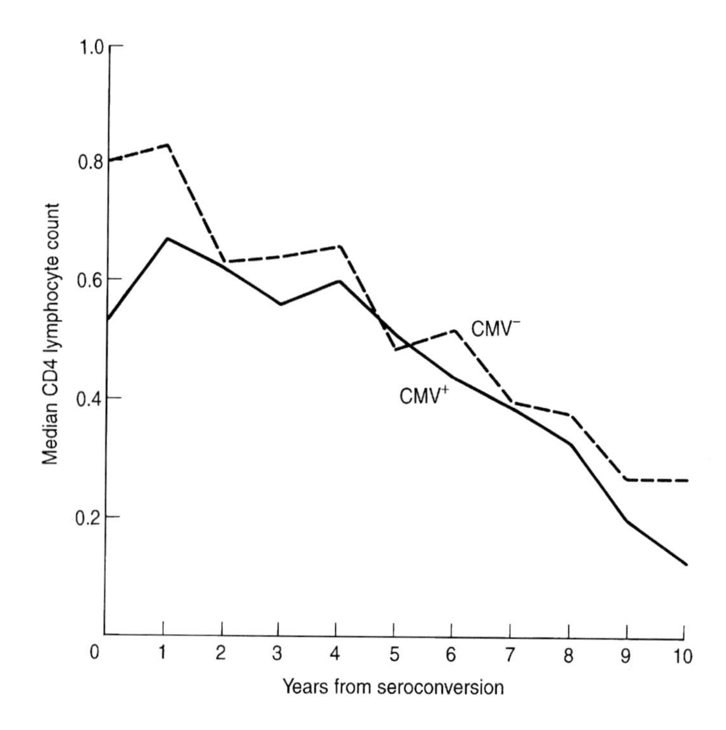

Figure 10.14 Decline in CD4+ lymphocyte counts from the time of HIV seroconversion by CMV serostatus. (Reproduced, with permission of Blackwell Scientific, from Webster A, Phillips AN, Lee CA, et al. CMV infection, CD4+ lymphocyte counts and the development of AIDS in HIV-1-infected haemophiliac patients. *Clinical & Experimental Immunology* 1992; **88**: 6).

Steroids are thought to modulate reticuloendothelial clearance of immune-complex coated platelets. In HIV associated thrombocytopenia, response is usually only partial and non-sustained once therapy has been stopped (Walsh et al, 1985; Abrams et al, 1986). There is concern that steroids may suppress cell mediated immunity, predisposing towards oropharyngeal candidiasis and possibly precipitating AIDS (Walsh et al, 1985; Abrams et al, 1986).

Zidovudine has been shown to elevate platelet counts in seropositive patients with ITP (Oskenhendler et al, 1987). The mechanism of action of zidovudine in HIV-associated thrombocytopenia is unknown. It has been suggested that the rapidity of the response reflects an inhibitory effect on reticuloendothelial function and reduced clearance of immune-complex coated platelets (Hymes et al, 1988). Zidovudine can produce a good response and has the advantage that it can be taken orally, has anti-HIV activity and is well tolerated in asymptomatic HIV positive patients (Lim et al, 1990).

Splenectomy has been considered to be the definitive treatment for non-HIV autoimmune thrombocytopenia and it has also been shown to be very effective in the treatment of HIV associated thrombocytopenia. Leissinger and Andes (1992) have reported complete responses in all four of four haemophilic patients undergoing splenectomy for severe ITP. They also reviewed the literature dealing with the management of seropositive haemophilic patients with ITP: the permanent response rate to splenectomy approaches 90% (Table 10.3). This compares favourably to results reported in more than 100 non-haemophilic seropositive patients with ITP in which there was an 80–90% permanent response rate to splenectomy. Danazol has also been used in haemophilic patients but is of minimal benefit (Oskenhendler et al, 1987).

Interferon has been used in treatment although the mechanism of action is unknown and there have been few reports of its use (Ellis et al, 1987; Taillan et al, 1988; Lim et al, 1990).

Thus haemophilic patients with thrombocytopenia present difficult management problems because of the double coagulopathy. Intravenous gammaglobulin is useful in the short term, particularly because up to 20% of cases remit spontaneously. Zidovudine should be the treatment of first choice, because it can be taken orally, is well tolerated in asymptomatic individuals and has anti-HIV activity. Interferon may be a suitable alternative if zidovudine is ineffective and splenectomy is the final alternative.

Table 10.3 Summary of reported responses to splenectomy in haemophilia patients with HIV-ITP

Reference	No. of patients	Age range (years)	Response to splenectomy			Median follow-up (months)
			CR	PR	NR	
Ratnoff et al (1983)	1	22	1	0	0	NA
Lim et al (1990)	3	6–26	2	1	0	NA
Beard & Savidge (1988)	5	13–37	4	1	0	12
Kim et al (1989)	4	18–64	4	0	0	12
Leissinger & Andes (1992)	4	11–33	4	0	0	36
Total	17	6–64	15	2	0	–

CR, platelet count maintained greater than 100 000/mm^3; PR, platelet count maintained at asymptomatic levels and greater than 50 000/mm^3; NR, platelet count less than 50 000/mm^3; ITP, immune thrombocytopenic purpura. (Reproduced, with permission, from Leissinger & Andes, 1992)

Liver disease and HIV

Haemophilic patients who were infected with HIV as a result of treatment with unheated clotting factor concentrates must also have been infected with hepatitis C (HCV). There is increasing evidence that liver disease is more severe when there is co-infection (Eyster et al, 1993; Telfer et al, 1994). Eyster and colleagues studied 236 haemophilic patients of whom 44% were co-infected with HIV and HCV and in these patients hepatomegaly, splenomegaly and elevation of transaminases were more common (Table 10.4). Among co-infected individuals with HIV infection superimposed on HCV infection, a palpable liver was 2.3 times (95% CI 1.2, 4.1) more likely and a palpable spleen 2.5 times (95% CI 1.3, 4.9) more likely compared with HCV only-infected subjects (Table 10.5). The cumulative incidence of liver failure was 42% over 27 years, and 10 years after HIV infection the cumulative incidence of liver failure was 17%. In contrast the cumulative incidence of AIDS in co-infected individuals was 31% at 10 years (Fig. 10.15). Telfer et al (1994) have also shown in 112 co-infected patients that HIV seropositivity is associated with an increased risk of raised transaminases, portal hypertension and liver failure. Viral replication of

Table 10.4 Prevalence of HIV and HCV infection among subjects with haemophilia by conditions associated with liver disease

Condition, [a]*n*[b] (%)	HCV–/ HIV– (%)	HCV–/ HIV+ (%)	HCV+/ HIV– (%)	HCV+/ HIV+ (%)
Hepatomegaly				
Present, 65 (37)	9	0	17	74
Absent, 110 (63)	35	1	31	33
Splenomegaly				
Present, 57 (33)	2	0	16	82
Absent, 115 (67)	38	1	31	31
Transaminase elevation				
Present, 82 (39)	2	0	38	60
Absent, 130 (61)	45	1	19	35

[a]Heptomegaly, liver palpable at least 2 cm below right costal margin; splenomegaly, palpable spleen; elevated transaminase, aspartate aminotransferase at least twice normal on at least two occasions 6 months apart.
[b]Excluded are subjects who had not received any type of blood products, and for hepatomegaly or splenomegaly, those missing annual examinations. Proportions may not total to 100% because of rounding.
(Reproduced, with permission from Eyster ME, Diamondstone LS, Lien, JM, et al, Natural history of hepatitis C virus infection in multitransfused hemophiliacs: effect of coinfection with human immunodeficiency virus. The Multicenter Hemophilia Cohort Study, *Journal of Acquired Immune Deficiency Syndromes* 1993; **6**: 602).

Table 10.5 Relationship of hepatitis C virus (HCV) and human immunodeficiency virus (HIV) status to conditions associated with liver disease: age-adjusted relative risk (95% CI) by infection status[a]

Condition	HCV+/HIV− vs. HCV−/HIV−	HCV+/HIV+ vs. HCV+/HIV−	HCV+/HIV+ vs. HCV−/HIV−
Hepatomegaly	1.6 (0.6, 3.8)	2.3 (1.2, 4.1)	3.2 (1.3, 7.7)
Splenomegaly	4.1 (1.1, 15.2)	2.5 (1.3, 4.9)	8.4 (2.2, 32.2)
Transaminitis	4.6 (1.7, 12.8)	1.0 (0.7, 1.5)	3.7 (1.3, 10.8)

[a]Excluded are subjects who had not received any type of blood products and subjects missing annual examinations.
(Reproduced, with permission from Eyster ME, Diamondstone LS, Lien, JM, et al, Natural history of hepatitis C virus infection in multitransfused hemophiliacs: effect of coinfection with human immunodeficiency virus. The Multicenter Hemophilia Cohort Study, *Journal of Acquired Immune Deficiency Syndromes* 1993; **6**: 602)

HCV is increased in the presence of HIV (probably because of immune deficiency). From 1978 to 1993 concentrations of hepatitis C RNA in coinfected haemophilic patients increased 58 times compared to a trebling in those infected with HCV alone (Eyster et al, 1994; Fig. 10.16). In a large London haemophilia centre 11 HIV-infected individuals died in liver failure (Lee et al, 1995). Eyster et al (1994), suggest that as more effective therapies are developed for HIV disease, more attention will need to be paid to the diagnosis and treatment of underlying HCV disease in people with haemophilia.

Sexual transmission and having children

It has been shown that 10–15% of regular female sexual partners of HIV-infected men with haemophilia become infected with HIV (Goedert et al, 1989). However in spite of their risk of HIV infection people choose to have children (Goldman et al, 1992). This study describes 12 couples who had 14 children conceived after the father was infected with HIV. Although five couples had conceived a child before the HIV antibody test was available and thus before the father's seropositivity was known, the majority of children were conceived when the parents were fully aware of the risks. In this small study all 14 children were shown to be HIV negative and to be healthy physically and mentally. However, 11 of 12 female partners remained HIV negative. The details of the fathers at the time of conception are shown in the Table 10.6.

In a follow-up study of HIV negative female partners of HIV-infected men with haemophilia knowledge of HIV status appeared to influence childbearing decisions; of 47 couples, 29 (62%) wanted more children, but only five attempted to

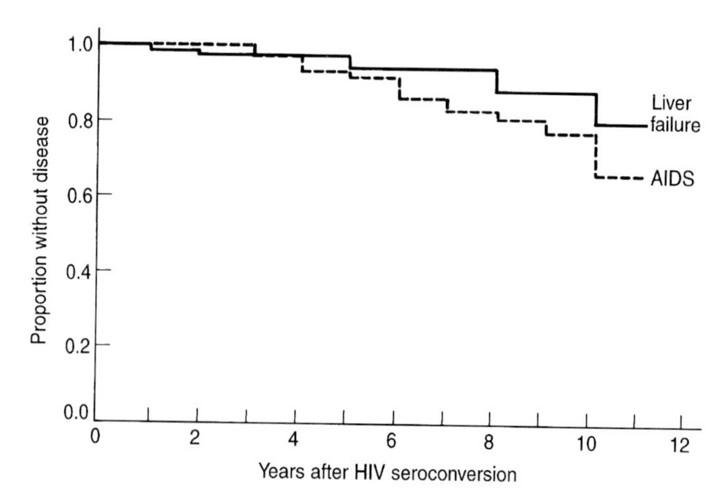

Figure 10.15 Kaplan–Meier actuarial analysis comparing cumulative incidence of liver failure and AIDS following HIV seroconversion among 97 HCV-infected subjects. (Reproduced, with permission, from Eyster ME, Diamondstone LS, Lien JM, et al. Natural history of hepatitis C virus infection in multitransfused haemophiliacs: effect of coinfection with HIV. The Multicenter Hemophilia Cohort Study. *Journal of Acquired Immune Deficiency Syndromes* 1993; **6**: 602.)

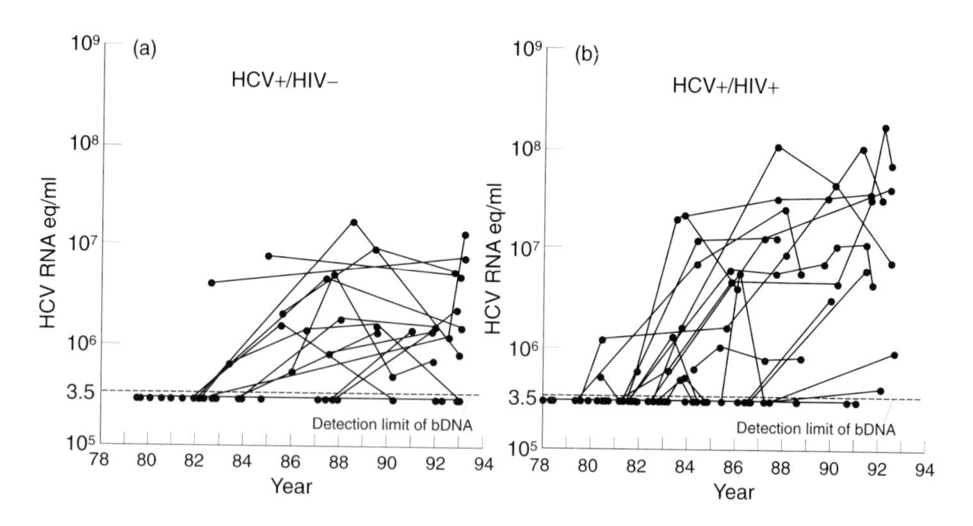

Figure 10.16 Serial HCV RNA levels on (a) 17 HCV^+/HIV^- subjects and (b) 17 HCV^+/HIV^+ subjects. (Reproduced, with permission, from Eyster *et al. Blood* 1994, **84**: p. 1020.)

Table 10.6 Father's details at time of conception

Child no.	Father's age (years)	CD4 lymphocyte count (× 10^9/l)	Length of HIV seropositivity (years)
1	33.8	–	2.0
2	26.7	0.6	3.4
3	31.8	–	0.9
4	31.1	–	2.5
5	25.3	–	1.0
6	30.1	0.27	3.7
7	37.7	0.56	3.5
8	22.8	0.36	2.7
9	33.9	–	3.0
10	26.1	1.13	5.9
11	25.6	0.94	3.5
12	28.0	0.36	10.0
13	25.0	0.40	6.0
14	27.0	0.34	7.7
Median	28.0		3.0
Range	22.8–37.7		0.9–10.0

(Reproduced, with permission, from Goldman et al, Children of HIV positive haemophiliac men. *Arch Dis Child* 1993, **68**: 133–134).

conceive after learning of the male partner's status. Furthermore couples who were aware of the man's HIV infection had substantially fewer acts of unprotected intercourse (median 3 vs. 26 per month) (Dublin, 1992). Options for safe parenting for the HIV-infected haemophiliac include adoption, foster parenting, and artificial insemination using sperm from a healthy donor (MMWR, 1990). Artificial insemination with processed semen from the HIV infected partner has unknown safety and efficacy (Semprini 1993). However in some cultures where women are valued for child bearing women face immense pressures to procreate and may find adherence to risk reduction guidelines extremely difficult (Goldman 1993).

Incidence of lymphomas and other cancers

Non-Hodgkin's lymphoma (NHL) and Kaposi's sarcoma have been found to be more common in HIV infection and the incidence of NHL is also increased in congenital immunodeficiencies and iatrogenic immunosuppression (Hoover & Fraumeni 1973; Filipovich et al, 1980). The National Cancer Institute have used the Multicenter Hemophilia Cohort to examine cancer incidence in individuals with haemophilia (Rabkin et al, 1992). Of 1065 haemophilic patients infected with HIV, there were 12 cases of NHL and two cases of Kaposi's sarcoma. The Kaposi's sarcoma occurred in a homosexual man and a person from the mediterranean region – presumably this tumour was related to risk factors other than haemophilia. The 12 cases of HIV-associated NHL were all intermediate or high grade (Table 10.7). Ten of these 12 tumours (83%) were extranodal, but only one was localized to the central nervous system. In addition to the known AIDS-related cancers, the HIV-positive patients had experienced two cases of basal cell carcinoma of the skin and eight other cancers in the same period since October 1982. The observed cases of NHL were 24 (95% CI, 13–43) times the expected numbers. The incidence of NHL increased exponentially with increasing duration of HIV infection and progression of immune deficiency. Activation of Epstein-Barr virus may be an important event in preceding lymphomagenesis. The incidence of NHL in the HIV-positive patients also increased with age. Thus the lymphoma incidence in haemophilic individuals is only partially explained by immunosuppression. It is likely that as improvements in therapy of HIV infection prolong survival there will be increases in the numbers of HIV-associated lymphoma.

The effect of clotting factor concentrate on CD4 slope

Clotting factor concentrates differ in the viral inactivation procedure used as well as the level of purity achieved. Presently available concentrates include intermediate purity products, with a specific activity of 1–50 u/mg, high-purity products made using chromatography and with a specific activity of 100–2000 u/mg, and very high-purity products made using monoclonal technology, with a specific activity of 2000–3000 u/mg. Several clinical studies suggested that monoclonal purified products had a beneficial effect on the decline of CD4 count in HIV-positive haemophilic patients (Brettler et al, 1989; Fukutake et al, 1990; Goldsmith et al, 1991). None of these studies had a control population. However, deBiasi et al, (1991) showed convincingly that there was a significant improvement in the decline of CD4 count in patients treated with monoclonal-purified product compared to those treated with intermediate product. A further randomised study comparing the use of monoclonal purified product with intermediate-purity concentrate has demonstrated stabilization of CD4 counts in those receiving the high-purity product and falling CD4 counts in patients on intermediate-purity products (Seremetis et al, 1993) (Fig. 10.17). A retrospective analysis of a large cohort of HIV-infected haemophiliacs has also demonstrated that those receiving high-purity concentrates had a slower decline of CD4 lymphocytes than those receiving intermediate-purity concentrates (Hilgartner et al, 1993). It would seem, however, that this beneficial effect is not shown by chromatographically purified concentrates (Mannucci, 1992) but recombinant factor VIII does show a

Table 10.7 Frequencies of incident cancers in 1065 HIV-positive (+) and 636 HIV-negative (–) Haemophilia patients, October 1982 to March 1991

Morphological classification	HIV +	HIV –
Non-Hodgkin's lymphoma		
Immunoblastic	1	—
Burkitt's lymphoma	2	—
Small non-cleaved cell, non Burkitt's lymphoma	2[a]	—
High-grade lymphoma, not otherwise specified	2	—
Large-cell diffuse T-cell lymphoma of uncertain	4	
classification	1[b]	—
Kaposi's sarcoma	2	—
Hodgkin's disease		
Nodular sclerosis	1	1
Mixed cellularity	1	—
Melanoma	1	1
Lymphoblastic leukaemia	1	—
Lung carcinoma	1	1
Oropharyngeal carcinoma	2	—
Cervical carcinoma in situ	1	—
Bladder carcinoma	—	1
Ependymoma	—	1
Basal cell carcinoma of the skin	2	3

HIV, human immunodeficiency virus.
[a]Includes one tumour that may have been polyclonal.
[b]Lymphoepithelioid non-Hodgkin's lymphoma vs. Hodgkin's disease.
(Reproduced, with permission, from Rabkin CS, Hilgartner MW, Hedberg KW, et al, *Journal of the American Medical Association* 1992; **276**: 1090).

stabilization of the CD4 count (Mannucci et al, 1994). A retrospective study in 37 patients has shown an improvement in CD4+ decline following a switch to monoclonal product (Sabin et al, 1994). Since it has been demonstrated that survival is dependent on CD4 rather than length of time from seroconversion (Phillips et al, 1992), it is likely that the stabilization of CD4 counts seen following treatment with high-purity products will translate into decreased morbidity and improved survival.

Prophylactic and antiviral therapy for HIV disease

Antiviral Therapy

In 1985 zidovudine was found to have in vitro activity against HIV. The first large clinical trial initiated in February 1986 in patients with advanced HIV

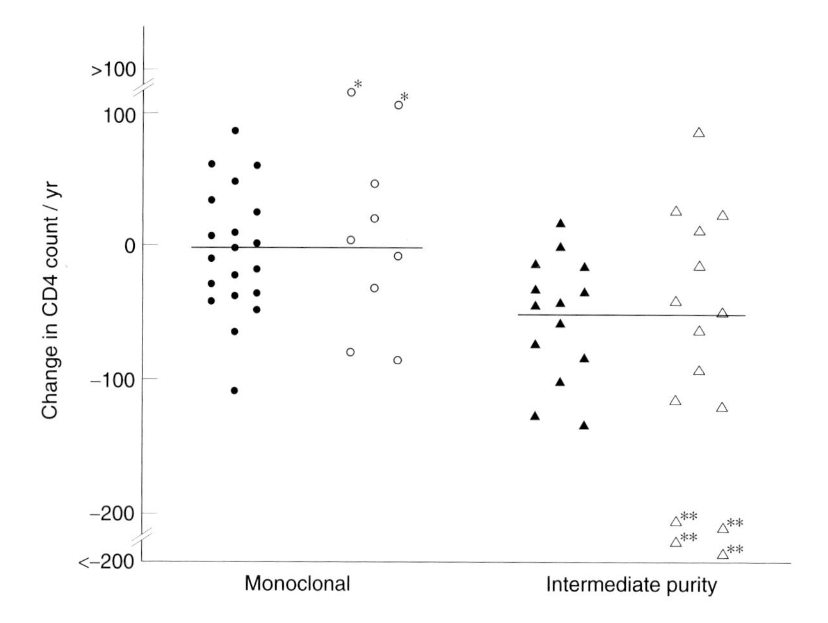

Figure 10.17 Individual change-rates in CD4 counts. ●, ○, monoclonal antibody purified product, 3 years in study (●) or not (○); ▲, △, intermediate product, 3 years in study (▲) or not (△). ⋆, values not to scale, of + 168 and + 296; ⋆⋆, values not to scale, of − 220, − 260, − 304 and − 410. Slope calculated for all available data, indicated by horizontal line. (Reproduced, with permission, from *Lancet* 1993; **324**: 701).

disease was stopped by the safety monitoring board after 7 months because there was a significant survival benefit for those receiving zidovudine. The drug was approved in 1987 by the Food and Drug Administratiion (FDA) for use in advanced disease (Fischl et al, 1987). The efficacy of zidovudine has been shown for a variety of clinical and laboratory parameters including prolongation of survival, delay of the occurrence of an AIDS-defining diagnosis, reduction of the incidence of opportunistic infections, stabilization of weight, improved performance, reversal of HIV-associated thrombocytopenia, stabilization of early-to-moderate HIV-associated dementia, increase in CD4 count, and reduction in viral burden by quantitative culture or measurement of p24 antigen (Sande et al, 1993).

Although there is proven in vitro and clinical activity of zidovudine there remains considerable debate about when to start therapy (Bartlett 1993). However, in the light of published results from therapeutic trials it is possible to establish some guidelines (Sande et al, 1993). The first study of early therapy

Table 10.8 Antiretroviral therapy for HIV-infected adults: recommendations from the 1993 NIAID state-of-the-art conference

Clinical status	$CD4^+$ range, cell count $\times 10^9$/l	Recommendation
	No previous antiretroviral therapy	
Asymptomatic	>0.50	No therapy
Asymptomatic	0.20–0.50	Zidovudine or no therapy
Symptomatic	0.20–0.50	Zidovudine
Asymptomatic	<0.20	Zidovudine
Symptomatic	<0.20	Zidovudine
	Previous antiretroviral therapy	
Stable	⩾0.30	Continue zidovudine
Stable	⩾0.30	Continue zidovudine or change to didanosine
Progressing	0.05–0.50	Change to didanosine or zalcitabine
Progressing	<0.05	Change to didanosine or zalcitabine
	Intolerant to zidovudine	
Stable or progressing	<0.05	Change to didanosine or zalcitabine

HIV, human immunodeficiency virus; NIAID, National Institute of Allergy and Infectious Diseases.
(Reproduced, with permission, from Sande MA, Carpenter CC, Cobbs CG, et al, *Journal of the American Medical Association* 1993; **270**: 2583–2589 © 1993 American Medical Association.)

was that of the AIDS Clinical Trials Group (ACTG 019) initiated in July 1987 with 3200 asymptomatic patients who were randomly assigned to receive low-dose zidovudine (500 mg/day), high-dose zidovudine (1500 mg/day), or placebo (Volberding et al, 1990). The interim analysis after 2 years showed a statistically significant delay in the progression of disease in patients with baseline CD4 counts below 500/μl who received zidovudine. On the basis of these results the FDA approved zidovudine in a dose of 500 mg/day for those with a CD4 count of < 500/μl. However there was some concern that the benefit observed in 4% of the cohort might not be extended to the other 96%.

Table 10.9 Recommendations for when to initiate treatment

Status	Recommendation
Symptomatic HIV disease[a]	Therapy recommended for all patients
Asymptomatic, CD4 cell count $<0.50 \times 10^9$/l	Therapy recommended[b]
Asymptomatic, CD4 cell count $<0.50 \times 10^9$/l	Therapy recommended for patients with >30 000–50 000 HIV RNA copies/ml or rapidly declining CD4 cell counts Therapy should be considered for patients with >5000–10 000 HIV RNA copies/ml

[a]Symptomatic human immunodeficiency virus (HIV) disease includes symptoms such as recurrent mucosal candidiasis, oral hairy leukoplakia, and chronic and unexplained fever, night sweats, and weight loss.
[b]Some would defer therapy in a subset of patients with stable CD4 cell counts between 0.35 and 0.50×10^9/l and plasma HIV RNA levels consistently below 5000–10 000 copies/ml
(Reproduced, with permission, from *Journal of the American Medical Association* 1996; **276**: 149.)

Table 10.10 Recommendations for initial therapy regimens

Zidovudine/didanosine, or zidovudine/zalcitabine, or zidovudine/lamivudine, or didanosine monotherapy[a]	If a protease inhibitor is added to a nucleoside analogue-containing regimen, the choice of protease inhibitor should be based primarily on antiretroviral potency and secondarily on other considerations as described in the text[b]

[a]Didanosine monotherapy may be less effective as initial therapy in patients with more advanced human immunodeficiency virus (HIV) disease. Other possible non-zidovudine containing regimens include didanosine/stavudine, stavudine/lamivudine, and stavudine monotherapy, although these regimens are less well studied.
[b]Antiretroviral potency refers to plasma HIV RNA and CD4 cell count responses associated with these drugs at approved doses and with currently available formulations.
(Reproduced with permission, from *Journal of the American Medical Association*, 1996; 276; 150.)

Table 10.11 Some selected options for changing therapy owing to treatment failure or drug intolerance[a]

Initial regimen	Subsequent regimen options
Treatment failure	
Zidovudine	Zidovudine/didanosine ± protease inhibitor
	Zidovudine/lamivudine ± protease inhibitor
	Didanosine ± protease inhibitor
	Didanosine/stavudine ± protease inhibitor
Didanosine	Zidovudine/lamivudine ± protease inhibitor
	Zidovudine/didanosine/protease inhibitor
	Stavudine/protease inhibitor
Zidovudine/didanosine	Zidovudine/lamivudine ± protease inhibitor
	Stavudine/protease inhibitor
Zidovudine/zalcitabine	Zidovudine/lamivudine ± protease inhibitor
	Stavudine/protease inhibitor
	Didanosine/protease inhibitor
Zidovudine/lamivudine	Didanosine/protease inhibitor
	Stavudine/protease inhibitor
	Didanosine/stavudine
	Lamivudine/stavudine
Drug Intolerance[c]	
Zidovudine[b]	Didanosine
	Didanosine/stavudine
	Lamivudine/stavudine
	Stavudine
Didanosine	Zidovudine/lamivudine
	Lamivudine/stavudine
	Stavudine/protease inhibitor
Zidovudine/zalcitabine	
Intolerance to zidovudine	Didanosine
	Didanosine/protease inhibitor
	Didanosine/stavudine
	Stavudine/protease inhibitor
Intolerance to zalcitabine	Zidovudine/zalcitabine ± protease inhibitor
Zidovudine/lamivudine	Didanosine/protease inhibitor
	Stavudine/protease inhibitor
	Didanosine/stavudine

[a]For patients whose initial regimen includes a protease inhibitor, subsequent regimens should include at least two new drugs chosen from among nucleoside analogues, nonnucleoside reverse transcriptase inhibitors (if available), and protease inhibitors (one should be selected for which there is likely to be little or no cross-resistance to the initial protease inhibitor).
[b]Considered a suboptimal regimen: all patients on zidovudine monotherapy should be reevaluated.
[c]A protease inhibitor could be added to the nucleoside analogue regimens listed (Reproduced, with permission, from *Journal of American Medical Association* 1996; **276**: 151).

Table 10.12 Agents currently available or under study for HIV antiretroviral chemotherapy with common dose regimens

Nucleoside analogue reverse transcriptase inhibitors
AZT (zidovudine): 200 mg t.d.s. or 250 mg b.d.
DDI (didanosine): 125–200 mg b.d.
DDC (zalcitabine): 0.75 mg t.d.s.
D4T (stavudine): 30–40 mg b.d.
3TC (lamivudine): 150 mg b.d.
Non-nucleoside analogue reverse transcriptase inhibitors
Nevirapine: 200 mg b.d.
Delavirdine: 300–400 mg t.d.s.
Loviride: 100 mg t.d.s.
Protease inhibitors
Saquinavir: 600 mg t.d.s.
Ritonavir: 600 mg b.d.
Indinavir: 800 mg every 8 hours
Nelfinavir: to be determined

(Reproduced, with permission, from *Medicine*, 1996;**24: 145.)**

In contrast the Anglo-French Concorde study has shown that long-term monotherapy with zidovudine during the asymptomatic phase of HIV infection does not prolong life or significantly reduce the incidence of opportunistic infection. This was a large study of approximately 2000 individuals over 3 years and therefore has the advantage of a large number of end-points (Concorde Coordinating Committee, 1994).

Meta analysis of several studies, does suggest that there is early benefit with zidovudine monotherapy in the prevention of opportunistic infection, which does not persist in the long term. Certainly when early disease events such as oral candidiasis, oral leukoplakia and herpes zoster are included as end-points it can be shown that zidovudine is of benefit for asymptomatic individuals with a CD4 count greater than 400/μl (Cooper et al, 1993). The advantages of early therapy with zidovudine include fewer side-effects and much less viral resistance. It may be that zidovudine monotherapy reduces viral load for only short periods and that early switching to other monotherapy is beneficial. Thus in the ACTG 116A, 116B/117 studies it has been shown that didanosine (DDI) and zidovudine are equivalent and that changing to DDI was beneficial.

A state of the art conference convened by the National Institute of Allergy and Infectious Disease has evaluated current information on the use of nucleoside analogue reverse transcriptase inhibitors (Sande et al, 1993; Table 10.8). These recommendations are for asymptomatic individuals who are zidovudine naive; those who are symptomatic but zidovudine naive; clinically stable patients who are tolerating zidovudine; patients experiencing clinical progression while on zidovudine; and those who are intolerant of antiretroviral therapy (Table 10.8).

Combinations of drugs of limited potency are likely to be more effective than monotherapy and there is evidence that combinations of various drugs with zidovudine do produce a more sustained fall in viral load and a more sustained rise in surrogate markers such as the CD4 count. At the present time although the role of antiretroviral drugs in symptomatic disease remains unchallenged, present indications suggest that combinations have greatest benefit for initial therapy.

Chemotherapy for HIV infection poses a challenge for the physician and increasingly therapeutic guidelines are being developed both in the USA and UK and these will need to be updated as new data continue to emerge (Carpenter et al, 1996) (Tables 10.9, 10.10, 10.11). During 1997 it is likely that a dozen or more licensed agents may be available for use, alone or in double or triple drug combinations (Table 10.12). Although clinical trial results are useful in guiding therapy, often studies are not comparable and patients may differ from those enrolled in clinical trials. In addition, many agents are approved for use before final study results are published. Therefore treatment must be individualized with decisions dependent on available drug options, disease stage, underlying conditions, and concomitant medications as well as the CD4 count and viral load.

Prophylaxis

During the first decade of the AIDS epidemic, treatment was directed toward the diagnosis and treatment of acute opportunistic infection. Gradually it was appreciated that prevention or prophylaxis was a more logical approach to the management of opportunistic infections. Prophylaxis was first developed for *Pneumocystis carinii pneumonia* (PCP) and has now been extended to other AIDS-related pathogens: *Toxoplasmosis*, *Mycobacterium avium* complex and fungal infections (Decker & Masur, 1994).

Prophylaxis against PCP should be offered to all patients with a CD4 count $< 200/\mu l$ when the risk of such infection increases. Co-trimoxazole given by mouth in a dose of 960 mg three times a week is the treatment of choice. At this dose the drug is generally well tolerated, rash (occurring in about 20% patients) being the most common unwanted effect. Pentamidine delivered through a nebulizer (eg Respigard II) is less effective than co-trimoxazole but may become necessary where co-trimoxazole is not tolerated.

Toxoplasmic encephalitis is one of the mst common and most treatable causes of central nervous system infections in HIV-infected patients. Most cases develop when the CD4 count is $<100/\mu l$. It has been shown that co-trimoxazole given for prophylaxis of PCP in a dose of 960 mg three times a week will also prevent toxoplasmosis.

Mycobacterium avium complex (MAC) occurs in 30–50% of HIV infected individuals but usually only when the CD4 count is less than $10–50/\mu l$. Rifabutin has been assessed in a large randomized trial. It has been recommended by a US Public Health Service Task Force published in the Morbidity and Mortality Weekly Report (MMWR) that rifabutin 300 mg by mouth daily should be given to patients with HIV infection who have a CD4 count <100/μl (Decker and Masur 1994).

It has been suggested that prophylactic isoniazid, 300 mg/day, is effective in preventing *Mycobacterium tuberculosis*. The recommendations from CDC as published by MMWR are that individuals who show a positive tuberculin reaction should be offered prophylaxis with isoniazid for 6–12 months (MMWR, 1993). However this becomes impossible to apply in countries such as the UK where Bacille-Calmette-Guérin (BCG) is given to teenagers. Furthermore the occurrence of Mycobacterium tuberculosis (MTB) at relatively high CD4 counts make this form of prophylaxis impracticable.

Clarithromycin 500 mg BD has been shown to be effective in a randomized placebo control trial to prevent MA (Pierce et al, 1996).

The use of triazoles continues to increase given the low toxicity. Recurrent oral and oesophageal candidiasis have led to increasing use of ketoconazole, fluconazole and more recently, itraconazole for long-term prophylaxis. However recent reports of resistant *Candida albicans* are becoming more frequent in patients receiving azoles. In patients with haemophilia a dose of 150 mg fluconazole weekly has proved beneficial (Lim et al, 1991a).

Life- or sight-threatening infection with CMV occurs in approximately 40% of HIV infected patients. While prophylaxis would appear to be a reasonable strategy in patients with positive CMV IgG, no evidence of end organ disease and CD4 counts <100/μl, there has been no drug available with sufficient convenience, low toxicity and efficacy to warrant widespread use. The use of acyclovir has been disappointing. A recent placebo controlled trial in HIV-infected patients with a CD4 count <150/μl failed to show a protective effect for CMV disease although there was a survival benefit, the cause of which is not understood (Youle et al, 1994).

The prophylaxis regimens for common pathogens are summarized in Table 10.13. The ability to suppress opportunistic infection has given a tremendous advance in the quality of care. However, as patients live longer with low CD4 counts they will inevitably develop new opportunistic processes. Moreover as prophylaxis is used more widely drug resistance will increase for each targeted pathogen.

Hepatitis and haemophilia

History

Transfusion associated jaundice was first recognized in the 1940s (Beeson, 1943; Spurling et al, 1946). It became an increasingly recognized complication of

Table 10.13 Drug regimens for prophylaxis of opportunistic infections

Opportunistic infection/ agent	Adult dose (mg)	Route	Dose interval
***Pneumocystis carinii* pneumonia**			
Trimethoprim-sulphamethoxazole	160/800	Oral	Daily
	160/800	Oral	Once/twice daily[b]
	80/40	Oral	Daily
Pentamidine	300[a]	Aerosol (Respigard)	Monthly
		Aerosol (Fisons)	Bi-weekly
Pyrimethamine-sulphadoxine	50/100	Oral	Bi-weekly
Dapsone	100	Oral	Daily[c]
Pyrimethamine-dapsone	75/100	Oral	Weekly
Toxoplasmic encephalitis			
Trimethoprim-sulphamethoxazole	160/800	Oral	Daily
Pyrimethamine-dapsone	75/200	Oral	Weekly
***Mycobacterium avium* complex**			
Rifabutin	300	Oral	Daily
Cytomegalovirus	None	None	None
Fungal			
Fluconazole	100–200	Oral	Daily
Mycobacterium tuberculosis			
Isoniazid	300	Oral	Daily[d]

[a]Load: five doses of 60 mg each 24–72 hours apart over 2 weeks, then 60 mg.
[b]Two or three days per week.
[c]In one or two or more divided doses.
[d]For 1 year
(Reproduced, with permission, from Decker & Masur, 1994.)

haemophilia treatment with the introduction of plasma product therapy in subsequent years (McMilllan et al, 1961). By the 1970s the rate of symptomatic acute hepatitis with jaundice was reported in 2–6% of treated haemophilic patients (Biggs, 1974). It was noted to occur particularly in patients who had previously received little or no treatment with blood products (Kasper & Kipnis 1972).

Hepatitis A virus

Hepatitis A virus (HAV) is only rarely transmitted by transfusion (Hollinger et al, 1983; Sheretz et al, 1984) and has formerly not been a problem for recipients of blood product therapy. However, outbreaks of hepatitis A have recently been reported from Italy (Mannucci, 1992), Germany (Gerritzen et al, 1992), the Republic of Ireland (Temperley, 1992) and Belgium (Peerlinck & Vermylen, 1993). All cases were associated with the use of a high purity factor VIII concentrate sterilized by solvent detergent (Octa V. I., Octapharma). A case control study conducted on the Italian cases has associated the outbreak to this product (Mannucci et al, 1989) but it has not been possible to produce the infection in animals by injecting them with the concentrate. Since HAV is non-enveloped, it and other non-enveloped viruses would not be inactivated by solvent/detergent. For this reason fractionators are introducing double inactivation procedures (Mannucci, 1993). A further outbreak of HAV has been associated with solvent detergent treated factor VIII (Alphanate) amongst patients with haemophilia in the USA (MMWR, 1996). These manufacturers are adding another virucidal step, heating at 80°C for 72 h.

Hepatitis B and delta infection

The Australia antigen, an antigen against which multitransfused haemophiliacs developed precipitating antibodies was reported in the mid-1960s by Blumberg (Blumberg et al, 1967). This led to the identification of the several specific serological markers that are now available for the characterization of hepatitis B virus (HBV) infection. The majority of intensively treated older haemophiliacs have serological evidence of previous HBV infection – over 90% in a series reported in our centre (Lee et al, 1985a). Most of these infections were acquired subclinically followed by acquired immunity as shown by the presence of core antibody. A small minority of infected patients have in the past become chronic carriers of HBsAg with or without antiHBe (Telfer et al, 1993). There is evidence that chronic carriers of HBsAg have a suppression of other viral infections, particularly HCV: so-called viral interference (Lim et al, 1991b; Dolan, 1995). The majority of intensively treated older haemophiliacs have serological evidence of previous HBV infection. A study from nine US regional haemophilia centres tested for markers of HBV during 1987 and 1988 (Troisi et al, 1993) showed evidence of previous HBV in 75 and 33%, and active HBsAg in 12 and 4% of HIV positive, negative individuals respectively. Thus HBV transmission to haemophiliacs has largely been stopped by the advances made in blood donor screening and concentrate sterilization, but since patients with bleeding disorders are at a higher risk of receiving unsterilized blood products hepatitis B vaccination is practised.

Hepatitis D virus (HDV, delta agent) requires the presence of HBV for its propagation. Therefore superinfection with HDV can occur in chronic HBV and coinfection in acute hepatitis B. Among individuals who receive multiple transfusions of blood and blood products, haemophiliacs have a high risk of acquiring HDV infection (Rizzetto et al, 1982; Jacobson et al, 1985). Rosina et al (1985) reported an anti-HD prevalence of 34% among 79 HBsAg-positive haemophiliacs who had received commercial clotting factor concentrates in Western Europe and the USA. The agent was clearly present in the UK volunteer donor population in the early 1980s; we have described a patient who seroconverted for anti-HDV following a single infusion of National Health Service (NHS) factor IX concentrate (Lee et al, 1985a).

Lemon et al (1991) conducted a prospective multicentre clinical study of HDV infection amongst haemophilic patients from the USA. HDV infection was defined by the presence of antibody or the presence of HDV RNA in those without antibody. HDV infection was associated with a past history of acute hepatitis and with evidence of chronic liver disease. Haemophilic patients with HDV were also shown to have rapidly progressive liver disease. Death occurred in 18% of HDV-positive individuals compared with 8% of those who were HDV negative (Table 10.14).

An interesting phenomenon of suppression of HCV by replication of HDV has been demonstrated (Eyster et al, 1995). Eight chronic carriers of HBsAg from a cohort of 99 patients with haemophilia co-infected with HIV and HCV were tested for antibody to HDV and quantitatively for HIV RNA, HCV RNA, and HDV RNA. HCV RNA was detected in only one of five patients with HDV infection. In contrast, all three without HDV had high levels of HCV RNA. This represents the well-known phenomenon of viral interference which occurs commonly between hepatitis viruses but is ill understood. It is unlikely that sterilized clotting factor concentrates continue to transmit HDV (Lee, 1992) but protection against HBV infection with vaccination will also provide protection.

Table 10.14 Mortality and hepatitis D status among HBsAg-positive haemophiliacs ($n = 60$)

	HDV RNA or anti-HD (+)	Anti-HD (–)
n	22	38
Mean follow-up (months)	26.7	26.3
Death	4 (18%)	3 (8%)
Hepatitis, fulminant	1 (5%)	—
Hepatitis, chronic	2 (9%)	—
AIDS-related	—	2 (5%)
Cancer (non-HCC)	—	1 (3%)
Heart disease	1 (5%)	—

HCC, hepatocellular carcinoma.
(Reproduced, with permission, from Zuckerman, 1993.)

Hepatitis C

Before the introduction of heat treatment of clotting factor concentrates in the mid-1980s, virtually 100% of patients who received a first exposure to clotting factor concentrate developed non-A non-B (NANB) hepatitis (Fletcher et al, 1983; Kernoff et al, 1985). This was formerly diagnosed by exclusion of hepatitis A, hepatitis B, CMV and Epstein-Barr virus. There were gross under-estimates of prevalence because many cases of acute and chronic NANB hepatitis were apparently asymptomatic. It was not until the isolation of the major blood-borne NANB agent designated hepatitis C virus (HCV) (Kuo et al, 1989) and the development of serological tests for HCV that estimates of incidence could be made. However, the first generation test that was directed against the C-100 epitope underestimated the problem in haemophilia. This was particularly the case in HIV positive haemophiliacs who must have been infected with HCV and when second-generation tests were used in these patients a much greater percentage showed HCV seropositivity (Fig. 10.18). Tedder et al (1991) tested sera from 21 patients who had received large amounts of unheated factor VIII concentrate and whereas antibodies to core epitopes of HCV were detected in 100% of the sera only 62% were anti-C100 positive. Furthermore, hepatitis C viraemia was demonstrated in 90% of the patients by polymerase chain reaction (PCR) amplification of the 5′ untranslated region of the HCV genome. Watson et al (1992) have also shown that almost all HCV-infected patients have evidence of ongoing viral replication.

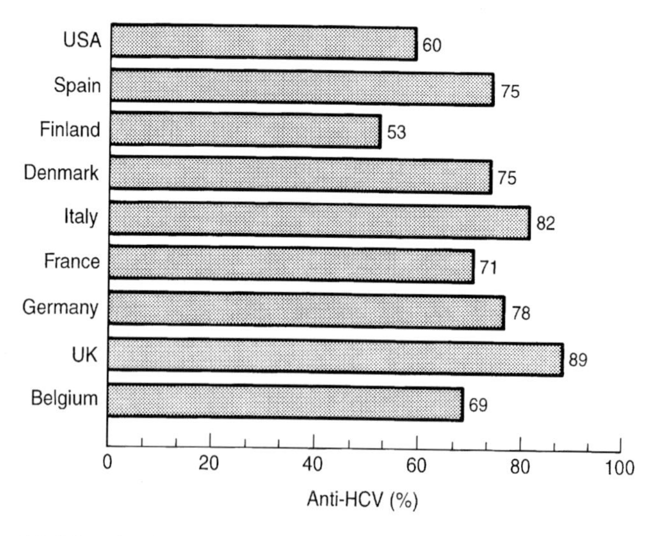

Figure 10.18 Anti-HCV in haemophilia patients worldwide. (Reproduced, with permission, from Zuckerman AJ (Ed.) *Viral Hepatitis*. Edinburgh: Churchill Livingstone, 1993 p. 505).

Table 10.15 Incubation period and time to seroconversion following first exposure of eight hemophiliacs studied within 6 weeks of disease onset.

Incubation (weeks)	Time to seroconversion (weeks)	
	anti-p22	anti-C100-3
2.0	6.5	14.6
2.1	4.4	4.4
2.9	3.7	3.7
3.3	6.0	12.7
3.9	4.4	12.8
4.0	11.6	12.3
6.1	8.2	22.8
8.4	9.3	9.3

(Reproduced, with permission, form the *International Monitor on Hemophilia* 1993; **1:** 29).

It has been possible using retrospective sera to follow the events in acute HCV infection. Amongst a series of 58 patients who developed NANB hepatitis following a first exposure to clotting factor concentrate (Kernoff et al, 1985) the median time to aspartate transaminase elevation (AST) was 4 weeks (range 1–7) and to anti-C100 seroconversion 11 weeks (range 7.5–14.5) (Lim et al, 1991b). In the same group of patients Dourakis et al (1992) have shown that time to anti-p22 (core) seroconversion was 6.25 weeks with a range of 3.7–11.6 weeks (Table 10.15). These intervals to seroconversion are much shorter than prospectively followed transfusion recipients (Alter et al, 1989). The shorter period may reflect a higher inoculum of transmitted virus in pooled concentrates compared with single blood donor units.

It is not clear whether all patients who have been infected with HCV remain viraemic. Garson et al (1990) have shown three temporal patterns of viraemia in haemophilic patients who had a clear episode of HCV following treatment with unsterilized factor VIII: transient viraemia in acutely resolving hepatitis C; viraemia lasting for several years in chronic hepatitis C; and intermittent viraemia in chronic hepatitis C.

In a study by Mauser-Bunschoten et al (1995), viraemia, as assessed by detection of HCV-RNA by cDNA polymerase chain reaction, in 277 haemophilic patients showed that 225 were positive. Viraemia was not found in 52 negative anti-HCV patients, while 182 of 225 (81%) anti-HCV positive patients had detectable viraemia. None of the 39 nonviraemic patients with anti-HCV (17%) had serum ALT levels high enough to be indicative of hepatitis. Only 8 out of 39 (21%) non-viraemic patients with anti-HCV antibodies had slight ALT elevations. Furthermore, significantly more patients (158 out of 177, 89%) with HCV viraemia had elevated ALT values than did patients without viraemia.

Significantly and persistent high ALT levels were found in 78 out of 177(44%) viraemic patients. The authors conclude that nonviraemic HCV-infected patients without elevated ALT levels, about 20% of anti-HCV positive patients, may be considered to have cleared the virus, thus resolving the HCV infection.

HCV genotypes

Several distinct genotypes of HCV whose distributions show regional and ethnic variation have been identified. It has been suggested that biological variations between genotypes may explain some of the differences in the severity and clinical course of HCV infection and that some genotypes may be more or less responsive to interferon therapy (Dusheiko et al, 1994). For the most part, in Northern Europe and North America types 1, 2 and 3 predominate, type 4 is the principal genotype found in the Middle East, Central and North Africa, while type 5 is the predominant variant in South Africa.

In haemophilic patients in Edinburgh, the distribution of genotypes was similar to that found in Scottish blood donors (Jarvis et al, 1994) (Fig. 10.19). These investigators found that over a period of 10 years there was a change in genotype and serotype in 9 of 29 patients.

Eyster and Hatzakis (1996) showed the distribution of genotypes in haemophilic patients compared to the US population. There was a much higher proportion of genotype 3 (Table 10.16). Furthermore, changes in genotype over time occurred in 58% and this was more common in the presence of HIV.

In a study in Belgium, HCV genotype 1b was found predominant in both

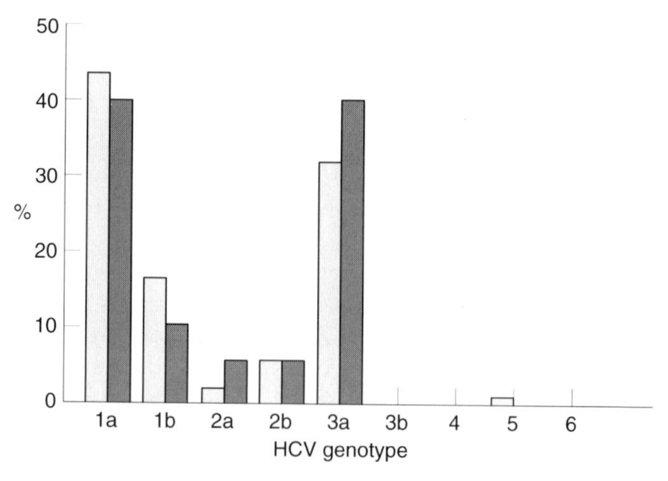

Figure 10.19 HCV genotype distribution in non-commercially treated haemophiliacs (■) and blood donors (□) from Scotland. (Reproduced, with permission, from *Haemophilia* 1995, **1** (suppl 4): 3.)

Table 10.16 Prevalence of Genotypes

	HIV+ n = 17	HIV– n = 14	Total n = 31	U.S. Population[a] Estimates *n* = 139
1a	6 (35%)	4 (29%)	10 (32%)	37.4%
1b	2 (12%)	2 (14%)	4 (13%)	37.4%
2	1 (6%)	1 (7)	2 (6.5%)	10.8%
3	6 (35%)	7 (50%)	13 (42%)	5.8%
4a	1 (6%)	0	1 (3.2%)	not detected
Mixed	1 (6%)	0	1 (3.2%)	0.7%

[a]Chronic HCV patients from FL, MO and CA.
(Reproduced, with permission, from *Gastroenterology* 1996; **110**: A 1187).

haemophilia patients and the general population, but in the haemophilic patients double infection with two genotypes occurred as well as a relatively high infection with type 2 and 3 (Sheng et al, 1995).

It is interesting that in Japan where patients with haemophilia have been treated with concentrates derived from US donors, the predominant genotype in patients with haemophilia was 1a whereas for the general population of Japanese patients type 1b was the most common (Suou et al, 1996).

In a comprehensive study of hepatitis C virus (HCV) genotype and its clinical significance (Telfer et al, 1995), 189 HCV RNA-positive patients were typed by restriction fragment length polymorphism (RIFL) in an amplified segment of the 5′ non-coding region of the HCV genome. This showed a distribution of genotype 1 in 121 (64%), type 2 in 23 (12%), type 3 in 36 (19%), type 4 in 3 (2%) and type 5 in 2 (1%) with mixed infection in 3 (2%). Type 1 was associated with higher HCV RNA levels and with a poor response to interferon. Progression to hepatic failure was more common in type 1 than type 3 and this was statistically significant (Fig. 10.20).

It has also been shown that HCV genotype 1 has an accelerating effect on HIV progression compared to other genotypes (Sabin et al, 1997) (Fig. 10.21).

It is possible that as well as changes of genotype occurring spontaneously over time in haemophilic patients there may be a change with treatment. In a study of 25 patients who were treated with α-interferon, in a 6-month observational period before treatment 3 out of 25 (12%) patients changed genotype and following treatment the change occurred in 10 out of 25 (40%) patients (Devereux et al, 1995). Most patients who underwent changes in genotype responded to treatment: the response to treatment in 7 out of 10(70%) was incomplete, and in 5 out of 10 (50%) it was complete. In contrast, in only 1 out of 15 patients (7%) without a change in genotype was there a complete response to interferon treatment. Most patients who showed a complete clinical response, 6 out of 25 (25%), were of genotype 2 or 3. It is likely that the

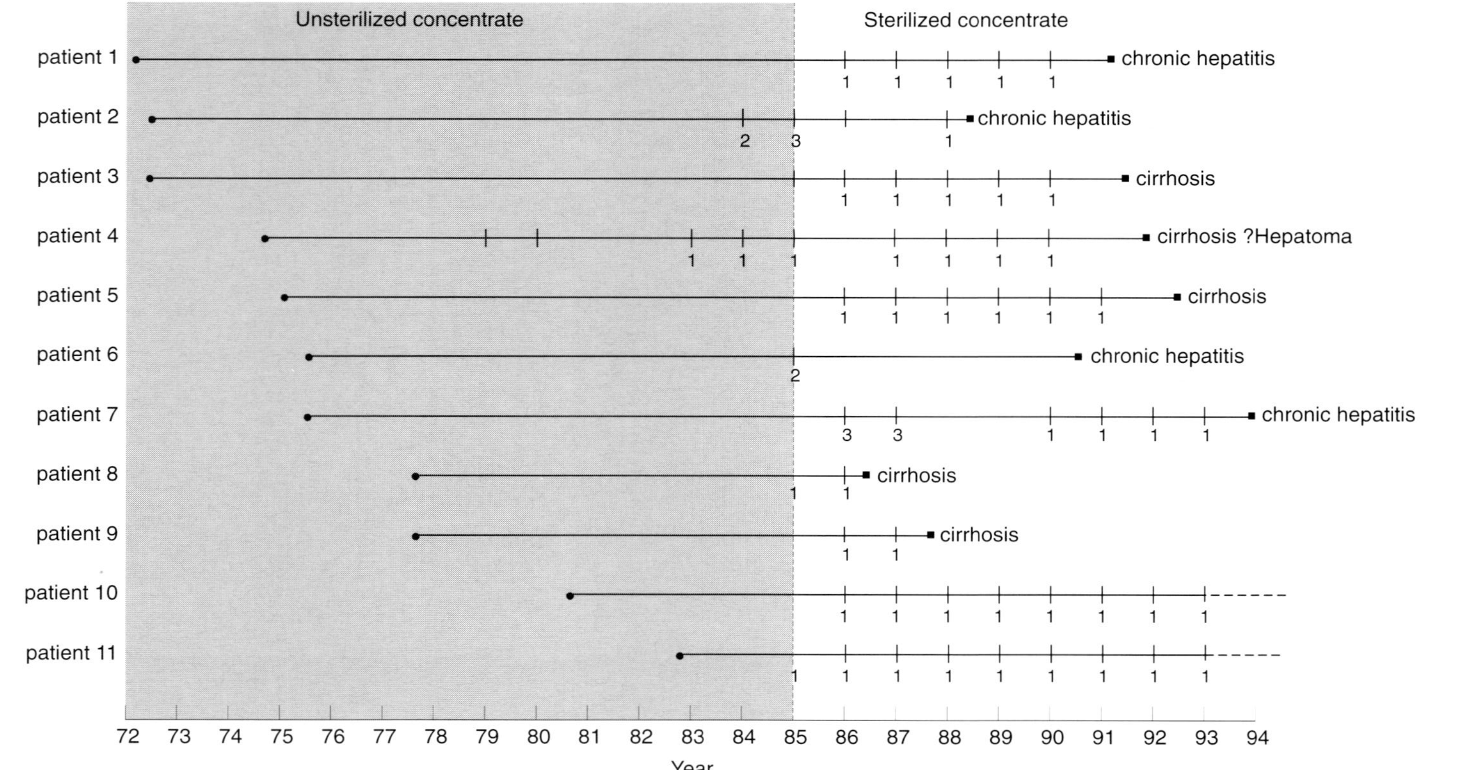

Figure 10.20 Longitudinal follow-up of HCV genotype in 11 patients with postmortem histological findings. First exposure to large donor pool coagulation factor concentrate. ■, death; +, HCV RNA positive; –, HCV RNA negative; 1, 2, 3, HCV genotype. (Reproduced, with permission, from *Thrombosis and Haemostasis* 1995, **75**: 1259.

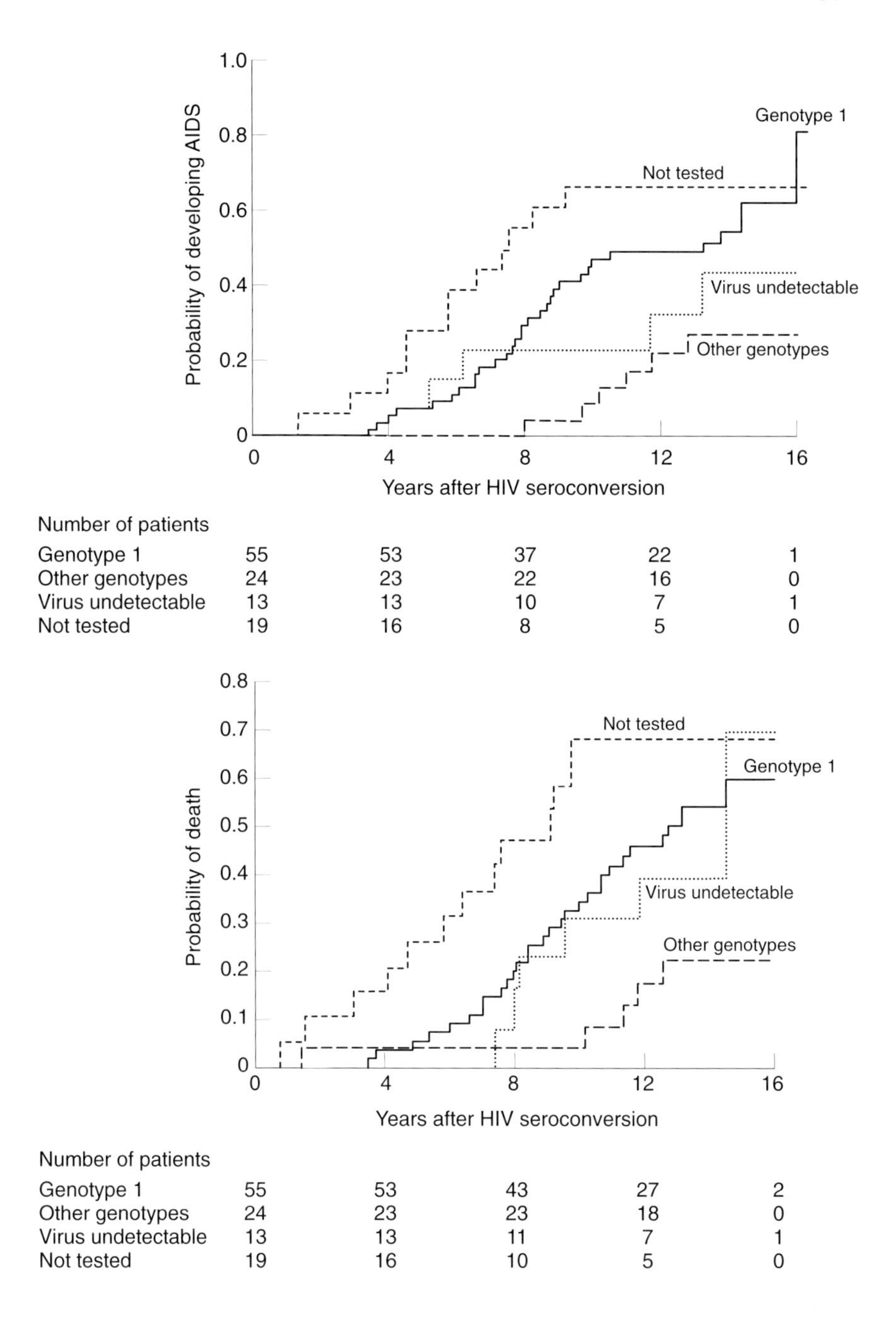

Figure 10.21 Kaplan–Meier plots showing progression to AIDS and death by number of years after HIV seroconversion stratified by HCV genotype test result. (Reproduced, with permission, from *Journal of Infectious Diseases*, 1997; **175**: 166.)

observation of change in genotype after interferon as well as association with response is attributable to a change in the prevalent genotype rather than a change caused by mutation. Infection with more than one genotype of HCV in haemophilic patients may account for the poorer response to interferon compared to other groups (Telfer et al, 1995).

Essential mixed cryoglobulinaemia has been reported to occur in association with HCV (Pascual et al, 1990; Casato et al, 1991). We have reported a patient who developed cryoglobulinaemia in association with vasculitis, arthritis and nephritis following a first exposure to clotting factor concentrate. This coincided with acute hepatitis, which has since been serologically proven to be hepatitis C (Lee et al, 1985c).

Several studies have shown that the transmission of HCV to partners of haemophiliacs is low (Schulman & Grillner, 1990; Eyster et al, 1991; Kolho et al, 1991, Widell et al, 1991, Lee et al, 1992, Brettler et al, 1992). In many of these studies there are additional risk factors, e.g. drug use. However, even though the prevalence of anti-HCV antibodies in female partners of haemophiliacs is low, it remains higher than that observed among blood donors. Thus the importance of condom use has to be stressed when a sexual partner is anti-HCV positive.

Multiple viral infections

Multiple viral infections may occur in haemophilic patients. As a result, complex viral interactions develop and it is sometimes difficult to disentangle the modulating influences of different hepatotropic viruses. Fig. 10.22 shows acute HCV and HBV infection in a patient who received a first exposure to NHS factor IX concentrate (Lee, 1985b; patient 4 of Lim et al, 1991b). In this patient the level of anti-C100 declined at the onset of HBV infection and there was a delay in the appearance of serological markers to HBV. This is the phenomenon of viral interference previously observed in experimental animals. In a cohort of 42 anti-HCV positive haemophiliacs the five who were also HBsAg positive were HCV reverse transcriptase/PCR negative compared with the 4 out of 37 (11%) anti-HCV positive haemophiliacs who were HBsAg negative (Hanley, 1993) (Table 10.17). This was thought to represent the effect of HBV replication inhibiting the replication of HCV. Watson et al (1992) have shown negative or indeterminate HCV serology in two HBsAg positive carriers with haemophilia. This correlates with a finding of a decreased prevalence of anti-HCV in HBsAg-positive patients with hepatocellular carcinoma and cirrhosis (Tanaka et al, 1991). All these studies show that concurrent infection with HCV and HBV interfere with the replication of the respective viruses one upon another.

A further example of viral interaction is shown in Fig. 10.23. This patient was first exposed to factor VIII concentrate in 1976 when he developed acute 'non-B' hepatitis. He continued to receive factor VIII and in 1977 had a presumed subclinical attack of HBV infection that resulted in him becoming a HBsAg/HBeAg positive carrier. In early 1980, he seroconverted from HBeAg

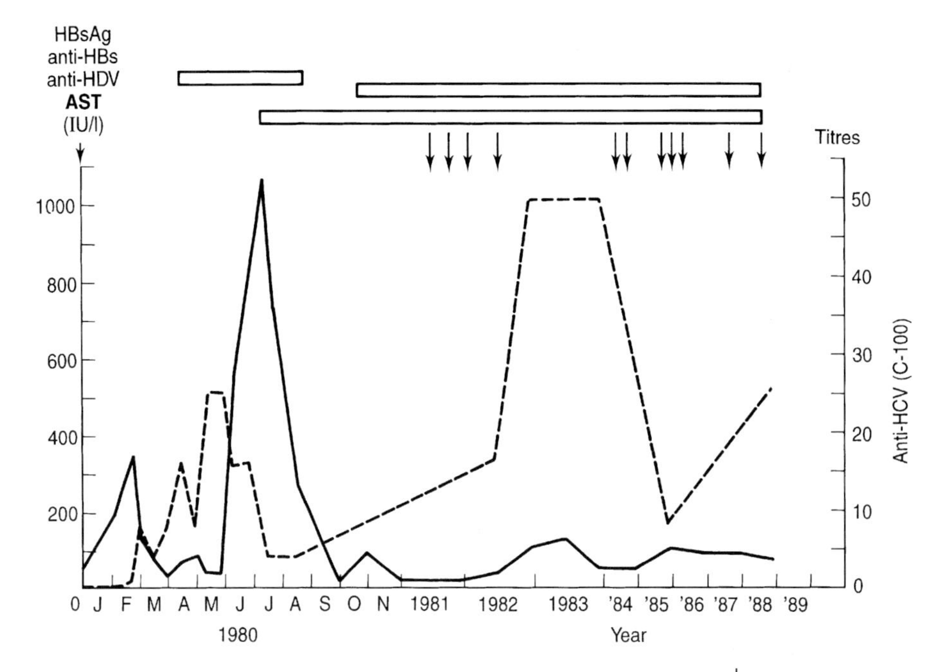

Figure 10.22 Viral interference. ——, AST; ······, Anti-HCV; ↓, F/IX concentrate. (Reproduced, with permission, from Zuckerman, AJ (Ed.) *Viral Hepatitis*. Edinburgh: Churchill Livingstone, 1993).

Table 10.17 Effects of HBV and HIV co-infection on detection of HCV RNA in a cohort of 42 anti-HCV positive haemophiliacs

	n	No. (%) RT/PCR negative	*p**
HBsAg			
Positive	5	5 (100)	0.0001
Negative	37	4 (11)	
Total	42	9 (21)	
Anti-HIV			
Positive	11	2 (8)	0.564
Negative	31	7 (23)	
Total	42	9 (21)	

*Two-tailed Fisher's exact test. RT/PCR, reverse transcriptase/polymerase chain reaction.

(Reproduced, with permission, from Hanley JP, Dolan G, Day S, et al. Interaction of hepatitis B and hepatitis C infection in haemophilia. *British Journal of Haematology* 1993; **85**: 611.)

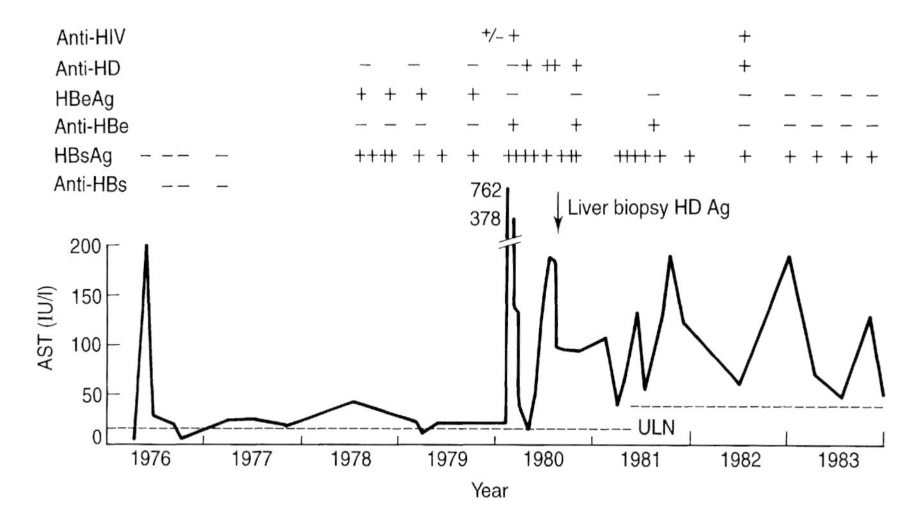

Figure 10.23 The relationship between HBV and delta agent in a patient with haemophilia A. ULN, upper limit of normal. (Reproduced, with permission, from Zuckerman, AJ (Ed.) *Viral Hepatitis*. Edinburgh: Churchill Livingstone, 1993).

to antiHBe and this was accompanied by a severe exacerbation of the hepatitis that was attributed to clearance of virus from infected hepatocytes. Retrospective testing showed that anti-HDV became detectable shortly after this episode and it seems likely that the exacerbation was due to HDV superinfection. It may also be relevant that the patient seroconverted to anti-HIV at the onset of the exacerbation of hepatitis. Hatzakis et al (1987) have shown a prevalence of 1.2% of concurrent HBsAg, anti-HD and anti-HIV in a population of 247 studied Greek haemophiliacs. They point out that the prognosis for such patients is unknown. In a report by Eyster et al (1994) the natural history of HCV in 156 haemophilic patients of whom 98 (63%) were HIV seropositive was reported. Eleven patients developed hepatic decompensation and the risk in anti-HIV positive individuals was three times higher than in anti-HIV negative patients and was estimated as 42% after 27 years' exposure.

In a similar retrospective study 11 of 255 patients developed hepatic decompensation. The risk was 11% at 20 years after first treatment with large donor pool clotting factor concentrate (Telfer et al, 1994). Anti-HIV positive patients were 21 times more likely to develop this complication than HIV-negative individuals. There was also a significant association with p24 antigenaemia and with a declining CD4 count. It is possible that the immunosuppressive effects of HIV infection facilitate HCV replication and mutation thus resulting in a higher viral load and increased liver damage. This is certainly supported by the finding of increased HCV replication with time from HIV seroconversion (Eyster et al, 1995).

Hepatocellular carcinoma

Approximately 50–90% of multitransfused haemophilic patients show abnormalities of serum transaminases and therefore evidence of chronic liver disease. It has been estimated that 30% show evidence of cirrhosis (Lee and Kernoff, 1990; Triger and Preston, 1990). In non-haemophilic patients there is clear evidence that patients with cirrhosis are at risk of developing hepatocellular carcinoma (HCC).

Colombo et al (1991) carried out a questionnaire-based survey among large haemophilia centres worldwide in order to obtain more information on the incidence of HCC in haemophilia. In a survey of 89 centres comprising 11 801 patients, 10 cases of HCC were identified (Table 10.18). This represented a crude rate of HCC of 3.2/1 000 000 patients per year. This was at least 30 times higher than the corresponding background incidence of this tumour in the countries of origin of the patients: USA, Germany and Italy. The epidemiological, clinical and serological characteristics and outcome of the 10 patients with HCC are shown in Table 10.18. Four of the ten patients had a history of heavy alcohol consumption. The average incubation period for transfusion-associated HCC is thought to be 20–30 years (Kiyosawa et al, 1990). Since transfusion transmitted hepatitis was relatively low until the 1970s, when commercial clotting factor concentrates were used on a large scale (Lee and Kernoff 1990), HCC is likely to occur in increasing numbers in this patient group.

Treatment

Hoofnagle et al (1986) first showed that alpha interferon had a beneficial effect on aminotransferases and liver histology in post-transfusion NANB hepatitis. Several large randomized trials have confirmed these findings (Davis et al, 1989, Di Bisceglie et al, 1989) but none of these studies included patients with haemophilia. Makris et al (1991) showed in haemophilic patients that 50% showed normalization of transaminases and improvement of liver histology after treatment with low-dose recombinant alpha interferon. In this study 10 patients received three MU subcutaneously thrice weekly for a year and eight were untreated. Biopsies were performed at entry on 20 patients and on 17 patients on conclusion of the study. Biopsy appearances in the treated group of patients were significantly improved compared with controls. It is interesting that improvement in liver histology was also noted in three HIV antibody patients since the progression of HCV liver disease may be accelerated in the presence of HIV (Martin et al, 1989; Eyster et al, 1993). We have also shown that haemophilic patients infected with HCV respond to interferon treatment and that co-infected individuals have a lower response rate (Telfer et al, 1994).

There are potential hazards of performing liver biopsies in haemophilic patients as well as the high cost of clotting factor concentrate required to cover the pro-

Table 10.18 Epidemiological and clinical characteristics and outcome of 10 patients with hepatocellular carcinoma (HCC)

Case	Centre	Patient age (years)	Serum markers				Liver cirrhosis	Alcohol abuse	Presenting symptoms	Tumour characteristics	Therapy	Present status
			HBsAg	Anti-HCV	Anti-HIV	AFP (ng/ml)						
1	Worcester, MA, USA	74	Pos	NA	Pos	NA	Yes	Yes	None[a]	Diffuse	None	Dead[c]
2	Padua, Italy	46	Pos	NA	Neg	1060	Yes	NA	Abdominal pain	Multifocal	None	Dead
3	Padua, Italy	51	Pos	NA	Neg	171	Yes	NA	Ascites	Multifocal	None	Dead
4	Miami, FL, USA	56	Neg	Pos	Pos	1399	Yes	No	Abdominal pain	Unifocal	Cisplatin	Dead
5	Milan, Italy	55	Neg	Pos	Pos	NA	Yes	No	Jaundice	Unifocal	None	Dead
6	Venice, Italy	39	Neg	Neg	Neg	25	Yes	Yes	Jaundice	Multifocal	None	Dead[c]
7	Frankfurt, Germany	49	Pos	Pos	Neg	1200	Yes	Yes	None	Multifocal	OLT	Alive
8	Frankfurt, Germany	52	Neg	Pos	Pos	807	Yes	No	None	Unifocal	Resection	Alive
9	Providence, RI, USA	49	NA	NA	NA	NA	NA	Yes	None	Lung metastases	None	Dead
10	Chapel Hill, NC, USA	42	Pos	NA	NA	NA	Yes	No	None[b]	Multifocal	None	Dead

NA, information not available; OLT orthotopic liver.
[a]These patients also had anti-HD.
[b]In these patients HCC was incidentally diagnosed at autopsy.
[c]These patients died of causes other than HCC, which was incidentally discovered at autopsy.
(Reproduced with permission, from Zuckerman, 1993).

cedure (Lee, 1997). Thus, even though histological examination of the liver is the ideal method of assessing response to treatment with interferon, it is unlikely to be performed routinely in haemophilic patients. Further trials are required to establish the ideal dose, frequency of administration and length of treatment with interferon.

It is possible that in the multiviral-infected patient, interferon may stop replication of more than one virus. For the haemophilic patient on home treatment it is possible to administer interferon intravenously (Lee et al, 1989).

Ribavirin, a guanosine analogue, is the first drug to offer a potentially effective oral treatment for chronic hepatitis C (Reichard et al, 1991). Multicentre trials, including haemophilic patients, are near completion. It is likely that further trials will be designed to evaluate combination therapy with alpha interferon in the hope of providing a cure for some individuals with chronic HCV disease.

Liver transplantation

Liver transplantation in patients with haemophilia not only reverses the liver failure but also the coagulation defect (Bontempo et al, 1987). It is likely that the hepatocyte is the site of synthesis of factor VIII:C because it contains messenger RNA (Wion et al, 1985). Amongst four patients reported by Bontempo et al (1987) the synthesis of factor VIII occurred as early as 6 hours after the establishment of circulation through the new liver. Orthotopic liver transplantation has been used to treat haemophilia A (Gibas et al, 1988), haemophilia B (Merion et al, 1988) and combined haemophilia A and B (Delorme et al, 1990). In all these cases the transfusion related liver disease and the coagulation defect have been reversed by transplantation. However, the application of liver transplantation to the haemophilic population is complicated by the high prevalence of HIV disease. Rubin et al (1987) reported that five of 10 non-haemophilic recipients of a liver transplant who were, or became, anti-HIV positive died of infection shortly after transplantation, an early mortality rate that was much higher than in HIV-negative individuals.

Thus it is likely that liver transplantation will become common in the management and treatment of end-stage liver disease in haemophilia (Lee, 1997). The cost-benefit is obvious: after transplantation the liver functions and the haemophilia is cured. Even if the patient has HIV infection and the transplant becomes infected with HCV, he can expect a much better quality of life, as well as saving perhaps £30 000 a year in clotting factor concentrate.

Hepatitis A vaccination

In order to protect susceptible patients against hepatitis A, vaccination with hepatitis A vaccine is being recommended. There is accumulating evidence that haemophilic patients respond well in spite of the need to give the vaccine by the subcutaneous route, apart from those who are immunocompromised with HIV infection (Wilde et al, 1995; Zuckerman et al, 1996).

Hepatitis B vaccination

Although advances have been made in blood donor screening and concentrate sterilization, haemophilic patients continue to be at above average risk of contracting hepatitis B infection. This is not only because of the residual risk of concentrates but also because other therapeutic products such as cryoprecipitate and the cellular components of blood cannot be effectively sterilized. Vaccination is therefore mandatory for all patients without serological evidence of immunity.

Current vaccines are either derived from the plasma of HBsAg carriers or are produced by recombinant technology in yeast. In view of the bleeding disorder, subcutaneous administration is preferred and is well tolerated (Desmyter et al, 1983; Mannucci et al, 1989; Miller et al, 1989). A study using yeast recombinant vaccine in haemophiliacs has shown that this is immunogenic (Mannucci et al, 1988) with seroconversion rates similar to those for plasma derived vaccines.

Although it was initially thought that a protective level of anti-HBs would usually be retained for at least 5 years' evidence from haemophiliacs and other groups indicates that it may be lost much earlier. Those infected with HIV respond to vaccine with a lower initial anti-HBs titre and/or lose anti-HBs more quickly (Zanetti et al, 1986; Drake et al, 1987; Miller et al, 1989). The duration of antibody response is dependent on initial peak anti-HBs titres. In a series of 67 anti HIV negative haemophiliacs there was a progressive decline in titres but anti-HBs was still detectable after 4 years (Mannucci et al, 1989). It was extrapolated that patients with less than maximal antibody titre would need vaccinating every 5–6 years and those with greater than maximal antibody response could wait until 10–12 years. In a further study of 167 haemophilic patients it was estimated that the median time for anti-HBs levels to fall to 100 iu/l was between 36 and 42 months, with a shorter period for older or HIV-negative infected patients (Table 10.19) (Pillay et al, 1994).

It is important to note that anti-HIV seropositive patients known to have previously been anti-HBc positive remain at risk of acquiring HBV infection by transfusion. Williams et al (1988) reported acute hepatitis B in 11 of 27 haemophilic boys who received a common batch of factor VIII. Two previously immune children who were also HIV positive became infected with HBV.

Patients with severe bleeding disorders should be vaccinated soon after diagnosis because in spite of sterilization, concentrates can still be infectious (Mannucci et al, 1988). In newly diagnosed infants, immunization should be started immediately after birth.

Table 10.19 Estimated time for hepatitis B surface antibody levels in vaccine responses to decline to 100 iu l^{-1}

Group		Median (months)	Maximum estimated time (months)	*p* value[a]
Sex	Male	38.5	152.2	
	Female	13.7	177.0	0.18
Age group (years)	⩽ 15	51.2	152.2	
	16–30	20.6	122.6	
	> 30	30.9	53.0	0.03
Disorder	Factor VIII < 2%	20.0	152.2	
	Factor VIII > 2%	37.4	122.6	
	Factor IX	49.8	67.4	
	Other/not known	38.2	117.0	0.66
Hepatitis B core antibody	–ve	37.2	152.2	
	+ve	20.6	67.4	0.27
HIV antibody	–ve	40.4	152.2	
	+ve	18.0	61.7	0.05
Method of vaccination	Intradermal	23.5	68.7	
	Subcutaneous	38.9	152.2	0.35

Data collected on 90 individuals.
[a]*p* value based on a Wilcoxon test where the comparison is between two groups, or a Kruskal–Wallis test where the comparison is between more than two groups.
(Reproduced, with permission, from Pillay et al, 1993).

Hepatitis G (HGV)

Two unique flavivirus–like genomes, have been isolated from a tamarin (Simons et al, 1995). The original isolate was from a 34-year-old surgeon (GB) with acute, icteric hepatitis that was subsequently passed through tamarins. It is likely that there are three agents: GBV-B (a tamarin virus), GBV-A (a human virus) and GBV-C, which has been detected in two patients who developed anaemia after transfusion. These viruses have been detected in all areas of the world and the frequency ranges from 2% in blood donors to 14% in multiply transfused individuals. Another virus hepatitis G virus (HGV) has been isolated which may be identical to HGBV-C (Alter et al, 1996). Seroprevalence studies have shown the virus to be present in 46% of injecting drug users, 22% of dialysis patients, 10% of haemophilic patients and 16% of multitransfused patients (Adamson et al, 1995).

It has been shown that despite the high level of HGV contamination of unsterilized clotting factor concentrates, the recipients do not have a high level of persistent infection as shown by PCR (Jarvis et al, 1996). A report of detection of antibodies to a putative HGV envelope protein has suggested that only a minority of individuals infected with HGV become carriers whereas the majority develop antibody (Tacke et al, 1997).

Parvovirus

Human parvovirus B19, is a serum virus which was first found in asymptomatic blood donors (Cossart et al, 1975). It was subsequently shown that it was widely transmitted to haemophilic patients by clotting factor concentrates (Azzi et al, 1992; Schwart et al, 1991; Corsi et al, 1988; Morfini et al, 1992). B19 is a non-enveloped virus which is thermoresistant and the currently used methods of virus inactivation by solvent detergent, or by dry heating, seem to be ineffective in destroying these particles. A recent study evaluated the seroprevalence of parvovirus B19 in 22 HIV- and HCV-negative haemophiliacs who were treated exclusively with clotting factor concentrates which were considered safe with respect to HIV and HCV transmission (Flores et al, 1995). Whereas there was a 32% prevalence of parvovirus seropositivity in controls, there was a 77% seropositivity to parvovirus in patients treated with clotting factor concentrate. These results show that haemophilic patients have a higher seroprevalence of B19 than a normal population. Parvovirus B19 infection is common and occurs worldwide. There is a three- to four-year epidemic cycle with a seasonal peak in the first half of each year. Around 50% of blood donors have IgG antibody from past infection so one strategy to avoid parvovirus infection might be to choose blood donors who were IgG positive or an alternative would be to screen blood donors for B19 DNA by PCR.

Acute infection with parvovirus causes minor febrile illness. However, transient aplastic crises or chronic anaemia may occur, particularly in patients with haemoglobinopathies. Disturbances of consciousness and hepatic dysfunction have also been described. It is usually suggested that this is only a risk for immunosuppressed patients. However, an immunocompetent adult with haemophilia has been reported with a pancytopaenia and septicaemia secondary to treatment with a heated clotting factor concentrate (Yee et al, 1995). A further immunocompetent 11 year old has also been described who developed a severe disorder associated with severe neurological disturbance following parvovirus infection secondary to treatment with factor VIII concentrate (Coumau et al, 1996). Of greatest concern is the occurrence of parvovirus infection during pregnancy when it can result in miscarriage or hydrops foetalis. Thus for the carrier of haemophilia, the argument for the use of recombinant clotting factor concentrate is compelling. In a study where B19 DNA in 25 clotting factor concentrates, prepared by a variety of procedures of purification and activation were assessed using dot blot hybridization assays and nested PCR, 9 out of 25 products were positive

(Zakrzewska et al, 1992). However the presence of B19 DNA in clotting factor concentrates does not necessarily indicate a risk of infection with parvovirus. Therefore, this cannot be recommended as a screening method yet.

Creutzfeldt-Jakob disease

Creutzfeldt-Jakob disease (CJD) is a rapidly developing degenerative disease of the central nervous system characterized by dementia, multifocal myoclonus and periodic triphasic discharges on EEG. On October 18, 1994, the American Red Cross reported to the FDA that a 64-year-old blood donor had died of CJD. He had donated more than 90 times over a period of 30 years, and plasma from his donations was often pooled to make plasma derivatives. Baxter and the American Red Cross initiated voluntary withdrawal of implicated lots of IVIg, factor VIII, albumin and plasma protein fraction on November 17, 1994. In November 1994, haemophilia treaters in New York also notified patients who had received implicated lots of factor VIII.

The concerns about the transmissibility of CJD by transfusion have been fuelled by the work of Manuelidis et al (1985) who inoculated buffy coat cells from the peripheral blood of two CJD patients into the brains of rodents which resulted in spongiform degeneration. It is thought that the disease is caused by an infectious protein or prion which induces conformational changes in normal plasma membrane protein (DeArmond & Prusiner, 1995).

Various investigators have examined the possibility of CJD transmission by blood transfusion. The frequency of blood transfusions or donations did not differ between CJD cases and matched controls in a prospective study of the transfusion histories among 202 CJD cases (Esmonde et al, 1993).

Furthermore, the Medline database contains 1485 references on CJD and 6385 references on haemophilia between January 1976 and October 1994 (Adamson et al, 1995). None of these references links CJD and haemophilia. An extensive review of mortality data at CDC by L Schonberger has not revealed a single CJD death in an individual with a clotting disorder.

Unfortunately, because of the long incubation period of CJD, which may be 30 years, there will be a long period of time before more definitive answers are available as to the transmission by blood products.

References

Abrams DI, Kiprov DD, Goedert JJ, Sarngadharan MG, Gallo RC. Antibodies to human T-lymphotropic virus type III and development of the acquired immunodeficiency syndrome in homosexual men presenting with immune thrombocytopenia. *Annals of Internal Medicine* 1986; **104**: 47

Adamson JW, Blaine Hollinger F, et al. Challenges to transfusion medicine: infection and immunologic complications of blood transfusion. *Education Programme of ASH* (Seattle) 1995 pp. 82–92.

Allain JP, Laurian Y, Paul DA, et al. Long-term evaluation of HIV antigen and antibodies to p24 and gp41 in patients with hemophilia. Potential clinical importance. *New England Journal of Medicine* 1987; **317**: 1114.

Alter HJ, Purcell RH, Shih JW, Melpolder JC, Houghton M, Choo QL. Detection of antibody to hepatitis C virus in prospectively followed transfusion recipients with acute and chronic non-A, non-B hepatitis. *New England Journal of Medicine* 1989; **321**: 1494.

Alter MJ, Gallagher M, Morris T, et al. Epidemiology of non-A-non-E hepatitis. In: Rizzetto M, ed. Proceedings of the 9th Triennial International Symposium on Viral Hepatitis and Liver Disease, Rome, Italy, April 21–25. 1996.

Aronstam A, Congard B, Evans DI, et al. HIV infection in haemophilia–a European cohort. *Archives of Disease in Childhood* 1993; **68**: 521.

Azzi A, Ciappi S, Zakvrzewska K, et al. Human parvovirus B 19 infection in hemophiliacs first induced with two high-purity, virally attenuated factor VIII concentrates. *American Journal of Hematology* 1992; **39**: 228.

Bartlett JG. Zidovudine now or later? [editorial]. *New England Journal of Medicine* 1993; **329**: 351.

Beard J, Savidge GF. High-dose intravenous immunoglobulin and splenectomy for the treatment of HIV-related immune thrombocytopenia in patients with severe haemophilia. *British Journal of Haematology* 1988; **68**: 303.

Beeson PB. Jaundice occurring one to four months after transfusion of blood or plasma. *Journal of the American Medical Association* 1943; **121**: 1332.

Biggs R. Jaundice and antibodies directed against factors 8 and 9 in patients treated for haemophilia or Christmas disease in the United Kingdom. *British Journal of Haematology* 1974; **26**: 313.

Blumberg BS, Gerstley BJS, Hungerford DA, et al. A serum antigen (Australia antigen) in Down's syndrome, leukaemia and hepatitis. *Annals of Internal Medicine* 1967; **66**: 924.

Bontempo FA, Lewis JH, Gorenc TJ, Spero JA, Ragni MV, Scott JP. Liver transplantation in hemophilia A. *Blood* 1987; **69**: 1721.

Brettler DB, Forsberg AD, Levine PH, et al. Factor VIII:C concentrate purified from plasma using monoclonal antibodies: human studies. *Blood* 1989; **73**: 1859.

Brettler DB, Mannucci PM, Gringeri A, et al. The low risk of hepatitis C virus transmission among sexual partners of hepatitis C-infected hemophilic males: an international, multicenter study. *Blood* 1992; **80**: 540.

Carpenter CCJ, Fischl MA, Hammer SM, et al. Consensus statement. Antiretroviral therapy for HIV infection in 1996. *JAMA* 1996; **276**: 146.

Casato M, Taliani G, Pucillo LP, Goffredo F, Lagana B, Bonomo L. Cryoglobulinaemia and hepatitis C virus. *Lancet* 1991; **337**: 1047.

Centers for Disease Control. Pneumocystis carinii pneumonia among persons with haemophilia A. *Morbidity and Mortality Weekly Report* 1982; **31**: 365.

Centers for Disease Control. HIV-1 infection and artificial insemination with processed semen. *Morbidity and Mortality Weekly Report* 1990; **39**: 255.

Centers for Disease Control. Tuberculosis control laws – United States, 1993. Recommendations of the Advisory Council for the Elimination of Tuberculosis (ACET). *Morbidity and Mortality Weekly Report* 1993; **42**: 1–28.

Centers for Disease Control. Hepatitis A among persons with hemophilia who received clotting factor concentrate – United States, September-December 1995. *Morbidity and Mortality Weekly Report* 1996; **45**: 29.

Cheingsong-Popov R, Panagiotidi C, Bowcock S, Aronstam A, Wadsworth J. Relation between humoral responses to HIV gag and env proteins at seroconversion and clinical outcome of HIV infection. *British Medical Journal* 1991; **302**: 23.

Chorba TL, Holman RC, Strine TW, et al. Changes in longevity and causes of death among persons with hemophilia A. *American Journal of Hematology* 1994; **45**: 112.

Colombo M, Mannucci PM, Brettler DB, et al. Hepatocellular carcinoma in hemophilia. *American Journal of Hematology* 1991; **37**: 243.

Concorde co-ordinating committee. Concorde: MRC/ANRS randomised double-blind controlled trial of immediate and deferred zidovudine in symptom-free HIV infection. *Lancet* 1994; **343**: 871.

Cooper DA, Gatell JM, Kroon S, et al. Zidovudine in persons with asymptomatic HIV infection and CD4+ cell counts greater than 400 per cubic millimeter. The European-Australian Collaborative Group. *New England Journal of Medicine* 1993; **329**: 297.

Corsi B, Azzi A, Morfini N, et al. Humanparvovirus infection in haemophiliacs first infused with treated clotting factor concentrates. *Journal of Medical Virology* 1988; **25**: 165–170.

Cossart YE, Field AM, Cant B, et al. Parvovirus-like particles in human sera. *Lancet* 1975; 72.

Coumau E, Peynet J, Harzic M, et al. Severe parvovirus B19 infection in an immunocompetent hemophiliac-A child. *Archives de Pediatrie* 1996; **3**: 35.

Cuthbert RJ, Ludlam CA, Tucker J, Steel CM, Beatson D, Rebus S. Five year prospective study of HIV infection in the Edinburgh haemophiliac cohort. *British Medical Journal* 1990; **301**: 956.

Darby SC, Rizza CR, Doll R, Spooner RJ, Stratton IM, Thakrar B. Incidence of AIDS and excess of mortality associated with HIV in haemophiliacs in the United Kingdom: report on behalf of the directors of haemophilia centres in the United Kingdom. *British Medical Journal* 1989; **298**: 1064.

Darby SC, Ewart DW, Giangrande PLF, et al. Mortality before and after HIV infection in the complete UK population of haemophiliacs. *Nature* 1995; **377**: 79.

Davis GL, Balart LA, Schiff ER, et al. Treatment of chronic hepatitis C with recombinant interferon alfa. A multicenter randomized, controlled trial. Hepatitis Interventional Therapy Group. *New England Journal of Medicine* 1989; **321**: 1501.

DeArmond SJ, Prusiner SB. Etiology and pathogenesis of prion diseases. *American Journal of Pathology* 1995; **146**: 785.

DeBiasi R, Rocino A, Miraglia E, et al. The impact of a very high purity Factor VIII concentrate on the immune system of human immunodeficiency virus-infected haemophiliacs: a randomised, prospective, two-year comparison with an intermediate purity concentrate. *Blood* 1991; **78**: 1919.

Decker CF, Masur H. Current status of prophylaxis for opportunistic infections in HIV-infected patients. *AIDS* 1994; **8**: 11.

Delorme MA, Adams PC, Grant D, Ghent CN, Walker IR, Wall WJ. Orthotopic liver transplantation in a patient with combined hemophilia A and B. *American Journal of Hematology* 1990; **33**: 136.

Desmyter J, Colaert J, Verstraete M, Vermylen J. Hepatitis B vaccination of hemophiliacs. *Scandinavian Journal of Infectious Diseases – Supplementum* 1983; **38**: 42.

Devereux H, Telfer P, Dusheiko G, et al. Hepatitis C genotypes in haemophilic patients treated with alpha-interferon. *Journal of Medical Virology* 1995; **45**: 284.

Di Bisceglie AM, Martin P, Kassianides C, et al. Recombinant interferon alfa therapy for chronic hepatitis C. A randomized, double-blind, placebo-controlled trial. *New England Journal of Medicine* 1989; **321**: 1506.

Dolan G. Viral interference in haemophilia. *Haemophilia* 1995; 1 (suppl 4): 13.

Dourakis S, Brown J, Kumar U, et al. Serological response and detection of viraemia in acute hepatitis C virus infection. *Journal of Hepatology* 1992; **14**: 370.

Drake JH, Parmley RT, Britton HA. Loss of hepatitis B antibody in human immunodeficiency virus-positive hemophilia patients. *Pediatric Infectious Disease Journal* 1987; **6**: 1051.

Dublin S, Rosenberg PS, Goedert JJ, et al. Patterns and predictors of high-risk sexual behaviour in female partners of HIV-infected men with hemophilia. *AIDS* 1992; **6**: 475.

Dusheiko G, Schmilovitz-Weiss H, Brown D, et al. Hepatitis C virus genotypes: an investigation of type-specific differences in geographic origin and disease. *Hepatology* 1994; **19**: 13.

Ellis ME, Neal KR, Leen CL, Newland AC. Alfa-2a recombinant interferon in HIV associated thrombocytopenia. *British Medical Journal* 1987; **295**: 1519.

Esmonde TFG, Will RG, Slattery JM, et al. Creutzfeld-Jakob disease and blood transfusion. *Lancet* 1993; **341**: 205.

Eyster ME, Hatzakis A. HCV genotypes in multitransfused hemophiliacs. *Gastroenterology*. 1996; **110**: A1187.
Eyster ME, Gail MH, Ballard JO, Al-Mondhiry H, Goedert JJ. Natural history of human immunodeficiency virus infections in hemophiliacs: effects of T-cell subsets, platelet counts, and age. *Annals of Internal Medicine* 1987; **107**: 1.
Eyster ME, Ballard JO, Gail MH, Drummond JE, Goedert JJ. Predictive markers for the acquired immunodeficiency syndrome (AIDS) in hemophiliacs: persistence of p24 antigen and low T4 cell count. *Annals of Internal Medicine* 1989; **110**: 963.
Eyster ME, Alter HJ, Aledort LM, Quan S, Hatzakis A, Goedert JJ. Heterosexual co-transmission of hepatitis C virus (HCV) and human immunodeficiency virus (HIV). *Annals of Internal Medicine* 1991; **115**: 764.
Eyster ME, Diamondstone LS, Lien JM, Ehmann WC, Quan S, Goedert JJ. Natural history of hepatitis C virus infection in multitransfused hemophiliacs: effect of coinfection with human immunodeficiency virus. The Multicenter Hemophilia Cohort Study. *Journal of Acquired Immune Deficiency Syndromes* 1993; **6**: 602.
Eyster ME, Fried MW, Di Bisceglie AM, et al. Increasing hepatitis C virus RNA levels in haemophiliacs: relationship to human immunodeficiency virus infection and liver disease. *Blood* 1994; **84**: 1020.
Eyster ME, Sanders JC, Battegay M, et al. Suppression of hepatitis C virus (HCV) replication by hepatitis D virus (HDV) in HIV-infected hemophiliacs with chronic Hepatitis B and C. *Digestive Diseases and Sciences*. 1995; **40**: 1583.
Filipovich AH, Spector BD, Kersey J. Immunodeficiency in humans as a risk factor in the development of malignancy. *Preventive Medicine* 1980; **9**: 252.
Fischl MA, Richman DD, Grieco MH, et al. The efficacy of azidothymidine (AZT) in the treatment of patients with AIDS and AIDS-related complex. A double-blind, placebo-controlled trial. *New England Journal of Medicine* 1987; **317**: 185.
Fletcher ML, Trowell JM, Craske J, Pavier K, Rizza CR. Non-A non-B hepatitis after transfusion of factor VIII in infrequently treated patients. *British Medical Journal* 1983; **287**: 1754.
Flores G, Juarez JC, Montoro JB, et al. Seroprevalence of parvovirus B 19, cytomegalovirus, hepatitis A virus and hepatitis E virus antibodies in haemophiliacs treated exclusively with clotting factor concentrates considered safe against human immunodeficiency and hepatitis C viruses. *Haemophilia* 1995; **1**: 115.
Fukutake K, Hada M, Ikematsu S, et al. Multicenter study on the influence of long-term continuous use of ultrapurified factor VIII preparation on the immunological status of HIV-infected and non-infected hemophilia A patients (Abstract). *XIXth International Congress of the World Federation of Hemophilia* 1990.
Garson JA, Tuke PW, Makris M, Briggs M, Machin SJ, Preston FE. Demonstration of viraemia patterns in haemophiliacs treated with hepatitis-C-virus-contaminated factor VIII concentrates. *Lancet* 1990; **336**: 1022.
Gerritzen A, Schneweis KE, Brackmann HH, Oldenburg J, Hanfland P, Caspari G. Acute hepatitis A in haemophiliacs. *Lancet* 1992; **340**: 1231.
Gibas A, Dienstag JL, Schafer AI, et al. Cure of hemophilia A by orthotopic liver transplantation. *Gastroenterology* 1988; **95**: 192.
Goedert JJ, Kessler CM, Aledort LM, et al. A prospective study of human immunodeficiency virus type 1 infection and the development of AIDS in subjects with hemophilia [see comments]. *New England Journal of Medicine* 1989; **321**: 1141.
Goldman E, Lee C, Miller R, Kernoff P, Morris-Smith J, Taylor B. Children of HIV positive haemophilic men. *Archives of Disease in Childhood* 1993, **68**: 133–134.
Goldman E, Miller R, Lee CA. Counselling HIV positive haemophilic men who wish to have children. *British Medical Journal* 1992; **304**: 829.
Goldman E, Miller R, Lee CA. A family with HIV and haemophilia. *AIDS Care* 1993; **5**: 79.
Goldsmith JM, Deutsche J, Tang M, et al. CD4 cells in HIV-1 infected hemophiliacs: effect of factor VIII concentrates. *Thrombosis and Haemostasis* 1991; **66**: 415.
Hanley JP, Dolan G, Day S, Skidmore SJ, Irving WL. Interaction of hepatitis B and hepatitis C infection in haemophilia. *British Journal of Haematology* 1993; **85**: 611.
Hatzakis A, Hadziyannis S, Maclure M, Louizou C, Yannitsiotis A. Concurrent hepatitis B, delta and human immunodeficiency virus infection in hemophiliacs [letter]. *Thrombosis & Haemostasis* 1987; **58**: 791.

Hilgartner MW, Buckley JD, Openskalski EA, et al. Purity of factor VIII concentrates and serial CD4 counts. *Lancet* 1993; **341**: 1373.
Hollinger FB, Khan NC, Oefinger PE, et al. Posttransfusion hepatitis type A. *JAMA* 1983; **250**: 2313.
Hoofnagle JH, Mullen KD, Jones DB, et al. Treatment of chronic non-A,non-B hepatitis with recombinant human alpha interferon. A preliminary report. *New England Journal of Medicine* 1986; **315**: 1575.
Hoover R, Fraumeni JF, Jr. Risk of cancer in renal-transplant recipients. *Lancet* 1973; **2**: 55.
Hymes KB, Greene JB, Karpatkin S. The effect of azidothymidine on HIV-related thrombocytopenia. *New England Journal of Medicine* 1988; **318**: 516.
Jacobson IM, Dienstag JL, Werner BG, Brettler DB, Levine PH. Epidemiology and clinical impact of hepatitis D virus (delta) infection. *Hepatology* 1985; **5**: 188.
Jarvis LM, Watson HG, McOmish F, Peutherer JF, Ludlam CA, Simmonds P. Frequent reinfection and reactivation of hepatitis C virus genotypes in multitransfused hemophiliacs. *Journal of Infectious Diseases*. 1994; **170**: 1018.
Jarvis LM, Davidson F, Hanley JP, et al. Low-frequency of persistent infection with HGV or GBV-C in hemophiliacs and other plasma product users. *Hepatology* 1996; **24**: 49.
Karpatkin S. Immunologic thrombocytopenic purpura in HIV-seropositive homosexuals, narcotic addicts and hemophiliacs. *Seminars in Hematology* 1988; **25**: 219.
Kasper CK, Kipnis SA. Hepatitis and clotting-factor concentrates. *Journal of the American Medical Association* 1972; **221**: 510.
Kernoff PB, Lee CA, Karayiannis P, Thomas HC. High risk of non-A non-B hepatitis after a first exposure to volunteer or commercial clotting factor concentrates: effects of prophylactic immune serum globulin. *British Journal of Haematology* 1985; **60**: 469.
Kiyosawa K, Sodeyama T, Tanaka E, et al. Interrelationship of blood transfusion, non-A, non-B hepatitis and hepatocellular carcinoma: analysis by detection of antibody to hepatitis C virus. *Hepatology* 1990; **12**: 671.
Kolho E, Naukkarinen R, Ebeling F, Rasi V, Ikkala E, Krusius T. Transmission of hepatitis C virus to sexual partners of seropositive patients with bleeding disorders: a rare event. *Scandinavian Journal of Infectious Diseases* 1991; **23**: 667.
Kuo G, Choo QL, Alter HJ, et al. An assay for circulating antibodies to a major etiologic virus of human non-A, non-B hepatitis. *Science* 1989; **244**: 362.
Lee CA. Coagulation factor replacement therapy. In Hoffbrand AV, Brenner MK (eds): *Recent Advances in Haematology* 6. Edinburgh: Churchill Livingstone, 1992.
Lee CA. Investigation of chronic hepatitis C infection in individuals with haemophilia. *British Journal of Haematology* 1997; **96**: 424.
Lee CA. Hope for haemophilia patient with hepatitis. *Gut* 1997, **3**: 887–888.
Lee CA, Kernoff PB. Viral hepatitis and haemophilia. *British Medical Bulletin* 1990; **46**: 408.
Lee CA, Bofill M, Janossy G, Thomas HC, Rizza CR, Kernoff PB. Relationships between blood product exposure and immunological abnormalities in English haemophiliacs. *British Journal of Haematology* 1985a; **60**: 161.
Lee CA, Kernoff PB, Karayiannis P, Farci P, Thomas HC. Interactions between hepatotropic viruses in patients with haemophilia. *Journal of Hepatology* 1985; **1**: 379.
Lee CA, Kernoff PB, Peters DK. Cryoglobulinaemia in haemophilia. *British Medical Journal* 1985c; **290**: 1947.
Lee CA, Phillips A, Elford J, Miller EJ, Bofill M, Griffiths PD. The natural history of human immunodeficiency virus infection in a haemophilic cohort. *British Journal of Haematology* 1989; **73**: 228.
Lee CA, Webster A, Griffiths PD, Kernoff PB. Symptomless HIV infection after more than ten years [letter]. *Lancet* 1990; **335**: 425.
Lee C, Chrispeels J, Telfer P, Dusheiko G. Hepatitis C antibody profile in adults with haemophilia and their sexual partners [letter]. *British Journal of Haematology* 1992; **81**: 133.
Lee CA, Sabin CA, Phillips AN, et al. Morbidity and mortality from transfusion-transmitted disease in haemophilia. *Lancet* 1995; **345**: 1309.
Leissinger CA, Andes WA. Role of splenectomy in the management of hemophilic patients with human immunodeficiency virus-associated immunopathic thrombocytopenic purpura. *American Journal of Hematology* 1992; **40**: 207.

Lemon SM, Becherer PR, Wang JG, et al. Hepatitis delta infection among multiply-transfused hemophiliacs. *Progress in Clinical & Biological Research* 1991; **364**: 351.
Lever AM, Brook MG, Yap I, Thomas HC. Treatment of thrombocytopenia with alpha interferon. *British Medical Journal* 1987; **295**: 1519.
Lim SG, Lee CA, Kernoff PB. The treatment of HIV associated thrombocytopenia in haemophiliacs. *Clinical & Laboratory Haematology* 1990; **12**: 237.
Lim SG, Lee CA, Hales M, O'Doherty M, Winter M, Kernoff PB. Fluconazole for oro-pharyngeal candidiasis in anti-HIV positive haemophiliacs. *Alimentary Pharmacology & Therapeutics* 1991a; **5**: 199.
Lim SG, Lee CA, Charman H, Tilsed G, Griffiths PD, Kernoff PB. Hepatitis C antibody assay in a longitudinal study of haemophiliacs. *British Journal of Haematology* 1991b; **78**: 398.
Makris M, Preston FE, Triger DR, Underwood JC, Westlake L, Adelman MI. A randomized controlled trial of recombinant interferon-alpha in chronic hepatitis C in hemophiliacs. *Blood* 1991; **78**: 1672.
Mannucci PM. Outbreak of hepatitis A among Italian patients with haemophilia. *Lancet* 1992; **339**: 819.
Mannucci PM. Modern treatment of haemophilia: from the shadows toward the light. *Thrombosis and Haemostasis* 1993; **70**: 17.
Mannucci PM. The choice of plasma-derived clotting factor concentrates. *Baillières Clinical Haematology* 1996; **9**: 273.
Mannucci PM, Gringeri A, Morfini M, et al. Immunogenicity of a recombinant hepatitis B vaccine in hemophiliacs. *American Journal of Hematology* 1988; **29**: 211.
Mannucci PM, Zanetti AR, Gringeri A, et al. Long-term immunogenicity of a plasma-derived hepatitis B vaccine in HIV seropositive and HIV seronegative hemophiliacs. *Archives of Internal Medicine* 1989; **149**: 1333.
Mannucci PM, Brettler DB, Aledort LM, et al. Immune status of human immunodeficiency virus seropositive and seronegative hemophiliacs infused for 3.5 years with recombinant factor VIII. *Blood* 1994; **83**: 1958.
Manuelidis EE, Kim JH, Mericangas JR, et al. Transmission to animals of Creutzfeld-Jakob Disease from human blood. *Lancet* 1985; **ii**: 896.
Martin P, Di Bisceglie AM, Kassianides C, Lisker-Melman M, Hoofnagle JH. Rapidly progressive non-A, non-B hepatitis in patients with human immunodeficiency virus infection. *Gastroenterology* 1989; **97**: 1559.
Mauser-Bunschoten EP, Bresters D, van Drimmelen AAJ, et al. Hepatitis C infection and viremia in Dutch hemophilia patients. *Journal of Medical Virology*. 1995; **45**: 241.
McMillan CW, Diamond LK, Surgenor DM. Treatment of classic haemophilia: the use of fibrinogen rich in factor VIII for haemorrhage and for surgery. *New England Journal of Medicine* 1961; **265**: 277.
Mellors JW, Rinaldo CR, Gupta P, et al. Prognosis in HIV-1 infection predicted by the quantity of virus in plasma. *Science* 1996; **272**: 1167.
Merion RM, Delius RE, Campbell DA, Jr., Turcotte JG. Orthotopic liver transplantation totally corrects factor IX deficiency in hemophilia B. *Surgery* 1988; **104**: 929.
Miller EJ, Lee CA, Karayiannis P, Holmes S, Thomas HC, Kernoff PB. Immune response of patients with congenital coagulation disorders to hepatitis B vaccine: suboptimal response and human immunodeficiency virus infection. *Journal of Medical Virology* 1989; **28**: 96.
Morfini M, Longo G, Rossi Ferrini P, et al. Hypoplastic anemia in a hemophiliac first infused with a solvent/detergent treated factor VIII concentrate: the role of human B 19 parvovirus. *American Journal of Hematology* 1992; **39**: 149.
O'Brien TR, Blattner WA, Waters D, et al. Serum HIV-1 RNA levels and time to development of AIDS in the multicenter hemophilia cohort study. *JAMA* 1996; **276**: 105.
Oksenhendler E, Bierling P, Farcet JP, Rabian C, Seligmann M, Clauvel JP. Response to therapy in 37 patients with HIV-related thrombocytopenic purpura. *British Journal of Haematology* 1987; **66**: 491.
Pascual M, Perrin L, Giostra E, Schifferli JA. Hepatitis C virus in patients with cryo-globulinemia type II. *Journal of Infectious Diseases* 1990; **162**: 569.
Pasi KJ, Ononye C, Jenkins PV, Sabin CA, Lee CA. Analysis of CKR5 mutants in HIV infected haemophilic patients and HIV exposed but uninfected haemophilic patients. *Blood* 1996; 88 (10 suppl 1): 654a.

Peerlinck K, Vermylen J. Acute hepatitis A in patients with haemophilia A [letter]. *Lancet* 1993; **341**: 179.
Phillips A, Lee CA, Elford J, et al. Prediction of progression to AIDS by analysis of CD4 lymphocyte counts in a haemophilic cohort. *AIDS* 1989; **3**: 737.
Phillips AN, Lee CA, Elford J, et al. Serial CD4 lymphocyte counts and development of AIDS. *Lancet* 1991a; **337**: 389.
Phillips AN, Lee CA, Elford J, Webster A, Janossy G, Griffiths PD. p24 antigenaemia, CD4 lymphocyte counts and the development of AIDS. *AIDS* 1991b; **5**: 1217.
Phillips AN, Lee CA, Elford J, et al. More rapid progression to AIDS in older HIV-infected people: the role of CD4+ T-cell counts. *Journal of Acquired Immune Deficiency Syndromes* 1991c; **4**: 970.
Phillips AN, Elford J, Sabin C, et al. Immunodeficiency and the risk of death in HIV infection. *Journal of the American Medical Association* 1992; **268**: 2662.
Phillips AN, Sabin CA, Elford J, Bofill M, Lee CA, Janossy G. CD8 lymphocyte counts and serum immunoglobulin A levels early in HIV infection as predictors of CD4 lymphocyte depletion during 8 years of follow-up. *AIDS* 1993; **7**: 975.
Phillips AN, Sabin CA, Elford J, et al. Use of CD4 lymphocyte count to predict long term survival free of AIDS after HIV infection. *British Medical Journal* 1994; **309**: 309.
Pierce M, Crampton S, Henry D, et al. A randomized trial of clarithromycin as prophylaxis against disseminated Mycobacterium avium complex infection in patients with advanced acquired immunodeficiency syndrome. *New England Journal of Medicine* 1996; **335**: 384.
Pillay D, Pereira C, Sabin C, et al. A long-term follow up of hepatitis B vaccination in patients with congenital clotting disorders. *Vaccine* 1994; **12**: 978.
Pottage JC, Jr, Benson CA, Spear JB, Landay AL, Kessler HA. Treatment of human immunodeficiency virus-related thrombocytopenia with zidovudine. *Journal of the American Medical Association* 1988; **260**: 3045.
Rabkin CS, Hilgartner MW, Hedberg KW, et al. Incidence of lymphomas and other cancers in HIV-infected and HIV-uninfected patients with hemophilia. *Journal of the American Medical Association* 1992; **267**: 1090.
Ragni MV, Bontempo FA, Myers DJ, Kiss JE, Oral A. Hemorrhagic sequelae of immune thrombocytopenic purpura in human immunodeficiency virus-infected hemophiliacs. *Blood* 1990; **75**: 1267.
Ratner L. Human immunodeficiency virus-associated autoimmune thrombocytopenic purpura: a review. *American Journal of Medicine* 1989; **86**: 194.
Ratnoff OD, Menitove JE, Aster RH, Lederman MM. Coincident classic hemophilia and "idiopathic" thrombocytopenic purpura in patients under treatment with concentrates of antihemophilic factor (factor VIII). *New England Journal of Medicine* 1983; **308**: 439.
Reichard O, Andersson J, Schvarcz R, Weiland O. Ribavirin treatment for chronic hepatitis C. *Lancet* 1991; **337**: 1058.
Rizzetto M, Morello C, Mannucci PM, et al. Delta infection and liver disease in hemophilic carriers of hepatitis B surface antigen. *Journal of Infectious Diseases* 1982; **145**: 18.
Rosina F, Saracco G, Rizzetto M. Risk of post-transfusion infection with the hepatitis delta virus. A multicenter study. *New England Journal of Medicine* 1985; **312**: 1488.
Rubin RH, Jenkins RL, Shaw BW, et al. The acquired immunodeficiency syndrome and transplantation. *Transplantation* 1987; **44**: 1.
Sabin C, Pasi J, Phillips A, et al. CD4+ counts before and after switching to monoclonal high-purity factor III concentrate in HIV-infected haemophilic patients. *Thrombosis and Haemostasis* 1994; **72**: 214.
Sabin CA, Telfer P, Phillips AN. The association between hepatitis C virus (HCV) genotype and human immunodeficiency virus (HIV) disease progression in a cohort of hemophilic men. *Journal of Infectious Diseases* 1997; **175**: 164.
Sahmoud T, Laurian Y, Garzengel C, et al. Progression to AIDS in French haemophiliacs association with HLA-B35. *AIDS* 1993; **7**: 497.
Sande MA, Carpenter CC, Cobbs CG, Holmes KK, Sanford JP. Antiretroviral therapy for adult HIV-infected patients. Recommendations from a state-of-the-art conference. National Institute of Allergy and Infectious Diseases State-of-the-Art Panel on Anti-Retroviral Therapy for Adult HIV-Infected Patients. *Journal of the American Medical Association* 1993; **270**: 2583.
Savona S, Nardi MA, Lennette ET, Karpatkin S. Thrombocytopenic purpura in narcotics addicts. *Annals of Internal Medicine* 1985; **102**: 737.

Schulman S, Grillner L. Antibodies against hepatitis C in a population of Swedish haemophiliacs and heterosexual partners. *Scandinavian Journal of Infectious Diseases* 1990; **22**: 393.

Schwart TF, Roggendorf M, Hottentrager B, et al. Removal of parvovirus B 19 from contaminated factor VIII during fractionation. *Journal of Medical Virology* 1991; **35**: 28.

Semprini AE. Insemination of HIV-negative women with processed semen of HIV-positive partners. *Lancet* 1993; **341**: 1343.

Seremetis S, Aledort LM, Bergman G, et al. Three-year randomised study of high-purity or intermediate purity factor VIII concentrates in symptom-free HIV-seropositive haemophiliacs: effects on immune status. *Lancet* 1993; **342**: 700.

Sheng L, Willems M, Peerlinck K, et al. Hepatitis C virus genotypes in Belgian hemophiliacs. *Journal of Medical Virology* 1995; **45**: 211.

Sherertz RJ, Russell BA, Reuman PD. Transmission of hepatitis A by transfusion of blood products. *Archives of Internal Medicine* 1984; **144**: 1579–1580.

Simmonds P, Beatson D, Cuthbert RJ, et al. Determinants of HIV disease progression: six-year longitudinal study in the Edinburgh haemophilia/HIV cohort. *Lancet* 1991; **338**: 1159.

Simons JN, Leary TP, Dawson GJ, et al. Isolation of novel virus-like sequences associated with human hepatitis. *Nature Medicine* 1995; **1**: 564.

Spurling N, Shone J, Vaughan J. The incidence, incubation period and symptomatology of homologous serum jaundice. *British Medical Journal* 1946; **2**: 409.

Steel CM, Ludlam CA, Beatson D, et al. HLA haplotype A1 B8 DR3 as a risk factor for HIV-related disease. *Lancet* 1988; **1**: 1185.

Strickler RB, Abrams DI, Corash L, Shuman MA. Target platelet antigen in homosexual men with immune thrombocytopenia (retracted by Shuman MA, Corash L, Hittelman KJ. In: New England Journal of Medicine 1991; **325**: 487). *New England Journal of Medicine* 1985; **313**: 1375.

Suou T, Kawatani T, Nishikawa K, et al. High prevalence of hepatitis C virus genotype 1a in Japanese hemophiliacs. *International Hepatology Communications* 1996; **4**: 301.

Tacke M, Kiyosawa K, Stark K, et al. Detection of antibodies to a putative hepatitis G virus envelope protein. *Lancet* 1997; **349**: 318.

Taillan B, Fuzibet JG, Pesce A, Vinti H, Sanderson F, Dujardin P. Alpha-interferon in thrombocytopenic purpura. *Lancet* 1988; **2**: 170.

Tanaka K, Hirohata T, Koga S, et al. Hepatitis C and hepatitis B in the aetiology of hepatocellular carcinoma in the Japanese population. *Cancer Research* 1991; **51**: 2842.

Tedder RS, Briggs M, Ring C, et al. Hepatitis C antibody profile and viraemia prevalence in adults with severe haemophilia. *British Journal of Haematology* 1991; **79**: 512.

Telfer PT, Devereux HL, Goldman E, et al. Prevalence of HIV and hepatitis C virus infection in sexual partners of haemophilic patients. *British Journal of Haematology* 1993; 84 (suppl 1):58.

Telfer P, Sabin C, Devereux H, et al. The progression of HCV-associated liver disease in a cohort of haemophilic patients. *British Journal of Haematology* 1994; **87**: 555.

Telfer PT, Devereux H, Savage K, et al. Chronic hepatitis C virus infection in haemophilic patients: clinical significance of viral genotype. *Thrombosis and Haemostasis.* 1995; **74**: 1259.

Temperley IJ, Cotter KP, Walsh TJ, Power J, Hillary IB. Clotting factors and hepatitis A. *Lancet* 1992; **340**: 1466.

Triger DR, Preston FE. Chronic liver disease in haemophiliacs. [Review]. *British Journal of Haematology* 1990; **74**: 241.

Troisi CL, Hollinger FB, Hoots WK, et al. A multicenter study of viral hepatitis in a United States hemophilic population. *Blood.* 1993; **81**: 412.

Volberding PA, Lagakos SW, Koch MA, et al. Zidovudine in asymptomatic human immunodeficiency virus infection. A controlled trial in persons with fewer than 500 CD4-positive cells per cubic millimeter. The AIDS Clinical Trials Group of the National Institute of Allergy and Infectious Diseases. *New England Journal of Medicine* 1990; **322**: 941.

Walsh C, Krigel R, Lennette E, Karpatkin S. Thrombocytopenia in homosexual patients. Prognosis, response to therapy, and prevalence of antibody to the retrovirus associated with the acquired immunodeficiency syndrome. *Annals of Internal Medicine* 1985; **103**: 542.

Watson HG, Ludlam CA, Rebus S, Zhang LQ, Peutherer JF, Simmonds P. Use of several second generation serological assays to determine the true prevalence of hepatitis C virus infection in haemophiliacs treated with non-virus inactivated factor VIII and IX concentrates. *British Journal of Haematology* 1992; **80**: 514.
Webster A, Lee CA, Cook DG, Grundy JE, Emery VC, Kernoff PB. Cytomegalovirus infection and progression towards AIDS in haemophiliacs with human immunodeficiency virus infection. *Lancet* 1989; **2**: 63.
Webster A, Phillips AN, Lee CA, Janossy G, Kernoff PB, Griffiths PD. Cytomegalovirus (CMV) infection, CD4+ lymphocyte counts and the development of AIDS in HIV-1-infected haemophiliac patients. *Clinical & Experimental Immunology* 1992; **88**: 6.
Widell A, Hansson BG, Berntorp E, et al. Antibody to a hepatitis C virus related protein among patients at high risk for hepatitis B. *Scandinavian Journal of Infectious Diseases* 1991; **23**: 19.
Wilde JT, Rymes N, Skidmore S, et al. Hepatitis A immunization in HIV-infected haemophilic patients. *Haemophilia* 1995; **1**: 196.
Williams MD, Boxall EH, Hill FG. Change in immune response to hepatitis B in boys with haemophilia. *Journal of Medical Virology* 1988; **25**: 317.
Wion KL, Kelly D, Summerfield JA, Tuddenham EG, Lawn RM. Distribution of factor VIII mRNA and antigen in human liver and other tissues. *Nature* 1985; **317**: 726.
Yee TT, Lee CA, Pasi KJ, et al. Life-threatening human parvovirus B 19 infection in immuno-competent haemophilia. *Lancet* 1995; **345**: 794.
Youle MS, Gazzard BG, Johnson MA, et al. Effects of high-dose oral acyclovir on herpes virus disease and survival in patients with advanced HIV disease: a double-blind, placebo-controlled study. *AIDS* 1994; **8**: 641.
Zakrzewska K, Azzi A, Patou G, et al. Human parvovirus B 19 in clotting factor concentrates: B 19 DNA detection by the nested polymerase chain reaction. *British Journal of Haematology* 1992; **81**: 407.
Zanetti AR, Mannucci PM, Tanzi E, et al. Hepatitis B vaccination of 113 hemophiliacs: lower antibody response in anti-LAV/HTLV-III-positive patients. *American Journal of Hematology* 1986; **23**: 339.
Zuckerman JN, Moore S, Smith J, et al. A study to assess the immunogenicity, reactogenicity and safety of hepatitis A vaccine administered subcutaneously to patients with congenital coagulation disorders. *Haemophilia* 1996; **2**: 235.

11 Inhibitors and their Management

HAROLD R. ROBERTS

Introduction

The major obstacle to the treatment of haemophilia A and B at the present time is the development of neutralizing antibodies (inhibitors) against factor VIII and factor IX, respectively. These inhibitors, when present in sufficient concentrations, render conventional replacement therapy ineffective. Even in low titre, they require higher doses of clotting factor to achieve haemostasis. There is increasing interest in understanding the pathogenesis and treatment of inhibitors because of their frequency, their cost, and the fact that they not only complicate therapy but frequently do not respond to any of the current therapeutic manoeuvres. A greater understanding of inhibitors is particularly needed, given the recent possibilities of gene therapy for both haemophilia A and B.

This chapter will be devoted to a discussion of the aetiology, pathogenesis, diagnosis and treatment of antibodies against factor VIII and factor IX that develop in patients with haemophilia A and B, respectively. The development of anti-factor VIII antibodies in non-haemophilic patients will also be discussed briefly.

Inhibitors Against Factor VIII in Patients with Classic Haemophilia (Haemophilia A)

Definition and characterization

Inhibitor development in haemophilia A patients has been recognized since 1941, when Lawrence and Johnson (1941) published the first report. The majority of

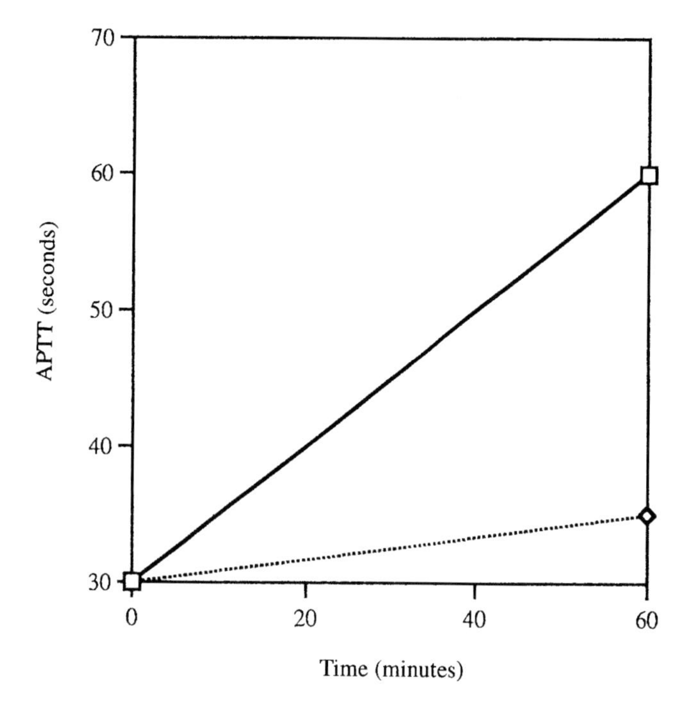

Figure 11.1 The APTT of inhibitor plasma incubated with normal pooled plasma at 37 °C for 1 hour (solid line) in comparison to control plasma without an inhibitor (dashed line). Note how the inhibitor plasma causes prolongation of the APTT over time at 37 °C incubation. This is what is meant by the antibody reacting in a time- and temperature-dependent manner.

antibodies develop in severely affected patients who have been previously treated and who have little or no circulating factor VIII antigen.

Factor VIII inhibitors are usually IgG immunoglobulins, with a few noted to be IgM or IgA (Fulcher et al, 1987; Sanchez-Cuenca et al, 1990). Of the IgG inhibitors, approximately 50% are restricted to the IgG_4 isotype with the rest being a combination of two or more subclasses, usually IgG_4 with one of the other subclasses. Rarely are these antibodies IgG_2 or IgG_3 only. Light chains are usually kappa, but can be lambda or a combination of both. Because the majority of these antibodies are of the IgG_4 isotype, they do not fix complement and do not result in serum sickness. The antigen–antibody complexes formed are non-precipitating.

An interesting and unique characteristic of anti-factor VIII antibodies is their dependence upon time and temperature in their interaction with factor VIII (Biggs et al, 1972b) (Fig. 11.1). They can be best identified by their ability to neutralize factor VIII at 37 °C after 1–2 hours of incubation. Why these antibodies have such distinctive requirements is not completely understood.

Two types of anti-factor VIII antibodies have been described based on the kinetics of their inactivation of factor VIII. Most of them will completely inhibit factor VIII activity in vitro when present in excess. These are so-called type I antibodies that exhibit second-order kinetics, i.e. there is a linear relationship between antibody concentration and residual factor VIII after incubation (Biggs et al, 1972b). Inhibitors occur at various times after infusion of factor VIII concentrates and they are, for all practical purposes, alloantibodies elicited by exposure to what the body interprets as a foreign antigen. In a few patients, the anti-factor VIII antibodies will not completely inactivate factor VIII in vitro, and exhibit complex kinetics. These have been labelled type II antibodies, which, in contrast to type I antibodies, do not exhibit a linear relationship between the antibody concentration and residual factor VIII activity (Biggs et al, 1972a). The majority of anti-factor VIII antibodies that exhibit type II kinetics are autoantibodies that develop spontaneously in non-haemophilic patients, but they have also been described in haemophilia patients. Despite the difference in kinetics between anti-factor VIII alloantibodies and autoantibodies, both are predominantly of the IgG_4 subclass.

Specific amino acid sequences responsible for the antigenic nature of the factor VIII molecule vary and, in most cases, have not been completely elucidated. However, studies have shown the A2 and C2 domains in factor VIII to contain epitopes that most often react with alloantibodies (Fulcher et al, 1985; Scandella

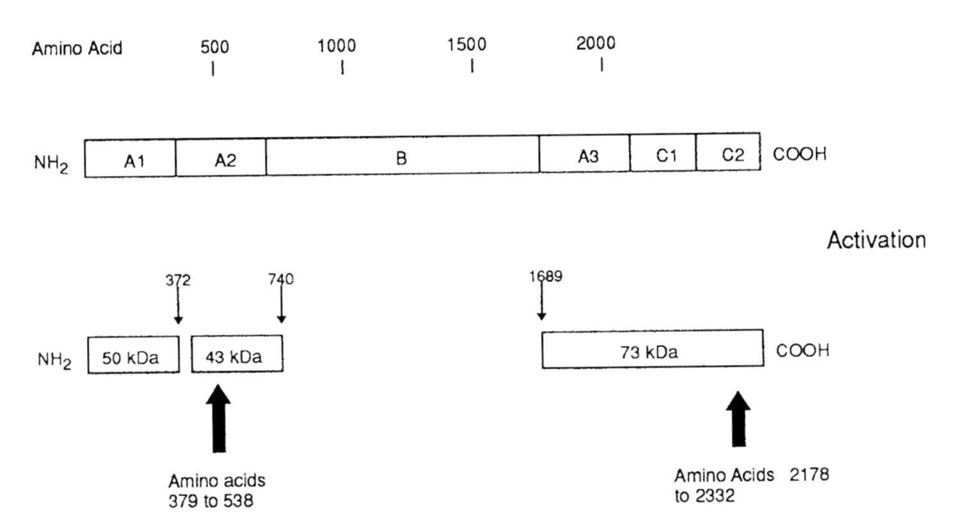

Figure 11.2 A schematic representation of factor VIII and the cleavage that occurs upon thrombin activation. The top figure is the factor VIII molecule prior to activation. In the bottom figure the dark arrows depict the regions in the A2 and C2 domains that are epitopes for the majority of antibodies. Also note that the B domain is no longer present in the activated factor VIII molecule. This accounts for the fact that antibodies to epitopes in this domain are non-neutralizing.

et al, 1988, 1989; Lubahn et al, 1989) (Fig. 11.2). Antibodies that react with the A2 domain in the heavy chain recognize a region in the amino-terminus between amino acid residues 379 and 538. Antibodies that react with the C2 domain in the light chain recognize a region in the carboxy-terminus between amino acid residues 2178 and 2332. Arai and colleagues (1989) have also demonstrated that several light chain specific antibodies could prevent the interaction of factor VIII with phospholipid surfaces. These data support other evidence demonstrating that the light chain is the site of interaction of factor VIII with membrane surfaces. Less frequently, antibodies recognize epitopes on the A1, A3 and C1 domains. Most of the antibodies reacting with the A and C domains neutralize factor VIII activity. However, not all antibodies recognizing epitopes in these domains are inhibitory. The frequency of occurrence of non-neutralizing antibodies is not known because they do not interfere with function and they are not searched for. Antibodies have also been described that recognize epitopes on the B domain, but these do not neutralize factor VIII activity, since the B domain is not necessary for factor VIII activity.

Lubahn et al (1990) have compared the inhibitors found in their patients with a different population of patients described by Fulcher et al (1987, 1988) and report that antibodies from the two populations differ in that one has a larger population of antibodies recognizing a 43 kD fragment in the A2 domain. The reasons for the different epitopes from the two populations are not clear but may be due to genetic, technical or other differences not yet identified.

It is of interest that there is some stability in the antibody population of affected patients. For example, Fulcher et al (1987, 1988) have shown that the factor VIII fragment recognized by a given patient's antibody remained the same over a long period of observation. On the other hand, Fulcher et al (1988) have convincingly demonstrated that a patient's antibody population may change over time and recognize distinctively different epitopes. Again, the factors influencing stability or instability of epitope recognition sites by the anti-factor VIII antibodies are not completely understood. Scandella et al (1993) have recently confirmed that changes in epitope specificity can occur over time. Nilsson et al (1990) have also shown that antibody populations change; after induction of immune tolerance, for example, neutralizing antibodies may disappear, but non-inhibitory antibodies against factor VIII can still be detected.

Incidence and risk factors for inhibitor development

One of the first studies of the incidence of inhibitors in haemophilia A was reported by McMillan and colleagues (1988), who found an incidence of 8 per 1000 patient years of observation. Since then the reported incidence of inhibitor development in haemophilia A patients has varied widely from 5 to over 50% in various studies. Recent literature suggests that among severely affected patients who are most at risk, the incidence may be underestimated. Ehrenforth and co-workers (1992) found an overall incidence of 24% in all haemophilia A patients, but an incidence of 52% when only severely affected patients were studied.

The importance of disease severity in inhibitor development is evident in a survey conducted by Gill (1984) on a large group of haemophilia A patients with inhibitors. In this group of inhibitor patients, 80% had severe disease (<1% factor VIII activity), 15% had moderate disease (1–3% factor VIII activity) and 4% had a mild disorder (>4% factor VIII activity). Other risk factors for development of inhibitors include age and cumulative treatment. In heavily treated children, 50% of inhibitors develop by the age of 20 years and 71% by the age of 30 years (McMillan et al, 1988).

The risk for development of inhibitors increases as the number of treatments increases. In a cooperative study of the natural history of inhibitors, it was found that anti-factor VIII antibodies developed after 8 to 250 cumulative days of exposure to factor VIII concentrates (McMillan et al, 1988). Most patients who develop high-titre inhibitors usually do so more rapidly after less than 90 exposure days to factor VIII (Kasper, 1973; McMillan, 1984; McMillan et al, 1988).

The method of purification of factor may also play a role in development of alloantibodies. An interesting observation in 1993 by Peerlinck and colleagues described a higher than normal incidence of inhibitor development in haemophilia A patients from Belgium treated with a particular intermediate-purity factor VIII product prepared by the Dutch Red Cross. In this study, the incidence of clinically important inhibitor development with this particular product among heavily pretreated individuals was 31 per 1000 patient years of observation. This incidence was significantly higher than the control group of patients who received a solvent detergent treated factor VIII product, none of whom developed an inhibitor. A similar finding was noted in The Netherlands in association with the same type of factor VIII concentrate used in Belgium. In this report a 4.5-fold increase in inhibitor development was noted in multiply transfused haemophilia A patients (Rosendaal et al, 1993). Interestingly, when this product was removed from use, the occurrence of new inhibitors decreased. These two reports are the first convincing evidence that the method of manufacture of factor VIII plays a role in the development of anti-factor VIII antibodies.

Some early data had suggested that ultra-pure factor VIII may be associated with an increased risk of inhibitor development, but the reports cited above make *all* factor VIII products, whether of low or high purity, suspect for causing inhibitors (Bell et al, 1990; Kessler and Sachse, 1990). More recent data, using ultra-pure factor VIII products (including recombinant factor VIII) in previously untreated patients, suggest that inhibitors occur more commonly than previously thought, perhaps because of better detection of transient or low-level inhibitors that disappear following continuous treatment with factor VIII (Addiego et al, 1990, 1993; Lusher et al, 1993). In a recent review, Hoyer (1993) reports that the frequency of inhibitors using recombinant product may be slightly increased, but there is no evidence as yet that the cumulative risk is increased. At this point, it is clear that it will require a longer period of close

Table 11.1 Occurrence of inhibitors in haemophilia A brother pairs

Inhibitor Combination	Observed occurrence	Expected occurrence
Both brothers with anti-factor VIII inhibitor	6	2.3
Only one of two brothers with inhibitor	5	12.3
Neither brother with inhibitor	20	16.3

observation of patients receiving new factor VIII products before the true incidence of inhibitors can be determined.

There is evidence suggesting a genetic predisposition to development of inhibitors. A study by Frommel and Allain looked at pairs of brothers with haemophilia A (Frommel and Allain, 1977; Frommel et al, 1977). In this study they found a higher number of brother pairs who were both antibody positive than one would expect from random chance. A study performed by Lubahn et al (1990) showing a higher than expected occurrence of inhibitors in brother pairs is shown in Table 11.1. Several studies have been done to determine if HLA antigens are associated with an increased risk of developing an inhibitor, and none has been found. However, there may be a negative correlation between the HLA-Cw5 antigen and the development of an inhibitor (Aly et al, 1990).

The type of genetic defect may also have an influence on the development of inhibitors in haemophilia A (Gitschier et al, 1985). Patients with anti-factor VIII antibodies studied so far have had gene defects ranging from gross gene deletions to point mutations and insertions. Some of the same point mutations have been found in both inhibitor and non-inhibitor patients. Also, deletions described in inhibitor patients are found throughout all the exons of the factor VIII gene, and there has been no readily identifiable difference between inhibitor and non-inhibitor patients. Still there seems to be some correlation between the type of gene defect and the likelihood of anti-factor VIII antibody development, since approximately 50% of haemophilia A patients who have gene deletions develop antibodies (Gitschier, 1989). Whereas the presence or absence of dysfunctional factor VIII antigen has not been determined in all inhibitor patients, the general consensus is that those patients who are antigen negative are more likely to develop inhibitors. It is clear, however, that some patients who are antigen positive also develop inhibitors.

In spite of all the work done to date on inhibitor development in haemophilia A, it is still not possible to predict accurately those patients at risk for development of antibodies. Patients can, however, be stratified into high-risk categories if: they are severely affected; have a family history of inhibitor development;

Table 11.2 Risk factors for the development of anti-factor VIII antibodies in haemophilia A patients

- Disease severity: 80% of haemophilia A patients with inhibitors have <1% factor VIII activity
- Exposure to factor VIII concentrates: the majority of high-titre inhibitors develop after <90 days of exposure to factor VIII
- Genetic factors
  - (a) Family history of inhibitor development
  - (b) Negative correlation with HLA Cw5 antigen
  - (c) Molecular defects: especially gene deletions and nonsense point mutations resulting in patients without factor VIII antigen
- Method of purification of factor VIII concentrate

have been exposed to factor VIII replacement therapy; and if their molecular defect results in a lack of factor VIII antigen (Table 11.2).

Clinical manifestations

Haemophilia A patients with inhibitors have bleeding episodes similar to patients without inhibitors. Both experience spontaneous haemorrhages characterized by haemarthroses and soft-tissue haemorrhages. There is some debate about whether the presence of an inhibitor increases the frequency of bleeding episodes. Some believe that this does indeed happen. In our experience, however, the presence of an inhibitor does not result in an increased frequency of haemorrhagic episodes, although it does render management much more difficult. Since patients with inhibitors respond poorly to therapeutic interventions, morbidity and mortality are increased.

The majority of patients with haemophilia develop high-titre inhibitors, arbitrarily defined as > 10 Bethesda units (Bu) after challenge with factor VIII. In some patients, titres will fall during periods when they are not exposed to factor VIII, but the inhibitor titre will frequently increase dramatically in a brisk anamnestic response. This usually occurs within 5–7 days after re-exposure to factor VIII. These patients are referred to as "high responders". The cut-off for inhibitor titres that distinguishes high responders from low responders varies according to definitions used by different investigators.

It should be emphasized that a "high responder" patient may present with an inhibitor titre that is undetectable if the patient has not received a transfusion of factor VIII in a long time. High-responder patients whose initial inhibitor titre is low can often be identified by a history of a previous high titre. In other high-responder patients the inhibitor titre will always be high, even after prolonged avoidance of factor VIII concentrates.

A minority of haemophilia patients with anti-factor VIII antibodies are termed "low responders". Low responders have antibody titres of <10 Bethesda units and do not exhibit an anamnestic response when rechallenged with factor VIII. Occasionally, patients who have been low responders for some time can convert to a high responder.

Laboratory findings

An inhibitor is detected by mixing the patient's plasma 1:1 with normal plasma and performing an activated partial thromboplastin time (APTT) on the mixture at zero time and after incubation at 37°C for 1–2 hours. In the presence of an inhibitor, the APTT on the mixture will be prolonged, rather than corrected, as would be the case if an inhibitor were not present. When the inhibitor is present in high titre, the APTT at zero time will often be prolonged, but sometimes the inhibitor can be detected only after incubation at 37°C. While this pattern of time and temperature dependence is highly suspicious for a factor VIII inhibitor, it is best to make certain that the inhibitor is specific for factor VIII. This can be done by adding an appropriate dilution of inhibitor plasma to normal plasma, incubating for a period and determining the level of residual factor VIII as well as other factors in the intrinsic pathway such as IX, XI and XII. If the inhibitor is specific for factor VIII, only factor VIII will be decreased in the normal plasma and other clotting factors will be normal, provided that an appropriate dilution of inhibitor plasma is added. If the antibody to factor VIII is present in excess (i.e. not sufficiently diluted) it will inhibit factor VIII in the substrate plasmas used to assay other clotting factors, causing them to be spuriously low. Making sure that the inhibitor is specific for factor VIII and that it is time and temperature dependent will distinguish a factor VIII inhibitor from a lupus anticoagulant and other inhibitors. The prothrombin time (PT) is, of course, normal in the presence of a factor VIII inhibitor.

Since both alloantibodies and autoantibodies against factor VIII interact with factor VIII in a time and temperature dependent manner, these characteristics are used when quantitating the inhibitor titre. Inhibitors are quantitated by mixing equal volumes of patient inhibitor plasma with a source of factor VIII, followed by incubation of the mixture at 37°C for a specified period of time. The units derived from this type of assay are arbitrary. Two similar procedures are primarily used to quantitate inhibitors. The Bethesda method, used mainly in the USA, employs pooled plasma as a source of factor VIII and an incubation time of 2 hours. The New Oxford method uses factor VIII concentrate instead of pooled plasma and requires a 4-hour incubation instead of 2 hours. One Bethesda unit is, by definition, the amount of anti-factor VIII antibody necessary to inhibit 50% of the factor VIII in a 1:1 mix of appropriately diluted patient plasma and normal pooled plasma after incubation at 37 °C for 2 hours. Therefore, if a 1 : 100 dilution of patient plasma reduces factor VIII activity in normal plasma by 50%, the Bethesda titre will be 100 units. One New Oxford unit is, by definition, the amount of antibody necessary to inhibit 50% of the added factor VIII concentrate after incubation at 37 °C for 4 hours. Because of the different sources of factor used for these two assays, the units of inhibition are not equal or completely interchangeable. However, one New Oxford unit is roughly equivalent to 0.8 Bethesda units (Austen et al, 1982).

Treatment

General overview of the products available

Acutely, treatment in haemophilia A patients with inhibitors is aimed at stopping haemorrhage rather than decreasing the inhibitor titre. The products used for haemostasis in haemophilia A patients include prothrombin complex concentrates, activated prothrombin complex concentrates, human factor VIII in higher than normal doses, porcine factor VIII, and recombinant factor VIIa. Other agents have been tried, e.g. factor Xa–phospholipid complexes and tissue factor apoprotein, but these agents are highly experimental and not generally available so they will not be considered further.

Prothrombin complex concentrates and activated prothrombin complex concentrates are used in haemophilia A patients with anti-factor VIII antibodies because of their so-called inhibitor "bypassing" properties. Prothrombin complex concentrates contain varying amounts of all of the vitamin K-dependent clotting factors, including factors II, VII, IX and X plus small amounts of activated forms of these factors. Several companies presently make prothrombin complex concentrates, and the concentration of the vitamin K-dependent factors varies depending upon the method of manufacture (Table 11.3). The efficacy of prothrombin complex concentrates is difficult to assess because their effectiveness rests on subjective impressions of the patient and treating physician and not on a reliable laboratory measure of haemostatic efficacy. Based on the response in haemarthroses, it is estimated that 40–50% of bleeding episodes derive some benefit from prothrombin complex concentrates (Lusher et al, 1980; Sjamsoedin et al, 1981). In addition to the usual prothrombin complex concentrates, "activated" prothrombin complex concentrates are also available (Table 11.3). In the latter there is intentional "controlled activation" of the vitamin K-dependent clotting proteins. After activation, these products contain variable amounts of activated factors VII, IX and X, which is dependent on each company's formulation and processing. It is estimated that 65% of haemophilia A patients with inhibitors who are treated with activated prothrombin complex concentrates derive some benefit (Lusher et al, 1980; Sjamsoedin et al, 1981). Unfortunately, like prothrombin complex concentrates, there is no way to monitor the efficacy of these products with a laboratory test.

Table 11.3 Prothrombin complex concentrates and their use in patients with inhibitors

Product (manufacturer)	Use in inhibitors	Risk of viral transmission		Association with thrombosis	Units of protein per 100 units of factor IX			
		Hepatitis	HIV		II	VII	IX	X
Prothrombin complex concentrates								
Bebulin VH (Immuno)	Yes	No	No	No	120	13	100	139
Proplex T (Baxter-Hyland)	Yes	?	No	Yes	50	400	100	50
Profilnine HT (Alpha)	Yes	Yes	No	Yes	148	11	100	64
Konyne 80 (Cutter)	Yes	No	No	Yes	100	20	100	140
Ultrapure factor IX								
AlphaNine	No	None reported	No	No	<5	<5	100	<20
Mononine (Rorer)	No	None reported	No	No	<1	<1	100	<1
Activated prothrombin complex concentrates								
Autoplex (Baxter Hyland)	Yes	No	No	Yes	Variable amount of factors II, VII and X and activated factors VIIa, IXa and Xa			
Feiba (Immuno)	Yes	No	No	Yes				

A 1980 survey on the treatment of inhibitor patients with prothrombin complex concentrates suggested that most clinicians saw the greatest benefit from doses ranging from 26 to 75 units/kg of body weight, although clinical efficacy was not always evident after the initial dose (Blatt et al, 1980). Unfortunately, some of these products are associated with several side-effects, including minor local problems such as phlebitis at the intravenous site, or more severe systemic effects including thrombosis and disseminated intravascular coagulation.

Human factor VIII concentrates are available as both intermediate-purity and ultrapure products, including recombinant factor VIII. All factor VIII products can be used in very high doses in selected patients with inhibitors. Because of the problems with viral contamination during the early 1980s, many clinicians prefer to use ultrapure factor VIII products in an attempt to prevent transmission of human immunodeficiency virus (HIV), hepatitis, or other as yet unknown pathogens in previously untreated or minimally treated individuals.

Porcine factor VIII has a high degree of homology with human factor VIII but it possesses a much higher potency than the human material, which makes it a particularly effective agent in the treatment of factor VIII inhibitors. Human anti-factor VIII antibodies from haemophilia A patients have about a 25% cross-reactivity rate with porcine factor VIII. Porcine factor VIII is associated with allergic reactions in some individuals and may require the concomitant use of prednisone.

Recently, recombinant human factor VIIa (rFVIIa) has been used successfully in haemophilia A and B patients with inhibitors on a compassionate basis (Hedner and Glazer, 1992). Many of the patients treated with rFVIIa had life- or limb-threatening haemorrhages that had not responded to all other approved treatment alternatives. Some of these patients were able to undergo emergency surgical procedures with very good results. The dose of rFVIIa to obtain haemostasis was 70–100 μg/kg of body weight. This product must be administered every 2–4 hours to maintain haemostasis. Adverse side-effects clearly attributed to rFVIIa are almost non-existent. There are reports of only two patients who experienced mild cardiovascular events, but both patients had underlying diseases predisposing them to cardiovascular complications. There was initial concern that rFVIIa might predispose patients to disseminated intravascular coagulation. However, only one patient, who had other high-risk factors for this condition, has been reported.

None of the factor VIII bypassing agents are as effective as factor VIII would be if it could be used. Nevertheless, when the inhibitor titre is so high that neither human nor porcine factor VIII can be used successfully, the bypassing agents become valuable adjuncts in the treatment of these patients.

Treatment of "minor" haemorrhages in low-responder patients

Whereas many low-responder patients can be treated with high doses of human or porcine factor VIII, one modality of treatment for minor haemorrhages in

Table 11.4 Treatment of inhibitors in haemophilia A patients

Type of patient	Initial titre	Minor haemorrhage	Major haemorrhage
High responder	<10 BU	Recombinant factor VIIa; prothrombin complex concentrates; activated prothrombin complex concentrates	Human factor VIII; recombinant factor VIIa; porcine factor VIII, prothrombin complex concentrates; activated prothrombin complex concentrates
High responder	>10 BU	Recombinant factor VIIa; prothrombin complex concentrates; activated prothrombin complex concentrates	Porcine factor VIII; recombinant factor VIIIa; prothrombin complex concentrates; activated prothrombin complex concentrates; exchange + high-dose factor VIII
Low responder	<10 BU	Recombinant factor VIIa; prothrombin complex concentrates; activated prothrombin complex concentrates	High-dose human factor VIII; recombinant factor VIIa; porcine factor VIII, activated prothrombin complex concentrates

BU, Bethesda units.

these patients is prothrombin complex concentrates (Table 11.4). The use of prothrombin complex concentrates as opposed to high doses of human or porcine factor VIII is based on the belief that low-responder patients may convert to a high-responder status when treated with factor VIII. Thus, mild or minor haemorrhages are treated with bypassing agents. Doses of prothrombin complex concentrates of up to 75 units/kg body weight every 8–12 hours are usually effective. Unfortunately, the response may not be evident until several doses have been administered. If no response is seen after three or more doses of prothrombin complex concentrates then activated prothrombin complex concentrates can be tried. Activated prothrombin complex concentrates are administered at doses of 75–100 units/kg body weight every 8–12 hours for several doses. Again, response may be delayed until several doses have been administered. If and when recombinant factor VIIa becomes available, this would represent the treatment of choice in some centres. The usual dose of recombinant factor VIIa is 75–100 μg/kg body weight every 2–4 hours.

Treatment of "major" haemorrhage in low-response inhibitor patients

When patients with low-response inhibitors (<10 Bethesda units and no anamnestic response) experience major haemorrhagic episodes, they should be treated immediately with high doses of human factor VIII or porcine factor VIII as first-line agents (Table 11.4). The initial dose should be sufficient to neutralize the antibody and result in free circulating factor VIII. Subsequent doses are given to maintain free factor VIII levels until haemorrhage is controlled. In our experience with patients who have less than 10 Bethesda units of antibody, an arbitrary bolus dose of 10 000–15 000 units of human factor VIII concentrate is given, followed by 1000 units per hour by continuous infusion. If measurable factor VIII levels are obtained after the bolus infusion, this usually indicates that the inhibitor can be neutralized. Human factor VIII can be continued at 1000 units per hour until a satisfactory increase in factor VIII levels is attained. The infusion can be adjusted to maintain therapeutic factor VIII levels. If no measurable factor VIII levels are attainable, human factor VIII is stopped and porcine factor VIII is administered. The dose of porcine factor VIII usually begins at 50–100 units/kg of body weight but may require several hundred units per kilogram to neutralize the antibody and attain adequate factor VIII blood levels. If no measurable factor VIII levels are obtained with human or porcine factor VIII, prothrombin complex concentrates, activated prothrombin complex concentrates or recombinant factor VIIa (when available) represent viable alternatives. Unfortunately, in a life-threatening haemorrhage, there may not be sufficient time to wait for a response from these secondary measures. In patients with life-threatening haemorrhage when time is critical, exchange transfusions sufficient to reduce the antibody titre to levels that permit the use of human or porcine factor VIII should be attempted.

Treatment of "minor" haemorrhage in a high-response inhibitor patient

Patients with Bethesda inhibitor titres of >10 Bethesda units who present with minor haemorrhages can be treated with prothrombin complex concentrates or activated prothrombin complex concentrates in doses described previously (Table 11.4). They should be observed for several doses to see if a response is obtained. Again, recombinant factor VIIa in doses described above might be preferred in some centres if it were available. Patients with high-response inhibitors who have an initial titre that is low will usually respond to high doses of human factor VIII. However, this is not used for minor haemorrhage because of the rapid anamnestic response that will occur upon re-exposure to human factor VIII concentrates. When this occurs the patient may be refractory to factor VIII should a major haemorrhagic episode occur.

Treatment of "major" haemorrhage in high-response haemophilia A inhibitor patients

In high-response inhibitor patients who present with initial Bethesda titres of <10 Bethesda units, major haemorrhages can be treated with high doses of human factor VIII even though an anamnestic response will occur in 4–7 days (Table 11.4). These patients should be treated with human factor VIII in a similar manner to low-response inhibitor patients with a bolus of 10 000–15 000 units of human factor VIII followed by an infusion of 1000 units per hour. Human factor VIII can be continued as long as adequate factor VIII levels are attained. If a measurable factor VIII level is not obtained with human factor VIII, porcine factor VIII in doses ranging from 100 units to several hundred units per kilogram body weight is the next option as long as the patient's inhibitor does not cross-react with the porcine material. When neither of these measures is effective, prothrombin complex concentrates, activated prothrombin complex concentrates and high-dose human or porcine factor VIII infusion with or without exchange transfusions represent therapeutic alternatives.

In patients who present with life-threatening haemorrhage who have Bethesda titres >10 Bethesda units, porcine factor VIII represents first-line treatment. Even though porcine factor VIII is often highly effective, the patient's antibody may cross-react with it initially or, alternatively, the patient may develop neutralizing antibodies to it after 4–7 days of therapy. If porcine factor VIII is not effective in patients with high-titre inhibitors, other measures such as prothrombin complex concentrates, activated prothrombin complex concentrates, recombinant factor VIIa or exchange transfusion pheresis with high-dose factor VIII infusion may be attempted.

Therapeutic manoeuvres to lower antibody titres

Several treatment options have been reported that are aimed not at controlling haemorrhage but at suppressing or lowering the antibody titre so that patients can again be treated with factor VIII concentrates. These include induction of immune tolerance, protein A plasmapheresis to remove antibody, cytotoxic therapy to suppress antibody, and anti-idiotype antibodies to neutralize anti-factor VIII antibodies.

The most commonly used treatment for suppression of antibody production is induction of immune tolerance. In an attempt to suppress anti-factor VIII antibody production the inhibitor patient is given daily infusions of factor VIII over several months. Induction of tolerance seems to be most effective when begun soon after recognition of the presence of an inhibitor, but inhibitors of long standing can still be eradicated by high-dose regimens such as the Brackmann protocol (Brackmann, 1986). In the literature there are reports of efficacy with both high-dose factor VIII regimens of 100 units/kg of body weight twice a day, and low-dose factor VIII regimens of 25–50 units/kg of body weight per day. Examples of high- and low-dose regimens are shown in Table 11.5. In our experience a high-dose factor VIII regimen is required in those patients who have high-titre inhibitors. Human factor VIII is administered according to this regimen until the inhibitor disappears and the factor VIII half-life is restored to normal. The biggest drawbacks to induction of immune tolerance are the cost of the factor VIII and the time and support required over months or even a year or more of continuous therapy. Nilsson and colleagues

Table 11.5 Examples of tolerance protocols for haemophilia A inhibitor patients

Immune tolerance protocols	Dose	Initial response
High-dose regimen		
Brackmann (modified)	100 units/kg FVIII twice a day until antibody titre 1 unit. Then 150 units/kg FVIII per day until FVIII half-life normal	In 16 of 21 patients, titre fell to <1 unit
Low-dose regimens		
Kasper	50 units/kg FVIII per day	9 of 12 patients responded
Netherlands protocol	25 units/kg FVIII per day	11 of 18 patients responded

FVIII, factor VIII.

(1988) have shown an added benefit with the addition of immunosuppressives such as cyclophosphamide and intravenous gamma globulin to the regimen of factor VIII infusions. In patients with initially high antibody titres, protein A plasmapheresis is included. This protocol has been termed the Malmö regimen.

Plasmapheresis can be used to remove anti-factor VIII antibodies from the circulation so that factor VIII infusions can be given. Protein A columns have been added to routine plasmapheresis in an attempt to improve the efficacy. This is possible because protein A has a high affinity for IgG, especially IgG subclasses 1, 2 and 4. Since most anti-factor VIII antibodies in haemophilia A are of the IgG_4 subclass, the protein A readily binds the antibody, effectively removing it from circulation. Gjorstrup and colleagues (1991) have been able to show a 50% reduction in plasma IgG after a single pheresis on haemophilia A patients with inhibitors. After three plasma exchanges the haemophilia A patients had reduction of their anti-factor VIII antibody level by 70–90%, thus allowing treatment with factor VIII concentrates. Unfortunately, the inhibitor returned in high titre between exchanges due to movement of extravascular IgG into the intravascular compartment.

Cytotoxic drugs alone are rarely effective in eliminating the inhibitor, as has been demonstrated by Nilsson et al (1973) in haemophilia B patients with inhibitors.

Work is now being done on anti-idiotype antibodies which bind to epitopes on the variable region of antibodies. Interest in this area was prompted by the observation that in some haemophilic brother pairs only one brother had an inhibitor and the other brother had anti-idiotype antibodies which were thought to suppress development of anti-factor VIII antibodies (Frommel, 1984; Moffat et al, 1989). Some patients with spontaneous anti-factor VIII antibodies seem to suppress their immune response with anti-idiotype antibodies (Sultan et al, 1987; Tiarks et al, 1989). De la Fuente and Hoyer (1984) have reported 11 patients who had partial neutralization of their anti-factor VIII antibodies by a polyclonal rabbit anti-idiotype antibody. While this approach may be promising, it is likely that the number of different anti-idiotypes necessary may make this approach cumbersome or even impractical.

Inhibitors in Haemophilia B Patients

Anti-factor IX antibodies are similar to anti-factor VIII antibodies in many ways. Like factor VIII antibodies, anti-factor IX antibodies are typically IgG, usually of the IgG_4 subclass. Inhibitors in haemophilia B patients, as in haemophilia A, also seem to have a familial predisposition. The genetic defects leading to antigen-negative haemophilia B, particularly gene deletions, constitute a risk factor for development of anti-factor IX antibodies. Gross gene deletions have been found in 60% of haemophilia B patients who develop an inhibitor (Giannelli et al,

1983; Gitschier et al, 1985; Hassan et al, 1985). Other haemophilia B patients with inhibitors who do not have gene deletions have been studied and shown to have nonsense mutations and small nucleotide deletions (Matsushita et al, 1990; Green et al, 1989).

A notable distinction between haemophilia A and B is that, unlike anti-factor VIII antibodies which are time and temperature dependent, anti-factor IX antibodies are not.

Development of inhibitors in haemophilia B patients is much less common than in haemophilia A, with an overall incidence among all haemophilia B patients of 3%. The calculated incidence among severe haemophilia B patients is 7–10%, which is still much less common than in severe haemophilia A (Ehrenforth et al, 1992). Exactly why haemophilia B patients have a significantly lower incidence of inhibitor development is not understood since many of the risk factors such as severity and cumulative treatment are the same for haemophilia A and B. Perhaps the much smaller molecular size of factor IX compared with factor VIII presents fewer antigenic stimuli to the immune system.

Clinical manifestations

Haemophilia B patients with anti-factor IX inhibitors tend to have similar bleeding patterns as non-inhibitor patients except for an increased morbidity and mortality that occurs as a result of ineffective treatment. Such patients may be unresponsive to conventional doses of factor IX as well as several other therapeutic manoeuvres. As in haemophilia A, inhibitor patients with haemophilia B may be low responders or high responders.

Laboratory findings

Patients with inhibitors to factor IX will have a normal prothrombin time (PT) and a prolonged activated partial thromboplastin time (APTT). However, when their plasma is mixed with normal plasma, the APTT is prolonged and the inhibitor can be shown to be specific for factor IX in a manner similar to that described for factor VIII. Anti-factor IX antibodies are quantitated in an assay similar to the factor VIII Bethesda assay. Even though anti-factor IX antibodies are not time and temperature dependent, the factor IX Bethesda titre is usually performed by incubating the mixture of pooled plasma and patient inhibitor plasma at 37°C for 2 hours.

Treatment

Prothrombin complex concentrates and activated prothrombin complex concentrates have been the mainstay of treatment for haemophilia B patients with inhibitors. Recent approval of high-purity factor IX concentrates has provided a treatment option with less thrombotic risk for patients with an initial antibody titre of less than 10 Bethesda units. Factor VIIIa is also effective.

Recently, a factor IX product prepared by recombinant DNA techniques has been approved in the USA and this can be used in patients with haemophilia B.

Treatment of haemophilia B patients with low-response inhibitors

Low-response inhibitors in haemophilia B patients were previously treated with prothrombin complex concentrates. However, purified factor IX concentrates are now available and can be given in high dose to neutralize the antibody (Table 11.6). Purified factor IX products are an improvement since they have not been associated with the thrombotic risks seen with prothrombin complex concentrates. Since all factor concentrates presently in use for haemophilia B patients with inhibitors contain factor IX, they all have the potential of converting a low responder into a high responder. Low-responder patients with inhibitors to factor IX could also be treated with recombinant factor VIIa when this product becomes available. In minor haemorrhages some physicians would consider it to be the treatment of choice since there would be no danger of converting a low responder to a high responder.

Treatment of major or minor haemorrhage in high-response inhibitors with an initial titre of <10 units

Treatment of major or minor haemorrhage in a high-response haemophilia B inhibitor patient whose initial titre is <10 units is best accomplished by the use of high doses of purified factor IX concentrates (Table 11.6). Doses sufficiently large to neutralize the antibody and then produce free factor IX blood levels should be administered. This may require >5000 units of pure factor IX. Prothrombin complex concentrates or activated prothrombin complex concentrates are also useful if the anti-factor IX antibody cannot be neutralized. Since all concentrates approved for use in haemophilia B inhibitor patients contain factor IX, an anamnestic response can be seen with the use of prothrombin complex concentrates or activated prothrombin complex concentrates. When available, recombinant factor VIIa would represent alternative therapy. The dose of recombinant factor VIIa for haemophilia B inhibitor patients is similar to that described in haemophilia A inhibitor patients.

Treatment of major or minor haemorrhages in haemophilia B patients with high-titre (>10 BU) inhibitors

In patients whose initial anti-factor IX antibody titre is >10 Bethesda units, the antibody cannot be overwhelmed with high doses of purified factor IX concentrates (Table 11.6). Prothrombin complex concentrates can be used first but some prefer to try activated prothrombin complex concentrates as the initial treatment. These agents are used in doses similar to those described for haemophilia A patients with inhibitors. Again, recombinant factor VIIa would be a viable treatment option as well.

If a life-threatening haemorrhagic event occurs and time is critical, exchange transfusion to lower the antibody titre can be combined with high-dose purified factor IX concentrates to raise factor IX blood levels.

Other treatments

Another option for the treatment of inhibitors in haemophilia B patients is suppression of anti-factor IX antibodies. In two haemophilia B patients, Nilsson et al (1973) gave large doses of factor IX concentrates concomitantly with cyclophosphamide (Table 11.6). In both of these patients the inhibitor disappeared transiently, but returned after 12 days in one and 3 months in the other. There are no other reports of induction of immune tolerance in haemophilia B

Table 11.6 Treatment of haemophilia B inhibitor patients

Type of patient	Initial titre	Therapy
High responder	<10 BU	High-dose purified factor IX; recombinant factor VIIa; prothrombin complex concentrates; activated prothrombin complex concentrates
High responder	>10 BU	Prothrombin complex concentrates; recombinant factor VIIa; activated prothrombin complex concentrates; exchange + high-dose factor IX; IV gamma globulin; Cytoxan
Low responder	<10 BU	High-dose purified factor IX; recombinant factor VIIa prothrombin complex concentrates; activated prothrombin complex concentrates

BU, Bethesda units; IV, intravenous.

patients with inhibitors. It would seem worthwhile, in view of the availability of highly purified factor IX concentrates, free of thrombotic risks and blood-borne infections, to set up a trial of induction of immune tolerance in haemophilia B patients.

Spontaneous Anti-factor VIII Antibodies in Non-haemophilic Patients

Acquired inhibitors to factor VIII in the non-haemophilic population are the most common spontaneous inhibitors to any coagulation factor. Still, these inhibitors are rare with an estimated incidence of one in one million. They are autoantibodies that develop in a variety of settings, although the majority (approximately 45%) develop in otherwise healthy individuals over the age of 50 years (Table 11.7). Among the elderly population, males and females are affected about equally. The remainder of autoantibodies against factor VIII are reported in patients with collagen vascular disorders such as rheumatoid arthritis, those with severe allergic reactions to drugs such as penicillin, chloramphenicol and phenytoin, and those with certain malignancies. They also occur in pregnant or postpartum women.

Recently, researchers have reported the presence of factor VIII neutralizing antibodies in the plasma of 17% of healthy blood donors screened at random (Algiman et al, 1992). These patients had no clinical sequelae of these antibodies, which were present in low titre (≤2 BU). There was no difference in the factor VIII levels between donors with antibodies and donors without antibodies. The relevance of these antibodies in the pathogenesis of spontaneous inhibitors to factor VIII which cause clinical haemorrhage is not yet understood.

Clinical manifestations

Patients usually present with spontaneous haemorrhage that is often more severe

Table 11.7 Groups at risk for development of spontaneous anti-factor VIII autoantibodies

- Idiopathic usually in healthy individuals >50 years of age
- History of collagen vascular disorders or other autoimmune disorders
- Severe allergic reaction to drugs, e.g. penicillin, chloramphenicol and phenytoin
- Malignancies, both lymphoproliferative, such as lymphomas, and solid tumours, such as prostatic carcinoma
- Pregnant and postpartum women

than in haemophilia patients with an inhibitor. An acquired inhibitor should be suspected in a patient with no prior history of bleeding who presents with an unexplained haemorrhage, in particular a dissecting haematoma. In a 1981 survey by Green and Lechner, 87% of patients identified with an autoantibody to factor VIII had a major bleeding episode and 22% died as a result of the inhibitor. In this survey Green and Lechner also found that about one-third of patients who received only supportive care had spontaneous remission of their inhibitors. Postpartum women were the group most likely to have remissions spontaneously or with only steroid therapy. The mean duration of these inhibitors prior to disappearance was 14 months.

Laboratory findings

Patients with autoantibodies to factor VIII present with a prolonged APTT but a normal PT. The patient sample can then be mixed 1 : 1 with normal plasma and the APTT repeated. In a true factor deficiency, the APTT should correct completely to normal after a 1 : 1 mix with normal plasma. The presence of an inhibitor should be suspected if the mixing study does not correct completely into the normal range. An incubated mixture with patient and normal plasma along with appropriate controls should always be performed at 37 °C for 1–2 hours since autoantibodies to factor VIII, like alloantibodies, are usually time and temperature dependent. However, anti-factor VIII inhibitors in non-haemophilic patients are often difficult to detect because of complex reaction kinetics which result in residual factor VIII in the incubation mixture. Occasionally a low-affinity inhibitor can be present even when the 1 : 1 mixing study corrects completely. Any patient who presents with a low factor VIII level, an acquired bleeding disorder, and who has a prolonged APTT should be suspected of having an anti-factor VIII autoantibody. As discussed previously, factor assays should be performed to define the presence of an inhibitor to a specific coagulation factor. Since high-titre anti-factor VIII antibodies can inhibit factor VIII in substrate plasma, assays for other clotting factors may initially be low. This issue can be resolved by performing factor assays on serial dilutions of patient plasma. If the antibody is specific, the factor it inhibits will remain low as the plasma is diluted but the factors not inhibited will correct as the antibody is diluted.

After determination of the presence of an autoantibody to factor VIII, a Bethesda or New Oxford assay should be performed to quantitate the titre of the antibody. As stated above, autoantibodies to factor VIII are usually type II, which do not completely inhibit factor VIII activity. This makes an accurate assessment of the titre difficult. Because of the kinetics of these antibodies the titre of the antibodies does not usually correlate with the severity of the bleed or the responsiveness to treatment.

Treatment

Because of the rarity of this disorder and the heterogeneity of the diseases associated with spontaneous inhibitors, it is difficult to make generalizations about the appropriate management. However, careful management of these patients is mandatory because if haemorrhage can be controlled, mortality can be avoided and the inhibitor will eventually disappear. Once these inhibitors remit it is extremely rare for them to return. Acutely, management is aimed at controlling haemorrhage, a goal that is often more difficult than in patients with haemophilia. Products such as recombinant factor VIIIa, prothrombin complex concentrates and activated prothrombin complex concentrates have been used with variable results. When patients do not respond to prothrombin complex concentrates or have life-threatening haemorrhages, porcine factor VIII should be used if the human antibody does not cross-react with the porcine product. Even when the autoantibody titre is very high, the cross-reactivity of the antibody with porcine factor VIII may be sufficiently low that infusion of porcine factor VIII will lead to excellent blood levels of factor VIII and haemostasis. In patients with a low-titre inhibitor, higher than usual doses of human factor VIII concentrates may result in haemostatic levels of factor VIII. Occasionally, the Bethesda titre does not aid in determination of how someone will respond to factor VIII concentrates. The inhibitor titre cannot be relied upon in calculating the amount of factor VIII necessary to obtain adequate blood levels.

Long-term management is aimed at suppression of the antibody. Many agents such as protein A plasmapheresis, steroids, cytotoxic agents and intravenous gamma globulin have been used. Unfortunately, the efficacy of suppressive therapy is difficult to evaluate because of the rarity of this disorder, the high mortality associated with this disorder, and the large number of patients who spontaneously recover without any treatment other than supportive care.

Intravenous gamma globulin has been used in many patients and should always be tried. This therapy is relatively free of risk and is often used as one of the initial treatment options. Prednisone as an immunosuppressive therapy is usually administered concomitantly with intravenous gamma globulin. In our experience, intravenous gamma globulin is given as 1 g/kg body weight per day for 2 days. If the patient cannot tolerate the volume of the intravenous IgG in the 2-day protocol, it is administered as 400 mg/kg body weight per day for 5 days.

The prednisone is usually begun at 2 mg/kg/day. Once a response is seen, the patients are tapered off the prednisone over several months. Unfortunately, while intravenous gamma globulin and prednisone appear to be beneficial, the effects are not immediate. Supportive care and treatment of bleeding episodes must be continued until the antibody disappears.

Cytotoxic therapy has the highest potential for adverse side-effects, especially in the elderly population most at risk for development of spontaneous inhibitors. However, these agents are useful especially in groups least likely to recover spontaneously, such as those with underlying collagen vascular disorders and underlying malignancies. Cyclophosphamide and azathioprine are the two agents most often used in this setting. Cyclophosphamide has been used in protocols both orally and intravenously, and both routes of administration seem to be effective.

Protein A plasmapheresis has been used because of the binding affinity that protein A has for IgG. While protein A pheresis may be effective transiently, it often fails (Gjorstrup et al, 1991).

References

Addiego JE, Gomperts E, Liu SL, et al. Treatment of hemophilia A with a highly purified factor VIII concentrate prepared by anti-FVIIIc immunoaffinity chromatography. *Thrombosis and Haemostasis* 1990; **64:** 232.

Addiego J, Kasper C, Abildgaard C, et al. Frequency of inhibitor development in haemophiliacs treated with low-purity factor VIII. *Lancet* 1993; **342:** 462.

Algiman M, Dietrich G, Nydegger UE, Boieldieu D, Sultan Y, Kazatchkine MD. Natural antibodies to factor VIII (anti-hemophilic factor) in healthy individuals. *Proceedings of the National Academy of Sciences USA* 1992; **89:** 3795.

Aly AM, Aledort LM, Lee TD, Hoyer LW. Histocompatibility antigen patterns in haemophilic patients with factor VIII antibodies. *British Journal of Haematology* 1990; **76:** 238.

Arai M, Scandella D, Hoyer LW. Molecular basis of factor VIII inhibition by human antibodies. Antibodies that bind to the factor VIII light chain prevent the interaction of factor VIII with phospholipid. *Journal of Clinical Investigation* 1989; **83:** 1978.

Austen DEG, Lechner K, Rizza CR, et al. A comparison of the Bethesda and New Oxford methods of factor VIII inhibitor assay. *Thrombosis and Hemostasis* 1982; **47:** 72.

Bell BA, Kurczynski EM, Bergman G. Inhibitors to monoclonal antibody purified factor VIII. *Lancet* 1990; **336:** 638.

Biggs R, Austen DEG, Denson KWE, Borrett R, Rizza CR II. Antibodies which give complex concentration graphs. *British Journal of Haematology* 1972a; **23:** 125.

Biggs R, Austen DEG, Denson KWE, Rizza CR, Borrett R. Mode of action of antibodies which destroy factor VIII. I. Antibodies which have second order concentration graphs. *British Journal of Haematology* 1972b; **23:** 137.

Blatt PM, Menache D, Roberts HR. A survey of the effectiveness of prothrombin complex concentrates in controlling hemorrhage in patients with hemophilia and anti-factor VIII antibodies. *Thrombosis and Haemostasis* 1980; **44:** 39.

Brackmann HH. Induced immunotolerance in factor VIII inhibitor patients. *Progress in Clinical and Biological Research* 1986; **150:** 181.

De La Fuente B, Hoyer LW. The idiotypic charteristics of human antibodies to factor VIII. *Blood* 1984; **64:** 672.

Ehrenforth S, Kreuz W, Scharrer I. Incidence of development of factor VIII and factor IX inhibitors in haemophiliacs. *Lancet* 1992; **339:** 594.

Frommel D. Anti-idiotypic suppression of antibodies to factor VIIIc. *Lancet* 1984; **ii:** 1210.

Frommel D, Allain JP. Genetic predisposition to develop factor VIII antibody in classic hemophilia. *Clinical Immunology and Immunopathology* 1977; **8:** 43.

Frommel D, Muller JY, Prou-Wartelle O, Allain JP. Possible linkage between the major histocompatibility complex and the immune response to factor VIII in classic hemophilia. *Vox Sang* 1977; **33:** 270.

Fulcher CA, Mahoney SdG, Roberts JR, Kasper CK, Zimmerman TS. Localization of human factor VIII inhibitor epitopes to two polypeptide fragments. *Proceedings of the National Academy of Sciences USA* 1985; **82:** 7728.

Fulcher CA, Mahoney SdG, Zimmerman TS. FVIII inhibitor IgG subclass and FVIII polypeptide specificity determined by immunoblotting. *Blood* 1987; **69:** 1475.

Fulcher CA, Mahoney SdG, Lechner K. Immunoblot analysis shows changes in factor VIII inhibitor chain specificity in factor VIII inhibitor patients over time. *Blood* 1988; **72:** 1348.

Giannelli F, Choo KH, Rees DJG, Boyd Y, Rizza CR, Brownlee GG. Gene deletions in patients with haemophilia B and anti-factor IX antibodies. *Nature* 1983; **303:** 181.

Gill FM. The natural history of factor VIII inhibitors in patients with hemophilia A. *Progress in Clinical and Biological Research* 1984; **150:** 19.

Gitschier J. Molecular genetics of hemophilia A. *Schweizenische Medizinische Wochenschrift* 1989; **119:** 1329.

Gitschier J, Wood WI, Tuddenham EGD, et al. Detection and sequence of mutations in the factor VIII gene of haemophiliacs. *Nature* 1985; **315:** 427.

Gjorstrup P, Berntorp E, Larsson L, Nilsson IM. Kinetic aspects of the removal of IgG and inhibitors in hemophiliacs using protein A immunoadsorption. *Vox Sang* 1991; **61:** 244.

Green D, Lechner K. A survey of 215 non-hemophilic patients with inhibitors to factor VIII. *Thrombosis and Hemostasis* 1981; **45:** 200.

Green PM, Bentley DR, Mibashan RS, Nilsson IM, Giannelli F. Molecular pathology of haemophilia B. *EMBO Journal* 1989; **8:** 1067.

Hassan HJ, Leonardi A, Guerriero R, et al. Hemophilia B with inhibitor: molecular analysis of the subtotal deletion of the factor IX gene. *Blood* 1985; **66:** 728.

Hedner U, Glazer S. Management of hemophilia patients with inhibitors. *Hematology/Oncology Clinics of North America* 1992; **6:** 1035.

Hoyer LW. Incidence of factor VIII inhibitors in patients with severe hemophilia A. In: Aledort LN, Hoyer LW, Lusher JM, Reisner HM, White II GC (Eds), *Inhibitors to Coagulation Factors* (1995) Chapel Hill, NC: Plenum.

Kasper CK. Incidence and course of inhibitors among patients with classic hemophilia. *Thrombosis et Diathesis Haemorrhagica* 1973; **30:** 263.

Kessler CM, Sachse K. Factor VIII: C inhibitor associated with monoclonal-antibody purified FVIII concentrate. *Lancet* 1990; **335:** 1403.

Lawrence JS, Johnson JB. The presence of a circulating anticoagulant in a male member of a hemophiliac family. *Transaction of the American Clinical Climatological Association* 1941; **57:** 223–231.

Lubahn BC, Ware J, Stafford DW, Reisner HM. Identification of a factor VIII epitope recognized by a human hemophilic inhibitor. *Blood* 1989; **73:** 497.

Lubahn BC, Reisner EG, Reisner HM. Genetic susceptibility to inhibitor formation in hemophilia A: related individuals develop antibodies to similar regions of F.VIII. *Blood* 1990; **76:** 427a (abstr.).

Lusher JM, Shapiro SS, Palascak JE, et al. Efficacy of prothrombin complex concentrates in hemophiliacs with antibodies for factor VIII. A multicenter trial. *New England Journal of Medicine* 1980; **303:** 421.

Lusher JM, Arkin S, Abildgaard CF, et al. Treatment with recombinant FVIII of previously untreated patients with hemophilia A. Safety, efficacy and development of inhibitors. *New England Journal of Medicine* 1993; **328:** 453.

Matsushita T, Tanimoto M, Yanamoto K, et al. DNA sequence analysis of three inhibitor-positive hemophilia B patients without gross gene deletion: identification of four novel mutations in factor IX gene. *Journal of Laboratory and Clinical Medicine* 1990; **116:** 492.

McMillan CW. Clinical patterns of hemophilic patients who develop inhibitors. In: Hoyer LW (Ed.), *Factor VIII Inhibitors*. New York: Alan R. Liss, 1984: 31.

McMillan C, Shapiro S, Whitehurst D, et al. The natural history of factor VIII: C inhibitors in patients with hemophilia A: a natural cooperative study. II. Observations on the initial development of factor VIII:C inhibitors. *Blood* 1988; **71:** 344.

Moffat EH, Furlong RA, Dannatt AHG, Bloom AL, Peake IR. Anti-idiotypes to factor VIII antibodies and their possible role in the pathogenesis and treatment of factor VIII inhibitors. *British Journal of Haematology* 1989; **71:** 85.

Nilsson IM, Hedner U, Bjorlin B. Suppression of factor IX antibody in hemophilia B by factor IX and cyclophosphamide. *Annals of Internal Medicine* 1973; **78:** 91.

Nilsson IM, Berntrop E, Zettervall O. Induction of immune tolerance in patients with hemophilia and antibodies to factor VIII by combined treatment with intravenous IgG, cyclophosphamide, and factor VIII. *New England Journal of Medicine* 1988; **318:** 947.

Nilsson IM, Berntorp E, Zettervall O, Dahlback B. Noncoagulation inhibitory factor VIII antibodies after induction of tolerance to factor VIII in hemophilia A patients. *Blood* 1990; **75:** 378.

Peerlinck K, Arnout J, Gilles JG, Saint-Remy JM, Vermylen J. A higher than expected incidence of factor VIII inhibitors in multitransfused haemophilia A patients treated with an intermediate purity pasteurized factor VIII concentrate. *Thrombosis and Haemostasis* 1993; **69:** 115.

Rosendaal FR, Nieuwenhuis HK, van den Berg HM, et al. A sudden increase in factor VIII inhibitor development in multitransfused hemophilia A patients in The Netherlands. *Blood* 1993; **81:** 2180.

Sanchez-Cuenca JM, Carmona E, Villanueva MJ, Aznar JA. Immunological characterization of factor VIII inhibitors by a sensitive micro-ELISA method. *Thrombosis Research* 1990; **57:** 897.

Scandella D, Mahoney SdG, Mattingly M, Roeder D, Timmons L, Fulcher CA. Epitope mapping of human factor VIII inhibitor antibodies by deletion analysis of factor VIII fragments expressed in *Escherichia coli. Proceedings of the National Academy of Sciences USA* 1988; **85:** 6152.

Scandella D, Mattingly M, Mahoney SdG, Fulcher CA. Localization of epitopes for human factor VIII inhibitor antibodies by immunoblotting and antibody neutralization. *Blood* 1989; **74:** 1618.

Scandella D, Kessler C, Esmon P, et al. Epitope specificity and functional characterization of factor VIII inhibitors. In: Aledort LN, Hoyer LW, Lusher JM, Reisner HM, White II GC (Eds), *Inhibitors to Coagulation Factors* (1995) Chapel Hill, NC: Plenum.

Sjamsoedin LJM, Heijnen L, Mauser-Bunshcoten EP, et al. The effect of activated prothrombin complex concentrates (FEIBA) on joint and muscle bleeding in patients with hemophilia A and antibodies to factor VIII. A randomised double-blind clinical trial. *New England Journal of Medicine* 1981; **305:** 717.

Sultan Y, Rossi F, Kazatchkine MD. Recovery from anti-VIII: C (antihemophilic factor) autoimmune disease is dependent on generation of anti-idiotypes against anti-VIII: C autoantibodies. *Proceedings of the National Academy of Sciences USA* 1987; **85:** 3150.

Tiarks CY, Pechet L, Humphreys RE. Development of anti-idiotypic antibodies in a patient with a factor VIII autoantibody. *American Journal of Hematology* 1989; **32:** 217.

12 Inherited Bleeding Disorders in Pregnancy

Isobel D. Walker and
Ian A. Greer

Introduction

Haemophilia A and Haemophilia B

The prevalence of haemophilia A in the UK is around 1–2 per 5000 male births. Haemophilia B is around 10 times less frequent (1–2 per 50 000 males). Females "carry" these X-linked recessive disorders. Female carriers usually inherit their abnormal gene for factor VIII (FVIII) or factor IX (FIX) from one or other of their parents – a haemophilic father or a mother who is herself a carrier. As female carriers usually have a normal gene on their other X chromosome, they generally have coagulation factor activity >50 iu/dl, which is adequate for normal haemostasis. Thus, the vast majority of female carriers of haemophilia A or haemophilia B do not have significant bleeding problems and, indeed, many carriers will remain undetected unless specifically sought. Troublesome bleeding may, however, occur in the minority of haemophilia carriers in whom clotting factor activity is <40 iu/dl. Unexpectedly low clotting factor activity may be the result of extreme lyonization, of coinheritance of a variant von Willebrand factor allele such as von Willebrand's disease Normandy or, very rarely, of coincidence with another chromosomal abnormality such as Turner's syndrome (XO). With the increasing success of patient associations the risk of homozygosity may rise but at present female haemophiliacs (as opposed to female haemophilia carriers) are distinctly rare.

Statistically, 50% of the male children of female carriers will have haemophilia and be at risk of serious bleeding; 100% of the daughters of haemophiliacs and 50% of the daughters of haemophilia carriers will be carriers who may in time bear haemophiliac sons and carrier daughters.

Von Willebrand's disease

Von Willebrand's disease is the most common clinically significant heritable abnormality of coagulation affecting women. It is very difficult to ascertain precisely the prevalence of all forms of von Willebrand's disease because it has a very wide spectrum of clinical presentation and, certainly in the past, many of the milder cases may not have been recognized. Von Willebrand's disease is more common than generally realized and its prevalence may be as high as 1% (Rodeghiero et al, 1987).

Von Willebrand factor synthesis is controlled by a gene situated on the short arm of chromosome 12; von Willebrand's disease is therefore an autosomally inherited disorder and both autosomal dominant and autosomal recessive forms are described. The most widely accepted classification of von Willebrand's disease depends on von Willebrand factor multimer characteristics dividing von Willebrand's disease into three major classes, denoted type I, type II and type III.

Type I von Willebrand's disease is the most common type, accounting for 70–75% of patients. It is characterized by a reduction in all forms of von Willebrand factor multimers, but the full range, including the highest molecular weight forms, remains detectable in the patient's plasma. Different systems of subclassifying type I von Willebrand's disease have been described. The inheritance of type I von Willebrand's disease is usually autosomal dominant but in some the inheritance is autosomal recessive and the heterozygotes are asymptomatic carriers. In non-pregnant patients with type I von Willebrand's disease the von Willebrand factor antigen is usually between 10 and 40 u/dl, equivalent to that of FVIII:C and roughly equivalent to the von Willebrand factor ristocetin co-factor activity. When patients with type I von Willebrand's disease are given desamino-8-D-arginine vasopressin (DDAVP) there is a rise in the concentration of all of the multimers and the bleeding time is usually shortened. The bleeding tendency in type I von Willebrand's disease is generally fairly mild.

The feature common to all type II subvariants is loss of the highest molecular weight von Willebrand factor multimers. The von Willebrand factor is functionally impaired and the bleeding time is usually prolonged. Factor VIII:C activity is equal to or greater than the von Willebrand factor antigen level. In non-pregnant patients both may be within the normal range or reduced. The von Willebrand factor ristocetin co-factor activity is usually significantly lower than the von Willebrand factor antigen level. Various subtypes of type II von Willebrand's disease are described. In type IIA there is loss of high molecular weight (HMW) forms of von Willebrand factor – predominantly low molecular weight (LMW) multimers are seen. Treatment with DDAVP results in an increase in the smaller, but not the larger, multimers and the bleeding time is usually not completely corrected. In type IIB von Willebrand's disease the multimer pattern again shows loss of large multimers but the intermediate and small forms are present. In these patients there is increased interaction between platelets and von Willebrand factor in the presence of ristocetin, the abnormal von Willebrand factor seeming to have enhanced reactivity with platelet glycoprotein 1b (GP1b). Patients with type IIB von Willebrand's disease frequently have mild to moderate thrombocytopenia. Infusion of DDAVP into these patients results in a transient appearance of larger multimers of von Willebrand factor but the bleeding time is not fully corrected and the platelet count falls further. DDAVP should therefore be avoided in patients with type IIB von Willebrand's disease.

Other subvariants of type II von Willebrand's disease are described and these are discussed elsewhere in this book. With the exception of the subvariants type IIC and type IIH, the inheritance of type II von Willebrand's disease is usually autosomal dominant. However, cases of recessive type IIA and type IIB have been described (Asakura et al, 1987; Donner et al, 1987). Bleeding in type II von Willebrand's disease (particularly type IIA von Willebrand's disease) tends to be more severe and episodes occur more frequently than in type I von Willebrand's disease.

Type III von Willebrand's disease is clinically the most severe. In these patients FVIII:C is very low (in the range 1–10 u/dl) and von Willebrand factor antigen is undetectable or very low (less than 5 u/dl). No multimers are seen. Patients have haemophilic-type lesions such as joint bleeds in addition to mucosal bleeding. Treatment with DDAVP has no effect in this type of von Willebrand's disease. Probably many type III von Willebrand's disease patients are homozygotes of recessively inherited von Willebrand's disease but some may be compound heterozygotes. The prevalence in the UK of type III von Willebrand's disease is approximately 1 in 10^6 but the condition is more prevalent in cultures where consanguinity is common. In general the parents are clinically unaffected or have a mild bleeding tendency only. The parents' von Willebrand factor levels may be at, or just below, the lower limits of normality. Obviously parents who produce a child with type III von Willebrand's disease require full investigation, follow-up and careful counselling with respect to the management of future pregnancies and the availability of prenatal diagnosis.

It is essential that, as far as possible, families with these heritable bleeding problems understand the genetic implications of their disorder. Counselling and care of females as well as males should be an integral part of the comprehensive care which must be widely and easily available to all families with inherited bleeding disorders.

Factor VIII Complex and Factor IX Changes in Pregnancy

Normal pregnancy is associated with major changes in haemostatic mechanisms: the concentration of many coagulation factors increasing and overall plasma fibrinolytic activity decreasing. The levels of the components of the FVIII complex, FVIII:C and von Willebrand factor antigen and activity, increase progressively from the first trimester (Fournie et al, 1981; Stirling et al, 1984). Factor VIII:C rises from a mean of 130 iu/dl in the first trimester to a mean of 212 iu/dl at term. Mean von Willebrand factor antigen levels are also around 130 iu/dl in the first trimester but much greater variability in the rise during pregnancy results in a higher mean von Willebrand factor antigen level at term, the mean at term being around 375 iu/dl (Hathaway and Bonnar, 1987). When comparisons of FVIII:C and von Willebrand factor antigen are made within individuals, the ratio of von Willebrand factor antigen to FVIII:C is around 1 or slightly less in uncomplicated pregnancies but may be raised and exceed unity in complicated pregnancy (e.g. in severe pre-eclampsia) where there is elevation of the von Willebrand factor antigen level (Caires et al, 1984) due to endothelial damage or dysfunction. von Willebrand factor activity rises to a mean of around 170 iu/dl in the second and third trimesters (Hathaway and Bonnar, 1987).

Haemophilia carriers and most women with von Willebrand's disease also show an increase in the components of the FVIII complex during pregnancy, FVIII:C and von Willebrand factor antigen and activity levels increasing sufficiently such that the majority do not suffer excessive bleeding. When bleeding does occur it happens more frequently postpartum than during pregnancy and is usually associated with a surgical delivery or with perineal or genital tract damage. Some patients with von Willebrand's disease show variable responses with lesser increases in their levels of FVIII:C and von Willebrand factor during pregnancy (Adashi, 1980; Hill et al, 1982; Ramsahoye et al, 1993) particularly those with low FVIII:C (<15 iu/dl) prior to delivery. Bleeding times shorten significantly in pregnancy in a minority of von Willebrand's disease patients (Conti et al, 1986; Ramsahoye et al, 1993). Furthermore, measurement of bleeding time, FVIII:C, von Willebrand factor antigen and von Willebrand factor activity are not always predictive of patients who will bleed (Lipton et al, 1982; Greer et al, 1991).

In general, patients with type I von Willebrand's disease do not bleed excessively during pregnancy. On the other hand type II and type III von Willebrand's disease patients do have an increased tendency to bleed, particularly postpartum. In type IIA von Willebrand's disease not all patients show a significant increase in HMW multimers of von Willebrand factor antigen during pregnancy (Takahashi, 1983). This may explain the relatively greater risk of pregnancy-associated haemorrhage in women with type IIA von Willebrand's disease than in women with type I von Willebrand's disease. Type IIB von Willebrand's disease patients may develop worsening thrombocytopenia during pregnancy.

Type III von Willebrand's disease patients show little or no increase in the FVIII complex levels and remain at significant risk of bleeding during pregnancy, delivery and postpartum.

Even though the vitamin K-dependent coagulation factors have many properties in common they do not all behave similarly during pregnancy. Factors VII and X show moderate increases to around 170 u/dl and 125 u/dl, respectively (Stirling et al, 1984) whilst the levels of prothrombin and FIX remain unchanged or show a slight rise only.

Carriers of haemophilia B may therefore have FIX levels substantially below normal even at the end of pregnancy (Briet et al, 1982; Greer et al, 1991).

Counselling and Family Planning

Families with heritable bleeding disorders should have easy access to information and counselling, including advice on contraception and family planning. Because over the past 7 or 8 years Haemophilia Centres have become heavily involved in the management of their patients with human immunodeficiency virus (HIV), family planning advice has sometimes been limited to advice about "safe sex" and the use of condoms. Whilst this remains essential, much broader counselling should be offered formally and informally to both males and females, patients and partners.

Planning families

Males with haemophilia do not transmit their disorder to their sons, but all of their daughters are obligate carriers. The female partners of haemophilic males should be carefully counselled and led to try to understand the possible conflicts and psychological stresses of mothering a daughter whose own reproductive ambitions will inevitably be clouded by the possible prospect of producing an affected male child. Some couples where the male has haemophilia, particularly if he is severely affected, may wish to avoid this situation and consider means of ensuring only male children are produced (e.g. by selective termination or in vitro fertilization, IVF) or in some instances may seek artificial insemination by a donor (DI).

Unfortunately, young female relatives of haemophiliacs often only consider investigation to establish their likelihood of being a haemophilia carrier when they have already committed themselves and are already pregnant or are in a relationship that is likely to lead to pregnancy. Although carrier testing for haemophilia B has become easier and can, if necessary, be done during pregnancy, in general, haemophilia carrier testing during pregnancy should be avoided if possible. Carrier testing should be performed much earlier, ideally at puberty, when the girl is old enough to understand the implications but before she is sexually active and certainly before her first pregnancy. Parents of possible carrier females should themselves be counselled and advised about the requirement to encourage their daughters to present themselves for early investigation. Girls whose close male relatives are severely affected may be more willing to seek investigation themselves than girls who are related to males with milder disease or whose only affected male relatives are more distant. Prior to commencing investigation the limitations of current carrier testing have to be fully discussed with the possible carrier and her family. A questionnaire survey of first-degree female relatives of 167 Finnish haemophilia A patients showed that these relatives considered haemophilia a "serious" disease. Most of these women were aware of the risk of carriership and of having an affected son, and 16% said they would definitely terminate a pregnancy where the fetus was a haemophilic male (Ranta et al, 1994). A further evaluation of experience of, and attitudes to, carrier detection and prenatal diagnosis was carried out among 549 potential and obligate carriers of haemophilia (Varekamp et al, 1990). Almost all considered carrier testing to be of value. Nearly 50% had been assessed for carrier status, but surprisingly 41% had not been tested and had not received information regarding the heredity of haemophilia. Women with severely affected relatives were more likely to have been tested for carriership. Lack of knowledge of possible carriership and a lack of awareness of the possibility of carrier testing appeared to be important factors for those women not having been tested. Almost a third of those surveyed favoured prenatal diagnosis with subsequent possibility of termination of pregnancy if the fetus was affected. In those women who would object to prenatal diagnosis, the main factor was that they did not consider haemophilia to be a disorder serious enough to justify abortion. These surveys highlight the need for counselling with regard to carriership and pregnancy and prenatal diagnosis as well as appropriate contraception.

Female carriers of haemophilia may feel isolated and under great stress. Usually their husband or partner's family will have had no previous contact with inherited bleeding disorders and may find it difficult to come to terms with the possibility of having a haemophilic child in the family. Whilst haemophilia carriers may be relatively better able to accept a carrier daughter than can the normal partner of a haemophilic man, they may find themselves emotionally devastated by irrational guilt feelings if they produce a severely affected son. If at all possible, all of these and other possible psychological stresses should be discussed openly and freely before pregnancy. Careful counselling on the availability and benefits and risks of prenatal diagnostic testing should be offered to couples before they embark on a first pregnancy.

Because, in general, von Willebrand's disease is a much milder disorder than haemophilia, counselling of affected women is less stressful. Nonetheless, family planning advice and genetic counselling is important for these women and may allay previously unexpressed fears about the risks to themselves during pregnancy and delivery and fears that their children may have a more major bleeding disorder.

In general, female carriers of haemophilia and women with von Willebrand's disease should be reviewed at regular intervals during their reproductive life, even if they remain asymptomatic. These review visits allow informal counselling and encourage the women to take a more positive attitude to carrier testing, family planning and prenatal diagnosis.

Contraception, menstrual problems and gynaecological surgery

The principles of contraception are essentially unchanged in the congenital coagulopathies and the methods of contraception used should be tailored to the patient's requirements. However, from the foregoing discussion it is clear that carriers and affected individuals, both male and female, should not find themselves in a situation of an unplanned pregnancy when many difficult decisions may have to be considered under constraints of time. Thus, contraception must be part of the package of care offered to such individuals. The range of contraception available will include barrier methods, the combined oestrogen and progesterone oral contraceptive pill and the progesterone-only pill, depot preparations such as Depo-Provera and Norplant, the intrauterine contraceptive device (IUCD) and male and female sterilization. No technique is absolutely contraindicated and the choice will largely be governed by factors other than the bleeding disorder per se. Where an individual may be a carrier of hepatitis B or HIV, barrier contraception should be used and it may also be useful to consider additional contraception, for example, the oral contraceptive pill if the couple feel that a pregnancy would be disastrous. Women with von Willebrand's disease frequently complain of heavy periods (Greer et al, 1991) and the combined oral contraceptive pill may be the ideal preparation in this situation to reduce heavy bleeding and offer contraception in parallel. In addition, the administration of oestrogen may increase the levels of von Willebrand factor antigen by stimulating its endothelial production. This may be useful in women with mild to moderate von Willebrand's disease (Alparin, 1982; Caller, 1984). As the IUCD can provoke increased menstrual blood loss it is largely unsuitable for patients with von Willebrand's disease. However, the progestogen-impregnated IUCDs that are beginning to be used in the treatment of menstrual problems may offer the benefits of IUCD usage without the excess risk of bleeding and this will virtually abolish heavy menstrual bleeding, at least in normal women. At present, however, there is essentially no experience of this preparation in women with von Willebrand's disease but clearly this is an agent that could be considered. Depot progesterone preparations may have a role to play but, in general, such intramuscular or implantable devices are likely to be unsuitable for the majority of patients with von Willebrand's disease because of the risk of haematoma. However, these devices and preparations may be satisfactory for women who are carriers of the haemophilias. Sterilization, either male or female, can also be offered if appropriate.

Operative procedures should not be undertaken lightly in such patients as even relatively minor procedures such as diagnostic curettage may result in substantial intra- or postoperative haemorrhage if appropriate haemostatic cover has not been obtained. Any operative therapy should be managed in association with the local Haemophilia Unit.

Antifibrinolytic agents such as tranexamic acid are also of value in the management of menorrhagia in these women (Aledort, 1991; Scott and Montgomery, 1993).

Pelvic haematomas within the broad ligament or into the ovaries, such as within a haemorrhagic corpus luteum, have also been reported in von Willebrand's disease (Greer et al, 1991) and it is important to consider such haemorrhagic problems in patients with von Willebrand's disease who have pelvic pain before embarking on a surgical procedure with its possible complications. Haematomas are best managed conservatively, where possible, with haemostatic products given to prevent further bleeding until a spontaneous resorption of the haematoma. If conservative treatment is unsuccessful, operative intervention may be required.

A further gynaecological problem is miscarriage in the first or second trimester. At this point the concentrations of the FVIII complex may not have increased satisfactorily to prevent haemorrhage (Sorosky et al, 1980; Punnonen et al, 1981).

In contrast to the high frequency of menorrhagia in women with von Willebrand's disease, carriers of haemophilia A do not have a high incidence of menorrhagia. In one recent review of 18 obligate carriers of haemophilia A (Greer et al, 1991), only four had sought gynaecological advice for menorrhagia and all four had had diagnostic curettage performed without complication. However, three of them had FVIII:C and von Willebrand factor concentrations within the normal range while the fourth who had a low concentration of FVIII:C (around 40 iu/dl) received haemostatic cover preoperatively. Furthermore, three of these women went on to have an abdominal hysterectomy, two without complications and the third with the complication of a vault haematoma requiring treatment with FVIII concentrate infusions over 1 week postoperatively. This patient's FVIII:C level was around 40 iu/dl. It has to be anticipated in carriers who have essentially normal levels of FVIII:C that there is no evidence of an excessive incidence of haemorrhagic problems in association with spontaneous abortion, uterine evacuation or sterilization. In a further study of bleeding symptoms in carriers of haemophilia A and B, Bunschoten et al (1988) found that the incidence of menorrhagia was not significantly different from a reference group of women, although they did report a higher risk of haemorrhage after surgical procedures. These authors have shown an association between the level of FVIII:C and bleeding risk by a logistic regression analysis.

In patients who are carriers of haemophilia B, baseline FIX concentrations are often significantly below the normal range (Greer et al, 1991). Just as in haemophilia A, these women may be more at risk of haemorrhage after surgical procedures and this is associated with the level of FIX (Bunschoten et al, 1988). High purity factor IX cover will be required for some of these carriers if major surgery is planned.

Pregnancy

Preconception counselling

Pregnancy planning should be encouraged and patients with haemophilia or von Willebrand's disease and carriers or potential carriers of haemophilia should seek specialist medical advice from their haematologist and if possible an obstetrician prior to conception. This is usually easiest achieved when the affected patient is female, but couples where the potential father has a heritable bleeding disorder should also be referred for prepregnancy counselling. At this stage the options for prenatal diagnosis may be discussed again and other aspects of the management of the planned pregnancy considered.

Women who may require blood product therapy and who are not already immune should be immunized against hepatitis B. Immunization should, if possible, be completed prior to conception, but if the patient is already pregnant immunization against hepatitis B is safe during pregnancy (although not ideal). Because of recent reports of outbreaks of hepatitis A in some haemophiliacs, immunization against hepatitis A is also currently offered to non-immune patients who may require blood products.

Management of pregnancy

Carriers or potential carriers of haemophilia A or B and women with von Willebrand's disease require review at a Haemophilia Centre throughout pregnancy so that their coagulation factor activity and, if appropriate, von Willebrand factor antigen and activity can be monitored. In carriers or potential carriers of haemophilia A or B where prenatal diagnostic tests have not been performed (currently in the UK the majority of carriers), information about the sex of the fetus is extremely useful in managing the pregnancy and ultimately the delivery. Modern ultrasound scanning equipment allows visualization of fetal external genitalia and offers a non-invasive method of identifying most male fetuses by about 18–20 weeks. It should be noted, however, that although the diagnosis of a male fetus on ultrasound is almost always correct, the diagnosis of a female fetus is less accurate.

Maternal coagulation factor activity and the levels of von Willebrand factor do not show a significant increase until the second trimester and in the case of FIX may not show any significant rise at all. Invasive procedures during pregnancy that may result in accidental maternal, fetal or placental haemorrhage therefore require careful consideration on an individual patient basis.

Patients and their partners should realize that even chorionic villous sampling (CVS) for prenatal diagnosis may be hazardous because of the risk of bleeding and CVS should be performed only after full discussion, not only of the perceived benefits but also of the risks. One possible way of avoiding risks of invasive procedures for prenatal diagnosis is to perform preimplantation diagnosis on pregnancies resulting from IVF. This involves removal of one or two cells from an eight-cell embryo at day 3 in vitro. This does not appear to adversely affect embryo development (Tarin and Handyside, 1993). Both polymerase chain reaction (PCR) and fluorescent in situ hybridization (FISH) have been used to sex human preimplantation embryos for X-linked disorders but FISH appears to be the better option (Veiga et al, 1994). Such a strategy may have a place in the haemophilias. The use of FISH to identify and transfer only female embryos in a haemophilia carrier with a successful twin pregnancy outcome has been reported (Veiga et al, 1994).

Spontaneous abortion, pregnancy termination or surgery during the first trimester may be complicated by serious maternal haemorrhage unless the levels of the FVIII complex or FIX are raised to around 40 iu/dl. Carriers of haemophilia B may remain at risk of bleeding throughout pregnancy and planned surgery, invasive procedures, miscarriage or other accidental bleeding must precipitate immediate reassessment of the patient's current FIX activity and if necessary replacement therapy.

Monitoring of coagulation factor activity and, if appropriate, von Willebrand factor throughout pregnancy and particularly in the last trimester provides opportunities for discussion about the management of delivery. A planned delivery date may be advisable if there is any concern that the levels of clotting factor or von Willebrand factor activity may be inadequate for haemostasis.

Management of delivery

In the absence of obstetric contraindication, vaginal delivery at term is usually preferred. However, early recourse to Caesarean section is recommended for carriers of haemophilia A or B with a known male fetus if the chance of an easy vaginal delivery is for any reason compromised. For all women with a heritable bleeding disorder, early Caesarean section should be considered if labour fails to progress steadily. If an operative or instrumental delivery does become necessary this should be performed by the most experienced member of staff available. Minimizing maternal genital tract or perineal trauma reduces the risk of postpartum bleeding.

Since fetal scalp electrodes and scalp vein sampling can cause massive haematomas, it would seem prudent to avoid them if the fetus may have von Willebrand's disease or in haemophilia carriers where the fetus is known to be male or its sex is not known. Likewise ventouse extraction should be avoided in a potentially affected fetus.

The need for an atraumatic delivery and the avoidance of difficult vaginal deliveries is emphasized by several reported series. In a 10-year retrospective study of 150 patients with haemophilia (Yoffe and Buchanan, 1988), eight of the infants developed central nervous system haemorrhage in the newborn period and over 60% of them had significant haematological sequelae. Other series have reported similar problems with intracranial haemorrhage (Bray and Luban, 1989; Kletzel et al, 1989) and traumatic vaginal delivery was implicated as a precipitant in the majority of infants with central nervous system haemorrhage.

Blood product therapy

Factor VIII:C levels usually rise during pregnancy and in general also increase significantly in haemophilia A carriers and in women with type I von Willebrand's disease. Practically it is useful to recheck coagulation factor activity in the last trimester at around 34–36 weeks gestation. Providing the FVIII:C activity exceeds 40 iu/dl, these women are unlikely to bleed excessively during normal delivery and blood product therapy is not usually necessary to cover an uncomplicated vaginal delivery. If, however, Caesarean section is planned or becomes necessary, FVIII:C activity should be in excess of 50 iu/dl. In some women this may require infusion of a high-purity plasma or recombinant FVIII concentrate. Occasionally haemophilia A carriers with very low FVIII:C activity do not raise their FVIII:C levels even to 40 iu/dl (Greer et al, 1991) and they may require infusion of FVIII concentrate to cover even an anticipated straightforward delivery.

Because FIX activity does not show as great a rise as FVIII:C during pregnancy, female carriers of haemophilia B may have levels of FIX inadequate for haemostasis even at term (Briet et al, 1982). It is essential that these women are reviewed at around 34–36 weeks gestation and their FIX levels rechecked. Carriers of haemophilia B more frequently require blood product therapy to cover delivery than do carriers of haemophilia A. For vaginal delivery FIX activity should be raised to 40 iu/dl and for Caesarean section to 50 iu/dl. High-purity FIX concentrate should be used as FIX concentrates containing factors II, VII and X are potentially thrombogenic.

In carriers of haemophilia A or B and in type I von Willebrand's disease, following delivery, FVIII:C and FIX levels should be maintained at about 40 iu/dl for at least 4–5 days – longer in the presence of bleeding or wound infection.

Frequently type IIA and type III von Willebrand's disease and occasionally type IIB von Willebrand's disease patients require blood product therapy to raise their FVIII:C and von Willebrand factor complex levels to cover delivery, even an uncomplicated vaginal delivery. Monitoring of FVIII:C and von Willebrand factor complex levels in the third trimester allows replacement therapy to be planned where necessary. Prophylactic infusion of FVIII concentrates containing significant amounts of the larger von Willebrand factor multimers, e.g. Haemate P (Centeon) or 8Y (Blood Products Laboratory) (UK Haemophilia Centre Directors 1997), should be commenced at the onset of labour aiming to raise the FVIII:C and von Willebrand factor activity levels above 40 iu/dl for vaginal delivery or above 50 iu/dl for Caesarean section. Levels must be maintained above 40 iu/dl for at least 4–5 days after delivery.

DDAVP infusion

Carriers of haemophilia A and some patients with type I or type IIA von Willebrand's disease show a rise in their factor VIII and von Willebrand factor complex levels in response to infusion of DDAVP. In non-pregnant patients DDAVP is frequently used to cover dental work or minor surgery, but because it is mildly oxytocic some haematologists and obstetricians prefer to avoid its use during ongoing pregnancy. It may, however, be useful immediately prior to or after delivery or following abortion or termination where a moderate rise in FVIII:C and von Willebrand factor complex is required for a few days only. After surgery DDAVP may cause water retention and hyponatraemia (Lowe et al, 1977). Indeed, maternal water retention provoking a grand-mal seizure has been reported (Chediak et al, 1986) with repeated therapy. It is recommended, therefore, that blood urea and electrolytes are monitored and excessive fluid input (e.g. dextrose infusions) are avoided. Because of the risk of causing platelet aggregation and thrombocytopenia due to binding of abnormal intermediate-sized von Willebrand factor multimers to the platelets (Rick et al, 1987), type IIB von Willebrand's disease patients must not be given DDAVP. The response to DDAVP is greater (von Willebrand factor (and FVIII:C) in normal pregnant women than in normal non-pregnant women (four-fold versus two-fold) (Davison et al, 1993)).

Analgesia

In all patients with defective haemostasis, intramuscular injections have to be avoided. If necessary, analgesia to cover delivery has therefore to be given subcutaneously or intravenously. There is no consensus on the safety or otherwise of epidural anaesthesia to cover delivery in patients with von Willebrand's disease or carriers of haemophilia but it has been suggested that providing the coagulation screen is normal, the Simplate bleeding time <10 minutes and the platelet count $>100 \times 10^9/l$, there should normally be no contraindication to inserting an epidural catheter (Letsky, 1991). The uncomplicated use of epidural anaesthesia in type I von Willebrand's disease has been reported (Milaskiewicz et al, 1990), but clearly such management must be carefully weighed up in terms of potential risks and benefits. Before removing the catheter a repeat coagulation screen and platelet count would seem prudent and in cases of elective surgery, spinal anaesthesia may offer a safer option.

Postpartum

Whilst excessive bleeding during carefully managed delivery is relatively uncommon in most carriers of haemophilia and in women with the common type I von Willebrand's disease and the type IIA variant, women with inherited abnormalities of the factor VIII and von Willebrand factor complex and in particular those who have variant (non-type I) forms of von Willebrand's disease are at risk of postpartum haemorrhage. It has been suggested that the increased risk of bleeding after delivery in these women is associated with rapidly falling levels of FVIII:C and von Willebrand factor complex postpartum (Krishnamurthy and Miotti, 1977). Several studies have reported severe bleeding after delivery in women with type IIA and type IIB von Willebrand's disease (Noller et al, 1973; Greer et al, 1991). In type IIA von Willebrand's disease it has been shown that although the levels of FVIII:C and von Willebrand factor antigen may rise during pregnancy, the large multimers of von Willebrand factor antigen do not appear in the blood and von Willebrand factor activity therefore remains low. It is very important that in patients with variant von Willebrand's disease (non-type I) products containing the larger von Willebrand factor multimers are used and that the response to the infusion is checked, not only in terms of the rise in FVIII:C but also in terms of von Willebrand factor activity. Providing FVIII:C and von Willebrand factor activity are raised above 40–50 iu/dl and maintained at these levels for 4–5 days, there should be no increased risk of postpartum haemorrhage.

At delivery a cord sample should be collected for investigation. Because some haemostatic factors are physiologically relatively reduced in neonates it may be difficult to exclude a mild to moderate inherited defect at birth (e.g. haemophilia B or von Willebrand's disease) and repeat examination at 3–6 months may be necessary. Intramuscular injections must be avoided in children of either sex with proven or possible von Willebrand's disease and in male children of haemophilia carriers (unless the baby is known to be unaffected). In these neonates, therefore, prophylactic vitamin K1 should be given orally and their general practitioner informed and asked to ensure that routine immunizations are given either subcutaneously or intradermally. In addition, immunization against hepatitis B should be considered. Both mother and baby should be reviewed at the Haemophilia Centre after discharge from the Maternity Unit.

References

Adashi EY. Lack of improvement in von Willebrand's disease during pregnancy. *New England Journal of Medicine* 1980; **303:** 1178.
Aledort LM. Treatment of von Willebrand's disease. *Mayo Clinic Proceedings* 1991; **66:** 841.
Alparin JB. Estrogens and surgery in women with von Willebrand's disease. *American Journal of Medicine* 1982; **73:** 367.
Asakura A, Harrison J, Gomperts E, Abildgaard C. Type IIA von Willebrand disease with probable autosomal recessive inheritance. *Blood* 1987; **69:** 1419–1420.
Bray GL, Lubon NL. Hemophilia presenting with intracranial hemorrhage. *American Journal of Diseases of Children* 1989; **141:** 1215–1217.
Briet E, Reismer HM, Blatt PM. Factor IX levels during pregnancy in a woman with haemophilia B. *Haemostasis* 1982; **11:** 87–89.
Bunschoten EM, van Houwelingen JC, Bisser EJMS, van Dijken PJ, Kik AJ, Sixma JJ. Bleeding symptoms in carriers of haemophilia A and B. *Thrombosis and Haemostasis* 1988; **59:** 349–352.
Caires D, Arocha-Pinango CL, Rodriguez S, Linares J. Factor VIIIR:Ag/factor VIII:C and their ratio in obstetrical cases. *Acta Obstetricia et Gynaecologica Scandinavica* 1984; **63:** 411–416.
Chediak JR, Albon GM, Maxey B. von Willebrand's disease and pregnancy: management during delivery and outcome of offspring. *American Journal of Obstetrics and Gynecology* 1986; **155:** 618–624.
Coller BS. von Willebrand's disease. In: Ratnoff OD, Forbes CD, (Eds), *Disorders of Haemostasis*. New York: Grune and Stratton, 1984: 241–269.
Conti M, Mori D, Conti E, Muggiasca ML, Mannucci PM. Pregnancy in women with different types of von Willebrand's disease. *Obstetrics and Gynecology* 1986; **68:** 282–285.
Davison JM, Shiells EA, Phillips PR, Barron WM, Lindheimer MD. Metabolic clearance of vasopressin and an analogue resistant to vasopressin are in human pregnancy. *American Journal of Physiology* 1993; **264:** F348–F353.
Donner M, Holmberg L, Nilsson IM. Type IIB von Willebrand's disease with probable autosomal recessive inheritance and presenting as thrombocytopenia in infancy. *British Journal of Haematology* 1987; **66:** 349–354.
Fournie A, Monrozies M, Pontonnier G, Boneu B, Bierme R. Factor VIII complex in normal pregnancy, pre-eclampsia and fetal growth retardation. *British Journal of Obstetrics and Gynaecology* 1981; **88:** 250–254.
Greer IA, Lowe GDO, Walker JJ, Forbes CD. Haemorrhagic problems in obstetrics and gynaecology in patients with congenital coagulopathies. *British Journal of Obstetrics and Gynaecology* 1991; **98:** 909–918.
Hathaway WE, Bonnar J. *Physiology of Coagulation in Pregnant Women and Newborn Infants.* New York: John Wiley, 1987: pp. 39–56.
Hill FGH, George J, Enayat MD. Changes in VIII:C, VIIIR:Ag, WF and ristocetin-induced platelet aggregation during pregnancy in women with von Willebrand's disease. *British Journal of Haematology* 1982; **50:** 691 (abstr.).
Kletzel M, Miller CH, Beaton DL, et al. Post-delivery head bleeding in hemophilic neonates: causes and management. *American Journal of Diseases of Children* 1989; **143:** 1107–1110.
Krishnamurthy M, Miotti AB. von Willebrand's disease and pregnancy. *Obsetetrics and Gynecology* 1977; **49:** 244–247.
Letsky EA. Haemostasis and epidural anaesthesia. *International Journal of Obstetric Anaesthetics* 1991; **1:** 51–54.
Lipton RA, Ayromlooi J, Coller BS. Severe von Willebrand's disease during labor and delivery. *Journal of the American Medical Association* 1982; **248:** 1355–1357.
Lowe GDO, Pettigrew A, Middleton S, Forbes CD, Prentice CRM. DDAVP in haemophilia. *Lancet* 1977; **ii:** 614 (letter).
Milaskiewicz RM, Holdcroft A, Letsky E. Epidural anaesthesia and von Willebrand's disease. *Anaesthesia* 1990; **45:** 462–464.

Noller KL, Bowie EJW, Kempers RG, Owen CA. von Willebrand's disease in pregnancy. *Obstetrics and Gynecology* 1973; **41:** 865–872.
Punnonen R, Nyman D, Gronroos N, Wallen O. von Willebrand's disease and pregnancy. *Acta Obstetrica et Gynaecologica Scandinavica* 1981; **60:** 507–509.
Ramsahoye BH, Davies SV, Dasani H, Pearson JF. Pregnancy in von Willebrand's disease. *Journal of Clinical Pathology* 1994; **47:** 569–570.
Ranta S, Lehesjoki AE, Peippo M, Kaariainen H. Hemophilia A: experiences and attitudes of mothers, sisters and daughters. *Pediatric Hematology and Oncology* 1994; **11:** 387–397.
Rick ME, Williams SB, McKeown LP. Thrombocytopenia associated with pregnancy in a patient with type IIB von Willebrand's disease. *Blood* 1987; **11:** 786–789.
Rodeghiero F, Castaman G, Dini E. Epidemiological investigation of the prevalence of von Willebrand's disease. *Blood* 1987; **69:** 454–459.
Scott JP, Montgomery RR. Therapy of von Willebrand's disease. *Seminars in Thrombosis and Haemostasis* 1993; **19:** 37.
Sorosky J, Klatsky A, Nobert GF, Burchill RC. von Willebrand's disease complicating 2nd trimester abortion. *Obstetrics and Gynecology* 1980; **55:** 253–254.
Stirling Y, Woolf L, North WRS, Seghatchian MJ, Meade TW. Haemostasis in normal pregnancy. *Thrombosis and Haemostasis* 1984; **52:** 176–182.
Takahashi N. Studies on the pathophysiology and treatment of von Willebrand's disease VI. Variant von Willebrand's disease complicating placenta praevia. *Thrombosis Research* 1983; **31:** 285–296.
Tarin JJ, Handyside AH. Embryo biopsy strategies for preimplantation diagnosis. *Fertility and Sterility* 1993; **59:** 943–952.
United Kingdom Haemophilia Centre Directors Organisation Executive Committee. Guidelines on therapeutic products to treat haemophilia and other hereditary coagulation disorders. *Haemophilia* 1997; **3**: 63–77.
Varekamp I, Suurmeijar TPBM, Brocker Vriends AMJT, et al. Carrier testing and prenatal diagnosis for hemophilia: experiences and attitudes of 549 potential and obligate carriers. *American Journal of Medical Genetics* 1990; **37:** 142–154.
Veiga A, Santalo J, Vidal F, et al. Twin pregnancy after preimplantation diagnosis for sex selection. *Human Reproduction* 1994; **9:** 2156–2159.
Yoffe G, Buchanan GR. Intracranial hemorrhage in newborn and young infants with haemophilia. *Journal of Pediatrics* 1988; **113:** 333–336.

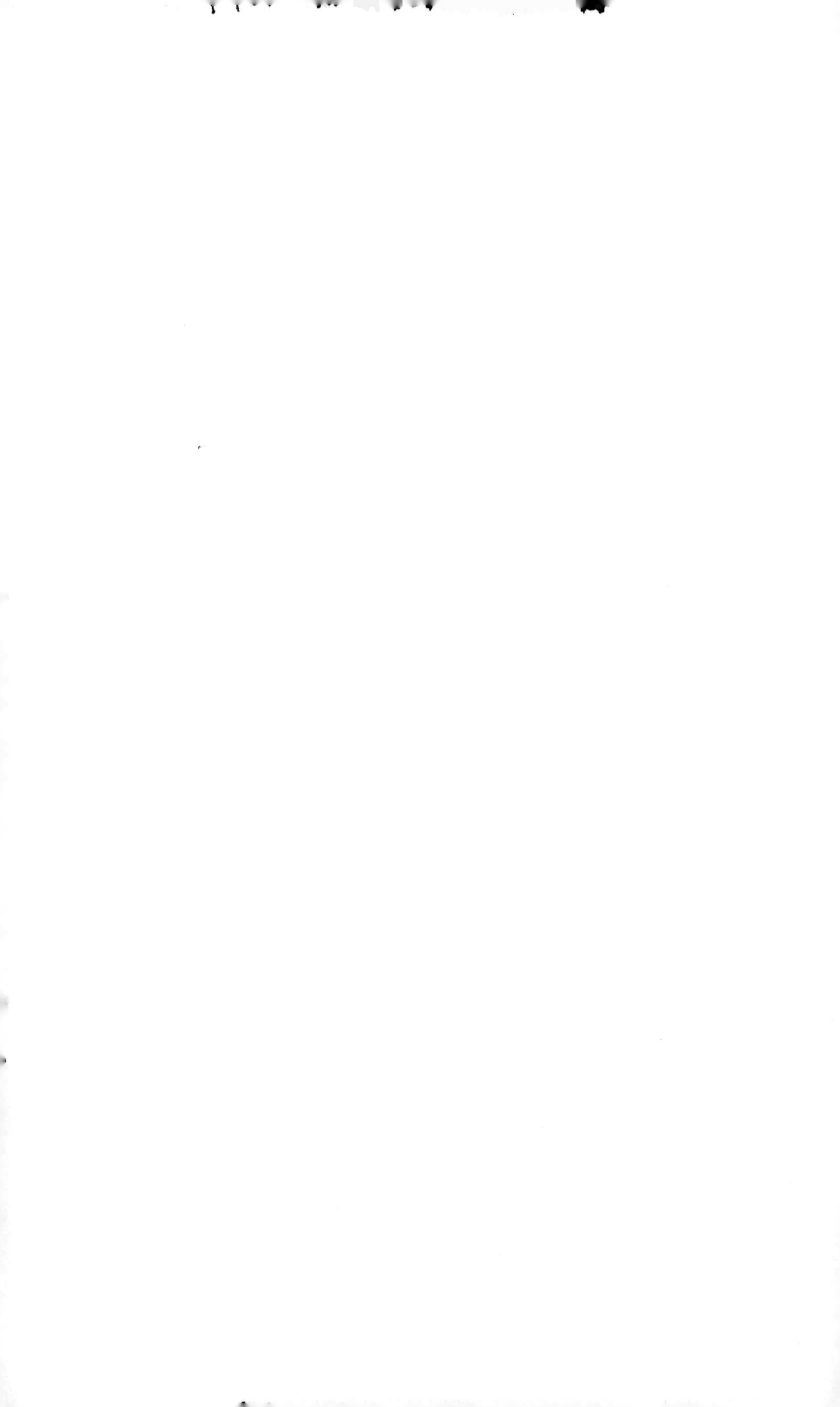

13

The Impact of Haemophilia on the Patient and Family

MARY L. FLETCHER

Introduction

There are two phenomena that should be taken into account when discussing the social implications of haemophilia. Haemophilia is a familial disease and any problems resulting from the disease will tend to involve the extended family. As a comparatively rare disease, few understand much about haemophilia except those that are in day-to-day contact with it (Markova et al, 1977).

The nature of social problems encountered by a person with haemophilia depend not only on the severity of his disease but also on his personality, his educational achievement and his position in society (Hjort, 1992). However, during the second half of the twentieth century there have been two significant events that have also had a major effect on the lives of those with haemophilia and also have had serious implications for their families and friends. The first event was the introduction of effective treatment with concentrated blood products. These began to be used in the 1960s and produced a great improvement in the quality of life of the patients and their families. In those countries able to afford the provision of adequate health care, the introduction of concentrated blood clotting factors led to an increase in life expectancy of haemophiliacs (Rizza and Spooner, 1983). Haemophilic men could then begin to expect to live to an old age, and instead of struggling to survive, could begin to think in terms of careers, marriage and retirement. Early treatment meant that acute bleeding episodes caused only short-term interruption to the lives of haemophiliacs (Seremetis and Aledort, 1994) and home treatment gave added freedom. Young haemophilic boys could look forward to a near normal life and they could expect to avoid the lasting restrictions of chronic pain and crippling, which has had serious social implications for older haemophilic men. With the help of their Haemophilia Centres, the majority of haemophilic men could manage their own lives and rarely had to turn to outside agencies to provide social support. For those haemophilic men who develop antibodies to factor VIII or

IX (Giangrande, 1994), the old social restrictions persist, and their bleeding problems may at times override all social considerations. Men who do have antibodies to factor VIII or IX are thus likely to need some social support.

Ironically it was a consequence of effective treatment that brought further undreamt-of social problems. Viral contamination of concentrates (see Chapter 10) caused enormous social problems for haemophilic men and their families and challenged even those with the most stable personalities, those who had attained high academic awards and those who had gained respect within their communities. In the world of haemophilia the risks of hepatitis as a consequence of transfusion therapy for bleeds had been recognized for over a decade. But during the 1970s the lay person perceived hepatitis to be a minor illness, and few were aware that a significant number of those infected would go on to develop chronic liver problems and consequential social problems. Human immunodeficiency virus (HIV) had a more dramatic impact and had serious social consequences (Darby et al, 1995). HIV attracted enormous media attention and because of this it affected the lives of all haemophiliacs, whether or not they were infected with HIV.

To meet the changing needs of the patients attending the Oxford Haemophilia Centre, we developed a pattern of care that incorporated the skills of specialist nurses, who had both community- and hospital-based experience. This enabled us to provide care and support for those with haemophilia, their families and partners, both at the hospital and in the patient's home. We were also able to develop good liaison with other health care workers, not only within the hospital complex, but also with the primary health care teams.

The Early Years

During the first year of his life the infant may have few bleeding problems, but this is more often than not followed by a difficult period when there is an increase in bleeding episodes as the infant begins to mobilize and explore and has opportunities when he can injure himself. At this stage of the child's development there are often many parental anxieties about haemophilia, which can be alleviated by support from specialist nurses and doctors at the Haemophilia Centre. In these early years any advice given about haemophilia should enable the parents to care for their child in as relaxed a way as possible whilst taking into account the dangers of haemorrhage.

However, haemophilia has implications on the whole family and in our experience the social consequences can be managed more easily if local primary health care teams are alerted to the possible problems. It is unlikely that most members of primary health care teams will have much knowledge of haemophilia and we have found that whilst some may welcome invitations to visit the regional Haemophilia Centre, others may find it more convenient to attend a talk on the disease at their local health centre. Haemophilia study days for general practitioners and community staff provide a useful opportunity when both the medical and social implications can be presented.

All families will experience difficulties following the birth of a severely affected haemophilic baby, but in families where there is no previous history of the disease (Chapter 2) such an event can be especially traumatic. In these cases any bruising on the baby will probably give rise to suspicions of abuse. Parents may have to undergo an unpleasant and stressful time as they find themselves under surveillance by health care professionals and social workers. In their desperation to find a reason for the bruising, these parents may frequently take their baby to their local doctor or hospital casualty department, and in doing so further increase the suspicions of concerned medical staff. Whilst being quizzed by one doubting professional after another, the parents can become so distraught with anxiety that paradoxically it comes as quite a relief when their baby is finally diagnosed as haemophilic.

Early infancy can be a very stressful time for any parents and the early life of babies with any congenital problem is a high-risk time for family breakdown. The parents of haemophilic babies have added stress because of the difficulty of recognizing a bleed in an infant who is unable tell them that he is in pain. Easy access to medical advice and support during these early years can relieve some of the stress, and help keep the family unit together. The overprotective parent, usually the mother (Jones, 1990), has always been a recognized phenomenon in families with a haemophilic child. Haemophilia nurses can provide valuable support for the parents and, if visits are made to the home, allow the mother to ask questions and address worries in a relaxed atmosphere. During this phase, advice and encouragement is vital to help parents gain confidence in their ability to care for their child.

Parents Groups are invaluable in helping the parents of a newly diagnosed haemophilic baby as they strive to come to terms with the implications of the diagnosis and the ensuing problems. The experiences of parents with older boys with haemophilia may help parents be less restrictive and combat any tendency towards overprotection. In our experience groups can provide useful support for the whole family; however, the groups should be focused on haemophilia and are most likely to be of benefit if set up by Haemophilia Centre staff or under the auspices of the Haemophilia Society. It should be remembered that some families will not want to attend group meetings and may prefer an introduction to another family, with similar problems to their own, whom they can meet on a casual basis or contact by phone. Non-haemophilic siblings may also benefit from such contacts and if they are able to talk to other children in similar families who understand their particular concerns.

When the young haemophilic child requires transfusions of factor VIII or IX, the treatment should be administered by someone who has expertise in the venepuncture of small babies and infants. If there are inept attempts at venepuncture during early childhood, this can have a negative effect, not only on the haemophilic child himself, but also on the parents. The child may become frightened and anxious for some time, making future treatment more difficult. The parents will become very distressed if they have to cope with a distraught child or a child who refuses to cooperate with doctors and nurses. If the parents become distressed at this stage it can lead to marital discord.

Early introduction of home treatment should be a common aim of those caring for the haemophilic child. If care was taken in venepuncture during his early infancy there will more likely be a trouble-free introduction to home treatment. Parents can start to give treatment at home as soon as the haemophilic boy has veins that present easy access, and he has learnt to have confidence in the ability of one of his parents to perform venepuncture (see Chapter 6). There is great variation in the age at which these factors come together; however, most boys will be on home treatment by the age of 5 years. Many families live some distance from specialist help provided by Haemophilia Centres, and visits to hospital can cause considerable disruption to family life, and become a drain on family finances. A well-established home transfusion regimen can bring a great reduction in the number of visits to the hospital and will usually herald a calmer period for the whole family. The financial burden, imposed by frequent visits to hospital, is also minimized and the family budget put under less strain.

Despite there being no new cases of HIV in the haemophilic population in the UK since 1986 (Darby et al, 1989), parents can still be worried about the possible risk of viral infection from transfusions. Some parents may hesitate to seek adequate factor replacement treatment for their child; this parental attitude is more likely to be found if the child is a mildly affected haemophiliac and only rarely needs transfusions of factor VIII or IX.

In most families it is the mother who will be the principal carer of a haemophilic boy and thus it is the mother who usually suffers the most stress. She should be encouraged to arrange some time on her own but may find it difficult to find a suitable person to look after her haemophilic son. A knowledgeable relative will often offer to look after the child or maybe a reciprocal arrangement can be made with another family with a haemophilic son. Nowadays mothers can have greater freedom as she can use mobile communication systems in order to keep in touch with those looking after her son. In the UK a scheme has been set up that will provide a free radio pager for the parents of boys with haemophilia.

Maternal Guilt

Mothers who are carriers of haemophilia feel guilty about many issues surrounding haemophilia. A carrier will feel guilt if she cannot give her husband a healthy son. If she decides to have no children, or to set a limit on the number of children she does have, she may feel she has failed in her duty as a wife.

The mother will at some stage blame herself for passing on haemophilia to her son and guilt can become a distressing problem, especially if she feels that other family members also blame her. Sometimes it is the husband who makes his wife feel guilty for passing on haemophilia to his son. Most grandparents give wholehearted support to a young family with a haemophilic infant and become well known at the Haemophilia Centre. However, it is not unknown for the reverse to happen and the grandparents, usually the in-laws, blame the wife of their son for giving birth to a disabled child. We have known of grandparents who have disowned a haemophilic grandson and others who have disowned their daughter-in-law, thus reinforcing any guilt she herself may already be feeling. The mother of a haemophilic infant may feel guilt at any distress caused by transfusion therapy. Perhaps the greatest guilt is felt by those who have given their child home treatment and in doing so injected them with material that has transmitted HIV or hepatitis. So much guilt can be cumulative and lead to psychiatric problems. Both guilt and family tensions surrounding these issues can precipitate marital discord, especially in families already struggling to cope with a haemophilic baby. Support and counselling should be available for all these mothers.

Siblings

The haemophilic boy and his mother may be the only family members who regularly visit the Haemophilia Centre but it should not be forgotten that there are social implications for any other children in the family. Siblings who do not have haemophilia can present with problems if they feel that they are not receiving enough love and attention, and jealousies may be exacerbated. Parents have to make choices, when a haemorrhage occurs, between the needs of their various children; it may be imperative for one or both parents to take, and stay with, the haemophilic child attending hospital, whilst the other siblings are left with alternative carers. Parents responding to the urgent needs of their haemophilic child may be the last to notice the problems of their other children. Haemophilia Centre staff can help if, whenever possible, they make a point of speaking specifically to the non-affected siblings. These problems may be exacerbated in households where a haemophiliac is terminally ill and other adults so occupied with the caring role that any non-affected children may have no opportunity to express their own feelings. Nurses, social workers or psychologists should be available to support these families.

The Extended Family

There are also social implications for other members of the extended family. Where there is a known history of haemophilia in a family, all the extended family members will be aware that any pregnancy within the family may herald the birth of a haemophiliac. They may all have strong views on termination of pregnancy; they may have old-fashioned ideas on the care and treatment of haemophilia. Grandparents may feel that as they have experienced the problems at first hand, that they have a duty to give advice, and find it hard to accept that a new mother may not want their advice. As already discussed, the grandparents can blame the mother for passing on haemophilia to their grandson. This can lead to a great deal of unhappiness within the extended family, a complete breakdown in the relationship with their daughter-in-law, and sometimes with their son too.

Education

Good management of his haemophilia should enable the haemophilic boy to develop to his full capacity and become a confident individual. Good liaison between his Haemophilia Centre staff and his teachers will promote a common understanding of his problems and expedite both his physical and intellectual development.

The haemophilic child will benefit from attending a playgroup or kindergarten. He will be able to mix with his peer group, giving him an opportunity to learn to cope on his own away from the watchful eye of his mother. A mother of a haemophilic boy may sometimes be reluctant to let her son venture out of her sight and may need some encouragement and support from Haemophilia Centre staff before allowing him to attend a pre-school group.

Kindergarten and pre-school groups should all accept a boy with haemophilia; however, they may hesitate to do so if they have no previous knowledge or experience of haemophilia. Any initial doubts can usually be allayed if a specialist nurse or doctor from the Haemophilia Centre contacts the organizers and offers advice. In our experience staff of pre-school groups are most worried about possible haemorrhage and how they would cope if they cannot immediately contact the boy's parents. They usually appreciate an offer from the mother to stay with her son for the first few days while he settles in and they assess his needs. If there should be a problem concerning his haemophilia they should be advised to contact the boy's parents in the first instance and be reassured that the parents will have the means to communicate with them. They should be given clear written instructions concerning the actions to take and the telephone number of the nearest haemophilia centre for use in emergencies.

Those responsible for running pre-school establishments might insist that they will require extra help in order to care for a boy with haemophilia, and that the extra costs thereby incurred might be prohibitive. It should be emphasized that if proper precautions have already been taken to minimize the risk of accidents, and if public health guidelines are adhered to, the only extra care needed will be if the boy has a bleed or is involved in an accident likely to cause a bleed when his parents should be called.

During his pre-school years the young child with severe haemophilia will have formed relationships outside his family group with his doctors and nurses at his Haemophilia Centre. He will be familiar with hospitals, which he will have learnt are places where he receives relief from pain and discomfort. He should have gained some confidence from these experiences which go some way to helping him overcome any social difficulties resulting from his haemophilia.

Before he starts his formal schooling, the parents of a haemophilic boy will often ask the staff of the Haemophilia Centre for advice on what information should be given to prospective teachers. During the last decade there have been anxious queries from teachers not only about the possibility of haemorrhage whilst at school, but also the concomitant risk of transmission of viral infections. Sometimes these anxieties have been prompted by the concerns of parents of other pupils or by school governors. They should be advised that they should take sensible hygiene precautions and wear gloves when coping with all episodes of bleeding from any child and that, if they do this, a boy with haemophilia should pose no special risk to staff, or other children, irrespective of his HIV or hepatitis C (HCV) status. However, this advice is not always sufficient to placate anxieties raised by adverse press reports and it not unknown for headmasters, school managers, teachers and parents of other pupils to believe that they have a right to know a haemophiliac's HIV or HCV status.

A haemophilic boy should be able to participate in most of the same educational activities as others of his age, but he may, at times, require special consideration. It should be explained to the teachers that by the time a haemophilic boy starts school he usually knows when to ask for help, and that by the time he leaves school he should be able to manage his haemophilia in most circumstances.

It is not uncommon for school teachers to ask for an extra helper to oversee the young haemophiliac whilst he is in the playground. In the UK the money for extra help can only be provided if a formal arrangement is made with the education authority. This requires "a statement of need". In this sense it is the needs of the child, not of the school, that are being assessed. The child for whom an assessment is made is categorized as disabled. Some parents do not want their haemophilic son so labelled. Haemophilia itself is no justification for issuing a "statement of need" and should not be an option, except for the most severely affected boy.

In those countries able to provide adequate treatment for haemophilia, the majority of haemophilic boys should be able to participate in mainstream education. Modern ideas of treatment and self-transfusion have brought about a change in medical and educational opinion on the most appropriate type of schooling for haemophilic boys. They are now less likely to suggest that a haemophiliac will benefit from attending a school designated for those with a physical disability.

Parents can now choose the most appropriate school for the scholastic needs of the individual child, maintain normal home life, and still ensure that he receives adequate treatment for his haemophilic problems.

National standards for education of all children are now set in many countries. In the UK all children must follow the National Curriculum during their years at school. A haemophilic boy, whose bleeding problems are well controlled, should be able to meet most of these standards, including the requirement for physical activities. Although a boy with haemophilia should be encouraged to participate in as many physical activities as possible, he will need to be excluded if he has a bleed or if the activity includes the possibility of injury to the head, violent body contact, or undue stress on a particular joint. Exclusions should include rugby, boxing, hockey and most of the martial arts (Jones, 1990). Encouragement should be given to activities that lead to the development of good general muscle tone and coordination. Prophylactic treatment allows the boy a greater choice of sport. The haemophilic boy, who has inhibitors to factor VIII, may have special problems and his particular needs should be assessed regularly by his doctors, teachers and parents. Teachers may require a letter from the Haemophilia Centre doctor, stating which activities should be prohibited and which avoided, especially when the boy has a bleed, and mentioning any other special considerations pertaining to his particular medical problems.

As the boy grows older, his teachers may worry not only about managing bleeding episodes, but also about the boy who conceals a bleed, either to enable him to continue with normal activities, or so that he can keep up with his peers. Some parents will wish to be informed if their son has a bleed at school; other parents will want the school to handle the problem "in loco parentis". Once a boy has learnt to give his own intravenous transfusions, his parents may arrange for him to keep a small quantity of factor VIII at school, and thus be able to give himself early treatment if a bleed should occur.

In many countries, including the UK, modern schools are designed to comply with regulations incorporating provision for disabled students. However, where the school buildings are older, there are often structural problems that cause physical barriers for a child with disabilities and the school may lack lifts or wheelchair access. Parents ought to enquire about access to classrooms and facilities before their son is enrolled at a new school. School managers may request information about a specific haemophiliac's particular disabilities, in order to assess the type of facilities needed, and to obtain funding for any improvements required. Head teachers may wish to ask for additional staff, particularly welfare assistants, and special equipment, in order to meet the educational needs of the child.

The haemophilic boy can gain great benefit if he participates in out-of-school activities, especially school trips, when he can begin to learn to cope away from the protective environment of his parents. Parents should ensure that those supervising each event are given clear written instructions detailing those activities that the haemophiliac should avoid, and what they should do if there is an accident. The older haemophilic boy should know how to treat routine bleeds himself and should take a relevant transfusion kit with him when he goes on excursions with the school.

Making friends with others in his peer group may be difficult for a boy with severe haemophilia. He may be self-conscious about his image if repeated bleeds have left him with a damaged joint; he may be teased because of his haemophilia; he may be taunted as a result of the intense publicity the media has given to homosexuality and HIV and the linking of these problems with haemophilia.

The friendships that a child makes within his peer group are an important aspect of school days: the child with haemophilia may find it difficult to form these friendships if frequent bleeds cause periods of interrupted schooling; prophylactic treatment should mean this is less of a problem in the future. Although boys with haemophilia will probably attend hospital outpatient departments regularly, they often have little opportunity to make friends with other haemophilic boys. Holidays specifically set up for boys with haemophilia go some way to alleviating this problem. In the UK such activity holidays are arranged by the Haemophilia Society and staffed by a doctor and a nurse with experience in caring for those with haemophilia. A few haemophilic boys with a severe bleeding tendency or inhibitors to factor VIII may still find that they have long spells in hospital during their school years; close liaison should be established between teachers at the hospital and at their school and the need for home tuition carefully monitored. Local education authorities may need some persuasion before they will provide home tuition and the parent and teachers will probably ask for support from their Haemophilia Centre when requesting such provision. Doctors may need to explain the special considerations needed by this particular group of haemophilic children.

Parents and teachers should be alert to the problem of bullying at school, which can be a problem for any child with a physical disability. If the school boy has a good relationship with his Haemophilia Centre staff he may be more willing to answer questions about bullying, at the hospital, a more neutral ground and removed from the school environment. Since HIV was given widespread publicity and those with haemophilia were known to be at risk of HIV, haemophilia has become associated, in the minds of many uninformed people, with homosexuality and drug abuse. Boys with haemophilia have reported discrimination by other pupils, and bullying does occur. We have found that liaison with the teachers and programmes of health education can, in most cases, resolve these problems; his classmates will rally round the haemophilic boy, and those who might have previously been bullies can provide protective support.

Careful consideration should be given to future careers long before the young person with haemophilia reaches his last year at school. Haemophilic boys who have problems either with damaged joints or frequent haemorrhagic episodes should be encouraged from an early age to plan for future jobs that avoid repetitive stress on specific damaged joints. Students should discuss their options with their careers officers bearing in mind that any traditionally male job of an unskilled nature is likely to be too arduous for those with haemophilia.

Transitions from school to work, and from home to living on his own, are often difficult times for those with haemophilia. Some find that a period of further education may not only make these transitions easier but can also be a passport to the lighter occupations most suited to those with haemophilia. By the time that they reach the stage of post-school education, most boys will have learnt to manage their own haemophilia, and are able to cope on their own away from their parents. If possible it would be wise to arrange further education at an establishment near to a large Haemophilia Centre to ensure continuity of care. The young student would benefit from an early visit to the new centre when he can organize his health care before he starts at college.

A handbook has been produced by the UK Haemophilia Society (1991) which describes the problems likely to occur during school days, and suggests how teachers should respond to these problems.

Adolescence

In the past it was unusual for those with haemophilia to have had much contact with people outside their family circle. In the early part of their life they may have received no treatment, or inadequate treatment with replacement factor; they may have had musculoskeletal problems that excluded them from taking part in many social activities; their circle of friends may have been small, limiting the choice of a female partner. Adequate treatment for bleeds should have left the present generation of adolescents with fewer problems but HIV infection has brought them a different set of problems. HIV is notorious for creating a marked change in physical appearance, but it is sometimes forgotten that haemophilia itself may have left a legacy of physical deformity. For whatever reason many young haemophilic men have to come to terms with the fact that they have a physical appearance which to them, and maybe to others, seems flawed and thus renders them less attractive to the opposite sex. Some of them may be unable to cope with these changes in their altered body image and may develop psychological disturbances or clinical depression. The younger patients find this particularly difficult and they may hide away from contact with their friends, just at the time that others in their age group are revelling in "good looks" and indulging in group activities. We have found that this is a serious problem for those who develop various forms of skin disease as a consequence of HIV disease. These patients will not only require help from a dermatologist but will also require advice on relationship problems.

Perhaps the most serious impact on adolescent sexuality has been the need for those with haemophilia to consider the implications of the transmission of HIV and HCV. The more thoughtful may be so sensitive to the consequences of their behaviour that they eschew any contact with the opposite sex; others become somewhat careless of their actions and have intercourse as frequently as possible with a multiplicity of partners; yet others feel an urgent need to marry and have children.

When seeking employment the adolescent must come to terms with the fact that his haemophilia, probably the most important aspect of his life to date, is now something that he cannot necessarily be open about, adding tension to an already nerve-racking time. He should be counselled to prepare himself well for an interview, to make sure he can explain his haemophilic problem accurately, that he can reassure a prospective employer that he is not a risk to other members of staff and that he can give himself any necessary treatment thus enabling him to maintain a good attendance record.

Marriage

Improvements in the treatment of haemophilia enable those with haemophilia to lead a near normal life and the majority of haemophilic men do find a partner, get married and most do have children. A few men with haemophilia decide not to father children in the knowledge that although their sons will be unaffected all their daughters will be carriers. On the other hand they may decide to have children as they believe that, by the time they have grandsons, treatment will be so effective that haemophilia will have become a minor problem.

The possibility of passing on viral infections has prevented some from entering into a long-term relationship. Psychological and practical considerations also impinge on married life of people with haemophilia. The balance of the marital relationship may often be uneven. The husband may be overdependent on his wife and he may resent this; the wife may be overinvolved in her caring role and she in her turn may resent her loss of freedom. At some stage in the marriage the wife may find herself the chief or only wage earner, she may have to go out to work, meet the needs of any children and also care for her haemophilic husband.

Physical disabilities and/or acute bleeds may limit sexual activity, and the couple may need to find alternative ways of expressing their sexuality. In our group of patients we have found that most do manage a successful sexual relationship, but that those who have physical limitation of movement do find that oral sex is easier to practise than vaginal intercourse. Sensitive counselling and practical advice should be offered to these couples to help them come to terms with their limitations and explore alternative ways of expressing their sexuality. If this advice is difficult to arrange through a Haemophilia Centre, the patient and his partner must be referred for experienced sexual relationship counselling.

Help for patients with sexual problems may be available locally and information can be obtained through Health Visitors, the Family Planning clinics, Relate (Marriage Guidance), or a society set up specifically to help with the sexual problems of the disabled (SPOD); this latter group is a useful source of information for doctors and nurses who care for haemophilic men. Local health education departments in the UK stock helpful leaflets.

Most adult haemophilic men who received blood products before 1986 (see Chapter 10) will now have either HIV or HCV infection and will be advised to think about using condoms to prevent transmission of virus to their partners. In a survey amongst married couples attending our haemophilia centre we found that it was not only the male but also the female partners who disliked the use of condoms. Some of these couples felt that their marriage was put at risk if either one of the partners insisted on using a condom. There is no doubt that those suggesting that they should use condoms are asking the haemophiliac and his wife to make difficult choices, and should not be surprised if some couples decided to practice unsafe sex, despite being fully aware of the risks involved.

Many of the haemophilic men choose wives from among their carers, and this can result in a marriage in which the balance of the marital relationship is uneven. The husband is too dependent on his wife and the wife too involved in her caring role. Either partner may feel uneasy with this variation from the normally accepted roles and there may be marital stress. Should her husband die, her reaction can vary from sheer relief as she is released from a caring role, or a profound grief from a double loss. The bereaved wife having had to take a leading role in family matters may be better prepared than most widows to manage her own life hereupon. Many widows prefer some initial bereavement support from Haemophilia Centre nurses; however, some might need long-term or more specialized support and require referral to other agencies. In the UK the charity "Cruse" has branches in most areas and specialize in offering support and counselling to widows. We have found that most of the bereaved do like to keep in touch with the Haemophilia Centre and bereaved parents are the mainstay of the "Friends" of our Centre.

Some wives may accompany their husbands when they visit their haemophilia centre, but some men like to keep their family life and haemophilia separate and as a result of this some wives and partners may feel neglected. We have found that it can be useful to organize groups for partners at the haemophilia centre. The partners, including some wives who had been married to a haemophiliac for many years, appreciate being able to learn about haemophilia, HIV and HCV from someone other than their husband.

Social Activities

Many people face the possibility of periods of unemployment and the possibility of an early retirement. Adults today are likely to have more time than previous generations for social activities. The haemophilic man is no exception and, because of his medical problems, will probably have more enforced leisure time than the average man of a similar age. He may be less likely to have been adequately prepared by previous experiences to be able to use this time to his best advantage. For future generations this may become less of a problem; with adequate treatment and prophylaxis (Nilsson, 1994), haemophilic men should be able to participate in many activities that have hitherto been inaccessible to them. Medicine is now embracing the concepts of holistic care and health promotion, emphasis being given to encourage physical activity in order to promote physical and mental well-being (Panicucci, 1993) and, in the case of haemophilic men, strong muscles. This enhanced physical state should enable them to take part in a wider variety of social activities and place them on more equal terms with their peer group.

Publicity given to HIV has led many of the general public to think that they can catch HIV from sporting contact with haemophiliacs. Haemophilic men with hepatitis or HIV should be advised to avoid all sport where injury could result in the transfer of blood. This is another reason for avoiding popular sports such as competitive football, rugby, boxing and the martial arts. It might seem obvious common sense but we have known of a mild haemophiliac who boxed for his university! Becoming proficient in a sporting activity can go a long way to compensating for lack of recognition in traditional sports. Many sports are now available for everyone and even the most disabled haemophiliac should find that there is an activity in which he can participate. Encouragement should be given to young haemophiliacs to take up sports that he can continue into adult life such as swimming, archery or sailing. Those with more severe handicaps can join local groups offering sport for the disabled.

Alcohol

A potential problem for those with haemophilia is alcohol abuse and this has serious consequences for those with hepatitis (see Chapter 10), for whom even a small amount of alcohol may be inadvisable. The social implications of not taking alcoholic drinks can be manifold; not only can it necessitate a change in the pattern of social activities but it can also have adverse effect for those in jobs where social drinking has become an accepted way of life. Alcohol abuse can easily become a problem for haemophiliacs at a relatively young age, especially for those who feel excluded from popular activities because of haemophilic problems. These young men may find that the easiest way to identify with others in their age group is in the pub, where they try to prove their masculinity by consuming large amounts of alcohol. Expert alcohol counselling should be arranged to help haemophilic men moderate their drinking habits.

Drug Abuse

Before transfusion therapy revolutionized the treatment of bleeding episodes, haemophiliacs suffered a considerable amount of pain which required treatment with strong analgesics. Some acquired a dependency on these prescribed drugs that may have lasted for several decades. Fewer young haemophilic men now become dependent on pain-relieving drugs but doctors should be aware that some can still become intolerant of their disabilities and begin to abuse analgesia. In their search for pain relief some may try a multiplicity of drugs and those with weak personalities can become part of the illegal drug scene, leading to serious social consequences, not only for themselves but also for their families. Others find out that there is a market on the streets for strong painkillers and can be tempted into selling prescribed analgesics. These patients must be alerted to the dangers of sharing syringes and needles and the need for the safe disposal of equipment used for home transfusions. Care for these patients should incorporate good liaison with both the general practitioner and social agencies. The use of cannabis has increased as young men with HIV find that it increases their appetite; many argue the need for legitimizing cannabis for use in these circumstances.

HIV

HIV brought public attention to haemophiliacs at the very time when they would have preferred to be anonymous. Their sex lives became a health education issue and a matter for public debate. They now found they were being linked, in the public mind, with members of other high-risk groups, and, moreover, that these groups tended to be seen to be on the fringes of society. In the past haemophiliacs may have been well known in their local communities, but after the advent of HIV some went out of their way to seek anonymity: they moved, avoided contact with neighbours and friends, and some changed jobs. This self-imposed isolation came at the very time that they needed more understanding and support. For many of them it was the first time in their lives that they had needed to seek social advice, and not wishing to have to disclose their HIV status they were reluctant to approach social agencies near their homes. They preferred to turn to their hospital environment and their haemophilia centres for advice and support.

In many countries, including the UK, the haemophiliacs were known to have HIV infection before public HIV prevention services were organized and haemophilia centre staff had to take on a health education role to ensure that the patients had adequate information and advice on safe sex practices. In our experience, young heterosexual couples sometimes only had a hazy idea of what constitutes risky sexual behaviour and some were unknowingly using sexual practices that put their partners at high risk of getting HIV. To enable us to counsel more effectively we decided to elucidate the problem by interviewing the female partners of 60 of our haemophilic men. We used a questionnaire to address specific questions about their sexual behaviour. We found that some practised anal intercourse regularly "like all other young couples do at first" or "not since we have known about HIV". Broaching the subject of sexual problems with both haemophilic men and their partners can provide an opportunity to reinforce safe sex practices and the use of condoms. We also found that the majority of the female partners do find it easier to talk to other females discussing sexual matters, as indeed do some of the males.

When HIV first infected the haemophilic men we found that married couples as well as single men welcomed an easily available supply of condoms. The married women were often worried that they might be identified in their local shop when asking for condoms. Privacy in small communities is difficult to maintain, and the wives of our patients worried that questions would be asked if they suddenly started buying condoms. This was a particular anxiety for those who had had hysterectomies, or those who had reached the menopause. The women felt that their neighbours would associated buying condoms as tantamount to saying "my husband has HIV". Despite the greater public awareness of the need for safe sexual activities and the greater public availability of condoms, those in small and isolated communities may still wish to maintain their privacy. Condoms should be made available at the Haemophilia Centres for those patients who have viral infections as a result of receiving contaminated blood products.

A young haemophilic boy who has been infected with HIV must receive counselling and advice on safe sex practices before he becomes sexually active. Puberty tends to start earlier in succeeding generations and so teenagers may have sexual intercourse at a correspondingly early age. If the boy is young his girlfriend may be young, possibly under the legal age for sexual intercourse, and her parents may wish for legal redress if they know she has been put at risk of contracting HIV. Counselling and practical advice should be offered, both to these young people and to their parents.

HIV infection often precipitates relationship problems. The fear of sexual transmission of HIV prevents some men from having any physical contact with their partners. In the early stages of the disease it may be skin problems, and later the severe weight loss, which alter the physical appearance (see Chapter 10) and make them fear that their partners will be repelled by their changed appearance. We have found that, although in these circumstances it is often the female partner who declines to have sexual intercourse, it may be the affected male who is the one who refuses. As a health prevention measure such a cessation of sexual intercourse may be ideal, but it can have a traumatic effect and disrupt a partnership at the very time the man affected by HIV needs comfort, support and someone to care about him. At the Oxford Haemophilia Centre we have organized group meetings for the partners of HIV-positive haemophilic men. These groups provide the partners with the opportunity to meet others with whom they could discuss common problems.

A dichotomy arises when those responsible for health protection measures issue dire public warnings of the consequences of HIV disease whilst other health professionals are trying to support and care for those already infected. In our experience these proclamations cause a great deal of anxiety, especially to the haemophilic men and their partners who may have been unwittingly engaged in unprotected sexual intercourse for many years. In a survey carried out at the Oxford Haemophilia Centre in 1989 and 1990 (unpublished) we found that although sexual activities in marriages at the time of seroconversion to HIV reflected those of the general population, the frequency of sexual intercourse and the use of unsafe practices were both reduced with passing time.

The drive to procreate is often strong in those with a life-threatening disease, and we have found that young haemophilic HIV-positive men and their wives do choose to have children, despite being fully aware of the danger of sexual transmission to the woman and maternal transmission to the fetus. Such pregnancies are an anxious time for the prospective parents. If there is an unplanned pregnancy the couple may have to make difficult decisions about the possible termination. If both the haemophilic husband and his wife are HIV positive and they still decide to have a baby, they will require sensitive support throughout a difficult period, at least until the final HIV status of the baby is known when the infant is about 18 months of age. HIV will complicate all the normal psychological problems of pregnancy and liaison will be needed between hospital departments to ensure that adequate support is provided. Some couples may decide not to take the risk of transmission of HIV to the woman or child and may ask about fertilization by donor. In the present economic climate it is unlikely that many HIV-positive haemophilic men and their partners will be able to take advantage of these expensive techniques. Similarly it is unlikely that adoption agencies will consider these couples as eligible candidates to adopt children. The screening tests for couples wishing to adopt are stringent, even without the added handicap of HIV infection.

Those haemophiliacs from communities where arranged marriages are the norm find that if they have HIV they will not be considered as suitable marriage partners. Patients with HCV or HIV may find that their religious customs prevent them from complying with optimum dietary advice. Physicians should also be aware that some of their patients may be taking large quantities of non-proprietary medicines and herbal concoctions. Guidelines set out for caring for the dying HIV-infected patient and for the handling of dead bodies can be contrary to ethnic or religious customs and may cause consternation and distress amongst grieving relatives.

An unexpected phenomenon within the haemophilic population has been the guilt, felt by some HIV-negative patients, as they watch one friend after another become progressively ill and die. We have known some who have developed psychiatric conditions which, although more often than not are of a minor nature, can be of such severity that the patient requires hospital admission. Other HIV-negative patients have felt excluded from the major concern in the haemophilic world. Some have felt jealousy of the ex gratia payment given to

HIV-positive men. This jealousy is often found amongst those who have more severe disabilities and latterly by an increasing number of those who have hepatitis.

The law of averages decrees that some haemophilic men will be homosexual. These men, irrespective of their HIV status, often feel guilt concerning both HIV and their sexual orientation, and will need advice and support in order to cope with their particular problems. It should not be assumed that they will turn to homosexual groups for this help.

Those doctors responsible for the running of the Haemophilia Centres should be aware of a potential risk of discrimination. Some haemophiliacs and some parents of haemophilic children blame the homosexual community for the spread of HIV. This attitude is not uncommon among bereaved parents, especially when the deceased haemophilic son was young. Heterosexual men may sometimes feel very uncomfortable if they are admitted to hospital wards that are predominately the preserve of homosexual men. This can have a negative effect on the haemophilic man, especially if he is unwell, worried or frightened.

Public interest in HIV and the possible discrimination is a fear felt by all haemophilic men and, as a consequence, they are very wary of giving information to anyone about their haemophilia or HIV status. This obviously creates difficulties when doctors and nurses need to communicate with health care workers and staff from other agencies who may think that they have a need to know a client's HIV status. Care needs to be taken when giving any certification of medical diagnosis to people not bound by strict laws of confidentiality. It should also be remembered that once a death is registered, the death certificates go into the the public domain and can be obtained and read by anyone.

HIV counselling services have been set up in many countries to offer support to those with HIV infection. In the UK money was allocated by the Government for HIV counselling. We found a reluctance amongst our patients to accept formal counselling, especially from agencies detached from their haemophilia centre. Haemophilic men from an early age have learnt to cope with serious health problems and most feel in control of their own lives; they may therefore resent the implication that once they have HIV infection that they must have "counselling". Most of them, however, were happy to talk to doctors and nurses whom they already knew. At our Haemophilia Centre we incorporated counselling into the general care of the patient, and made sure that at each visit to the Centre there was an opportunity for them to talk to an experienced member of staff. Patients who required specialist support were referred to the appropriate psychologist or psychiatrist. In the 1980s 54 of our patients took part in a psychological and neuropsychiatric assessment organized by our local department of psychiatry (Catalan et al, 1988). This research provided an additional opportunity for discussing HIV and personal problems and in a way that the patients found acceptable.

Since the appearance of HIV, haemophiliacs have tended to be less open about their problems. Some haemophilic men go to extraordinary lengths to keep their haemophilia a secret: some may hide their factor VIII and may not allow anyone to see venepuncture performed; others have home treatment supplies delivered to a relative's house so that the neighbours will not see it delivered. Letters sent from the hospital or the Haemophilia Society are directed elsewhere, in case any identification on the outside of the envelope can be recognized by neighbours and the connection made between their house and haemophilia or HIV. Some of those with haemophilia have cancelled their membership of the Haemophilia Society for this reason; some feel that they cannot support fund-raising or social events concerned with the Haemophilia Centre as they wish to remain anonymous.

Hepatitis

Although hepatitis virus B (HBV) has had social implications for haemophiliacs for several decades, it is only comparatively recently that it has been possible to test for HCV (see Chapter 10). Hepatitis C (HCV) has been shown to have infected those who have had blood products before 1986 and the majority of haemophiliacs over the age of 10 years now have to face the social consequences of infection, the unpredictability of the course of the disease, and the possibility of heterosexual transmission (Hallam et al, 1993). Once again advice has been sought by patients before research has confirmed the exact nature of the problem, giving rise to anxiety amongst those affected and their partners. The majority of adult haemophiliacs must consider using safe sex practices.

HCV has not received such intense media coverage as did the advent of HIV a decade ago, and as a consequence has so far led to fewer social problems. When making the previous financial award for English haemophilic patients with HIV infection, the presiding judge took into account the fact that these patients were all likely to have HCV infection as well. Those accepting these payments signed a statement that precludes them from making further claims for HCV. Many of those who have HCV infection, but who are not also infected with HIV, feel that they too should receive financial recompense.

Partners

We have found that although the haemophilic man may get support from his Haemophilia Centre staff, his partner may have had no opportunity to learn about haemophilia, HIV or HCV. Haemophiliacs can sometimes be reticent when passing on information to their partners about both haemophilia and viral infections; they fear that the severity of their problems may frighten partners and cause the break-up of the relationship. This is especially true when the relationship is relatively new and in our experience it is not unknown for a couple to have started a sexual relationship before the girl is told that her partner has HIV infection.

Carriers

Some, if not all, family members will be known at least informally to staff at Haemophilia Centres and this network of concerned family members will alert the staff to the needs of the carrier girls, and make it possible to arrange early counselling. A girl who knows that she carries a haemophilia gene should be encouraged to bring her partner to her local Haemophilia Centre, so that they can talk to an experienced member of the Haemophilia Centre staff. They should be given accurate information about haemophilia, its mode of transmission and possible treatments. It should not be assumed that a carrier necessarily has some understanding of the inheritance of haemophilia or of the problems that a haemophilic baby will present. A haemophilic father may have hidden the severity of his problems from his children, and some daughters may have only a sketchy knowledge of the amount of care needed by a haemophilic child.

The facilities for antenatal diagnosis should be discussed so that the couple may give thought to any religious or moral differences that may arise in the context of possible termination of pregnancy. We have known of cases where problems have arisen because a partner is a Jehovah's Witness. In one such family, with a known history of severe haemophilia A, a carrier's fiancé said he would refuse to give his permission for any antenatal diagnostic investigations or for any blood products to be given to any child that he might father: the engagement ended.

Once a carrier has a pregnancy confirmed she and her partner will have to decide whether to have antenatal investigations and if the fetus is haemophilic, they may want to consider the possibility of terminating the pregnancy. Because haemophilia is a familial disease, many of the girl's relatives will have strong views and will consider as open for family debate subjects that should be for private discussion between the couple concerned. These are all onerous decisions, but are particularly so for a carrier of haemophilia who may have watched her father or brother suffer or even die of haemophilia, HIV or hepatitis. It should be remembered that any dogmatic advice given before conception can make it difficult for a couple to return for support from their Haemophilia Centre, or to seek early antenatal care.

Employment

The choice of employment for those with haemophilia should be considered with care. The vagaries of world economies has brought unemployment to many countries and for haemophilic men the chances of finding employment become more difficult. In times of high unemployment there may also be fewer choices available for those with haemophilia, and employers, with plenty of applicants to choose from, will be less likely to employ someone with a disability. They may need to accept unsuitable jobs, with a consequential deleterious effect on their musculoskeletal system. Haemophiliacs should be advised to avoid those occupations that demand heavy manual labour, carry a high risk of injury, involve repetition likely to cause strain on particular joints or muscles, or are carried out in wet or damp conditions. Traditionally haemophiliacs were predominantly trained to do physically undemanding work, such as tailoring and office work, but many men feel their masculinity is threatened if they are expected to undertake such light work. Technological advances have brought changes in the types of job available and there is now a greater selection of employment suitable for those with haemophilia. The degree of severity of the bleeding problem will probably be the deciding factor when considering suitable employment: the milder the haemophilia problem, the greater the choice. There are some occupations that are obviously unsuitable for all those with bleeding problems such as the armed services and the emergency services. However, these rules are often flouted and those with haemophilia can be successfully employed in a wide range of jobs that others, including their medical advisers, think are inappropriate occupations.

Common sense might suggest that employers should be told that a candidate has haemophilia before he starts work but it should be remembered that most prospective employers will have little knowledge of haemophilia and, if there are other candidates, would probably be wary of accepting a man with haemophilia. A haemophiliac may find it easier to talk about his haemophilia to the doctor undertaking a pre-employment medical examination. In our experience we have found that many haemophiliacs wait until they start work, or at least until they have been at work for some time, before they tell their employer that they have haemophilia. However, there is always a possibility of accidental injury and a haemophiliac would be prudent to inform a responsible person at their workplace that they have a bleeding problem.

Haemophiliacs may feel that discrimination in the workplace might occur not only because of their haemophilia, but as a consequence of the publicity surrounding HIV and the idea, held by the uneducated, that there is a link between haemophilia and homosexuality. We know of one young haemophiliac who decided not to tell anyone either that he was haemophilic or that he had HIV. He went to the interview, and as the job involved quality control for food production, he was asked to attend a medical. He was examined by the doctor and passed as "A1" fit. He was a severe haemophiliac, with some muscle wasting, some joint deformity, and with venepuncture marks on his forearms which might have led many a lay person to suppose that he was a drug addict. He was offered the job. Two years later he decided to tell selected members of staff about his medical condition. Changes in working conditions began to arise and his job became untenable. He decided to change to another employer. We have seen other instances of the working environment being changed so that it becomes awkward for a haemophiliac to cope. One crippled haemophiliac was asked to move to an upstairs office. There was no apparent good reason for this change; the haemophilic man felt it must be due to his haemophilia and the possible link with HIV. He was indeed HIV positive but had not told anyone at his workplace; he thought that they might have suspected that he had AIDS. He did not wish to take any action fearing the publicity this might provoke so he asked for retirement on health grounds. In most countries with competitive economies there will always need to be some consideration given to those with disabilities and governments respond with varying legislation to prevent discrimination in the workplace. It is unlikely that a haemophilic man suffering from discrimination will want to risk notoriety by seeking legal redress.

Job security is threatened during times of high unemployment and those with haemophilia will be disinclined to take time off work to attend hospital appointments. If there is some flexibility in clinic hours, and if home treatment supplies can be delivered to their home or a nearby hospital, it will be easier for those who struggle to cope with disability, and may be of crucial assistance if they are to continue working.

From time to time employers may require a doctor to confirm disability and need. It can be useful if a note is added emphasizing the relatively few changes that may be needed to enable the haemophilic man to be a good employee. If there are problems at the workplace due to haemophilia or ill health, a specialist nurse or occupational therapist can give advice that may enhance the working environment and minimize future bleeding episodes. We have found that most of our patients are reluctant to ask for this sort of help as they fear it draws attention to their disability and is unlikely to be appreciated by employers.

In the UK each locality has a Disablement Employment Adviser (DEA) who has a responsibility to find employment for those with disabilities. Enquiries should be made at the Job Centre or Employment office. The DEA may suggest that a man with haemophilia should register as a disabled person. Many haemophilic men do not wish to register as "a disabled person", and for most there may be few benefits in doing so at present. Changes in government policy may confer some advantages of registering as disabled at some future stage in their working life, and patients should be encouraged to keep up to date with any new legislation.

There are other special facilities available through the UK Manpower Services Commission (MSC) for giving assistance to disabled people in employment, of which the most useful are help with the cost of travel to work and the modification of equipment. Employers have a duty to provide a car parking space near to the place of work for all employees who are registered disabled. A helpful booklet, published by the MSC, for prospective employers gives information about the employment of men with haemophilia.

During their working lives the vast majority of men with haemophilia are going to have bleeds that are severe enough to require periods away from work, and they will also need to visit their Haemophilia Centre for outpatient appointments. Like most people living and trying to work with chronic ill health or physical disability, they will often sacrifice their holiday entitlement in order to avoid sick leave. This can lead to tiredness and loss of concentration, accidents and more bleeds. There often comes a time in early middle age when the disabilities due to haemophilia demand a greater effort, and a job becomes too arduous. They may have more frequent episodes of haemorrhage into certain joints due to repetitive work. They may have used up their quota of sick leave. Such considerations may prompt a haemophilic man to consider a change to part-time work or to ask for early retirement. Most haemophiliacs will benefit from discussing these issues with their doctors and nurses and may seek some extra support at this time. For some, early retirement comes as a relief and heralds a new phase with fewer bleeding episodes; for others it has a negative effect as they seem to need the continuing incentive of working in order to cope with their musculoskeletal problems or to maintain their psychological well-being.

Housing

The person with severe haemophilia will be able to manage his condition more easily if he lives near a major Haemophilia Centre, and patients often tend to move closer to these centres. In the UK, some local housing departments have designated officials who can give help and advice on housing moves for those with medical problems. There are limitations on housing options because those with haemophilia may have difficulties in obtaining mortgages; however, in our experience all those who wished to own a house do manage to get the finance to do so. Housing can present problems, at any age, either as a result of musculoskeletal problems or because of social difficulties. The musculoskeletal disabilities are likely to increase with age and at some stage the haemophiliac will probably require ground floor accommodation or modifications to existing housing. In the UK advice is available through the local social services departments, which often have a designated occupational therapist experienced in housing problems of the physically disabled. In many areas grants are available for specified modifications; however, there is no mandatory funding and applications for assistance for financial help need to be made on an individual basis.

Holidays

In the past many haemophiliacs have limited their choice of holidays to their own countries and to those places with special provision for those with disabilities. Self-administration of factor VIII has widened the choices and many young and adventurous haemophiliacs will now travel the world with a few bottles of factor hidden in their rucksacks. It is perhaps prudent to choose locations with reasonable access to haemophilia centres and to take sufficient supplies of home treatment. Every haemophiliac travelling away from his home area should carry a letter from his haemophilia doctor, stating his factor VIII level and outlining his main medical problems. Haemophilia centres and national societies should be able to provide a list of the addresses of haemophilia centres throughout the world. All those with severe haemophilia travelling abroad should take supplies for self-administration of factor VIII and a custom declaration form confirming that he requires injections to treat his haemophilia. Insurance for foreign travel for those with haemophilia can be expensive. It is unlikely that haemophilia would be covered by any of the standard insurance policies provided by travel companies. Those needing insurance should be advised to make enquiries through their national haemophilia society. Additional problems arise for those with HIV infection who wish to travel to some countries for which an entry visa is required and in these cases there may be restriction on the length of stay. Those travelling by air may be required to produce medical confirmation of their fitness to fly.

Financial Implications

Government policies on health care in any country have a direct effect on individuals suffering from chronic disease and changes in these policies can have financial implications for both the affected person and his family. In the UK the policy to shift the care of the chronic sick from hospitals to the community has placed much of the cost of caring onto family budgets and added an extra burden for families caring for the long-term sick and disabled. As already discussed, initiatives by the government in the UK have helped HIV-positive haemophilic men, by giving them ex gratia payments to cover the extra costs incurred as a consequence of HIV. However haemophiliacs who do not have HIV may also require help with financial problems. The main source of financial assistance in the UK comes from state benefits. The benefits which doctors will be aware of are those that require a doctor's confirmation of ill health. A basic knowledge of some of the provisions that are available will enable a doctor to prompt his patient to claim benefit to which he may be entitled. Some patients will be hesitant to ask for "charity" but will be relieved to learn that their doctor thinks it is "OK" to apply for a benefit that is related to health needs.

Patients with haemophilia are likely to have short periods of incapacity due to acute bleeds, for which they will require sick certificates. For patients with haemophilia a request for a sicknote can often herald long periods of incapacity leading to financial difficulties and they should be reffered for social support. In the UK the Department of Social Services (DSS) provides a comprehensive range of benefits for those who are unable to work through disability or ill health (Disability Rights Handbook, 1995). These benefits are beset by complicated rules and regulations and claimants will probably require help in completing the forms to claim those benefits to which they are entitled. The patient is more likely to receive the benefits to which he is entitled if his doctor gives a clear and simple explanation of the problems specific to haemophiliacs and, where applicable, potential problems of strain on a damaged joint or the debilitating effects of HIV and HCV. Claims for entitlement are now usually assessed by clerical officers with little medical knowledge, hence the need for clarity.

In addition to statutory state benefits, there are organizations in the UK that have a specific remit to assist those with haemophilia. The national office of the Haemophilia Society will try to respond to requests for financial assistance but it does not have a large reserve of funds. Requests for grants will be considered if the applicant can show that the need is directly related to haemophilia; each request is means tested and there is limit of £500 for any one application. In some regions there are also local groups of the Haemophilia Society which are able to provide small cash grants of up to £50. The Society successfully campaigned for financial recompense for haemophiliacs affected by HIV. The process of litigation was traumatic for everyone involved: the haemophilic patient, his family and the Haemophilia Centre staff. The government responded by agreeing to an ex gratia award and set up a second agency, named the Macfarlane Trust, to distribute the money. The first awards were given to all those people with haemophilia who had become infected with HIV from contaminated blood products. The Macfarlane Trust also provides continuing financial support for those on low incomes or those who need help with the costs incurred for nursing care for those with illness attributable to HIV. The Haemophilia Society is campaigning for financial recompense for those with haemophilia who have HCV but do not have HIV.

Other Charities

Local charities are often pleased to help, and contact can be made directly or advice sought from Haemophilia Centres or local Social Work departments. In the UK, other national charities will sometimes provide assistance for those with haemophilia, especially in the case of children. The Roald Dahl Foundation has been established to give financial aid to children with haematological diseases, and gives sympathetic attention to applications for financial help from families with a haemophilic child. A severely affected haemophilic child with multiple problems may qualify for help from the "Family Fund" (Rowntree Trust).

Travel to Hospital

Travelling to and from hospital can be costly and patients who find this a burden should seek help. Travel costs can also pose problems for families visiting haemophiliacs when they are in hospital. Each hospital department should have a notice displayed informing the patients of help available for travel costs. Local charities will sometimes help with the cost of getting to and from hospital and some hospitals have their own charitable funds to help with this problem.

Final Considerations

The social and economic implications that we have discussed in this chapter are not often always easily resolved by medical intervention. Nevertheless, there is much that can be achieved for the haemophilic patient and his family, if his doctor uses the skills of other health care workers and has a multidisciplinary approach to the care of his patient at the Haemophilia Centre. It should be remembered that taking time to listen to a patient is of paramount importance and can help the patient gain the strength and confidence to cope both with his haemophilia and social problems.

References

Catalan J, Klimes I, Bond A, Day A, Rizza CR. Psychological and neuropsychiatric assessment of haemophiliacs with HIV infection. *International AIDS Conference*, Stockholm: 1988.

Darby SC, Doll R, Rizza CR, Spooner RJD. Seropositivity for HIV in UK haemophiliacs: for AIDS group of the UK Haemophilia Centre Directors. *Philosophical Transactions of the Royal Society of London Series B* 1989; **325:** 179.

Darby SC, Ewart DW, Giangrande PLF, Dolim PJ, Spooner RJD, Rizza CR. Mortality before and after HIV infection in the complete UK population of haemophiliacs. *Nature* 1995; **377:** 7982.

Disability Rights Handbook, 20th edn. London: Disability Alliance Educational and Research Association, 1995.

Giangrande PLF. Inhibitory antibodies. In: *The Management of Musculoskeletal Problems in the Haemophilias*. Oxford: Oxford University Press, 1994: 71.

Hallam NF, Fletcher ML, Read SJ, Majid AM, Kurtz JB, Rizza CR. Low risk of sexual transmission of hepatitis C virus. *Journal of Medical Virology* 1993; **40:** 251.

Hjort PF. The haemophiliac in the society. *Thrombosis Research* 1992; **67:** 339.
Jones P. *Living with Haemophilia*, 3rd ed. Tunbridge Wells: Castle House Publications, 1990.
Markova I, Lockyer R, Forbes CD. Haemophilia: a survey on social issues. *Health Bulletin* 1977; **35:** 177.
Nilsson IM. Prophylactic treatment of haemophilia A and B: current and future perspectives. *Science and Medicine* 1994; 121.
Panicucci F. Sport with haemophilia. *Proceedings of Meeting University of Pisa* 1993: 32.
Rizza CR, Spooner R. Treatment of haemophilia and related disorders in Britain and Northern Ireland during 1976–80: report of the *Directors of haemophilia centres in the United Kingdom. British Medical Journal* 1983; **286:** 929.
Seremetis SV, Aledort LM. *The Management of Musculoskeletal Problems in the Haemophilias.* Oxford: Oxford University Press, 1994: 265.
UK Haemophilia Society. *Treating Children with Bleeding Disorders.* London: UK Haemophilia Society, 1991.

14

Development of a National Database to Provide Information for the Planning of Care of Patients with Congenital Blood Coagulation Defects

Rosemary J.D. Spooner
and Charles R. Rizza

Background

In the UK the concept of treating haemophilia patients at special centres originated in 1950 when the Medical Research Council (MRC) set up a committee to consider the medical and social problems of patients with haemophilia. By 1955 the MRC had drawn up a list of 19 Centres where special facilities for the treatment and study of haemophiliacs were available. At that time the main concern of the Centres was to establish the diagnosis of haemophilia, issue the patient with an identity card and enter the patient's name into both the local Centre's register of patients and into the central register held by the MRC. Little treatment was available to haemophiliacs, apart from blood and plasma transfusions, although work was already underway in the UK to produce concentrated blood clotting factors from animals for clinical use (Macfarlane et al, 1954; Bidwell, 1955a,b). By 1957 a limited amount of freeze-dried factor VIII concentrate made from human plasma was also available (Kekwick and Wolf, 1957) and in 1961 factor IX concentrate was produced and used to treat haemophilia B (Christmas disease) patients (Biggs et al, 1961). In 1964 the introduction of cryoprecipitate greatly improved the treatment available to haemophilia A patients and other patients with factor VIII deficiency (Pool and Shannon, 1965). Freeze-dried concentrated factor VIII was still in short supply, so cryoprecipitate, which was easier and cheaper to produce and could be produced by most blood transfusion centres, came to be widely used throughout the UK.

In 1964 the responsibility for overseeing the organization of haemophilia care passed from the MRC to the Ministry of Health. The greater availability of freeze-dried concentrates and cryoprecipitate led to an improvement in treatment, in particular many more Centres were able to provide emergency treatment at short notice and to carry out major surgery safely. It therefore became necessary to review the organization of haemophilia care and to define the function of haemophilia centres.

In 1968 the Ministry of Health issued its health memorandum HM68(8) concerning "Arrangements for the care of persons suffering from haemophilia and related disorders". This memorandum contained a list of 36 Haemophilia Diagnostic and Registration Centres that would be prepared to take responsibility for the care of those suffering from haemophilia and related disorders in addition to the essential function of diagnosis, registration and the issue of haemophilia cards. Three of the 36 Centres (Oxford, Manchester and Sheffield) were designated as Special Treatment Centres to undertake major surgical treatment of patients with coagulation defects and to be available for consultation about all dangerous lesions in the patients.

In October 1968 Directors of all the UK Haemophilia Centres were invited to a meeting in Oxford to mark the opening of Oxford Haemophilia Centre's new buildings and at that meeting it was agreed that regular meetings of the Directors would be of value and give an opportunity to discuss a wide range of topics relating to patient care. It was also agreed that the Directors should send data regarding the patients they treated from 1969 onwards for the next 2–3 years to Oxford for collation and analysis on their behalf. Dr (later Professor) E.K. Blackburn was appointed as Chairman of the UK Haemophilia Centre Directors' Organization (UKHCDO) (as it is now known). Although the UKHCDO was in effect founded in 1968, it was very much an ad hoc organization with no funding from central government and it was not until 1991 that a Constitution was drawn up.

Since 1968, the Directors have met at least once a year to discuss matters specifically of interest in the management of haemophilia and to review the results of their surveys. In addition a Steering Committee, made up of the directors of the larger Centres, meets at least twice a year. Oxford Haemophilia Centre (OHC) has acted as the Secretariat for the UKHCDO since 1968, arranging meetings, circulating information of interest to all Directors and providing annual reports on the data that have been collated and analysed on behalf of the UKHCDO. There has been a large increase in the number of Haemophilia Centres, from 36 in 1968 to 103 today, and the type of information collected has expanded considerably. There is considerable variation in the number of patients treated annually by individual Haemophilia Centres, as is shown in Fig. 14.1, from which it will be seen that one-third of all Centres treated fewer than 10 patients in 1980 and two-thirds treated less than 20. Only six Centres treated more than 100 patients in the year (Rizza and Spooner, 1983). The pattern of distribution of patients being treated by Centres has not changed significantly since 1980.

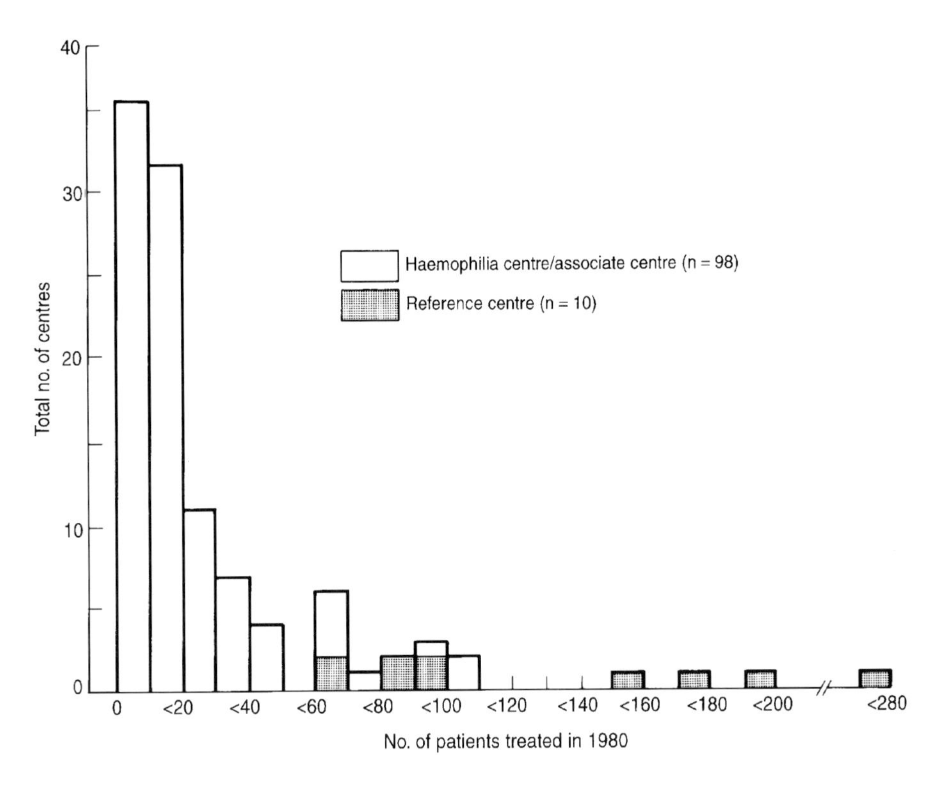

Figure 14.1 Number of patients treated during 1980 at haemophilia centres in the UK. (Reproduced from Rizza and Spooner, 1983, with permission.)

In the early 1970s the Department of Health reviewed the organization of haemophilia care in the UK and after discussion with the Haemophilia Centre Directors a document (HC76(4)) was issued in 1976, setting out the revised criteria for the designation of Haemophilia Centres and the services they were expected to provide for the patients. Appended to HC(76)4 was a list of 52 Haemophilia Centres, some having been designated as a result of being identified as providing a service to haemophiliacs in the UKHCDO's 1975 survey of hospitals not at that time recognized as Haemophilia Centres (Biggs and Spooner, 1978). Three types of centre were designated: Haemophilia Reference Centres, Haemophilia Centres and Associate Haemophilia Centres. Each of the Reference Centres was responsible for the provision of an advisory clinical and laboratory service to the individual haemophilia centres in their area (referred to as a "supraregion"). An appendix was attached to HC(76)4 listing 46 Centres in England and Wales, one Centre in Northern Ireland and Five Centres in Scotland but the designation of the individual Centres as either Reference Centre, Centre or Associate Centre was not disclosed in the document. In fact there were seven Reference Centres (six in England and one in Wales). At that time Northern

Ireland was included in the Oxford supraregion and Scotland elected to have a different way of organizing haemophilia care, although in practice there were two Reference Centres in Scotland. All haemophilia centres, irrespective of category, were expected to provide 24-hour emergency treatment for patients with haemophilia. The Directors of all 52 Haemophilia Centres agreed to send information to OHC regarding all haemophilia A and haemophilia B patients they knew (including patients who were not treated with blood products) and also, from 1976 onwards, details of treated von Willebrand's disease patients and treated carriers of haemophilia A or B. At that time information was not collected on von Willebrand's disease patients or carriers who had not received treatment. With the expansion of the arrangements for the care of haemophilic patients and improvement in registration, the number of patients known to have haemophilia A or haemophilia B steadily increased.

In 1993 the NHS Management Executive issued new Guidelines (HSG(93)30) entitled "Provision of haemophilia treatment and care", which had been drawn up after consultation with the UKHCDO Steering Committee and the Haemophilia Society. The three-tier system of Haemophilia Reference Centres, Centres and Associate Centres was replaced by the introduction of two types of Centre (Comprehensive Care Centres and Haemophilia Centres). The services that the two types of centre were expected to provide were set out in the document. All the existing Reference Centres became Comprehensive Care Centres and the UKHCDO Steering Committee (now called Executive Committee) set up a system for auditing these Centres, along with additional Centres that fulfilled the criteria for becoming Comprehensive Care Centres. This has resulted in the recognition of 24 Centres as Comprehensive Care Centres and 79 Centres as Haemophilia Treatment Centres.

Method and Organization of Data Collection

After the 1968 meeting of Directors, survey forms were drawn up by the Secretariat and approved by the Directors and the MRC, which was at that time funding a Research Laboratory within OHC. These early surveys gathered information only on haemophilia A and haemophilia B patients. The forms were designed for Centres to record personal details of the patients who had been treated in the relevant year. The details sought included name, date of birth, sex, coagulation defect, severity of coagulation defect, date of death, the type and amount of materials the patients received each time they were treated, the reason for the treatment, details of the incidence of jaundice, and if factor VIII or factor IX antibodies had been found, not found or not tested for. As no computing facilities were available in 1969 a manual system of data storage was set up. A system was devised to identify each individual patient by a diagnostic code number (1 for haemophilia A patients, 2 for haemophilia B patients) followed by a unique four digit number and the Centres were allocated with identification numbers so that the patients' names and the location of the Centres were used as little as possible, thereby helping to maintain confidentiality.

The survey forms were distributed at the beginning of each year to all Haemophilia Centre Directors, filled in at the Centres and returned as soon as possible to the Secretariat for collation and analysis. Some Centres had difficulties in completing the forms as they were short of staff or did not have adequate record-keeping facilities. In these instances a member of the staff of the Secretariat answered queries by telephone or letter and offered to visit the Centre to assist with the completion of the forms and advise (if required) on how the records system at the centre could be modified or improved. The offer was usually accepted and over the years many Centres have been visited. When the number of Centres increased, newly recognized Centres sometimes requested a short visit to clarify matters that were concerning them.

The original survey forms were used for only 2 years as experience with their use indicated that some changes were necessary. The greatest problem Directors experienced was with giving detailed information about every event for which the patient required treatment, so the main modification of the survey forms in 1971 was to cease to ask for details of each treatment and ask only for the total amount of each type of material the patient received during the year.

Although initially it was envisaged that the collation and analysis of UKHCDO data would be for only 2–3 years, this work has continued. The data forms have changed considerably over the years and the type of information has greatly expanded to keep abreast with current clinical practice and adverse events (such as AIDS). The scope of the survey work has also widened to include details of patients with von Willebrand's disease, carriers of haemophilia A or haemophilia B who received treatment, acquired haemophilia A, factor VII deficiency, factor XIII deficiency, platelet defects and other rare congenital blood coagulation defects.

As the volume of data received from Centres increased, it was realized by the Secretariat that the collation and analysis of patient data was likely to continue and would expand further. To facilitate this work and allow for more flexibility with the data analysis, it was decided in 1977 that a computerized register of the patient details should be set up. This decision was approved by the Haemophilia Society whose members were particularly concerned about confidentiality of a centrally-held register. Arrangements were made with the Oxford Regional Computer Unit for computing facilities on a mainframe computer to be made available to OHC for this purpose. The data remained under the control of the Secretariat and rigid security arrangements were set up. The patient data held in the manual register were entered into the computerized register and from 1977 onwards all new registrations, deaths, development of antibodies to factor VIII or factor IX and a record of the types of materials each patient received annually have been entered into the computerized system. Notification of new registrations, deaths, changes in diagnosis, development of inhibitors and changes of the patient's name are sent to the Secretariat as the events occur throughout the year. New patient registrations are checked by the Secretariat to ensure that entries are not duplicates for patients already registered. If the patient's name and date of birth are very similar to those of a patient already in the register, enquiries are made with the registering Centre to verify the information that has been provided.

By computerizing the patient data it has been possible for the Secretariat to send back lists of the details to Centres for checking and to provide Centres with annual computerized lists of the patients they may have treated in any one year, with columns to be filled in to indicate which patients were treated, whether or not they had factor VIII or factor IX antibodies and type of treatment materials the patients received, thus considerably reducing the clerical work entailed in completing the annual survey forms (usually referred to by the UKHCDO as Annual Returns). Additional data lists, either hard copy or on diskette, can also be provided on request to Centres regarding their own patients when these are required for local purposes. The original manual register has been retained and is kept up-to-date as it provides a useful source of information to complement the computerized data.

Since 1977 the computing facilities have been extended to incorporate additional data, such as details of patients with the rarer blood coagulation defects, laboratory results for von Willebrand's disease patients, results of human immunodeficiency virus (HIV) tests and details of cases of hepatitis. Details of acquired immune deficiency syndrome (AIDS) cases are kept in a separate database file within OHC, in which the patients names are not entered.

Following a survey of all Haemophilia Centres in 1987 to check whether patients currently in the National Register, but not reported as having received treatment for several years, were currently attending their Haemophilia Centre for follow-up appointments, it became clear that Centres had lost trace of some of their patients. Moreover, for some patients who had died the Haemophilia Centre reporting the death did not have details of the cause of death. It was therefore decided early in 1988 to make arrangements with the Office of Population Censuses and Surveys (OPCS) for all the patients in the National Register to be "flagged" and for a copy of their death certificate, retrospective or prospective, to be forwarded to the Secretariat in confidence. It was also arranged for details of death to be obtained from the General Register Offices (GRO) in Edinburgh and Belfast. The "flagging" with OPCS and GRO has enabled the Secretariat to improve the accuracy of the mortality data held in the National register and to identify patients in the register who no longer live in the UK.

As the continued use of the mainframe computer was proving to be expensive and smaller computers with the capability of handling large amounts of data were becoming available, it was decided in 1994 to transfer the data from the mainframe computer to a file server located within OHC, with connected personal computers to enable the data to be entered, edited and analysed on site at OHC. With assistance from the Oxford Radcliffe Hospital's Information Technology Service Delivery Unit, the data were transferred from the mainframe computer to a file server located within OHC during 1995. The database remains the responsibility of the Secretariat and security and confidentiality of the data has been retained.

Some additional items have been included in the new computerized system, such as Soundex coding and a field to "flag" for specific Centres the records of patients they no longer see so that these patients will no longer appear on the Centre's lists but the patient's details are retained in the system and the records are not lost.

Further expansions of the type of data held are planned: for example, the UKHCDO aims to include information regarding hepatitis C (HCV) and whether genetic data are available for individual patients at their Haemophilia Centre. It is also hoped that the Secretariat will be able to collect the home address postcode for the patients so that the geographic location of the patients can be more accurately assessed. As new blood products become available these are added to the database.

The national data are held by the Secretariat in strictest confidence on behalf of the UKHCDO and according to the requirements of the Data Protection Act; the number of staff involved with this work has been kept to the minimum and has never exceeded four at any one time, all of whom have worked on a part-time basis on the national data and have other duties within OHC. The staff has remained unchanged over many years and one member still working at OHC was involved in the original setting up of the National Register, and remains responsible for the day-to-day running of the system and for collation and analysis of the data. No information regarding individual patients or Centres is disclosed to third parties without the consent of the Centre concerned.

Through the analysis of UKHCDO data it has been possible to identify the number of patients known to UK Haemophilia Centres, the number of patients requiring treatment, the total amount of treatment materials that the patients need annually and the complications that can arise. Before 1969 it was not known how many patients with haemophilia A or haemophilia B required treatment in any one year, how much material (blood products) they needed and where they were treated. Also it was not known how many deaths occurred or the cause of death, nor was it known how many patients developed antibodies against factors VIII or IX, and the number of patients who suffered from jaundice (hepatitis) following treatment with blood products was not clear although it had been known for many years that jaundice could occur 1–4 months after transfusion of blood or plasma (Beeson, 1943; Spurling et al, 1946).

The first reports published in the medical press resulting from collation and analysis of the Directors' data were on the incidence of jaundice and antibodies against factors VIII and IX (Biggs, 1974) and a report by the Medical Research Council's Blood Transfusion Research Committee Working Party on the Cryoprecipitate Method of Preparing AHF Concentrates (1974). These were followed by a report on "Haemophilia treatment in the United Kingdom from 1969 to 1974" (Biggs and Spooner, 1977). A more detailed account of the different kinds of information collected is given below.

Number of Patients with Blood Coagulation Defects

Although a register of patients with haemophilia had been kept by the MRC and the information in the register had not been analysed, it was thought during the 1960s that there were about 2000 haemophilia A patients in the UK (Macfarlane, 1966). Initially the UKHCDO collected information only on patients with haemophilia A or B who required treatment. It soon became clear that the patients moved around the UK frequently and sometimes an individual patient was treated at several different Centres in one year. It was therefore necessary to set up a register of patients in such a way that the statistics regarding patient numbers could be adjusted to allow for duplications. Over the 6-year period 1969–74, 2600 haemophilia A and 388 haemophilia B patients received treatment at Haemophilia Centres and 62 haemophilia A and nine haemophilia B patients were known to have died (Biggs and Spooner, 1977). As the data collected over this period only concerned patients who required treatment and the number of identified patients had already exceeded the 1966 estimate of the total number of haemophilia A patients in the UK, the UKHCDO decided in 1975 to try to get more accurate information by surveying all hospitals in the UK not recognized as Haemophilia Centres to see if they had treated haemophiliacs (Biggs and Spooner, 1978) and also, from 1976, to include in their National Register details of all patients with haemophilia known to the Haemophilia Centres, even if they had not required treatment from 1969 onwards.

By December 1980 there were 4321 patients with haemophilia A and 777 with haemophilia B known to the UKHCDO (Rizza and Spooner, 1983). Of the 4321 haemophilia A patients in the register 1903 (44%) were severely affected, (<2 iu/dl of factor VIII) and of the 777 patients with haemophilia B 276 (36%) were severely affected (<2 iu/dl of factor IX). The largest total number of patients for all levels of severity fell within the 10–19 years age group (962 haemophilia A patients and 168 haemophilia B patients). The number of patients aged 70 years or more was surprisingly high (121 haemophilia A patients and 28 haemophilia B patients), considering that these patients had lived for most of their lives during a time when treatment for haemophilia was limited to transfusions of whole blood or plasma, on demand treatment was not available and surgery when undertaken was extremely hazardous. Thirty haemophilia A patients and five haemophilia B patients aged 70 years or more were severely affected (<2 iu/dl). The number of moderately affected (2–10 iu/dl) and mildly affected (>10 iu/dl) patients in the register aged <5 years may be incomplete as haemophilia is not always diagnosed early in these patients unless there is a history of haemophilia in the family or the child experiences some severe trauma requiring hospital attendance. On 1 January 1993 a total of 6278 patients with haemophilia A or haemophilia B were known to the UKHCDO. Of the 6278 patients, 5135 (82%) were known to be alive and living in the UK, 937 (15%) were dead, 24 (0.4%) had emigrated and 182 (3%) had been lost to follow-up;

Table 14.1 Number of patients with rare blood coagulation defects known to UK Haemophilia Centres in 1992

Coagulation defect	Number of patients
Acquired haemophilia A	81
Acquired haemophilia B	1
Acquired von Willebrand's disease	13
Congenital fibrinogen deficiency	55
Congenital prothrombin deficiency	11
Factor V deficiency	28
Factor VII deficiency	93
Factor X deficiency	62
Factor XI (PTA) deficiency	327
Factor XII (Hageman) deficiency	236
Factor XIII (FSF) deficiency	23
Combined XI + XII deficiency	3
Combined II + VII + X deficiency	4
Combined V + VIII deficiency	15
Combined XI + VIII deficiency	6
Combined VIII + IX deficiency	1
Other combined defects	10
Antithrombin III defects	64
Platelet defects	375
Fletcher factor	7
Total	1415

(Data reproduced with permission of the UKHCDO.)

2448 of the patients were severely affected (<2 iu/dl), 2726 mildly–moderately affected and for 104 the severity of their defect was not known (Darby et al, 1995).

In 1984 the Directors decided to include in their national statistics details of patients with all known rare coagulation defects, including acquired haemophilia A, acquired haemophilia B and acquired von Willebrand's disease. The number of patients with the rare defects known to the UKHCDO in 1992 is given in Table 14.1 (Rizza and Spooner, 1994).

Amount of Materials Required to Treat the Patients

During the 1960s Directors of Haemophilia Centres in the UK were carrying out their work with inadequate supplies of human factor VIII concentrates and it was envisaged that it was likely that the supply would remain scarce for many years to come (Biggs, 1966). The development of a national database provided important information on the pattern of factor VIII usage in the UK and allowed comparison with other countries when information from the latter was available. By collating and analysing the information provided by all the Centres it was possible to provide evidence for the Department of Health, Blood Transfusion Service (BTS) and the UK fractionation laboratories (Blood Products Laboratory, now called Bio Products Laboratory (BPL), in Elstree, Herts., and the Protein Fractionation Centre (PFC) in Edinburgh) that the supply of factor VIII concentrates needed to be increased substantially if the patients were to be treated adequately. It also enabled the Secretariat to provide statistical information to Supraregional (Reference) Centre Directors and Regional Directors regarding the quantities and types of material used in their regions over several years, how these requirements were increasing and where the patients were treated within the region or supraregion.

Haemophilia A

The total amount of factor VIII units used to treat haemophilia A patients in the UK has risen from 6.9 million units in 1969 to 131.7 million units in 1992 (Fig. 14.2). Although the number of patients treated by UK Haemophilia Centres has also risen, from 1022 in 1969 to 2430 in 1992, the increased amount of factor VIII units used reflects mainly an increase in the treatment requirements of individual patients. The increase in demand for treatment is partly due to the introduction in the 1970s of home treatment, which is now well established, accounting for 60% of the total amount of factor VIII units used in 1992 (Rizza and Spooner, 1994) and to optimum treatment being set at higher dosage levels. There has also been an increase in the amount of factor VIII used to treat haemophilia A patients with inhibitors (factor VIII antibodies). During the early days of treatment for patients who had developed factor VIII antibodies, many physicians considered that the amount of blood products given should be limited and patients were not encouraged to seek treatment for minor bleeds. This policy has changed and these patients now receive treatment with an appropriate product more frequently and some patients receive large doses of concentrate to suppress their antibodies. Information on the types and amount of materials used to treat these patients has been included in the Annual Returns from Haemophilia Centres since 1977. The therapeutic materials used include human factor VIII concentrates, activated and non-activated human prothrombin complex concentrates and porcine factor VIII.

Von Willebrand's disease

In 1976, the first year information was collected on patients with von Willebrand's disease, 186 patients were treated and received a total of 796 000 units of factor VIII; 84% of the materials was cryoprecipitate. By 1992 the number of patients treated had risen to 273 and they received a total of 5 million units of factor VIII plus 304 000 units of von Willebrand factor concentrate. Cryoprecipitate accounted for less than 2% of the factor VIII units used (Rizza and Spooner, 1994).

Carriers of haemophilia A

Information has been collected since 1976 on carriers of haemophilia A who require treatment. In 1976 19 carriers of haemophilia A were treated and received a total of 57 000 units of factor VIII; 16 000 units (28%) was given as cryoprecipitate. In 1992 40 carriers of haemophilia A were treated and received 132 000 units of factor VIII concentrate (Rizza and Spooner, 1994).

Acquired haemophilia A

Acquired haemophilia A is a rare defect and in 1985, the first year that information regarding the treatment of acquired haemophilia A was collected, 11 patients were treated by Haemophilia Centres with 201 000 factor VIII units. In 1992, 25 patients were treated and they received a total of 532 000 factor VIII units, plus 275 000 units of porcine factor VIII, 426 000 Factor Eight Inhibitor Bypassing Activity (FEIBA) units, 58 000 units of NHS factor IX and 340 mg of recombinant factor VIIa (Rizza and Spooner, 1994). The increase in the number of patients with acquired haemophilia A may well reflect an increase in referral to Centres from other hospitals as the availability of treatment for these patients became more widely known.

Acquired von Willebrand's disease

Acquired von Willebrand's disease is also a rare defect. Information regarding these patients was first collated and analysed in 1985. In 1992, six patients received 734 000 factor VIII units from Haemophilia Centres, including one patient who was on home treatment (Rizza and Spooner, 1994).

Haemophilia B

The UKHCDO has collected information regarding the treatment of haemophilia B (Christmas disease) since 1969, when supplies of factor IX concentrate

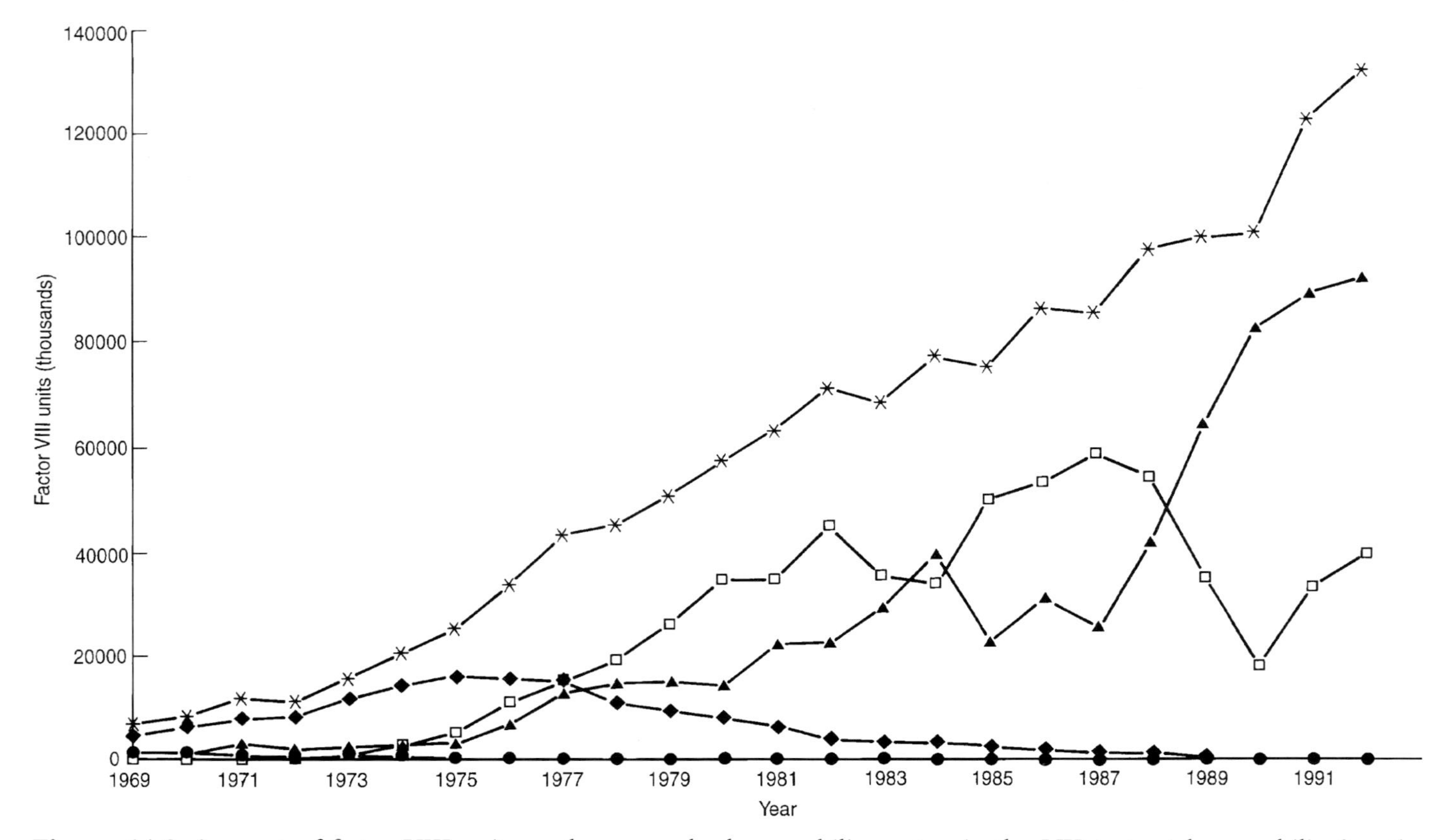

Figure 14.2 Amount of factor VIII units used per year by haemophilia centres in the UK to treat haemophilia A patients during 1969–1992. ●, plasma; ◆, cryoprecipitate; ▲, NHS factor VIII; □, commercial factor VIII; ✳, total. (Data reproduced with permission of the UKHCDO.)

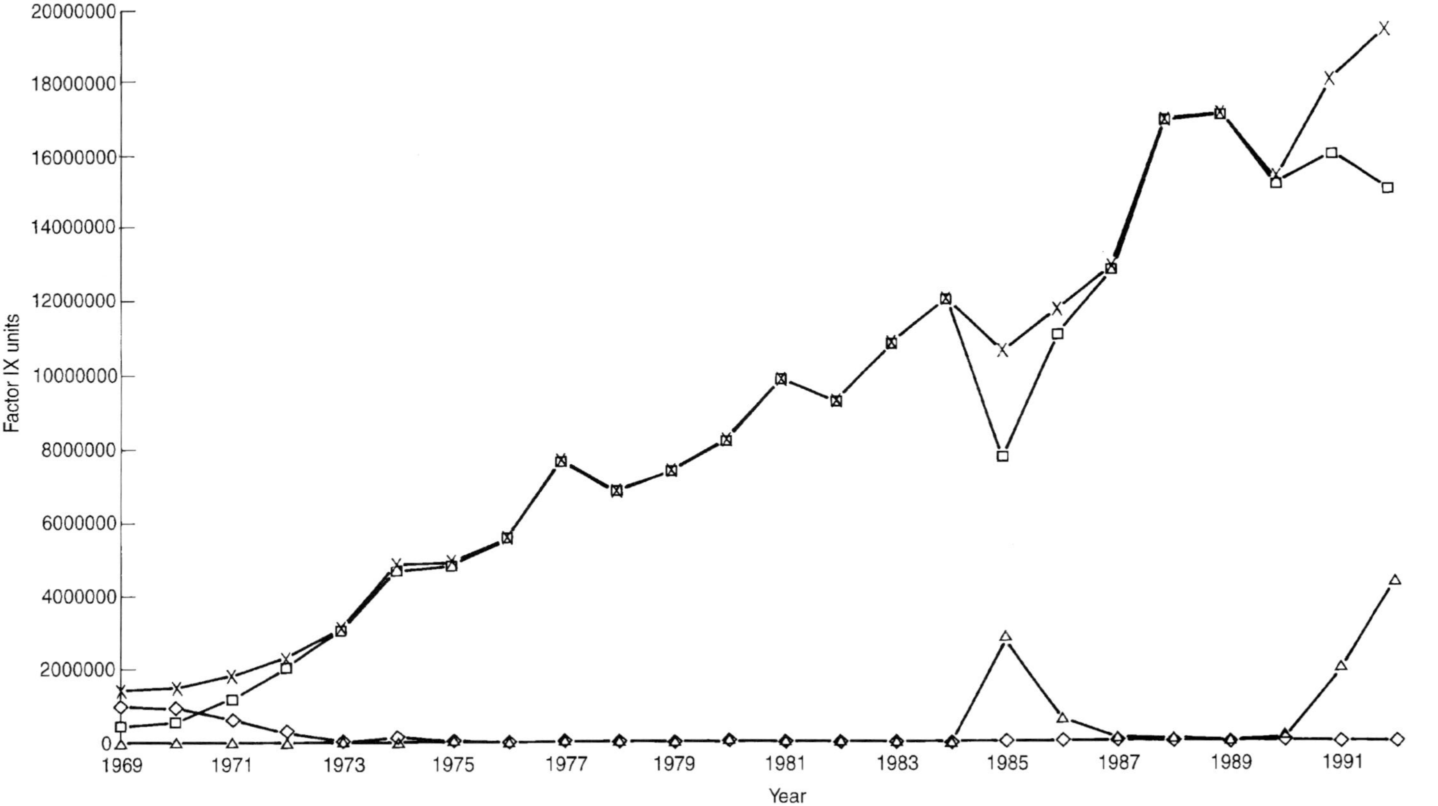

Figure 14.3 Amount of factor IX units used per year by haemophilia centres in the UK to treat haemophilia B patients during 1969–1992. ◇, plasma; □, NHS factor IX; △, commercial factor IX; X, total. (Data reproduced with permission of the UKHCDO.)

were not widely available and most patients were treated with plasma, the concentrate being reserved for the treatment of patients requiring surgery, dental extractions or patients having suffered some life-threatening trauma. The total amount of factor IX units used to treat haemophilia B (Christmas disease) patients has increased from 1.4 million factor IX units in 1969 to 19.4 million factor IX units in 1992 (Fig. 14.3). By 1979 factor IX concentrates were widely available and by 1991 plasma had ceased to be used for haemophilia B patients.

Carriers of haemophilia B

Information regarding the treatment of carriers of haemophilia B has been collected since 1976. Very few carriers of haemophilia B have required treatment: during 1976–1980 the number treated per year ranged from five to twelve patients. They were mainly treated with factor IX concentrates, though fresh frozen plasma was occasionally used. The total amount of factor IX used per year ranged from a total of 7000 to 115 000 factor IX units (Rizza and Spooner, 1983).

UKHCDO Working Parties

In 1977 the UKHCDO set up the first of its Working Parties to consider specific subjects that were topical at the time. The first three Working Parties were on hepatitis, home treatment and the treatment of patients who had factor VIII antibodies. Later on, Working Parties were set up to consider AIDS, recommendations on the choice of therapeutic materials, von Willebrand's disease, platelet defects, paediatrics, adverse events and genetics. The Working Parties were expected to last for only short periods while the matters of current interest were being investigated. The data held in the National Register have been used by the Working Parties as required and have provided them with detailed background information. The Working Party Chairmen report regularly to the UKHCDO's Steering Committee when they meet three to four times a year and to all the Directors at the UKHCDO Annual General Meeting and, when appropriate, publish papers in the medical press. The first paper published by a Working Party was on home treatment (Jones et al, 1978) and gave the results from two questionnaires regarding the number of patients on home treatment or in training for home treatment, the amount of material used by individual patients and the type of products used. The results of the HIV surveys were published by the AIDS Group of the UKHCDO in 1986 and 1988. The incidence of factor VIII inhibitors in 1990–1993 was published by the Inhibitor Working Party in 1995 (Colvin et al, 1995). The von Willebrand's disease Working Party published "Guidelines for the Diagnosis and Management of von Willebrand's Disease" in 1995.

The Adverse Events Working Party was set up in 1989. The Secretariat, on behalf of the Adverse Events Working Party (AEWP), sends out cards each quarter to every Haemophilia Centre to ask if there have been any adverse events during the previous 3 months or for confirmation that there was nothing to report if that was the case. The card lists the events specifically of interest to the UKHCDO, with a box for the centre to tick which (if any) events occurred. The events listed on the card at present are as follows:

Nothing to report	( )
HIV transmission	( )
Non-A, non-B or hepatitis C transmission	( )
Hepatitis B transmission	( )
New inhibitor	( )
Thrombotic event/DIC	( )
Transfusion reaction	( )
Other event (specify)	( )

The completed cards, including those with "nothing to report", are returned to the Secretariat as soon as possible. There is a note on the card to say that viral transmission events should also be notified as soon as possible after recognition to the Chairman of the Working Party who then contacts the Haemophilia Centre involved to obtain more details. Where appropriate he or she then notifies the Chairman of the Inhibitors Working Party or the Chairman of the Hepatitis Working Party. If the event is serious, details are passed to the Medicines Control Agency (MCA). This reporting system has received excellent support from the Haemophilia Centres and has enabled the UKHCDO to be better informed as to the incidence of adverse events; it is also useful to have the "nothing to report" returns as a control on the recording of incidents.

Complications of Treatment

The data collected by the UKHCDO have provided useful information regarding the incidence of jaundice/hepatitis, antibodies to factor VIII and factor IX and HIV/AIDS.

Hepatitis

During the period 1969–1974, 186 patients with haemophilia A who received blood products in the UK had 193 episodes of clinical jaundice, giving a mean incidence of 2.45% of the patients treated each year. For haemophilia B patients, the mean incidence of clinical jaundice was 1.67%. In addition some

Haemophilia Centre Directors reported patients who had abnormal liver function tests (LFTs) but who were not ill. Not all Haemophilia Centres had carried out LFTs on their patients so the incidence of abnormal LFTs in haemophiliacs could not be assessed in 1974. An outbreak of hepatitis associated with three batches of a commercial brand of freeze-dried factor VIII concentrate occurred in 1974 (Craske et al, 1975). Seven of these cases were of non-A/non-B hepatitis and four of hepatitis B. Two patients contracted both types of hepatitis. Over the period 1974–1976, the use of commercial factor VIII concentrates continued to increase and the overall incidence of acute hepatitis in haemophilia A patients rose to 3.5% in 1977.

In January 1977 the UKHCDO set up its Acute Hepatitis Working Party and a letter was published in the *Lancet* in November 1978 showing evidence for the existence of at least two types of factor VIII-associated non-A/non-B hepatitis (Craske et al, 1978); these findings were confirmed in 1983 (Fletcher et al, 1983).

Factor VIII/IX antibodies (inhibitors)

The development of factor VIII antibodies in haemophilia A patients is a serious complication of treatment. Fortunately the prevalence is not high and has remained at 6% of the number of patients known to the UKHCDO since 1976 (Rizza and Spooner, 1983). The number of new cases detected per year in 1969–1974 varied from 15 to 21 (Biggs and Spooner, 1977); in 1990–93 the incidence of new cases was less, ranging from four to 12 cases (Colvin et al, 1995). For haemophilia B patients the incidence of factor IX antibodies is less than 1% (Rizza and Spooner, 1983). The UKHCDO has closely checked their patients over the years when new types of blood products have been introduced and have not been able to attribute the development of antibodies to any particular product or fractionation method.

HIV/AIDS

In 1982 the UKHCDO became aware of the possibility that patients treated with blood products might develop AIDS and a system was set up for the reporting of clinical AIDS cases. At that time no tests were available for the detection of the virus causing AIDS but by 1985 a test for antibody to HIV had been developed and the computing facilities at OHC were extended to allow for the confidential recording of the results of the tests on haemophilic patients. It must be said here that in the early days of the HIV problem many Haemophilia Centre Directors were reluctant to send such sensitive information on their patients to a central register, even in coded form. In time this problem was overcome with the consent of the Directors, the patients and the Haemophilia Society.

A first survey of all haemophiliacs attending UK Haemophilia Centres showed that 896 (44%) of the haemophilia A patients tested and 20 (6%) of the haemophilia B patients tested were positive for HIV antibody (AIDS Group, 1986). By 1987, 1206 patients with haemophilia A or haemophilia B living in the UK had been identified as anti-HIV positive and 85 patients had developed AIDS (AIDS Group, 1989; Darby et al, 1989). Since 1987 more AIDS cases have been diagnosed but there have been no new HIV seroconversions. A study of the mortality of haemophiliacs in the UK is currently being undertaken on behalf of the UKHCDO and the first published report on the results of the study concerned mortality before and after HIV infection (Darby et al, 1995).

Number of Deaths and Causes of Death in the Haemophilic Population

Since 1969 Haemophilia Centre Directors have reported deaths of their patients to OHC, giving the date and cause. In 1969–74, 71 deaths were reported, the largest number being from intracranial bleeding (16). No information was given regarding the cause of death of 13 patients. The average age at death was 42.3 years for haemophilia A patients and 33.6 for haemophilia B patients (Biggs and Spooner, 1977). Eighty-nine patients with haemophilia A and 18 with haemophilia B died during 1976–80 (Rizza and Spooner, 1983). The average ages of the patients who died were 46.7 years for haemophilia A and 48.3 years for haemophilia B. Cerebral haemorrhage was again the most common cause of death in haemophilia A and accounted for 26 deaths (29%). With the appearance of HIV and AIDS in the UK the death rate of severely affected haemophiliacs rose steeply (Darby et al, 1995). During 1985–92 there were 403 deaths in HIV-seropositive patients, whereas 60 would have been predicted from rates in seronegatives, suggesting that 85% of the deaths in seropositive patients were due to HIV infection. Most of the excess deaths were certified as due to AIDS or to conditions recognized as being associated with AIDS.

Liaison of the UKHCDO's Secretariat with other Organizations

Over the years the Secretariat has, and still does, liaise with several organizations. The UK Haemophilia Society has been provided with much information and statistical data from the National Register and an annual statistical report is given to the World Federation of Haemophilia for inclusion in their compilation of haemophilia statistics throughout the world. Information has also been provided on several occasions to the World Health Organization, Council of

Europe for their coordinated blood transfusion research projects and to the Departments of Health in the UK. Information from the national database has been presented to the UK Fractionating Laboratories (BPL and PFC) to support the claim that there was the need for new products, such as factor VII concentrate and factor XIII concentrate, and the annual reports have helped the National Blood Transfusion Services to plan how much plasma is required for fractionation. Copies of the reports on the Annual Returns from Haemophilia Centres have been made available in recent years to the commercial companies manufacturing blood products. Only statistical information is given; information regarding specific patients or Haemophilia Centres is never divulged.

When the Public Health Laboratory Service Communicable Disease Surveillance Centre (CDSC) in Colindale, London, set up their system to collect information regarding AIDS cases, the Secretariat at OHC was asked if it would be possible for the information on haemophilic AIDS cases to be passed to them, in confidence, to ensure that they had notification of all the cases. The UKHCDO agreed to the data being passed on to CDSC, without the patients' names; the patients were identified by their National Register file number, date of birth and Soundex code (Mortimer and Salathiel, 1995). A system for the exchange of information was set up between the Secretariat in Oxford and CDSC in Colindale and works very well. In addition to the AIDS cases, information is exhanged on deaths of HIV-positive haemophiliacs and the information on all HIV-positive haemophiliacs has been exchanged and checked to ensure that the statistics regularly published by CDSC are as accurate as possible.

Conclusions

The UKHCDO's National Register provides data on the largest population of haemophilic patients on which documentation has been collected for more than 25 years without a break. By collating and analysing the data over this period of time it has been possible for the Directors to make projections of the amount of materials required to treat the patients and provide the information required to convince the fractionation laboratories in the UK (BPL and PFC) and the Department of Health that more funding was necessary if the patients were to receive the amount of treatment necessary for their well-being. This was particularly relevant when home treatment was introduced and when larger numbers of patients were requiring major orthopaedic operations as techniques such as total hip replacements were developed. As the National Register was already well established in 1982 it was not difficult for the Secretariat to extend the facilities to include data on AIDS cases and HIV. The detailed information about the type of blood products individual patients had received since 1977 made it possible for the AIDS Group to see whether prevalence of antibody to HIV varied with the type of blood products the patients received (AIDS Group,

1986). The recording of adverse events is a useful way for the Directors to be aware that problems can arise and to be alerted promptly should any new serious problem appear.

For a national register and data collection system to be set up, it is essential that the data be kept strictly confidential and that those contributing data are convinced that this is the case. It is also of the utmost importance that the Haemophilia Centres are the first to receive reports on their Annual Returns and that the data in the reports are not released for wider publication until the Directors have had a chance to discuss them. When such data are published it has been our practice to publish "on behalf of the UKHCDO", with acknowledgement made by name to those who have contributed data. In the early years of collation and analysis of UK data, it was important that someone from the Secretariat was always on hand to answer queries and was willing to visit Centres when required. Long-term commitment to the project of the staff in the secretariat has also played a significant part in the continued existence of a system adapted over many years to meet changing needs.

To create a National Haemophilia Database the essential requirements are:

1. Cooperation from Haemophilia Centre Directors and their staff.
2. Committed and knowledgeable staff at the Secretariat office.
3. Data should be held by the Secretariat strictly in confidence and should not be disclosed to third parties without the relevant Haemophilia Centre Director's consent.
4. Adequate flexible systems, both manual and computerized, for collation and analysis of the data.
5. Agreement with Haemophilia Centre Directors as to the type of data they wish to include in the database and which aspects of the data they would like to have collated and analysed.
6. The Haemophilia Centre Directors should receive regular reports on information obtained from the database and a report each year on the results of their Annual Returns.
7. Ad hoc reports required for a specific local purpose should, if possible, be provided.
8. Reports should not be published widely before the Directors have received the data.
9. Publications should be on behalf of the Directors and a list of the names of those who have contributed data should be included.
10. The system should be flexible enough to allow for expansion as and when necessary to include additional or new types of data.

Acknowledgements

We are most grateful to Mrs Patricia Wallace and Miss Sharon Osborne for secretarial and clerical assistance.

References

AIDS Group of the United Kingdom Haemophilia Centre Directors with the cooperation of the United Kingdom Haemophilia Centre Directors. Prevalence of antibody to HTLV-III in haemophiliacs in the United Kingdom. *British Medical Journal* 1986; **293:** 175.

AIDS Group of the United Kingdom Haemophilia Centre Directors with the cooperation of the UK Haemophilia Centre Directors. Seropositivity for HIV in UK haemophiliacs. *Philosophical Transactions of the Royal Society London Series B* 1989; **325:** 179.

AIDS Group of the United Kingdom Haemophilia Centre Directors with the cooperation of the United Kingdom Haemophilia Centre Directors. Prevalence of antibody to HIV in haemophiliacs in the United Kingdom: a second survey. *Clinical and Laboratory Haematology* 1988; **10**: 187.

Beeson PB. Jaundice occurring one to four months after transfusion of blood or plasma. Report of seven cases. *Journal of the American Medical Association* 1943; **121:** 1332.

Bidwell E. The purification of bovine antihaemophilic globulin. *British Journal of Haematology* 1955a; **1:** 35.

Bidwell E. The purification of antihaemophilic globulin from animal plasma. *British Journal of Haematology* 1955b; **1:** 386.

Biggs R. General conclusion about replacement therapy in haemophilia. In: Biggs R, Macfarlane RG (Eds), *Treatment of Haemophilia and other Coagulation Disorders.* Oxford: Blackwell Scientific, 1966.

Biggs R. Jaundice and antibodies directed against factors VIII and IX in patients treated for haemophilia or Christmas disease in the United Kingdom (on behalf of the Directors of 37 Haemophilia Centres in the United Kingdom). *British Journal of Haematology* 1974; **26:** 313.

Biggs R, Spooner RJD. Haemophilia treatment in the United Kingdom. From data collected by the Haemophilia Centre Directors of the United Kingdom. *British Journal of Haematology* 1977; **35:** 487.

Biggs R, Spooner RJD. National survey of haemophilia and Christmas disease patients in the United Kingdom. Report on behalf of the Haemophilia Reference Centre Directors of the U.K. *Lancet* 1978; **i:** 1143.

Biggs R, Bidwell E, Handley DA, et al. The preparation and assay of a Christmas-factor (factor IX) concentrate and its use in the treatment of two patients. *British Journal of Haematology* 1961; **7:** 349.

Colvin BT, Hay CRM, Hill FGH, Preston FE for the Inhibitor Working Party on behalf of the United Kingdom Haemophilia Centre Directors Organization. The incidence of factor VIII inhibitors in the United Kingdom, 1990–93. *British Journal of Haematology* 1995; **89:** 908.

Craske J, Dilling N, Stern D. An outbreak of hepatitis associated with intravenous injection of factor VIII concentrate. *Lancet* 1975; **ii:** 221.

Craske J, Spooner RJD, Vandervelde EM. Evidence for existence of at least two types of factor VIII-associated non-B transfusion hepatitis. *Lancet* 1978; **ii:** 1051.

Darby SC, Rizza CR, Doll R, Spooner RJD, Stratton LM, Thakrar B. Incidence of AIDS and excess of mortality associated with HIV in haemophiliacs in the United Kingdom: report on behalf of the directors of haemophilia centres in the United Kingdom. *British*

Medical Journal 1989; **298:** 1064.
Darby SC, Ewart DW, Giangrande PLF, Dolin PJ, Spooner RJD, Rizza CR on behalf of the UK Haemophilia Centre Directors Organization. Mortality before and after HIV infection in the complete UK population of haemophiliacs. *Nature* 1995; **377:** 79.
Fletcher ML, Trowell JM, Craske J, Pavier K, Rizza CR. Non-A non-B hepatitis after transfusion of factor VIII in infrequently treated patients. *British Medical Journal* 1983; **287:** 1754.
Jones P, Fearns M, Forbes C, Stuart J. Haemophilia A home therapy in the United Kingdom 1975–6. *British Medical Journal* 1978; **i:** 1447.
Kekwick RA, Wolf P. A concentrate of human antihaemophilic factor – its use in six cases of haemophilia. *Lancet* 1957; **i:** 647.
Macfarlane RG. Blood coagulation and haemostasis. In: Biggs R, Macfarlane RG (Eds), *Treatment of Haemophilia and other Coagulation Disorders*. Oxford: Blackwell Scientific, 1966.
Macfarlane RG, Biggs R, Bidwell E. Bovine antihaemophilic globulin in the treatment of haemophilia. *Lancet* 1954; **i:** 1316.
Medical Research Council's Blood Transfusion Research Committee Working Party on the Cryoprecipitate Method of Preparing AHF Concentrates. Factor VIII concentrates made in the United Kingdom and the treatment of haemophilia based on studies made during 1969–72. *British Journal of Haematology* 1974; **27:** 391.
Mortimer JY, Salathiel JA. "Soundex" codes of surnames provide confidentiality and accuracy in a national HIV database. *Communicable Disease Report* 1995; **5:** R183.
Pool JG, Shannon AE. Production of high-potency concentrates of anti-hemophilic globulin in a closed bag system. *New England Journal of Medicine* 1965; **273:** 1443.
Rizza CR, Spooner RJD. Treatment of haemophilia and related disorders in Britain and Northern Ireland during 1976–80: report on behalf of the directors of haemophilia centres in the United Kingdom. *British Medical Journal* 1983; **286:** 929.
Rizza CR, Spooner RJD. Report to UK Haemophilia Centre Directors on their Annual Returns for 1992. Oxford: Haemophilia Centre. UKHCDO 1994. Copies available from the UKHCDO's Administrative Secretary, Oxford Haemophilia Centre, Churchill Hospital, Oxford; price £5.00.
Spurling N, Shone J, Vaughan J. The incidence, incubation period and symptomatology of homologous serum jaundice. *British Medical Journal* 1946; **ii:** 409–412.
von Willebrand Working Party of the United Kingdom Haemophilia Centre Directors' Organisation. Guidelines for the Diagnosis and Management of the von Willebrand Disease. UKHCDO 1995. Copies available from the UKHCDO's Administrative Secretary, Oxford Haemophilia Centre, Churchill Hospital, Oxford; price £5.00.

15 Setting Standards of Care

PETER JONES

In 1992 the World Federation of Hemophilia (WFH, 1992) launched a strategic plan with the aim of encouraging the delivery of medical and psychosocial care to people with haemophilia and their families worldwide. On the cover of the WFH Decade Plan brochure are the photographs of two of my patients (Fig. 15.1). Thirty years divide these children. Both have severe haemophilia A without inhibitors. One has severe haemophilic arthropathy; the other boy is growing normally. The stark difference between them is due in part to the introduction of high-quality clotting factor concentrates, and in part to the introduction of comprehensive care. The majority of the world's haemophiliacs have neither, and the older picture is representative of their state of health *today*.

In a review of treatment at the Oxford Haemophilia Centre, Rosemary Biggs (1967) wrote that it was in 1938 that her colleague R.G. Macfarlane had "laid the foundation for modern therapy when he realised that the treatment of haemophilia could be rationalized only by understanding the physiology of normal clotting and haemostasis . . . there is in normal blood a factor . . . that is essential for the rapid activation of prothrombin and that this factor is at fault in haemophilia". In considering the setting of standards of care, these observations remain a valuable starting point. They emphasize the fact that care must always be based on the basic science of haemostasis and its control. This remains as true in these days of recombinant technology and gene therapy as it did then. An active coagulation laboratory with good quality control is the foundation on which all else is built.

The fate of patients with severe haemophilia at the time when Macfarlane started his work on haemostasis could hardly have been worse. In 1937 Birch reported her study of 98 patients and their affected relatives (Birch, 1937). Of 113 deaths, half were the result of bleeding after trivial injury, epistaxes or minor surgery. Most patients died in childhood, 82 before their 15th year, and only six people with severe haemophilia had survived their 40th birthday. In contrast, before the advent of disease associated with the hepatitis and human immunodeficiency viruses, the average life-span of the severely affected patient living in a developed country with access to factor VIII or IX concentrates was normal.

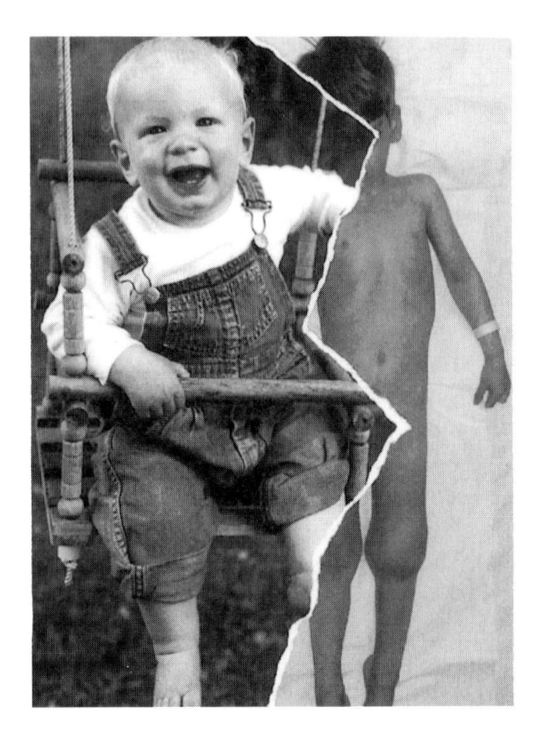

Figure 15.1 Two children with severe haemophilia A. The boy on the left benefits from modern therapy. The child on the right received inadequate replacement therapy 30 years ago.

It is the purpose of this chapter to review the elements of the management of haemophilia within an affected family, and to describe one approach to the prescription of treatment as part of the overall discipline of comprehensive care.

Optimum Care

In 1985, in his book *Haemophilic Bleeding* Aronstam introduced "a charter for haemophiliacs". He based it on the premise that it is reasonable to expect that everything possible will be done to maintain and improve the health of the person with haemophilia in physical, psychological and sociological terms. The key requirement of the charter was that the patient had access to someone with experience in the treatment of haemophilia. Backing him or her should be good laboratory facilities, counselling and cover for emergencies. There should be a specially designated area in the hospital to which patients could go for help at any time, without having to wait. Treatment and dosages should be tailored individually and, whenever possible, therapy should be given at home. Regular follow-up, physiotherapy, general health checks and surveillance for possible side-effects were essential. There should be immediate access to social work skills, genetic counselling and help for pain. Referral for specialist advice, especially orthopaedic advice, should be easy and there should be clear guidance on the management of complications of treatment, including inhibitors.

Jones (1990) extended this charter to answer the six basic needs of someone with haemophilia These remain:

- accurate diagnosis
- effective and safe treatment
- 24-hour cover
- regular follow-up
- expert counselling
- a good standard of communication about the disorder.

Accurate diagnosis

This is essential if the patient is to receive both the correct treatment and the genetic counselling appropriate to his or her disorder. Diagnosis is not simply the preserve of the coagulation laboratory, although accuracy and quality control here is crucial. It depends on the taking of a formal personal and family history (Table 15.1), with emphasis on the patient's response to trauma and the inheritance of the condition. Modern automated laboratory equipment and reagent kits make the differentiation of haemophilia A and B (Christmas disease) easy, at least in the developed world. However, differential diagnosis between haemophilia A and the various types of von Willebrand's disease still presents problems, especially when the disorder is mild. Multimeric analysis of von Willebrand's factor antigen demands the luxury of time and skilled workmanship unavailable in most laboratories.

In order to prescribe appropriate therapy, the severity of the disorder must be judged, and this may need repeated assays, together with transfusion experiments, to determine response and half-life. All the tests used must be subject to regular quality control using both in-house and external standards. Within the UK the National External Quality Assessment Scheme (NEQAS) system organized by the National Institute for Biological Standards and Control (NIBSC) provides a quality control programme for tests of coagulation and fibrinolysis. NEQAS works closely with the World Health Organization (WHO) and the Scientific and Standardization Committee (SSC) of the International Society on Thrombosis and Haemostasis (ISTH), one of the goals of which is to formulate international standards for nomenclature and methods.

Within the developing world things are far from being so easy and the majority of patients remain undiagnosed. In the absence of available, safe treatment, diagnosis may seem academic, but without it there can be no pressure on the medical, administrative and political authorities to provide even a modicum of care. And,

Table 15.1 The haemostatic history

1. Bruising
   - excessive/not excessive
   - spontaneous/always with trauma
   - superficial/deep
   - flat/raised
   - sites
2. Purpura
   - experienced/not experienced
     - cause, if known
   - site(s)
3. Haemarthroses
   - experienced/not experienced
     - cause, if known
   - site(s)
4. Epistaxes
   - experienced/not experienced
   - one or both nostrils
     - cause, if known
5. Gastrointestinal bleeding
   - haematemesis
   - melaena
     - cause, if known
6. Genitourinary
   - haematuria
   - menstruation:
     - cycle, duration periods, loss
     - pregnancies, postpartum haemorrhage(s)
7. Response to challenge:
   - (a) Cuts/trauma
     - duration of bleeding
       - normality of wound healing
   - (b) Dental extractions
     - duration of bleeding
     - secondary haemorrhage
     - whether abnormal bleeding inevitable
     - measures taken to control bleeding
   - (c) Intramuscular injections
     - haematoma formation
     - whether inevitable
   - (d) Surgery
     - type of operation
     - abnormal blood loss
     - persistent bleeding
     - secondary haemorrhage/haematoma
     - normality of wound healing
8. Any other evidence of abnormal haemorrhage.
   - neonatal/retroperitoneal/intracranial
9. Drug history
   - aspirin
   - non-steroidal anti-inflammatory agents
   - hormone therapy/replacement therapy (including contraceptive pill)
10. Family history of possible bleeding disorder

if the Decade Plan is to come to fruition, we must know where to target available resources, especially if cure becomes available with gene therapy or cell transplantation.

Whilst diagnosis and treatment may be lacking or even non-existent in countries generally considered to be developing in the context of their overall economies, it is overoptimistic to imagine that all those with haemophilia in richer nations receive a good standard of care. Poor people with chronic disorders can be locked into a system of deprivation and inappropriate care just as easily in a developed as in an undeveloped country. This is more likely to happen when there is a family history of severe haemophilia, repeated generations of a family not being able to provide adequate levels of financial support because

Table 15.2 Information that should be carried by a person with haemophilia, or by their parent or guardian

Patient details	
Name, address, telephone/fax number	
Diagnosis	
Resting clotting factor level	
Other diagnostic test results	
Blood group	
Inhibitor status – if positive:	high/low responder
	highest titre measured
Other health problems	
Recommended treatment	
Who to contact out of hours, and how	
Further information available from:	
Haemophilia Centre, address, telephone/fax number	
Family doctor, address, telephone/fax number	

their disorder prevents them from working. The converse is also true; richer individuals are able to escape to quality, usually private health care. This inverse relationship between morbidity or mortality and socioeconomic status has recently been emphasized by Pappas et al (1993). They have shown that, in the USA, the disparity between the death rates of poor and poorly educated people and those with higher incomes *increased* between 1960 and 1986. One of the most effective weapons that we have to ensure that those with severe haemophilia escape this trend is a system of audit, which is described in Chapter 16.

Once the diagnosis has been established and the resting level, if any, of the relevant factor in the bloodstream measured, the patient should be issued with written confirmation in the form of a card, which can be shown to doctors or dentists consulted in the future. Information on the card should be updated as treatment options change. Details of the information that should be recorded are shown in Table 15.2. In the UK a card prepared on behalf of the Department of Health is issued through officially recognized haemophilia centres. A similar card, which has the useful addition of a space for the patient's photograph, is available from the World Federation of Hemophilia. It is very important that all the information on the card is explained verbally to the patient and to his family. Illiteracy is widespread, and denial of illiteracy is common.

All patients and their families should be encouraged to join a Haemophilia Society or Foundation. A good society provides support, allows people to share problems and their solutions, and encourages good comprehensive care by continually updating members' knowledge of advances in therapy and, when necessary, representing patients' interests to their doctors.

Effective and safe treatment

Clotting factor concentrates are expensive and likely to remain so. This is partly because the companies concerned are, like all commercial companies, in business to make profits, and partly because the research and development involved in manufacture demands stringent quality control to remove viral contaminants. There is also a gross imbalance in the global market with less than a quarter of haemophiliacs having access to treatment. In addition, whilst presently available concentrates appear safe, there remain concerns about viral transmission (for instance the transmission of non-enveloped pathogens) and the stimulation of inhibitor formation. It is therefore imperative that the prescription of concentrates for a particular patient be both justified and closely monitored.

Whenever possible an alternative to concentrate should be used, the most appropriate for haemophilia A or von Willebrand's disease usually being desmopressin (deamino-8-D-arginine vasopressin; DDAVP) (Mannucci et al, 1977), which can now, for most purposes, be given intranasally. Desmopressin is only effective if the patient is able to make some endogenous factor VIII. It is therefore of value in people with mild haemophilia A or some types of von Willebrand's disease, notably type I. It is useless in people with other factor deficiencies, and is contraindicated in von Willebrand's disease type IIB because it causes thrombocytopenia. All those prescribed desmopressin should be warned of the danger of water intoxication if they do not restrict their fluid intake after a dose.

Within the developed world, patients with haemophilia B are relying increasingly on high-purity factor IX concentrates, which appear to carry a reduced risk of thromboembolism than the less pure prothrombin complex concentrates (Kasper 1973; Blatt et al, 1974; Mannucci et al, 1990; Gray et al, 1993). Both cryoprecipitate (for the treatment of factor VIII deficiency or afibrinogenaemia) and fresh frozen plasma (for the treatment of minor haemorrhage in haemophilia B) are no longer recommended because of the risk of viral transmission, but both are still the mainstay of therapy for people in developing countries with access to a bloodbank. New ways of removing enveloped viral contaminants, especially human imunodeficiency virus (HIV), using solvent detergent technology on these blood products should help to reduce or eliminate this threat.

Recently, attention has been focused on whether repeated exposure to exogenous protein within concentrates is safe, or whether it may cause a decline in immunity in multitransfused patients over time. There is, as yet, no convincing evidence that "pure" is better and, in particular, no evidence whatsoever of clinical disease as a result of long-term exposure to intermediate-purity products. Barrowcliffe (personal communication) has suggested that the terminology of "purity" be changed, partly because different manufacturers measure different things and partly because of the paradoxical situation in which some very pure products must have stabilizers for the otherwise fragile factor VIII molecule added. For instance, recombinant factor VIII presently has a human albumin stabilizer.

Whatever the eventual advantages or disadvantages of these products, one thing is clear. They are all more expensive than the intermediate-purity products, which are equally efficacious in the control of haemorrhage. Therefore, with the exception of patients infected with HIV for whom there is evidence of benefit, the case for use of high-purity concentrates remains unproven. From the viewpoint of finite world resources there is an additional argument for reserving their use. Despite great advances in conserving the yields of clotting factor in finished products, more source material is still required if the goal is higher "purity" and this may result in an overall shortage of factor VIII.

Twenty-four hour cover

Home therapy provides instantaneous access to treatment for most bleeds, but immediate help in hospital at any time must also be provided for haemorrhage that cannot be controlled, or which could threaten life and limb. A major part of the training for home therapy is the teaching of patients and their families to recognize when they must seek help. An obvious example of this is the care of head injury following which a hospital consultation, and often admission, is mandatory.

Families should have direct access to specialist help without the need to call a family doctor or to go via an Accident and Emergency (Casualty) department. This is because most doctors are unfamiliar with the treatment of haemophilia and may not appreciate how important it is to trust the patient's word that he is bleeding, despite the absence of physical signs.

Cover for holidays or business trips away from home is part of the 24-hour rule. Families should carry with them up-to-date details of their medication and any complications of their haemophilia, together with a supply of concentrate (or desmopressin) and, if intending to cross international frontiers, a note for Customs and Excise. They should also have knowledge of where to seek specialist help at their destination.

Finally, all those with haemophilia or a related disorder should wear identification with reference to the need for special help. Suitably inscribed "dog tags" or bracelets from Talisman or MedicAlert are widely available.

Regular follow-up

A commitment to regular follow-up is an essential part of the contract between the patient and his doctor at the haemophilia centre. Physical, social and psychological health should be checked regularly both in order to ensure that the prescribed treatment is working and to monitor that treatment for possible side-effects. All severely affected adults should be seen at least once a year, and all severely affected children at least every 6 months. In practice, most patients come to their local centre more frequently than this in order to ask questions and collect home therapy supplies.

Follow-up should, as a routine, include a full physical and musculoskeletal assessment, an opportunity for social assessment and a series of investigations. The exact nature of the latter will depend on the individual and on his or her exposure to blood products since they were last seen. Suggested requirements for follow-up are shown in Table 15.3. After follow-up some families like the reassurance of a letter about the results of the tests; others review progress at their next appointment. In the UK it is routine to write to the family doctor with results and recommendations.

Follow-up gives an opportunity for patients to ask questions and for staff to explain advances in therapy or news about side-effects. It is also the forum for a discussion about the individual use of factor concentrates and how this may be adjusted for the patient's benefit. In some cases these discussions are best held in the informality of the patient's home, especially when children are affected. More can often be achieved by friendly home visits by nurses and social workers from the centre than at formal follow-up in a hospital setting, which is intimidating to some patients and their relatives.

Expert counselling

The constellation of questions that arise in any family with haemophilia can only be answered by a team of people with experience both in the management of bleeding disorders and in special areas of expertise in medicine, surgery, nursing, physiotherapy and social work. The approach to haemophilia has to be multi-disciplinary; there is no place for consultation in isolation. This is especially relevant when genetic counselling is undertaken. It is useless to most couples to be told of the mathematical risks of giving birth to affected children without up-to-date knowledge of how the potential lives of such children could be affected by their disorder. This fact is recognized in the UK Health Service Guidelines, reproduced in Table 15.4.

Good communication

The multiple facets of haemophilia care require the closest possible communication between everyone concerned with treatment and advice. Poor communication will invariably lead to a fragmented haemophilia service. This can be very dangerous if, for instance, a surgeon proceeds without knowledge of the presence of an inhibitor, or the wrong blood product is given. Haemophilia is a rare disorder and a frightening one. Good communication helps both to inform and to reduce fear, allowing affected children to thrive and compete at school, and affected men to work normally.

A mark of the rapport existing in many centres as a result of good communication over the years is that the majority of patients with iatrogenic HIV infection still consult the doctors who probably prescribed the infected blood

Table 15.3 Assessment and investigations at routine follow-up of a patient with severe haemophilia

Date

Name

History since last assessment:

Bleeds:	Site(s) Frequency Cause (if known)
Pain:	Site(s) Severity Medication
Treatment:	On demand/prophylaxis Blood product used Total units used Who usually gives treatment Timing of treatment in relation to bleeds Efficacy Reactions/problems State of venous access Treatment other than blood products

General health

Dental health

Social health

Examination
General including height, weight, blood pressure, urinalysis, clinical abnormalities of liver, spleen, lymph nodes

Musculoskeletal including joint ranges, muscle power, gait, and evidence of arthropathy, synovitis, wasting

Investigations
Haemoglobin and indices
Total white cell count, differential
Platelet count
Immune function, CD4/8 counts
Liver function, ALT/AST
Vaccination status
Inhibitor screen
Radiology if indicated

Table 15.4 Provision of haemophilia treatment and care (adapted from Jones P, Haemophilia Home Therapy, 1980, London: Pitman Medical, pp. 132–134

Executive summary
This guidance sets out the background to haemophilia treatment and care, highlights the particular features and requirements of patients suffering from haemophilia and related conditions, and reminds National Health Service purchasers of the considerations that they will need to take into account in order to secure continuity of access to comprehensive treatment and care for these patients.

Action
Health Authorities will need to have regard to the considerations set out below in contracting for services to provide haemophilia treatment and care.

Background

The haemophilic condition
The haemophilic population in the UK comprises a group of patients whose medical management is both complex and costly. Some of the complexity arises because of the rarity of the condition, its lifelong nature, its variable severity and the fact that patients do not appear "ill" in the accepted sense of that term. It may not always be understood that the lack of prompt, appropriate treatment may lead to prolonged hospitalization and the misuse or even on occasion the wastage of expensive blood products.

Evolvement of the present mode of patient referral
Haemophilia patients have built up relationships with a chosen Centre for various reasons, and the Centre may not be within their home District. Haemophilia patients have tended to refer themselves directly to a particular haemophilia treatment centre, and have in many cases, though not universally, bypassed customary consultation with the general practitioner (family doctor) because of the specialized knowledge required for their treatment.

Considerations
Health Authorities will need to take into account in contracting for services for haemophilia patients that there are several particular considerations in securing the aim of access to comprehensive care:

- variability and severity of the haemophilic condition;
- complexity of the condition, which may require a diverse and complex range of services. Given the nature of the condition, the amount of treatment required by individual patients will be *unpredictable*;
- expertise in treatment of haemophilia patients is not uniformly available across the country;

Table 15.4 *Continued*

- the need for ease of access to supplies of blood products to support home treatment programmes;
- the prevalence of HIV, which is a significant problem in this group of patients, and the need for treatment and counselling for HIV-infected haemophilia patients;
- individuals may need little more than a review and access to blood products, but more sophisticated treatment will be required in many cases. As far as possible, Districts should plan for this through the contracting process in consultation with professional advisers. "Ad hoc" funding via extracontractual referrals is a poor alternative to proper service planning.

Contracts

Contracts should ensure that each patient has access to the services required to provide comprehensive care and will need to incorporate quality standards. Treatment can be provided by two types of haemophilia treatment centres, Comprehensive Care Centres and Haemophilia Centres, according to the services and facilities that they provide.

Access to the services required to provide comprehensive care can be secured either through a contract with a single Comprehensive Care Centre, or through contracts with a Haemophilia Centre and with a Comprehensive Care Centre for those services not available at the Haemophilia Centre.

The way in which access to these services is achieved will depend upon local facilities and the needs of individual patients. Contracts should secure access to comprehensive care on a planned basis. In view of the unpredictability of need and the potentially large cost involved, simple block contracts and Extracontractual Referrals (that is referrals for treatment of patients outwith the usual contracts drawn up by a particular hospital) may not be an appropriate form of contracting for haemophilia care. Purchasers are encouraged to move towards more sophisticated block or threshold contracts, which will take account of these considerations in contracting for haemophilia treatment and care, and to increase their use of cost and volume and cost per case contracts.

Medical audit

As part of the contracting process, health authorities will be seeking to obtain quality and cost-effective services for their haemophilia patients. The UK Regional Haemophilia Centre Directors' Organization has prepared a scheme of Medical Audit, which will play an important role in enabling all haemophilia treatment centres to maintain the highest standards of care.

products for them. The friendship and rapport that exists within haemophilia practice, despite all the problems of the past decade, should provide encouragement to those thinking of working with haemophilia. The discipline of contemporary medical management is tempered by enjoyment in most haemophilia centres; too great an emphasis on efficiency and economy can stifle the creativity and fun of working with one of the most infuriating but fascinating disorders in medicine.

Home Therapy

Much of modern haemophilia care is common sense. It is obviously more convenient for everyone – patient, family, doctor, schoolteacher, employer – when bleeds are treated quickly with minimal disturbance to everyday life. It is also in the best interests of the patient's health; bleeds treated before the appearance of physical signs stop quickly with the minimum of tissue damage. Bleeds treated late demand more and more frequent blood product and, when they recur in a major joint, inevitably result in haemophilic arthropathy.

Home therapy has economic advantages too. School or work is not disrupted, costs in travelling to and from hospital (which usually involve more than one person) are avoided, and there are savings for the hospital in terms of staff time and the use of facilities. Given all this, it now seems unbelievable that early attempts to introduce haemophilia home therapy were opposed on the grounds that lay people should not be taught to give themselves intravenous injections safely. The law of some countries, for example Italy and Spain, initially forbade self-injection, whilst in others physicians were reluctant to encourage home therapy because of the potential loss of earnings to themselves.

Nowadays home therapy is an essential component of comprehensive care. It has been placed within this context for a very good reason. It is as useless and potentially harmful to provide someone with haemophilia with a few boxes of concentrate and equipment and leave him to get on with it, as it is to give a diabetic a year's supply of insulin without the means to test his blood sugar levels. Good home therapy, like good diabetic therapy, requires discipline. Without it the patient and his family soon lose control of the disorder. Loss of control of haemophilia leads to crippling, handicap, and physical, social and psychological disadvantage. The criteria for home therapy are listed in Table 15.5. They are few in number and related mainly to the ability of a patient or his family to learn and maintain good venepuncture technique. When the disorder is mild and the need for treatment infrequent, there is little point in training for home therapy unless the home is geographically remote from the centre or the affected person travels widely in the course of his work.

Table 15.5 Criteria for home therapy

- Clinically severe, or moderately severe, haemophilia
- Adequate venous access
- Capable of techniques involved, including venepuncture and safe disposal of equipment
- Emotional acceptance of disorder
- Working knowledge of when to treat
- Relaxed relationship with centre staff
- Commitment to comprehensive care, including accurate record-keeping and regular follow-up

Documentation

The follow-up of severe haemophilia does not fit easily into the commonly used systems of medical record-keeping. The multiple bleeding episodes of the acute disorder, the long-term sequelae of the inadequately treated chronic disorder and the often unexpected demands imposed by the development of complications or surgery result in voluminous hospital and general practice records. Add to this the need for family studies and carrier detection and the unending psycho-social problems of some patients, and it is not surprising that routine haemophilia casenotes are, at best, indigestible and, at worst, indecipherable.

What is the information that is *essential* to record if someone with severe haemophilia is to receive the best possible treatment?

Inpatient records

It is important that the haemophilic patient is treated in exactly the same way as the non-haemophilic patient when hospital admission is indicated. It is tempting to skip the detailed medical history and examination of someone who is seen frequently as an outpatient. However, when this happens the patient is denied the scrutiny of the fresh mind and approach of the admitting doctor who may well uncover symptoms or signs of concurrent disease. The junior doctor is denied the opportunity of learning in depth about how people cope and adapt to the demands of chronic disease with acute exacerbations. The nursing staff are denied the full background information they need to ensure that the patient is nursed in safety.

When the approach of the admitting doctor is superficial, things are more likely to go wrong. An operation starts before laboratory proof of a good response to treatment. A wound is disturbed just before clotting factor infusion rather than just after. No-one notices the failure of response that heralds inhibitor formation until uncontrolled bleeding supervenes. Clear inpatient records with concise summaries are also needed both as historical documents useful in the long-term follow-up of patients and as essential tools in the retrospective analysis of side-effects and possible medico-legal work.

The detailed recording of replacement therapy during admission is made easier if a standard format for the recording of all treatment is adopted and used for outpatient and home therapy as well.

Outpatient records

Here, the essential information required can be divided into two categories: the recording of treatment of individual bleeds and the recording of follow-up examinations and investigations.

The treatment of bleeds

In 1979, on behalf of the World Federation of Hemophilia, I looked at the ways in which different clinics and families kept records of bleeds and replacement therapy (Jones, 1979). The most usual was the written diary or dated log, but

HAEMOPHILIA RECORD CARD

PATIENT'S SURNAME: FIRST NAME: DATE OF BIRTH:

HOME THERAPY: ☐ OUTPATIENT: ☐ INPATIENT: ☐

WHERE SEEN: HOSPITAL ☐ CLINIC/WARD: ☐

SITE(S) OF BLEED

JOINT	RIGHT	LEFT	MUSCLE	RIGHT	LEFT			
SHOULDER	☐	☐	UPPER ARM	☐	☐	GASTRO-INTESTINAL	☐	TICK IF BLEED CAUSED BY TRAUMA (INJURY) ☐
ELBOW	☐	☐	FOREARM	☐	☐	GENITO-URINARY	☐	
WRIST	☐	☐	ILIOPSOAS	☐	☐	HEAD INJURY/INTRACRANIAL	☐	
HAND	☐	☐	QUADRICEPS	☐	☐	LACERATION	☐	
HIP	☐	☐	HAMSTRINGS	☐	☐	OTHER	☐	
KNEE	☐	☐	CALF	☐	☐	DENTAL	☐	
ANKLE	☐	☐	OTHER	☐	☐	SURGICAL	☐	
FOOT	☐	☐						
OTHER	☐	☐	EPISTAXIS	☐	☐			

ADDITIONAL CLINICAL INFORMATION:

Figure 15.2 The front of the treatment card used by the Newcastle Haemophilia Centre (see text).

TICK IF TREATMENT PROPHYLACTIC

WAS THIS TREATMENT FOR A FRESH BLEEDING EPISODE? YES/NO

IF YES, TRANSFUSION GIVEN WITHIN: 1HR / 2 HRS / 12 HRS / > 12 HRS

BLOOD PRODUCT

NAME OF PRODUCT GIVEN	NO. OF VIALS	ACTUAL UNITS IN VIAL	DOSE IN UNITS	LOT/BATCH NUMBER	EXPIRY DATE (ON VIAL)

ADVERSE REACTION:

OTHER TREATMENT PRESCRIBED:	DOSE:	FREQUENCY:	DURATION:
CYKLOKAPRON DDAVP OTHER:			

CHECKED BY: (NAME IN BLOCK CAPITALS)	GIVEN BY: (NAME IN BLOCK CAPITALS)	OFFICE USE: ON COMPUTER: ON FLOWCHART:

Figure 15.3 The reverse of the treatment card used by the Newcastle Haemophilia Centre (see text).

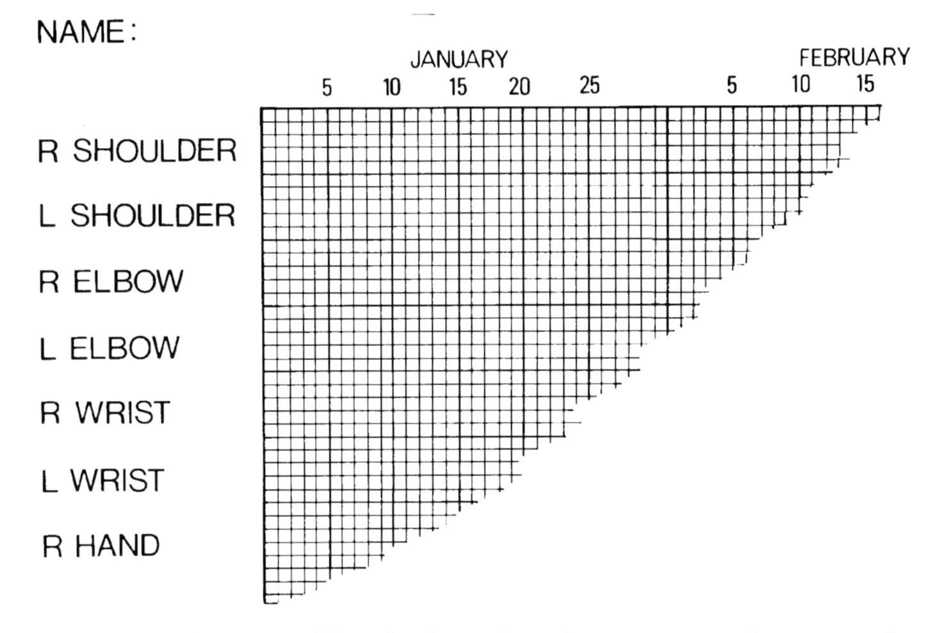

Figure 15.4 A corner of the calendar used to chart treatments given to a patient with haemophilia. Each treatment is entered as a vertical line: in the upper part of a particular day for morning therapy, in the lower part for afternoon therapy.

NAME: M.B. 4 yrs   YEAR: 1978

	January	February	March	April	May	June	July	August	September	October	November	December
R SHOULDER												
L SHOULDER												
R ELBOW												
L ELBOW												
R WRIST												
L WRIST												
R HAND												
L HAND												
R HIP												
L HIP												
R KNEE												
L KNEE												
R ANKLE												
L ANKLE												
R FOOT												
L FOOT							T					
MUSCLE					T R Forearm; Forearms				T L Calf			
DENTAL												
OTHER										T Head		
PROPHYLAXIS												

when it comes to assessing how well or how badly a patient is doing at follow-up consultations, which may be many months apart, the information in a written record can be very difficult to condense and interpret. It is also of little value as a teaching aid to affected children and, of course, useless to families with poor standards of literacy. For these reasons we have developed a system based on a checklist and a calendar rather than on a written description of each treatment.

The system consists of a card on which both clinical and treatment details are recorded, and a calendar that is filled in to provide a visual record of an individual's progress over time. The card is shown in Figures 15.2 and 15.3. It is coloured to differentiate it from other paperwork and the information it carries is easily transcribed for use in computer systems. It is used whenever treatment is given at home or in hospital and is completed by the person giving that treatment. People on home therapy can only obtain further supplies of clotting factor concentrate on receipt of their completed cards, which are checked by the nursing and secretarial staff of the Haemophilia Centre. Similar systems exist when supplies are provided by a home delivery service, an extension of comprehensive care increasingly used in countries like the USA where long distances separate families and their treatment centres. Examples of home infusion companies are Quantum Health Resources Inc. (USA) and Caremark (UK). Services like these are understandably popular with patients, but must not be allowed to take the place of comprehensive medical supervision and follow-up by centre staff experienced in the management of haemophilia.

The collective information available from these cards provides a record of:

- treated bleeds
- sites of bleeds
- timing of treatment
- timing in relationship to start of bleed
- number of treatments needed to stop bleeds
- type of treatment and doses used
- where treatment given
- person(s) giving treatment
- batch numbers and expiry dates of product(s) used
- concomitant treatment
- difficulties and short-term adverse reactions.

Figure 15.5 Treatments given in 1 year to a 4-year-old boy with severe haemophilia A. Reading from left to right, the first treatment was given on the morning of 20th January for a bleed in the left shoulder. The second was for a bleed in the right ankle on the morning of 2nd March. At the beginning of July a bleed into the left foot caused by trauma (T) had to be treated twice (morning and afternoon). The chart shows that the majority of bleeds were into the ankles, a typical pattern at this age. It also shows that all the joint bleeds stopped with one treatment, confirming that the correct dose of factor VIII was being prescribed.

NAME: L.A. 26 yrs   YEAR: 1978

	January	February	March	April	May	June	July	August	September	October	November	December
R SHOULDER												
L SHOULDER												
R ELBOW							3					
L ELBOW												
R WRIST												
L WRIST												
R HAND	T											T
L HAND												
R HIP												
L HIP												
R KNEE				3		3 3		3			3	
L KNEE												
R ANKLE												
L ANKLE												
R FOOT												
L FOOT					T		T					
MUSCLE				R Hamstring	R Thigh		3 L Biceps					
DENTAL												
OTHER												
PROPHYLAXIS.												

At follow-up a synopsis is available for comparison with previous personal and group records and for discussion with the patient and his family in the form of:

- amount of product used since last assessment (international units of VIII or IX)
- type of product used
- types and sites of bleeds
- timing of treatments.

Transcription of each treatment to a calendar chart (Figs 15.4–15.6) shows immediately where bleeds have occurred, whether they are stopping quickly on the dose of product previously prescribed, and whether there has been any targeting at a particular site. Annual calendars are easily understood by children and adults, and are especially useful in demonstrating changes for good or bad over time, both in the individual and by comparison with the charts of other patients. These are valuable in cases where the standards of literacy or understanding are poor. By laying the charts out on the consulting room floor in sequence, it is possible to "walk through the years" with the patient and his family in order to show them how changes in therapy affect bleeding patterns. One example of the value of this "visual audit" is its use in showing someone how prophylaxis can dramatically alter a bleeding pattern (Fig. 15.7).

Regular Follow-up and Family Support

With an incidence of 1 in 5000 males, haemophilia is a rare disorder unlikely to be seen by the average family doctor. The incidence of haemophilia B is some five times less than that for haemophilia A, and of severe von Willebrand's disease even lower. For this reason alone the care of someone with an inherited bleeding disorder should be based at a hospital centre rather than in the community. The staff of a haemophilia centre have immediate access to both the concentrates and other products needed for treatment and the laboratory and other resources needed to monitor that treatment. They also have up-to-date knowledge of the best treatment to recommend for each patient. This knowledge changes rapidly as new techniques are introduced to try and ensure

---

Figure 15.6 The treatment pattern in a 26-year-old man with severe haemophilia A. The right elbow and left knee were target joints in 1978. Several bleeds did not stop with a single dose of factor VIII, a particularly severe haemarthrosis of the right knee needing six treatments before it stopped. In October a left hip bleed required hospital admission (hatched area). In retrospect this patient would have benefited from prophylaxis.

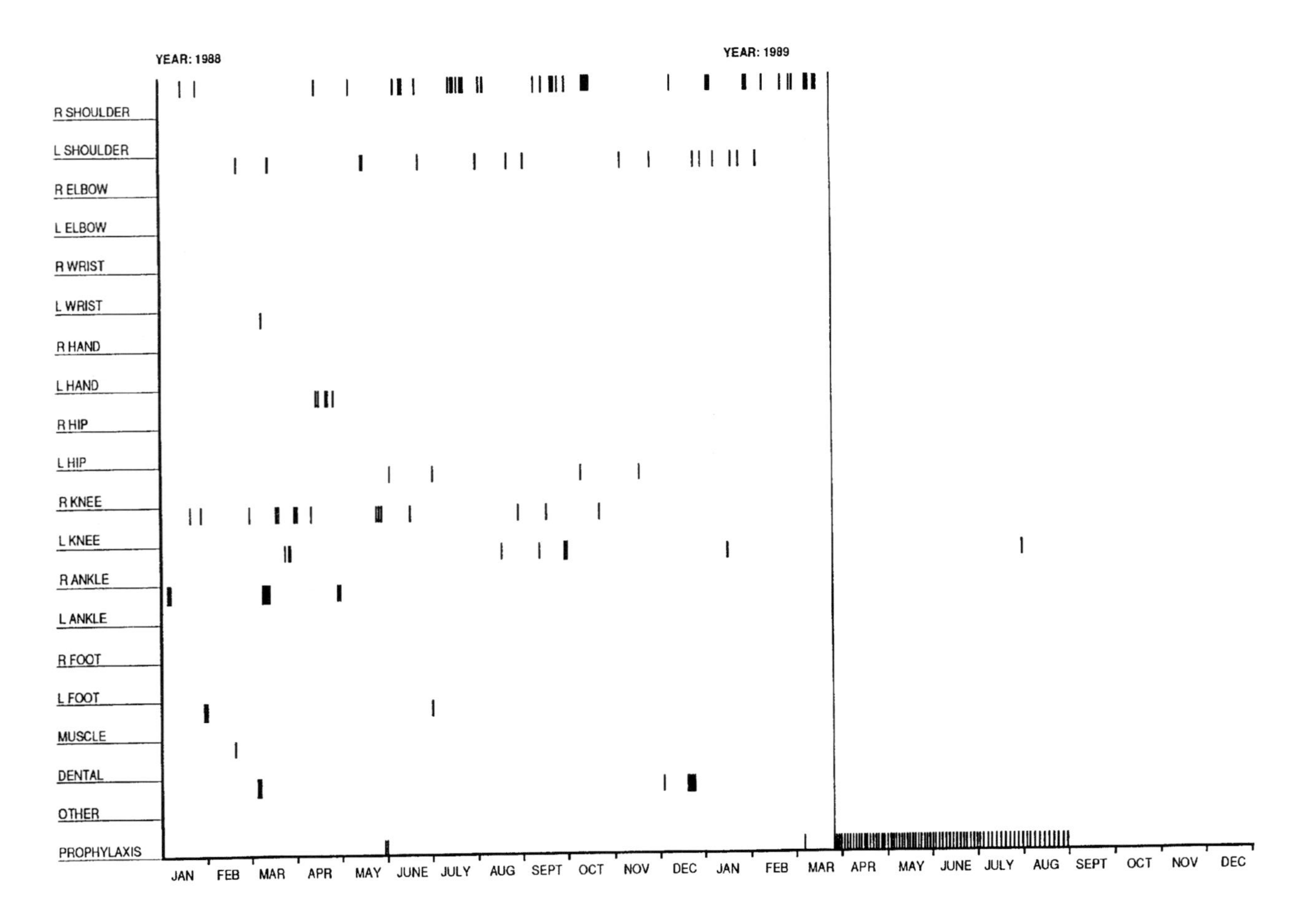
YEAR: 1988
YEAR: 1989
R SHOULDER
L SHOULDER
R ELBOW
L ELBOW
R WRIST
L WRIST
R HAND
L HAND
R HIP
L HIP
R KNEE
L KNEE
R ANKLE
L ANKLE
R FOOT
L FOOT
MUSCLE
DENTAL
OTHER
PROPHYLAXIS
JAN
FEB
MAR
APR
MAY
JUNE
JULY
AUG
SEPT
OCT
NOV
DEC
JAN
FEB
MAR
APR
MAY
JUNE
JULY
AUG
SEPT
OCT
NOV
DEC

the viral safety of blood products, and the overall safety of both blood and recombinant factor replacement therapy. The dual catastrophes of HIV and hepatitis contamination highlight how difficult this task can be both for the manufacturers and for the treaters.

Regular follow-up over the years inevitably leads to the establishment of friendship and emotional bonds between families and their centre. In general this bond is a good thing because it makes for informality and ease of approach. Most centres have an open door policy, encouraging people in difficulty to drop in at any time without the need for a formal appointment. Providing that this informality is subject to the objectivity of scrutiny by the professional staff of the centre, it is welcome. Abuses are rare and easily recognized, and should be discussed and resolved at weekly team meetings between the medical and other staff.

In many ways a busy haemophilia centre is like a general practice within the scientific setting of a hospital. The myriad problems that can present to any family at any time are coloured by the underlying bleeding disorder and therefore usually present to the centre rather than the general practitioner. Many can only be answered with specialist advice, and that is why the haemophilia team has to draw its expertise from a wide range of people, both in the hospital and in the community.

One of the possible structures for a comprehensive care centre providing support for haemophilic families is shown in Fig. 15.8. It relies for day-to-day management on a relatively small core team. It is essential that the people within this team are experienced in the care of severe haemophilia and are available without undue delay. Outwith the core team are a host of other experts and organizations, as diverse as blood transfusion services and head teachers, and dentists and housing officers. "Care for the carers" is usually a natural function of the core team rather than an outside agency, but help from others should be available if it is needed.

The requirements that need to be met by a centre providing comprehensive care have recently been formalized by the UK National Health Management Executive in association with the UK Haemophilia Centre Directors Organization (Health Service Guidelines, 1993; Table 15.6). The list forms a part of the document shown in Table 15.4. It is intended for managers and others with a responsibility for the provision of patient services. Although a part of the document is only applicable to the National Health Service, it is worth including in full because it provides a concise overview of what is needed to provide comprehensive care.

Figure 15.7 Calendar chart showing the effect of starting prophylaxis in March 1988. Prior to prophylaxis, multiple bleeds targeted major joints. This chart provides a graphic illustration of how haemophilic bleeding disrupts life, and has proved a valuable teaching tool when seeking financial support for haemophilia care.

Prophylaxis

At face value, prophylaxis seems to present the only logical approach to haemophilia care. If the relevant deficient or absent clotting factor is replaced by an active molecule, at the very least severe haemophilia is converted into a milder form. Spontaneous haemorrhage is avoided, and joint and muscle function is preserved. Haemophilic arthropathy and handicap in later life disappear.

Work in several countries, especially Sweden and the Netherlands, has shown conclusively that long-term prophylaxis works (Petrini et al, 1991; Nilsson et al, 1992). The results from individual centres using prophylaxis have now been supported by the findings of the international group looking at objective orthopaedic change associated with a variety of different dosage regimens over

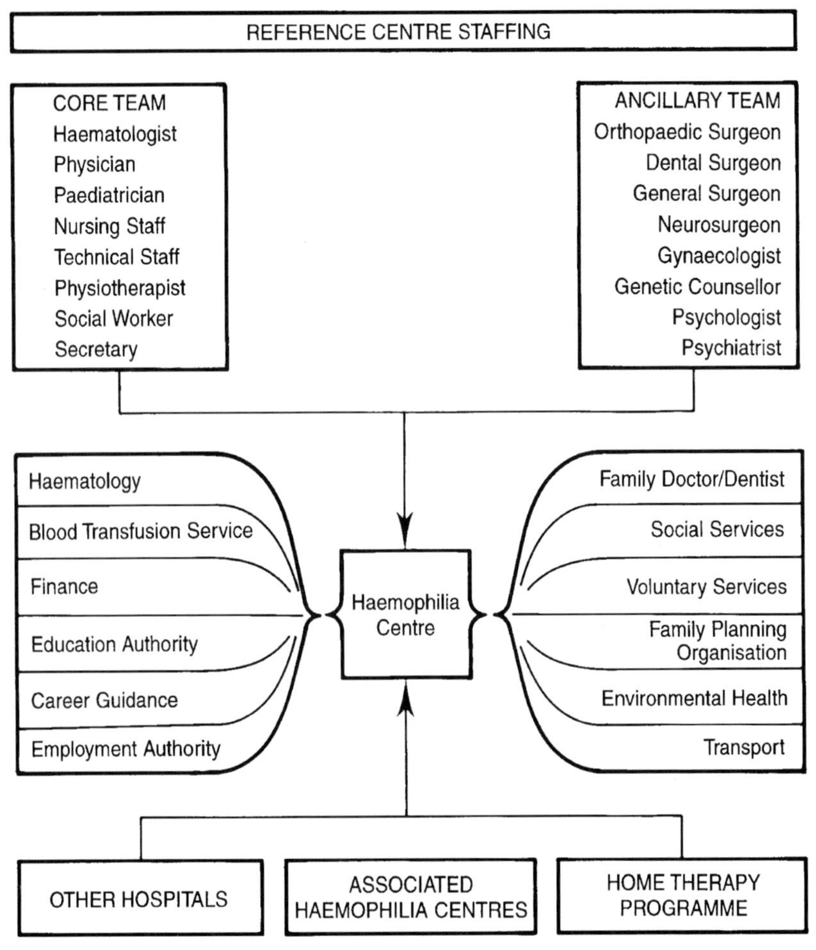

Figure 15.8 Haemophilia centre organization.

Table 15.6 Services provided by Haemophilia Centres

The Comprehensive Care Centre

A Comprehensive Care Centre normally provides treatment for 40 or more severely affected (less than 0.02 units of clotting factor present per millilitre of plasma) patients per year and needs to be able to provide all the following facilities:

(i) a clinical service provided by experienced staff for the treatment of patients with haemostatic disorders and their families at short notice at any time of the day or night

(ii) a laboratory service capable of carrying out all tests necessary for the definitive diagnosis of haemophilia and all common inherited haemorrhagic disorders, including the identification and assay of the relevant specific haemostatic factors. Further, capable of monitoring therapy and carrying out preliminary testing for inhibitors

(iii) where appropriate and indicated, to conduct in collaboration with other haemophilia treatment centres the further investigation of relatives of patients with haemophilia or other haemostatic disorders

(iv) an advisory service to patients and close relatives on matters specific to haemophilia. Advice should also be given to general practitioners (family doctors) as appropriate

(v) maintenance of satisfactory quality control and assurance for all laboratory tests offered in relation to clinical services, both by establishing appropriate internal procedures and by participation at the appropriate level in the UK National External Quality Assessment Scheme in Blood Coagulation (NEQAS), or other relevant approved external quality assessment schemes

(vi) maintenance of medical records; records must be maintained of all treatment administered and all adverse reactions reported. Special medical cards are to be issued and a register kept of all patients attending the centre

(vii) counselling in privacy of patients and their relatives

(viii) participation in appropriate clinical audit

(ix) where appropriate, to provide advice on and organization of home therapy programmes either individually or in collaboration with other haemophilia treatment centres

(x) the provision of prophylactic treatment programmes for patients with haemophilia and other haemostatic disorders

(xi) 24-hour advisory service to Haemophilia Centres and support to such Centres as appropriate

(xii) a specialist consultant service for all surgery including orthopaedic and dental, for infectious diseases (such as HIV and hepatitis) and paediatric care, and for genetic, HIV, social care and any other counselling services

(xiii) a reference laboratory service for Haemophilia Centres. The services should also include the diagnosis of atypical cases, genotypic analysis, the assay of inhibitors and other haemostatic factors, the diagnosis of hereditary platelet disorders, the supply of assay standards and reagents and, when requested, advice and recommendations concerning analytical procedures

(xiv) educational facilities for medical staff, nurses, medical laboratory scientific officers, counsellors and other personnel as required in order to promote optimal comprehensive care of patients

(xv) coordination of meetings and undertaking research programmes, including the conduct of clinical trials and to establish and participate in suitable Regional and National programmes of clinical audit.

The Haemophilia Centre

It would normally be expected that a Haemophilia Centre would provide services (i) to (ix) above.

a 5-year period. The conclusion of this, the Orthopedic Outcome Study (Aledort, 1994), was that patients on prophylaxis for more than 45 weeks a year had significantly fewer joint and total bleeding episodes, significantly less progression of radiological change over time and significantly fewer days lost from school or work than patients receiving on-demand replacement therapy. Why then do we not recommend that everyone with clinically severe haemophilia A or B is started on prophylaxis?

The first reason is financial. As Aledort has pointed out, the cost of long-term prophylaxis may be prohibitive. Most budget-holders still look at patient treatment in the short term and haemophilia costs usually head any hospital drug expenditure list. Administrators will have to be persuaded to think in the long term if prophylaxis is to be offered to all severely affected children. They need to know that early investment is worthwhile in terms of lower future expenditure on the control or repair of joint damage, and the costs of both physical and social handicap. This is a difficult challenge because a comprehensive look at both hospital and community expenditure is required if a true picture of the cost benefit ratio to the individual with severe haemophilia is to emerge.

Presumed increases in cost when prophylaxis is prescribed depend on an assumption that there will be an overall increase in the amount of therapeutic material used. However, dosages reported in studies of the effect of haemophilia A prophylaxis vary widely, from 500 to 6240 iu/kg of body weight/year. This means that a 10-year-old boy weighing 30 kg needs between 15 000 and 187 000 iu of factor VIII a year. This wide divergence was looked at in the Orthopedic Outcome Study, which concluded that a dosage of ≥2000 iu/kg/year (or, in the case of the 10 year old, 60 000 iu of factor VIII) produced the best results if given as regular prophylaxis to eliminate bleeding episodes. If prophylaxis is continued to 18 years, or beyond the years of growth, the total amount of factor VIII needed for a 70 kg man with severe haemophilia A is 140 000 iu per year.

In global terms the answer to whether long-term prophylaxis can be justified is more obvious. It is estimated that only 20% of people with haemophilia presently receive treatment and that the great majority of these live in developed countries. The reasons for this disparity are complex, but the main one is a lack of availability of replacement therapy at an affordable price. As pointed out earlier in this chapter, an increase in consumption within the wealthy nations will inevitably add to the problems of health care delivery in poorer countries. In the long term, cheap recombinant factor or the application of gene therapy may solve this imbalance. In the meantime can we justify the increase in demand required by prophylaxis?

Prophylaxis does not prolong life and there is little evidence that the quality of life is improved more than that of someone on well regulated, on-demand home therapy. If the aim is to prevent all joint damage, then prophylaxis must be started before the first joint bleed. In practice, this means that regular intravenous injections should start at around 2 years of age. It also means that the injections should continue at least until the risk of spontaneous haemarthroses is lowest, a time thought to coincide with cessation of growth, which in males occurs at around the age of 18 years.

The average number of bleeds occurring in someone with severe haemophilia is 35 per year. If the dosage is right and bleeds are treated promptly, most stop with one treatment (Jones, 1980). In contrast a patient on alternate-day prophylaxis requires 182 injections a year, together with the occasional treatment for a breakthrough or accidental bleed. Therefore, over the 16-year period taking him from infancy to adulthood, the youngster on prophylaxis presently has to have 182 × 16 = 2912 intravenous injections, in contrast to some 35 × 16 = 560 injections for somebody using on-demand home therapy. Of course, in reality the life of a growing boy with haemophilia is rarely as ordered as this, and the sums can give only a simplistic view. However, they do indicate a difference that is, in my experience, recognized by many families. Despite the proven advantages of prophylaxis in terms of prevention of arthritis in later life, many patients prefer the option of on-demand therapy. Regular injections are described as boring, an intrusion into everyday life, and a constant reminder of haemophilia, which they would prefer to forget about until treatment became necessary. This argument holds much less strongly for someone with haemophilia B who, because of the longer half-life of factor IX in comparison with that of factor VIII, usually only requires prophylactic injections at weekly intervals.

The need for haemophilia A patients on prophylaxis to inject themselves so often has led to a search for better methods of venous access and for ways in which the half-life of factor VIII can be extended. Presently, some doctors advocate the use of indwelling cannulas but, whilst long lines have proved very popular with some families, consensus opinion is that they are not without risk of infection and that this, together with the finite life of present devices, contraindicates their use in the majority of children for whom a more acceptable treatment option is available. If a reliable pump capable of constantly infusing low-dose prophylactic therapy becomes a reality, their views, and the problems associated with high rates of factor VIII consumption, will change.

Finally, a child started on prophylaxis before his first bleed grows up without any experience of haemophilia. If prophylaxis ceases he will not be able to recognize the aura that precedes the physical signs of a bleed and, as a consequence, unnecessary tissue damage will occur. The situation is analogous to the severely affected diabetic who has never experienced a hypoglycaemic episode, and therefore has no concept of the symptoms that warn him or her to seek help.

Summary

Within this chapter I have explained some of the ways in which comprehensive care might be used for the mutual benefit of people with haemophilia, their families and the members of staff working on their behalf in haemophilia centres.

Of course, there are many other approaches to optimum care. Anyone in doubt about which method or methods to use should ask the patients how they perceive the role of the medical and paramedical professions in their lives (Hopkins and Wallace, 1993). Their answers are sometimes surprising!

References

Aledort LM, Haschmeyer RH, Pettersson H, the Orthopaedic Outcome Study Group. A longitudinal study of orthopaedic outcomes for severe factor-VIII-deficient haemophiliacs. *Journal of Internal Medicine* 1994; **236**: 391–399.

Aronstam A. *Haemophilic Bleeding: Early Management at Home.* London: Baillière Tindall, 1985: 101–107.

Biggs R. Thirty years of haemophilia treatment in Oxford. *British Journal of Haematology* 1967; **13:** 452.

Birch CLaF. *Haemophilia, Clinical and Genetic Aspects.* Urbana: University of Illinois, 1937.

Blatt PM, Lundblad RL, Kingdon HS, et al. Thrombogenic materials in prothrombin complex concentrates. *Annuals of Internal Medicine* 1974; **81:** 766–770.

Gray E, Tubbs J, Cesmeli S, Barrowcliffe TW. Thrombogenicity of factor IX concentrates: in vitro and in vivo results. *Thrombosis and Haemostasis* 1993; **69:** 1285 (Abstr. 2655).

Health Service Guidelines. Provision of haemophilia treatment and care. Health Service Guidelines. NHS Management Executive, HSG (93) 30.

Hopkins A, Wallace P. *Measurement of Patients' Satisfaction with their Care.* London: Royal College of Physicians, 1993.

Jones P. *World Federation of Haemophilia: Hemophilia Medical Records and Data Collection.* Montreal: World Federation of Hemophilia, 1979.

Jones P (Ed.). *Haemophilia Home Therapy.* London: Pitman Medical, 1980.

Kasper CK. Postoperative thromboses in hemophilia B. *New England Journal of Medicine* 1973; **289**: 160.

Mannucci PM, Ruggeri ZM, Pareti FI, Capitanio A. Deamino-8-D-arginine vasopressin: a new pharmacological approach to the management of haemophilia and von Willebrand's disease. *Lancet* 1977; 869–872.

Mannucci PM, Bauer KA, Gringeri A, et al. Thrombin generation is not increased in the blood of haemophilia B patients after infusion of a purified factor IX concentrate. *Blood* 1990; **76:** 2540–2545.

Nilsson IM, Berntorp E, Löfquist T, Pettersson H. Twenty five years experience of prophylactic treatment in severe haemophilia A and B. *Journal of Internal Medicine* 1992; **232:** 25–32.

Pappas G, Queen S, Hadden W, Fisher G. The increasing disparity in mortality between socioeconomic groups in the United States, between 1960 and 1986. *New England Journal of Medicine* 1993; **329:** 103–109.

Petrini P, Lindvall N, Egberg N, Blombäck M. Prophylaxis with factor concentrates in preventing hemophilia arthropathy. *American Journal of Pediatric Hematology/Oncology* 1991; **13:** 280–287.

World Federation of Hemophilia. *Decade Plan.* Montreal: World Federation of Hemophilia, 1992.

16 Clinical Audit of Haemophilia Care

Gordon D.O. Lowe

Introduction

In the previous chapter, standards of haemophilia care were reviewed, and the issue of how to achieve and maintain such standards was addressed. Clinical (or medical) audit has been defined as "the systematic, critical analysis of the quality of medical care, including the procedures used for diagnosis and treatment, the use of resources, and the resulting outcome and quality of life for the patient" (Department of Health, 1989). In this review, the term *clinical* audit will be used in preference to *medical* audit. This terminology is increasingly used within the UK, reflecting the multidisciplinary nature of health care and hence the need for collaborative audit by all relevant health care professionals, and not only by medical practitioners.

It is important to distinguish *clinical* audit from *financial* audit. In financial audit, accountants check business accounts to check how money was received and how it was spent. Indeed, the term audit is derived from the Latin *audire* (to hear) because in Roman times such financial accounting was verbal rather than written (or more recently, computerized). This having been said, good-quality haemophilia care is expensive and has to compete for funding with other health care services for its share of limited financial resources. Hence the recommendations resulting from clinical audit exercises often have financial implications.

The importance of clinical audit has been increasingly realized and addressed in the last 10 years. During this time, the number of published clinical audits has grown exponentially; as a result new journals dealing solely with such reports have been established. Many audits have shown that standards of medical care were not being met in individual units, hospitals or geographical areas, and that there was considerable variation in practice between such units, hospitals or areas. As a result, pressure for the establishment of formal clinical audit programmes has come from health care providers (professional bodies), patients (their representative bodies), and health care organizers/purchasers (the World Health

Organization, national and regional health departments, and commercial purchasers of health care).

At an international level, the World Health Organization's Appropriate Health Care and Technology Programme included, as target 31: "By 1990, all Member States should have built effective mechanisms for ensuring the quality of patient care" (Hopkins, 1990). In the UK, this issue was addressed by the Department of Health (1989), which required that each health district must have in place by 1991 some system of clinical audit, and also by the Royal College of Physicians of London, which produced a useful review and guidelines (Hopkins, 1990).

As a result of these activities, several countries have developed a national network of clinical standard-setting and audit activity. For example, in Scotland the Department of Health established a Clinical Research and Audit Group (CRAG), which recommended the national development of clinical guidelines by health care professionals. This has been progressed by a national network of relevant professional bodies (colleges): the Scottish Intercollegiate Guidelines Network (SIGN) (Petrie et al, 1995). This body produces (or approves) evidence-based national guidelines, to be implemented by the development of local protocols (Petrie et al, 1995). Such protocols are used to develop standards, which provide the framework for clinical audit programmes. Such programmes are facilitated both nationally and locally (at health board and hospital levels) by clinical audit groups or committees.

Upon this background of international and national development of clinical audit, this chapter will review:

1. the nature of clinical audit,
2. the development of internal clinical audit within a haemophilia centre, and
3. the development of external (national) clinical audit programmes in Scotland and the UK since 1990. Brief descriptions of these developments have been published previously (Lowe, 1993; Clinical Haematology Task Force, 1994).

The Nature of Clinical Audit

As defined above, clinical audit addresses the quality of medical care *systematically*. There are three major categories of clinical care, which can be examined in turn, but which are inter-related.

Structure

This is the quantity and type of available resources, including health care staff and their facilities. For a haemophilia centre, appropriate staff will include health care professionals with expertise in all aspects of haemophilia care (haematology, general medicine, paediatrics, nursing, social work, genetics, psychology and counselling; physiotherapy, rheumatology/rehabilitation and orthopaedics; infective disease, HIV and hepatology; and dental and other surgery). Their facilities will include the haemophilia centre, clinics, wards and equipment. Structure is relatively easy to measure, and to set standards for. However, it is not the whole story; health care quality does not necessarily correlate with staff and facilities.

Process

This is what the health care staff do for the patient. For a haemophilia centre, documented activities include clinic visits for diagnosis, education and review of patients and carriers; results of examinations and actions taken; treatments (home and hospital); and hospital admissions and operations. As with structure, documentation of these activities in hospital records can be reviewed relatively easily, and standards set. However, again it is not the whole story; health care quality does not necessarily correlate with adequacy of documentation.

Outcome

This is the most relevant measure of quality of health care, but is the most difficult to measure. Measurable outcomes include mortality, disability, other complications of the disease or patient care, and measures of patient satisfaction. For a haemophilia centre, disability in adults from chronic arthritis may reflect bleeds in childhood before effective factor replacement prophylaxis or therapy became widely available in the 1970s, rather than reflecting quality of health care in recent years. Likewise, mortality and disability from human immunodeficiency virus (HIV) infection or chronic hepatitis B or C does not usually reflect adversely on historical compliance by haemophilia centres with standard medical practice of ensuring adequate factor replacement prophylaxis or therapy for potentially disabling or fatal bleeding. On the other hand, recent evidence strongly suggests that progressive arthritis and disability from haemophilic arthropathy in children with severe haemophilia is largely preventable by regular prophylaxis (see Chapter 6).

Clinical audit is not only systematic, but *critical*. This presents a problem for internal audit within specialized units such as haemophilia centres, in which specialized staff members may not only be the only "expert" in an aspect of haemophilia care in their geographic area, but also have a "strong" personality, whose advantage is dedication to development of a service to their patients, but whose disadvantage may be oversensitivity (or insensitivity) to local audit by persons with lesser expertise. Such issues prompt the need for nationally organized peer review of specialized units, including haemophilia centres.

Finally, clinical audit should not only be systematic and critical – it should be *effective in implementing change* (Fig. 16.1). To achieve this, audit requires

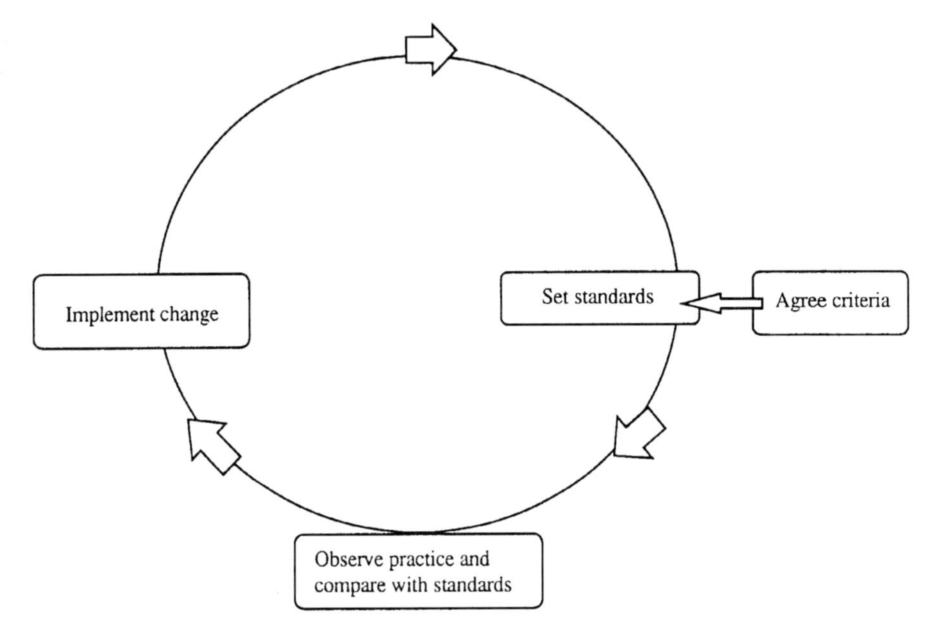

Figure 16.1 The audit cycle.

(a) standards, which are derived from review criteria, which are in turn derived from guidelines (Baker and Fraser, 1995); and (b) repeated audit programmes to assess whether change has occurred (Fig. 16.1). Baker and Fraser (1995) have pointed out that, in general, development of both audit and guidelines have progressed more rapidly than development of criteria and standards. This applies also to haemophilia care. Guidelines for haemophilia care have been developed both internationally (World Health Organization, 1991) and nationally, for example by the United Kingdom Regional Haemophilia Centre Directors' Organization (UKHCDO, 1992). As described below, the latter organization has also developed audit protocols. However, the development of review criteria and standards in haemophilia care remains at a relatively early stage.

Development of Internal Clinical Audit Within a Haemophilia Centre

The need for regular (often monthly for about an hour) formal internal clinical audit is now accepted by most medical units, including haematological units; haemophilia centres should not be an exception to this rule. Clinical audit meetings should be attended by all relevant clinical core staff, including juniors and students in training. Associated haemophilia centre staff (e.g. dental and other surgeons, HIV specialists, hepatologists or geneticists) might attend less frequently (e.g. 3- to 12-monthly), on occasions when their special aspect is addressed at audit meetings. To ensure attendance, the audit programme should be arranged and publicised to relevant personnel in advance (e.g. 6- to 12-monthly). The centre secretary is well placed to coordinate and publicise clinical audit meetings; to attend them, record attendance and take minutes; and to file minutes and produce an annual audit report for the hospital audit committee (and for external auditors: see below).

It is important to define an appropriate regular time and place for internal audit meetings so that as many staff as possible can attend and concentrate on audit without distraction from other activities. In a busy haemophilia centre, staff may have to take it in turns to answer the telephone and attend to patients while audit meetings progress. About 45–60 minutes is usually required to address issues seriously at an audit meeting. The provision of light refreshments can be an incentive to encourage attendance, as can an ongoing, circulated record of attendance by individual centre staff!

Suitable topics for a haematology centre might include (Clinical Haematology Task Force, 1994):

1. *Review of deaths or disasters.* These are clearly important outcomes. Hopefully such events are infrequent, and might be reviewed every 6–12 months.
2. *Audit of several randomly selected case records.* This is largely audit of process, requires little preparation, and can be very revealing! To be systematic, a proforma should be developed and completed (anonymously). As noted above, standards are under development, and will vary between countries, but questions might include the following.
   - Is the patient's bleeding disorder (or carrier status) clearly established, recorded in the centre records, and communicated to their general practitioner? Is the blood group recorded for patients with bleeding disorders?
   - Have they been reviewed in the last year (or the last 6 months for patients on home treatment or with hepatitis B or C infection; or the last 3 months for patients with HIV infection)?
   - If so, were relevant examinations and blood tests performed, and appropriate action taken on the results (including written information to the patient and general practitioner)?
   - Does current treatment accord with national/local guidelines?
   - Are treatment records up to date?
   - Are family investigations up to date?
   - Are clerical standards satisfactory (filing of reports, typing of discharge letters, etc.).
3. *Topic-based audit.* This is more time-consuming to perform, but probably the most educational type of audit. A specific topic is chosen (again usually process, but sometimes structure or outcome) and investigated in an adequate

random sample of patients, or possibly in the whole population. Possible topics might include:
- appointments at special clinics or counselling sessions (e.g. dental, genetic, hepatitis)
- screening for complications (e.g. inhibitors)
- compliance with a new guideline (local or national)
- prescriptions of analgesics for painful bleeds
- waiting times at clinics or at attendances for treatment
- patients' perceptions of specific aspects of haemophilia care.

4. *Prospective analysis of outcomes.* Increasing use of computerized databases in haemophilia centres should allow regular audit of outcomes, which might include:
   - prevention of joint damage by regular prophylaxis in children with severe haemophilia
   - prevention of blood-borne infections (through vaccination and use of low-risk products)
   - prevention of bleeding after surgery (including dental extraction) or delivery
   - prevention of complications of HIV and hepatitis C
   - audit of previous genetic counselling in mothers of recently born babies with severe haemophilia in families with a positive history.

Development of External (National) Clinical Audit Programmes in Scotland and the UK since 1990

As noted above, it can be difficult to organize local peer review because haemophilia care is highly specialized. In 1991, the Haemophilia Centre Directors in Scotland and Northern Ireland decided to pilot a national external clinical audit programme, in which haemophilia directors would audit each other. Each of the seven haemophilia centres was randomly assigned an external auditor from another centre, so that each centre was audited, and each supplied a director to audit another centre. For obvious reasons, no two centres were allowed to audit each other. A full day was agreed for each audit visit, at which the director of the audited centre was available.

The protocol used is shown in Table 16.1. It will be seen that the audit performed at the audit visit largely addressed structure and process; it addressed the standards defined in the currently available draft of the National Health Service (1993) directive on Haemophilia Care. One or two recent hospital admissions in the case records were also audited, using an audit form developed for medical admissions by the Royal College of Physicians of London (Hopkins, 1990).

In addition to the audit visit, the external auditor also assessed, as an outcome measure, patients' satisfaction with their care at the haemophilia centre. This

Table 16.1 Audit protocol – UK haemophilia centres 1992

1. **Patients' comments on centre**
The auditor should select at random up to 20 moderate-to-severely affected haemophiliacs from the confidential list provided by the audited haemophilia centre director, and mail the enclosed questionnaire (Table 16.2) with a covering letter and stamped addressed envelope, asking for a reply within 2 weeks. The list should then be destroyed. The auditors should incorporate patient comments in their report.

2. **Visit to centre**
The auditor should agree a date for this visit as soon as possible with the director of the audited centre, who should be available on this day. A full day will be required.
2.1 Inspection of coagulation laboratory
The auditor should record:
(a) The ability of the laboratory to carry out all tests necessary for definitive diagnosis of the haemophilias, including the identification and assay of specific haemostatic factors, platelet function abnormalities and inhibitors of haemostasis (where appropriate, in conjunction with other haemophilia centres)
(b) Out-of-hours availability of assays
(c) Quality control assurance – external (National External Quality Assurance Scheme (NEQAS)) participation and internal.
2.2 Inspection of clinical service and hospital records
(a) The clinical service cover provided (24-hour) and the experience of staff involved
(b) The facilities available for treatment and advice of patients and relatives
(c) The adequacy of documentation in hospital records (random selection of up to seven records of moderate or severe haemophiliacs, which should be available in the haemophilia centre on the day of audit):
   - type of disorder and level of relevant factor
   - family tree
   - outpatient clinic reviews: (i) adequate documentation? (ii) screening for inhibitors, hepatitis and HIV?
   - hospital admissions – use the Royal College of Physicians (RCP) of London form to audit one or two recent admissions
   - treatment given – amount and type of therapeutic products given in previous year (Oxford returns) and current year.

3. **Report**
The auditor should write a signed report (two to four A4 pages, plus RCP form) on his/her findings as outlined in the above protocol, including constructive comments as to how the service might be improved. The report should be sent in confidence to the audited centre director, and the auditor should keep one copy in confidence.

The author is grateful to the United Kingdom Haemophilia Centre Directors' Organization for permission to publish this audit protocol.

Table 16.2 Audit questionnaire to ascertain patients' comments on haemophilia centres

Audit Questionnaire – Haemophilia Centre

Dear

Thank you for agreeing to help us with the auditing of haemophilia care at your local haemophilia centre. Please return this questionnaire to me in the enclosed stamped addressed envelope. All your answers and comments will be treated in total confidence, and your name will not be divulged to any of your doctors. Please feel free to make any comments you wish.

Do you attend your haemophilia centre regularly?..

How satisfied are you with the following aspects of haemophilia care at your centre?

1. Treatment of bleeds:..
2. Reviews at clinics:..
3. Treatment and chronic joint and muscle problems, for example by physiotherapy:..
4. Counselling and answering your questions on haemophilia:.....................
5. Counselling and answering your questions on complications, such as HIV infection or hepatitis:..
6. Dentistry and other surgery:..
7. Arrangements for home treatment (if applicable):.......................................
8. Counselling and advice on employment, insurance, social work, school: ....

What improvements in care of haemophilia would you like to see at your centre?

....

....

What other comments would you like to make? ....

....

....

....

Thank you for your help. Please return the questionnaire to me in the next 2 weeks if possible.

Yours sincerely

The author is grateful to the United Kingdom Haemophilia Centre Directors' Organization for permission to publish this audit protocol.

appeared particularly important because, in many parts of the UK, patients had little choice but to attend their local haemophilia centre for treatment. Patient satisfaction was assessed by the auditor sending a confidential, anonymous questionnaire (Table 16.2) to a random selection of patients with moderate-to-severe haemophilia (or to mothers of such children) from a confidential list provided by the audited haemophilia centre director with their patients' permission. Patients (or mothers) were asked in a covering letter to reply to the auditor within 2 weeks, using a stamped addressed envelope supplied with the questionnaire. The auditors incorporated the patients' comments in their reports on the audit visit, which was sent in confidence to the audited centre director (Table 16.1).

The pilot study conducted in Scotland and Northern Ireland in 1991 was completed successfully, and was discussed at a subsequent meeting of Haemophilia Centre Directors in Scotland and Northern Ireland. While, in general, the delivery of health care by centres was judged to be of a reasonable standard, each auditor made constructive suggestions as to how the service might be improved. The main modification made to the protocol was to increase the number of mailed questionnaires from 10 to 20 (Table 16.1), because on average only 60% of patients returned questionnaires and it is important to have an adequate sample size to reflect the patients' opinions.

Following a report of this pilot study to the United Kingdom Haemophilia Centre Directors at their annual general meeting in October 1991, it was agreed to extend external (national) audit to the whole of the UK in 1991, using the same audit tools (Tables 16.1 and 16.2). Again this was completed successfully, and the UKHCDO has adopted participation in the national audit scheme as a requirement for accreditation of haemophilia centres. This is also in accordance with both National Health Service (1993) directives, and with the UK Haemophilia Society (1991) patients' charter. Currently, clinical audit of the larger Comprehensive Care Haemophilia Centres is envisaged as a 3-year cycle of UK activity. Regional audit of the smaller Haemophilia Centres in the UK has also been developed, as originally performed in Scotland and Northern Ireland. The original audit tools (Tables 16.1 and 16.2) are being developed, in line with development of national guidelines and standards, and with experience. To help "close the loop" of the audit cycle (Fig. 16.1), it is important that auditors are sent a copy of the previous audit report, so that changes in structure or process that address the recommendations of the previous report can be assessed. Audit also requires funding, and central funding for travel expenses of auditors was obtained by the UKHCDO from the National Health Service for the 1996 national audit programme.

The impact of external clinical audit upon haemophilia care remains to be assessed. It is to be hoped that the expenditure of both money and time will be justified by improved patient facilities, care and outcomes. At the very least, external audit reports can be used by haemophilia centre directors to argue the financial case to managers for improvements in staffing, facilities or other health care provision if extra resources are required. Experience to date suggests that an imminent external audit visit has a stimulating effect, especially on documentation! Comparison of different practices between haemophilia centres is also educational for both auditors and for the audited, promoting a fresh look at personal practice. Indeed, an inevitable consequence of inter-centre audit is the development of clinical care standards (Fig. 16.1).

A final question is: "What should be done if an external auditor finds serious deficiencies in care standards at a haemophilia centre, especially if these persist at a subsequent audit visit?" Following the practice of the UK National External Quality Assessment Scheme (NEQAS) for haematology laboratories, one suggestion is that the Chairperson of the body organizing the programme (e.g. a Haemophilia Centre Directors Organization), on being informed of a "persistent poor performer", contacts the centre director and offers assistance to improve performance. Again, further development of such procedures is required.

Conclusion

Clinical audit is here to stay, and it should be a requirement in haemophilia centres. The next few years should see progressive development of local and national audit programmes for haemophilia care, together with development of guidelines, standards, and an assessment of the effects of audit programmes.

The development of national, external clinical audit of haemophilia care may well be a model for audit of other regional specialist centres in medicine.

Acknowledgement

Development of external clinical audit programmes for haemophilia care in the UK involved the active participation of many of my fellow haemophilia centre directors, especially Drs Elizabeth Mayne (Belfast) and Christopher Ludlam (Edinburgh).

References

Baker R, Fraser RC. Development of review criteria: linking guidelines and assessment of quality. *British Medical Journal* 1995; **311:** 370–373.

Clinical Haematology Task Force, British Committee for Standards in Haematology. Medical audit: notes for haematologists. In: Wood, K (Ed.), *Standard Haematology Practice, 2*. Oxford: Blackwell Scientific, 1994; 261–277.

Department of Health. *Working for Patients*. London: Her Majesty's Stationery Office 1989.

UK Haemophilia Society. *The Essentials of Haemophilia Care*. London: UK Haemophilia Society 1991.

Hopkins A. *Measuring the Quality of Medical Care*. London: Royal College of Physicians 1990.

Lowe GDO. Clinical audit of haemophilia centres. *Bulletin of the UK Haemophilia Society* 1993; **April:** 6–8.
NHS Management Executive. Provision of haemophilia treatment and care. Health Service Guideline HSG(93) 30. London: Department of Health.
Petrie JC, Grimshaw JM, Bryson A. The Scottish Intercollegiate Guidelines Network Initiative: Getting Validated Guidelines into Local Practice. *Health Bulletin* 1995; **53:** 260–263.
United Kingdom Regional Haemophilia Centre Directors Committee. Recommendations on choice of therapeutic products for the treatment of patients with haemophilia A, haemophilia B and von Willebrand's disease. *Blood Coagulation and Fibrinolysis* 1992; **3:** 205–214.
World Health Organisation. Prevention and control of haemophilia. *Bulletin of the World Health Organisation* 1991; **69:** 17–26.

17 The Future

LOUIS M. ALEDORT

The incidence of haemophilia is the same throughout the world. How it is recognized, treated and supported varies markedly. The spectrum of diagnostic capabilities goes from none to elegant prenatal identification of the carrier state and in-utero detection of affected fetuses. The gap is wide when it comes to the level of government interest and/or knowledge of the disease as well as therapy. Many parts of the world have neither the capability of producing a native blood product nor any support for fractionated products. Many reading this have the luxury of outstanding comprehensive care problems supported in part or in whole by governmental agencies. If we are to have an impact on the future of haemophilia, we have an enormous responsibility to narrow this gap. This task is complicated, time consuming and requires dedicated personnel. The future work must be carried out in stages in order to achieve any success.

Initially, a nation has to recognize haemophilia as a priority. This may best be accomplished in a Third World country by linking it to other prevalent disorders, i.e. sickle cell anaemia and thalassaemia. Linkages are best made with other genetic and/or transfusion-dependent disorders. Another approach is to identify a prominent interested citizen who can champion the cause. Simultaneously, one has to identify or stimulate a health care professional to take on the task of haemophilia care. These persons can be trained within their World Health Organization (WHO) region as there are International Hemophilia Training Centres that can support the training of appropriate personnel. The World Federation of Hemophilia has put in place a "decade plan", which addresses this critical part of care throughout the world.

A more complex issue is the provision of blood replacement for the care of affected patients. Much has been written in this book regarding the miraculous scientific advances that have brought about the discovery of monoclonal and recombinant materials. Viral inactivation procedures have produced by far the safest products we have ever been able to transfuse (Mannucci and Colombo, 1988). However, these products are not without their substantial costs. Less than 5 years ago, factor VIII products cost as little as 10 cents (USA) per unit whereas today it is 60 cents to 1 dollar (USA).

Two possible mechanisms for providing product exist: the first is locally made cryoprecipitate, which offers considerable difficulty in most parts of the world that currently have no product. First and foremost is that organized blood delivery systems do not exist, and in places where they do exist, there may not be freezers for storage or distribution. In addition, many patients live far from urban centres, so that such a system is impracticable. Few countries can afford all the testing of donors to ensure safety from viruses such as hepatitis B or C, or human immunodeficiency virus (HIV). The blood supply would therefore be unsafe. The other more realistic potential is to supply viral-inactivated intermediate-purity product. Plasma supply is potentially unlimited. Technology exists for the rapid transfer of this material into lyophilized material. If the plasma were supplied free (voluntary) and centrally or regionally fractionated, unlimited supplies could be made available. There will also be a plethora of plasma available if recombinant factor VIII takes over a major portion of the western Europe and US marketplace. Through a well planned ("not-for-profit" or even "for-profit" enterprise) distribution programme, blood product could flow into these underdeveloped areas and provide the infrastructure for haemophilia care. This plan for the future, however, is in direct conflict with the WHO and the EEC plans regarding blood products (van Aken, 1992). They envision that each nation be self-sufficient for blood product; this implies blood collection and fractionation. Although an "ideal" in the minds of some, a more global approach makes it unrealistic. This philosophy would guarantee poor nations no therapy for haemophilia and leave large unused expensive fractionation potential in other parts of the world. Even now we see many examples of national interdependence with USA plasma fractionated in Europe, and USA Red Cross-collected plasma being fractionated by a different US agency. This makes for optimal utilization of technology and a final cost-effective product. An important future goal is to encourage the expansion of existing fractionation programmes or the initiation of a few new ones in order to take advantage of economy of scale. Each nation requiring blood product should be encouraged to campaign for human blood to produce affordable safe intermediate-purity product. Currently, high-purity product is too costly.

The diagnosis and treatment of haemophilia is very costly. The comprehensive team approach to this chronic disease, to be optimal, requires the involvement of a large number of skilled professionals (Gilbert and Aledort, 1977). Working together, they evaluate and plan for therapy, psychosocial well-being and, above all, the integration of the haemophiliac into society as a functioning person. Although all costs of this have never been accurately assessed, it is very expensive. Although these costs are high, it has been possible to measure the trade-offs. The rate of school and work attendance exceeds that of the general population. The percentage employed also exceeds the general population (Aledort and Brach, 1989). Studies from our centre and the Harvard School of Public Health reveal that one can quantify "productivity" based upon this comprehensive care model. It can now be shown that, by the patient's ability to work and earn the investment or "seed money" for their care rewards society because of financial return to the state. A healthier family unit results so that both parents can now enter the work force, rather than one remaining home

(Ross-Degnan et al, 1992). These studies underscore the reasons why governments should entertain the support of haemophilia care. The costs of the care system, however, pale in comparison with the costs of product that each patient requires in order to be allowed to achieve the above stated goals. In developed countries of the world, treatment per patient per annum varies from less than 500 u/kg/patient/year to greater than 2000 u/kg/patient/year. In terms of consumption of factor per capita in a nation, it ranges from 4 units in Denmark to 0.2 in Portugal (Kernoff, 1991). The differences are explained in several ways. One is that most countries treat their patients using an on-demand programme, i.e. treat when bleeding occurs, and a few countries, particularly those in Scandinavia (Nilsson et al, 1970) and Holland, have employed prophylactic regimens. In almost all of these nations, home care or self- or family-provided infusion is the standard of care. This latter approach, adopted since the 1970s, has been a major feature of comprehensive care, which allows for patient emancipation and the ability to make vital choices, including those of location and vocation.

Using these figures, for example, an average 70 kg adult, using only 1000 u/kg/year, would use 70 000 units every year. Current international pricing of high-purity factor VIII is at least 65 cents per unit. This is a requirement of 45 500 US dollars annually. These costs are in addition to those of the care system, hospitalizations, visits to an emergency room and reconstructive surgery when necessary. In our current global recession, even in countries where social security pays for all care, costs for haemophilia care are now coming under tight scrutiny. Although good data exist to show that replacement product given when bleeding occurs has markedly reduced hospitalizations and length of stay within the hospital, these arguments have not convinced all payers of health care. It becomes imperative that we continue to find innovative methods for health care economic research to continue to justify these high costs. I am convinced that they are justified, thus our task becomes complex and tedious yet absolutely necessary. These must include: productivity, decrease in current spending and reductions in future spending, including rehabilitation costs.

It is therefore imperative to keep these fiscal issues in mind as we embark on attempts to bring care for haemophilia patients to all parts of the world. It would be folly to think that all nations would not only give a high priority to haemophilia, but have the means to support it. A concerted effort, supported by hard data on the cost-effectiveness of care, will aid in this difficult task.

The recognition of acquired immune deficiency syndrome (AIDS) as a transfusion-transmitted disease and its extraordinarily high prevalence in haemophilia patients has received much publicity and offered many additional challenges in the management of this disorder. Ten years after the beginning of this epidemic we are left with a large number of HIV-infected persons. Most of these are well, many are ill and a large number require medication in an attempt to ameliorate this devastating disease. Several countries have offered reparations in the form of cash payments but most have essentially let the prevailing health care system deal with the issue. Reparations have not solved the underlying issue. As seen in the UK, an initial payment to families did not satisfy the infected patient, and a second payment was made. As the infection continues to be chronic in nature, and length of survival unpredictable, payments such as these will never suffice. We must develop a totally different strategy. A comprehensive programme is required to assure health care, psychosocial support for the patient and family, disability income for those who can no longer work and assistance for those without a support system. Until recently, few of these systems were in place for this group of patients. Many comprehensive haemophilia centres are now burdened with this enormous task and few, if any, have the support to provide these required services. Two other issues remain major problems for this infected cohort. One is that HIV has infected approximately 15% of their sexual partners (Smiley et al, 1988). This reality has had a major effect on long-established relationships and has threatened new ones. Revelation of haemophilia as well as HIV status threatens most new relationships. A significant consequence of this has been a substantial amount of sexual dysfunction. A major task for us is to be able to re-establish healthy marriages, without risking any further sexual transmission of HIV. There are no simple solutions. Several major projects are currently being funded in an attempt to provide methods of approaching this issue. For young unmarried haemophiliacs, in particular adolescents, the problem is far greater. Before HIV, our young haemophiliacs were more like most other people and could easily integrate into society. Now our infected young have to recognize that their blossoming sexuality has a special significance, and could lead to HIV transmission. This has caused havoc with this group of patients. Some have withdrawn totally, unable to establish intimacy or close friendships for fear of revealing their status. Others have sought and/or continue to engage in promiscuous, unprotected sexual activity. This group has the potential to infect a large number of uninformed, unsuspecting sexual partners. They are also the group least likely to be influenced by comprehensive case centre personnel or parents, but by peer groups. Getting this group to use condoms during sexual activity, unfortunately, has many connotations in our present world. There are religious bans on education about safer sex practices as well as on condom use. In addition, there are sexual partners who do not want condoms to be used, as the condom user is frequently questioned as to whether he is hiding a sexually transmitted disease. In addition, access and affordability of condoms are a real deterrent to their use. Although we have believed that education and information are key to changing behaviour in high-risk situations, the data tell us something quite different. Most of our patients know of the risks of the sexual transmission of HIV and how to prevent it. However, only 60% of our sexually active adolescents comply. Psychosocial research is critically needed to help us define ways to alter the behavior of these young infected males. We also need to find satisfactory pathways for them to reintegrate into their peer group, cope with their own growing sexuality, and maintain their self-esteem. This area is as critical a task for our haemophilia treaters as any they may have had to deal with in the past.

The second and final area of concern for our HIV-infected patients is the fact that family planning takes on a whole new meaning. In the past the major issue has been identifying the carrier, providing genetic information to the family and giving support to whatever decision was made. With advanced technology we were able to go further by carrying out intrauterine detection, and once again support the family in whatever decision they made regarding the outcome of the pregnancy. With all these skills and tools, we discovered two things: (a) the number of haemophiliacs being born was not substantially altered and (b) one-third of haemophiliacs born continue to be the result of new mutations in patients with no family history of haemophilia. HIV infection has dramatically altered the issues surrounding family planning.

During sexual intercourse a previously negative partner may seroconvert and if so 10–15% of her offspring may become infected (European Collaborative Study Group, 1992). The assumption that these facts inhibit families from attempting to have children is erroneous. It appears that many infected haemophiliacs and their wives are willing to take the risk for the sake of having a child. Even the use of artificial insemination by donor, in an attempt to reduce the likelihood of seroconversion, has not been successful (MMWR, 1990). The unpredictability of the outcome of the pregnancy raises substantial issues for the patient, his spouse and the clinic staff. The position of the staff must remain one of education as to risks and support for the decision of the patient and family. We need to encourage research into finding more satisfactory (if possible) ways for insemination without risk of infection: can one identify the non-infected sperm, is it possible to render semen non-infectious, and what are the key elements that determine the transmissibility of HIV to spouse and child? Although the National Cancer Institute (NCI) haemophilia HIV study group has sought such determinants, little has materialized that could help us with this serious issue.

As most viral illnesses have had little specific therapy, vaccines have been a major force in prevention of disease. Antibody titres derived from vaccines that approximate the coat of the virus have conferred immunity from direct viral exposure in susceptible animals. Early human studies of safety have led to the initiation in late 1992 of their use in already infected haemophiliacs in both the USA and Europe. We await the results of the impact of antibody production in response to vaccine in these infected patients.

The last 10 years have been focused on understanding the effects of infection with HIV, its staggering magnitude in this patient population and how to manage therapy. Enormous energy and financial resources have been provided to meet the need. Antiviral therapy has staved off AIDS in many patients so far, but even in combination with preventive therapy for opportunistic infections, thousands have developed AIDS and died. On the brighter side are the data from the NCI study group and corroborated by the National Heart Lung and Blood Institute of NIH; Transfusion Safety Study (NHLBI TSS) group that children exposed to HIV virus handle it far better, take substantially longer to destroy their T-cells and are far less likely to develop AIDS after 10 years (Goedert et al, 1989). This group continues to deserve careful scrutiny, in an attempt to determine those factors that are important for the development of AIDS.

The HIV virus does not stand alone as a major threat to those haemophiliacs treated before viral-attenuated products were available. Hepatitis C, affecting as many as 90% of patients exposed to blood products, has produced severe liver disease in at least 20–25% of them. This is either in the form of chronic active hepatitis or cirrhosis (Aledort et al, 1985). Those with cirrhosis frequently develop the classic complications of liver failure or portal hypertension; little can be offered to this group. However, a large number have disease that can respond to a new naturally occurring substance, α-interferon. Few studies have been carried out in haemophiliacs, but the literature in other patient groups is quite encouraging. If cirrhosis is not present, but substantial liver disease is, courses of α-interferon have produced substantial remissions (Aledort, 1993).

The problem of hepatitis C has become a major problem for patients with concomitant HIV infection. As HIV progresses, further liver damage occurs (Eyster et al, 1992). The use of antivirals, frequently associated with liver damage, may need to be discontinued because of severe liver disease progression. Careful evaluation of the use of α-interferon is needed in both singly and doubly infected haemophiliacs to evaluate its safety and efficacy. As more haemophiliacs are expected to have their HIV infection progress with time, we must be in a position of ameliorating this problem. Although liver transplantation has been reported to cure haemophilia (Delorme et al, 1990) and hepatitis C liver disease, there is no evidence that HIV can be helped by this procedure.

Despite the fact that HIV consumed us in the 1980s, the 1990s have brought us a large number of healthy children born with haemophilia. In our own health care region covering 28 620 643 people, there were 200 newborns recorded with haemophilia in the past 4 years. These children are quite fortunate in that they have been born in an era of extremely safe blood products. There has been no new HIV seroconversion reported since 1987 and hepatitis C is almost completely eradicated. Hepatitis B vaccine will prevent this viral agent from transmitting disease, and only a rare case of parvovirus infection has been reported (Morfini et al, 1992). Unfortunately, recent epidemics of hepatitis A cases have been reported (Peerlirck and Vermylen, 1993). Thus, these children and their families have a different outlook for the future. We must therefore refocus our attention on these children and their families. These new parents are as anxious about haemophilia as any have ever been. They require education as to the fundamental aspects of preventive health care, what can be expected, the genetics for family planning, appropriate vaccinations, early recognition of bleeding episodes, home care, schooling, sports, etc. All these basics that seem so simple have been lost because of the overwhelming issues of HIV. Staff burnout has led to a large turnover in personnel, so that few professionals knowledgeable about haemophilia care pre-HIV exist. What appears to be simple, I fear, will not be easy to reintegrate into our programmes. The incentives for doing so are great, in that there is great hope for these children to lead normal lives, to have these boys integrate into society and once again assume that they can reach the normal life-span that haemophiliacs had before HIV.

A critical goal for these young, uninfected haemophilia patients is to eradicate joint disease. It has been known for a long time that in haemophilic dogs, by correcting the clotting defect, all joint pathology would be prevented. In general, most of the therapy throughout the world is given on demand with dose regimens based upon estimates of an ideal treatment. Although prophylaxis is practised either intermittently or continuously in some countries, few data exist about the outcome of patients treated with a prophylactic regimen.

For decades, in Sweden, Nilsson and her co-workers (Nilsson et al, 1970) have been interested in and have used continuous prophylaxis as a method of treatment. The goal was to change the status of severe haemophiliacs to mild or moderate ones, thereby altering their long-term orthopaedic outcome.

Using this approach, Nilsson (1992) has described 25 years of experience with prophylaxis in 60 severe haemophiliacs (52 with factor VIII and eight with factor IX deficiency). The patients are divided into three groups based upon age and amount of therapy received. As expected, older patients were treated less heavily than children because factor was less available in the early years. Eventually, regimens were tailored to each patient to achieve baseline levels of at least 1%. Regimens were designed for very young patients beginning at age 1–2 years. Factor VIII-deficient patients were usually treated with 25–40 iu/kg three times weekly, and the same twice weekly for factor IX deficiency. End-points were orthopaedic joint and X-ray scores, bleeding episodes, lifestyle (time missed from work or school) and side-effects of treatments such as HIV, liver function, hepatitis C, inhibitors and immune function.

The most significant result was that patients who started young (less than 2 years of age receiving $1.7–9 \times 10^3$ iu/kg/year, always achieving pre-infusion levels of 1% or greater, recorded almost no bleeding episodes and maintained zero-zero scores in their joints for as long as 11 years of follow-up.

When young patients on continuous prophylaxis started early, as well as older ones who started later, with existing joint disease were compared with those who were treated on demand, all patients on prophylaxis fared better and maintained a lower joint and X-ray score. Current on-demand treatment regimens do not provide this level of joint preservation although many patients receive as much factor annually.

Many patients undergoing continued prophylaxis require a Portocath or Broviac to assure venous access. This type of access has been associated with complications such as infection. Patient acceptance may be a major deterrent. The requirement for large amounts of factor annually is a major problem. Several approaches need to be made in order to answer these two latter issues. Research must be carried out to analyze the cost-benefit ratio of such a programme. The lack of orthopaedic morbidity, access to work and school and the elimination of bleeding episodes require translation into fiscal terms. Such work is in progress and, when complete, will hopefully make a compelling story regarding support of such programmes. In addition, further studies, such as a randomized prospective study, are required to establish clearly the efficacy of such a prophylaxis regimen versus on-demand therapy. Another important future research area is the development of constant-infusion technologies for haemophiliacs. Chemotherapy, insulin and desferrioxamine have for some time been given by a constant-infusion technique. Taking advantage of the biological activity and half-life of factor VIII, it has been calculated that instead of 6000 units of factor per week, only 300 units would be required if a constant-infusion system were in place. This advance would have a substantial fiscal impact and make acceptance of such a programme more likely.

We have briefly discussed that current technology has brought us safer and high-purity products derived from human blood and now recombinant factor VIII. These higher-purity materials will also make continuous infusion more feasible. If all these studies support a programme of continued prophylaxis as both effective and feasible, it would markedly alter the way haemophilia care is delivered.

One cannot complete speculation as to the future without looking at two major advances: the introduction of recombinant factor and the promise of gene therapy. Over the past 3 years, two major fractionation companies have produced different recombinant factor VIII molecules that have been shown to have biological activity identical to human-derived factor VIII (Schwartz et al, 1990). They have been used successfully to treat bleeding episodes and major trauma or surgery. Complications in previously treated patients have been minimal. In large studies of previously untreated patients (PUPS), the record of viral safety for hepatitis B, hepatitis C and HIV is very good and no patient has developed any viral illness secondary to infusion. Outbreaks of hepatitis A from blood products and a rash of inhibitors in previously treated patients continue to temper our enthusiasm for technological advances (Van den Berg et al, 1992). However, a substantial and as yet unresolved question is whether recombinant materials lead to a higher prevalence of inhibitors. Currently in one PUP study 27% of the patients have developed an inhibitor to factor VIII (Lusher et al, 1993); in another study of much shorter duration, 17% (Bray, 1992) have developed inhibitors. The characteristics of the inhibitors are different from those usually seen because more than half are low-responding inhibitors. Almost all prior studies are not comparable, as they are either retrospective or of an incomparable prospective since they use different criteria and/or different methods of measuring the antibody titre. Epitope analysis of these inhibitors does not find them different from those associated with human-derived product. We have at present many safe, effective intermediate-purity as well as high-purity products to offer our patients. We have learned from bitter experience that we must be very cautious before embracing new therapeutic modalities lest we expose our patients to any potentially significant complications. The management of inhibitor patients, which is dealt with in Chapter 11, is a major problem when anamnestic or high-titred inhibitors occur. We must weigh the benefit–risk ratio before embracing any new therapy for PUPS.

Gene therapy, the concept of endowing a cell with information so it can produce a protein, is now possible and is in experimental design for haemophilia. Several companies are pursuing this and we hope that, in the future, patients may be the beneficiaries of this type of therapy. As with recombinant factor VIII, these proteins may lead to the production of antibodies. Whether this will impede their clinical application remains to be seen. However, future technology may be able to impede antibody production.

With safer products and the promise of "cures" for haemophilia, I suspect that the prevalence of haemophilia will continue to increase. As the ravages of transfusion-transmitted diseases pass, healthy uninfected young men will enter life as successful and integrated citizens, free from joint disease. We will find that any restraints for procreation will disappear. As these extraordinary events unfold, we as treaters have an even greater responsibility. We must ensure that our own health care systems, whether pluralistic or not, are prepared to implement these advances. Concerted data collection, lobbying efforts and articulate spokespersons must be ready to convince polycymakers that haemophilia is worthy of their attention. However, we must not forget those yet untreated and uneducated haemophiliacs, who constitute the majority of the world's haemophiliacs, and who must be given hope that they too shall have the same opportunity.

I dedicate the future to them hoping that our efforts may become their reality.

Acknowledgements

This study was supported in part by NIH Grant HL30567–03; National Heart, Lung and Blood Institute, Bethesda, Maryland; Health Services Administration Grant MCB–360001–04–01; Health and Human Services Grant HL–30567–02; the Regional Comprehensive Hemophilia Diagnostic and Treatment Center; the Margie Boas Fund; the International Hemophilia Training Center of the World Federation of Hemophilia; and the Polly Annenberg Levee Hematology Center, Department of Medicine, Mount Sinai School of Medicine of the City University of New York; a grant (5MO1 RR00071) for the Mount Sinai General Clinical Research Center from the National Center for Research Resources, National Institutes of Health.

References

Aledort LM. The consequences of chronic hepatitis C. A review article for the hematologist. *American Journal of Hematology* 1993; **44**(1): 29–37.

Aledort LM, Brach I. The cost of care for hemophiliacs. In: *Hemophilia in the Child and Adult*, 3rd edn. New York: Raven Press, 1989.

Aledort LM, Levine PH, Hilgartner M, et al. A study of liver biopsies and liver disease among hemophiliacs. *Blood* 1985; **66:** 367.

Bray G, for the Recombinate Study Group. Current status of clinical studies of recombinant factor VIII (Recombinate) in patients with hemophilia A. *Transfusion Medicine Reviews* 1992; **4:** 252.

Delorme MA, Adams PC, Grant D, Ghent CN, Walker IR, Wall WJ. Orthotopic liver transplantation in a patient with combined hemophilia A and B. *American Journal of Hematology* 1990; **33:** 136.
European Collaborative Study Group. Risk factor from mother to child in HIV-1. *Lancet* 1992; **339:** 1007.
Eyster ME, Diamond Stone LF, Lien JM, et al. Natural history of hepatitis C infection in multitransfused hemophiliacs: effects of coinfection with human immunodeficiency virus. *Journal of AIDS* 1993; **6:** 602–610.
Gilbert M, Aledort LM. Comprehensive care in hemophilia: a team approach. *Mt Sinai Journal of Medicine (New York)* 1977; **3:** 313.
Goedert JJ, Kessler CM, Aledort LM, et al. A prospective study of human immunodeficiency virus type 1 infection and the developments of AIDS in subjects with hemophilia. *New England Journal of Medicine* 1989; **321:** 1141.
Kernoff P. Current factor VIII usage related to self sufficiency: a European overview. *Royal Society of Medicine, Round Table Series* 1991; **25:** 4.
Lusher JM, Arkin S, Abildgaard CF, Schwartz RS, the Kogenate Study Group. Recombinant Factor VIII in Previously Untreated Patient Study Group. *New England Journal of Medicine* 1993; **328:** 453.
Mannucci PM, Colombo M. Virucidal treatment of clotting factor concentrates. *Lancet* 1988; **2:** 782.
Morfini M, Longo G, Ferrini R, et al. Hypoplastic anemia in a hemophiliac first infused with a solvent/detergent treated factor VIII concentrate: the role of human B19 parvovirus. *American Journal of Hematology* 1992; **39:** 149.
MMWR. HIV-1 infection and artificial insemination with processed semen. *Morbidity and Mortality Weekly Report* 1990; **39:** 249.
Nilsson IM. Twenty-five years' experience of prophylactic treatment in severe haemophilia A and B. *Journal of Internal Medicine* 1992; **232:** 25.
Nilsson IM, Blomback M, Ahlberg A. Our experience in Sweden with prophylaxis on haemophilia. In: *Proceedings of the 5th Congress of the World Federation of Hemophilia, Montreal 1968; Bibl Haematol.* Basel and New York: Karger, 1970:111.
Peerlinck K, Vermylen J. Acute hepatitis A in patients with haemophilia A. *Lancet* 1993; **341:** 179.
Ross-Degnan D, Soumerai SB, Avorn J, Bohn RL, Bright R, Aledort LM. Hemophilia Home Treatment: Economic Analysis and Implications for Health Policy. *International Journal of Technology Assessment in Health Care* 1995; **11**(2): 327–344.
Schwartz R, Abildgaard CF, Aledort LM, et al. Human recombinant DNA-derived antihemophilic factor (factor VIII) in the treatment of hemophilia A. *New England Journal of Medicine* 1990; **323:** 1800.
Smiley ML, White GC, Becherer P, et al. Transmission of HIV to sexual partners in hemophiliacs. *American Journal of Hematology* 1988; **28:** 27.
Van Aken WG. European self-sufficiency of plasma products. *XX World Federation of Hemophilia Abstracts* 1992; **128:** 250.
Van den Berg HM, Mauser-Bunschoten E, Roosendaal G. The development of inhibitors to factor VIII in multitransfused hemophilia A patients. *XX International Congress of the WFH Abstracts* 1992; **352:** 179.

Index

Page numbers in *italic* refer to illustrations and tables; **bold** page numbers indicate a main discussion.